Hair and Hair Disorders
Diagnosis and Management

Hair and Hair Disorders

Diagnosis and Management

Chief Editor

S Sacchidanand MD DVD DHA FRCP (Glasgow)
Registrar (Evaluation)
Rajiv Gandhi University of Health Sciences
Former Professor and Head
Department of Dermatology, STD and Leprosy
Bangalore Medical College and Research Institute
Bengaluru, Karnataka, India

Co-editors

Savitha AS MD DNB FRGUHS (Dermatosurgery)
Senior Resident
Department of Dermatology, STD and Leprosy
Victoria Hospital
Bangalore Medical College and Research Institute
Bengaluru, Karnataka, India

Lakshmi DV DVD FRGUHS (Pediatric Dermatology)
Senior Resident
Department of Dermatology, STD and Leprosy
Victoria Hospital
Bangalore Medical College and Research Institute
Bengaluru, Karnataka, India

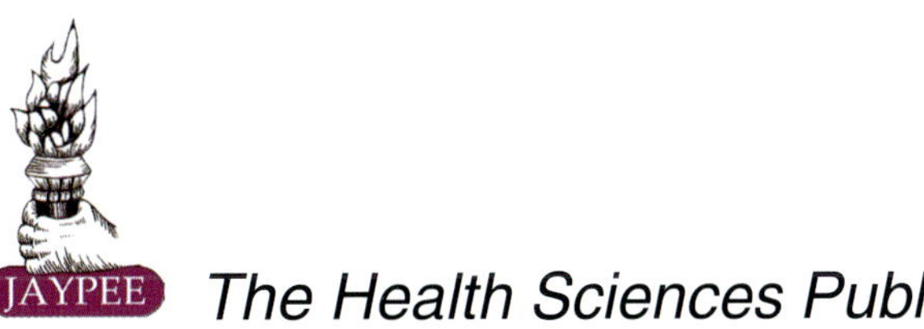

New Delhi | London | Philadelphia | Panama

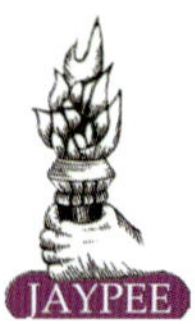

Jaypee Brothers Medical Publishers (P) Ltd

Headquarters

Jaypee Brothers Medical Publishers (P) Ltd
4838/24, Ansari Road, Daryaganj
New Delhi 110 002, India
Phone: +91-11-43574357
Fax: +91-11-43574314
Email: jaypee@jaypeebrothers.com

Overseas Offices

J.P. Medical Ltd
83, Victoria Street, London
SW1H 0HW (UK)
Phone: +44 20 3170 8910
Fax: +44 (0)20 3008 6180
Email: info@jpmedpub.com

Jaypee-Highlights Medical Publishers Inc
City of Knowledge, Bld. 237, Clayton
Panama City, Panama
Phone: +1 507-301-0496
Fax: +1 507-301-0499
Email: cservice@jphmedical.com

Jaypee Medical Inc
The Bourse
111 South Independence Mall East
Suite 835, Philadelphia, PA 19106, USA
Phone: +1 267-519-9789
Email: jpmed.us@gmail.com

Jaypee Brothers Medical Publishers (P) Ltd
17/1-B Babar Road, Block-B, Shaymali
Mohammadpur, Dhaka-1207
Bangladesh
Mobile: +08801912003485
Email: jaypeedhaka@gmail.com

Jaypee Brothers Medical Publishers (P) Ltd
Bhotahity, Kathmandu
Nepal
Phone: +977-9741283608
Email: kathmandu@jaypeebrothers.com

Website: www.jaypeebrothers.com
Website: www.jaypeedigital.com

Inquiries for bulk sales may be solicited at: jaypee@jaypeebrothers.com

Hair and Hair Disorders: Diagnosis and Management

First Edition: **2015**

ISBN 978-93-5152-340-6

Printed at Replika Press Pvt. Ltd.

Contributors

Anil Abraham MD FAAD FRCP (Glasgow)
Professor
Department of Dermatology STD and Leprosy
St Johns Medical College and Research Center
Bengaluru, Karnataka, India

Anoosha P MD
Consultant Dermatologist
Vee Care DermatoPlastic, Skin, Hair, Laser and
Day Plastic Surgery Clinic
Chennai, Tamil Nadu, India

Aparna Palit MD
Professor
Department of Dermatology, STD and Leprosy
Sri BM Patil Medical College
BLDE University
Bijapur, Karnataka, India

Archana L DVD
(Fellow in Medical Cosmetology)
Department of Dermatology, STD and Leprosy
Bangalore Medical College and
Research Institute
Bengaluru, Karnataka, India

Arun C Inamadar MD, DVD
Professor and Head
Department of Dermatology, STD and Leprosy
Sri BM Patil Medical College
BLDE University
Bijapur, Karnataka, India

Asha GS MD FRGUHS (Dermatosurgery)
Assistant Professor
Department of Dermatology, STD and Leprosy
Victoria Hospital
Bangalore Medical College and
Research Institute
Bengaluru, Karnataka, India

Ashok Kumar Jaiswal MD
Professor and Head
Department of Dermatology, Venereology and Leprosy
Dr BR Ambedkar Medical College
Bengaluru, Karnataka, India

C Janaki MD DD
Professor
Department of Dermatology
Madras Medical College
Chennai, Tamil Nadu, India

D Dinesh Kumar MD
Consultant Dermatologist
Vee Care DermatoPlastic, Skin, Hair, Laser and
Day Plastic Surgery Clinic
Chennai, Tamil Nadu, India

Divya Gorur MD
(Fellow in Dermatosurgery)
Victoria Hospital
Department of Dermatology, STD and Leprosy
Bangalore Medical College and Research Institute
Bengaluru, Karnataka, India

Dolly Gupta MD FIDS Certified in Trichology (USA)
Consultant Dermatologist and Hair Transplant Surgeon
MEDICA Super-specialty Hospital
Kolkata, West Bengal, India

Eshini Perera MBBS
Faculty of Medicine
Dentistry and Health Sciences
The University of Melbourne
Victoria, Australia

Eswari L MD
Assistant Professor (Fellow in Dermatosurgery)
Department of Dermatology, STD and Leprosy
Bangalore Medical College and Research Institute
Bengaluru, Karnataka, India

G Sentamil Selvi MD DD PhD
Professor and Head (Retired)
Department of Dermatology, STD and Leprosy
Madras Medical College
Chennai, Tamil Nadu, India

KC Nischal MD
Consultant Dermatologist
Nirmal Skin and Hair Clinic
Senior Consultant and Associate Manager
Medical Services
Kaya Skin Clinic
Bengaluru, Karnataka, India

Lakshmi DV DVD FRGUHS (Pediatric Dermatology)
Senior Resident, Victoria Hospital
Department of Dermatology, STD and Leprosy
Bangalore Medical College and Research Institute
Bengaluru, Karnataka, India

Leelavathy B MD FRGUHS (Medical Cosmetology)
Associate Professor and Head
Department of Dermatology, STD and Leprosy
Bowring and Lady Curzon Hospital
Bangalore Medical College and Research Institute
Bengaluru, Karnataka, India

Malavika Kohli MD DVD DNB
Director, Skin Secrets
Jaslok Hospital and Research Center
Breach Candy Hospital Trust
Mumbai, Maharashtra, India

Manjunath Shenoy M MD DNB
Professor and Head
Department of Dermatology, STD and Leprosy
Yenepoya Medical College, Deralakatte
Yenepoya University
Mangalore, Karnataka, India

Manoj Khanna MS MCh (Plastic Surgery) FICS (USA)
Fellowship (Cosmetic Surgery) (USA)
Consultant Plastic Surgeon
Enhance Aesthetic and Cosmetic Studios Pvt Ltd
Kolkota, West Bengal, India

Maya Vedamurthy MD FRCP (Glasgow)
Consultant Dermatologist
Anna Nagar, Chennai, Tamil Nadu, India

Neelima Sharma DVD
Consultant Dermatologist
Banaswadi, Bengaluru, Karnataka, India

Prabhakar M Sangolli MD DVD
Former Associate Professor
Dr BR Ambedkar Medical College
Consultant Dermatologist
Skin Care Center
Bengaluru, Karnataka, India

R Madhu MD (Derm) DCH
Senior Assistant Professor
Department of Dermatology (Mycology)
Madras Medical College
Chennai, Tamil Nadu, India

Raghini Ghiya MD
Consultant Dermatologist and Hair Transplant Surgeon
Siddharth Clinic
Surat, Gujarat, India

Rajiv Sharad Joshi MD DVD DNB
Consultant Dermatologist
PD Hinduja Hospital
Mumbai, Maharashtra, India

Ralph M Trüeb MD
Professor
Center for Dermatology and Hair Diseases
Wallisellen, Switzerland

Rodney Sinclair MD FACD
Epworth Hospital, Melbourne
Victoria, Australia

S Sacchidanand MD DVD DHA FRCP (Glasgow)
Registrar (Evaluation)
Rajiv Gandhi University of Health Sciences
Former Professor and Head
Department of Dermatology, STD and Leprosy
Bangalore Medical College and Research Institute
Bengaluru, Karnataka, India

Sanjeev J Aurangabadkar MD
Consultant Dermatologist
Skin and Laser Clinic
Hyderabad, Andhra Pradesh, India

Savitha AS MD DNB FRGUHS (Dermatosurgery)
Senior Resident
Victoria Hospital
Department of Dermatology, STD and Leprosy
Bangalore Medical College and Research Institute
Bengaluru, Karnataka, India

Shashikumar BM MD
Associate Professor
Department of Dermatology, STD and Leprosy
Mandya Institute of Medical Sciences
Mandya, Karnataka, India

Sheena Bansal MD
Consultant Dermatologist
Skin Essence
Kanpur, Uttar Pradesh, India

Shilpa K MD FRGUHS (Dermatosurgery)
Assistant Professor
Victoria Hospital
Department of Dermatology, STD and Leprosy
Bangalore Medical College and Research Institute
Bengaluru, Karnataka, India

Shrutakirthi D Shenoi MD DVD
Professor and Head
Department of Dermatology, STD and Leprosy
Kasturba Medical College
Manipal University
Manipal, Karnataka, India

Smitha Prabhu MD
Department of Dermatology, STD and Leprosy
Kasturba Medical College
Manipal University
Manipal, Karnataka, India

Sudhir Nayak UK MD
Assistant Professor
Department of Dermatology, STD and Leprosy
Kasturba Medical College
Manipal University
Manipal, Karnataka, India

TS Nagesh MD DNB
Associate Professor
Department of Dermatology, STD and Leprosy
Sapthagiri Institute of Medical Sciences and Research Center
Bengaluru, Karnataka, India

Urmila Nischal MD
Consultant Dermatologist
Nirmal Skin and Hair Clinic
Bengaluru, Karnataka, India

Venkataram Mysore DVD MD DNB DipRCPath (Lond) FRCP (Glasgow)
Consultant Dermatologist
Dermatopathologist and Hair Transplant Surgeon
Director
Venkat Charmalaya—Center for Advanced Dermatology and PG Teaching Center
Bengaluru, Karnataka, India

Vishalakshi S Pandit MD
Assistant Professor
Department of Dermatology, STD and Leprosy
Sri BM Patil Medical College
BLDE University
Bijapur, Karnataka, India

Preface

"To study medicine without books is to sail an uncharted sea; while to study books without patients is not to go to sea at all."

—***William Osler***

"Trichology" refers to study of "hair-related disorders". It is an upcoming branch of dermatology as 10–20% of dermatological out-patients present with hair-related problems. There is an ocean of opportunities for research work in hair-related disorders due to paucity of literature in this subspecialty and also need for a updated book that would throw light on management of hair-related conditions.

Hence, to fill up this void, we have planned to bring out a comprehensive textbook on hair and its related diseases in its entirety.

In the first edition of the book, we have aimed to provide an extensive data on hair-related disorders to complement the details available in major textbooks in the field of dermatology. We assure that the work has been sufficiently researched and hopefully would merit further editions. The various sections are based on presenting symptoms and signs, differential diagnosis, therapeutics and surgical modalities highlighted with text boxes and illustrations. Recent advances in the field of trichology have prompted the management of hair and hair disorders enormously, and this is reflected in the descriptions in the relevant sections.

We hope that this treatise will provide the knowledge and confidence to clinicians and postgraduates to untangle the locks of hair and scalp disorders.

We acknowledge the contribution of Sumedha Ballal, Divya Gorur, Chitrika, Shruti C, Varsha Shetty, Kumar Abhishek, Pushpa KR, Shalini, Maheshwari, Amina Asfiya and Linda Robert towards this project.

S Sacchidanand
Savitha AS
Lakshmi DV

Contents

1

Evolution of Hair

Lakshmi DV, S Sacchidanand

"It is not the strongest or the most intelligent who will survive but those who can best manage change."

—*Charles Darwin*

Introduction

Human skin is the most visible aspect of the human phenotype, characterized by a vast range of genetically determined skin colors and an enhanced ability to dissipate body heat. With time, it has undergone numerous adaptive structural changes that give it strength, resilience and sensitivity. One such component of skin is the human hair, performing a range of functions from insulation, protection against sunlight, enhancement of cutaneous sensations and ornamentation.

Convergent Evolution

The origin and early evolutionary history of hair is not clear, but there are several hypothetical models. It has been observed that the hair in humans and the feather follicle in birds have adopted a similar developmental pattern consisting of a proximal to distal growth mode and invagination of the epidermis to form follicles.[1]

The evolution of endothermy has driven the convergent evolution of hair and feather follicles, both forming multiple localized growth units with stem cells protected in the proximal follicle.[1] The topological arrangement allows them to elongate, moult and regenerate without structural constraints. This autonomy to regenerate its own hair cycle, is a characteristic feature of human hair, a consequence of changes in gene regulatory networks of corneous proteins **(Box 1.1)**.

Box 1.1: Convergent evolution: Feather—hair follicle

- Evolution of endothermy has driven evolution of hair and feather follicles
- Characteristic topological arrangement
- Autonomy to regenerate its own hair cycle

Scale as a Basal State for Hair Follicle

When reptiles established themselves on land, their integuments had to adapt to the challenges of terrestrial life by developing barriers which can prevent water loss, protect against ultraviolet (UV) irradiation and act as mechanical shields to provide protection against the rigors of terrestrial life. Once these basic needs were met, different types of reptilian scales evolved in the Mesozoic period to serve different functions and adapt diverse species to different niches. As amniotes evolved towards endothermy, skin appendages related to heat conservation appeared. Hairs and feathers evolved from Therapsid and Sauropsid reptiles, respectively, as a result of convergent evolution.[1]

Vertebrate skin appendages such as scales, feathers, hairs and teeth appear to be different, but share a number of common developmental pathways, such as the Hedgehog, bone morphogenetic protein (BMP) and Wnt signaling pathways.[1] Variation and innovation in developmental processes are thought to be key mechanisms for forming different types of skin appendages. The evolution of feathers and hairs possibly began from scales present in early reptiles in which the modulation and re-organization of gene regulatory networks led to new forms of skin appendages.

Box 1.2: Proposed hypothesis of hair origin

- Maderson's hypothesis
- Dhouailly and Sun hypothesis
- Alibardi's hypothesis

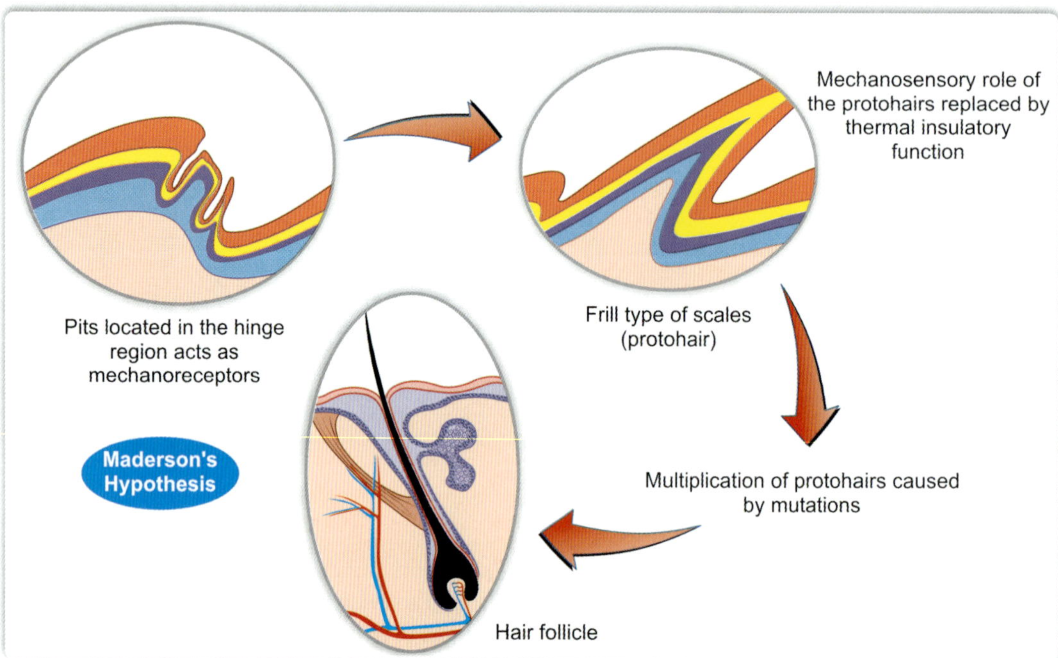

Fig. 1.1: Schematic representation of Maderson's hypothesis of origin of hair follicle

Several hypotheses have been proposed regarding the origin of hair **(Box 1.2)**. Maderson hypothesized that hairs arose from reptilian sensory appendages of the mechanoreceptor type (pit organ) that were located in the hinge region of ancient reptiles **(Figure 1.1)**.[1,2] Morphologically, the structure of the pits is reminiscent of a follicle, based on the invagination of the epidermis and the adjacent dermal structure. However, real dermal papillae with characteristics analogous to those of hairs, or even feathers, have not been demonstrated in these reptiles. Frill type of scales also possess follicle like structures, but the pit forms the follicle like structure from part of a scale. However, the cell behavior of pit formation, such as cell proliferation and regeneration, is totally unknown. The mechano-sensory role of the proto-hairs may have been gradually replaced by thermal insulatory function and contributed to successful endothermy. The multiplication of protohairs caused by mutations, has lead to the increase of hair density which could provide improved mechanical protection and insulatory function.

Dhouailly and Sun (1989) have proposed a different model **(Figure 1.2)**. The tongue is considered as one of the integuments. By comparing the topology and keratin types of scales and hairs with those of filiform and papillar taste buds, they suggested that gradual changes in the expression of keratins in the inner surface of the scale epidermis might have led to a transformation of the scale structure from a hemi-cylindrical form to the more completely cylindrical structure found in hairs. This progression could have been the origin of hair follicle invagination.[1,3]

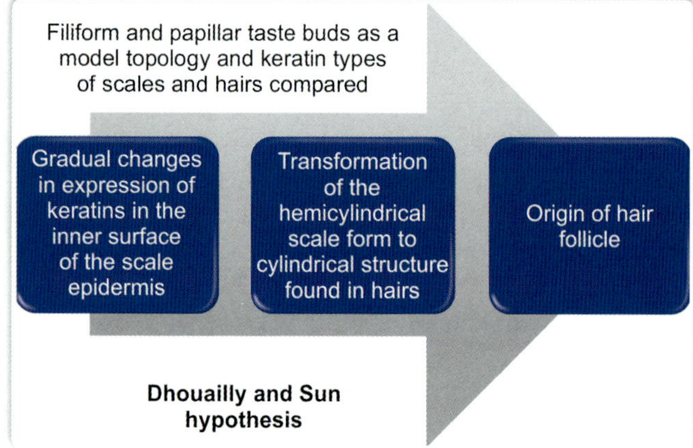

Fig. 1.2: Schematic representation of Dhouailly and Sun hypothesis of origin of hair follicle

Alibardi hypothesized that the progressive reduction of the outer surface of reptilian scales has restricted the morphogenetically active dermis previously associated to these areas, into smaller "niches", forming cell condensations indicated as dermal papillae. Hairs are derived from an invagination of the morphogenetically active mesenchyme near hinge regions of scales of reptilian ancestors (synapsids), which led to the formation of the dermal papilla associated with hair **(Box 1.3)**.[1,4]

Box 1.3: Synapsids

Morphogenetically active mesenchyme in hinge regions of scales of reptilian ancestors which form dermal papilla

Molecular Evolution of α- and β-keratin (Figure 1.3)

There are two main types of intermediate filament proteins in vertebrate keratinocytes: α- and β-keratins. Reptiles and birds have both α- and β-keratins while mammals only have α-keratins. Studies have indicated that basic amniotes possessed a common ancestral protein rich in glycine and proline sequences that diversified in the evolutive lineage. In reptiles and birds, β-keratins were formed, while in mammals high-glycine and high-sulfur proteins developed for this purpose. Both are small proteins that associate with α-keratins to make a very hard corneous material, utilized for hard scales, claws, hairs, horns, etc. In chickens and lizards, the α-keratin produced was found in their claws, but in mammals it was used to produce hair.[5]

Relative Hairlessness in Humans

Typically, mammals have dense fur that covers the entire body. Humans, however, have noticeably thinner, more translucent hair than other mammals.[6] Alan Rogers suggests that humans once were covered with hair similar to that of their closest relatives: apes. However, as humans migrated out of Africa, into areas with cooler climate such as Europe they needed a way to absorb UV radiation from the sun. As skin color adapted and got lighter, so did the amount of hair on the body.[7] The loss of hair was an adaptation to the less frequent sun exposure and colder temperatures to assist the body in absorbing UV rays from the sun (The cooling device hypothesis) **(Box 1.4)**.

Jablonski postulates that increasing body size (allometric theory), in conjunction with intensified hunting during the day at the equator, gave rise to a greater need to rapidly drive out heat (Diurnal hunter hypothesis) **(Box 1.5)**.[7,10,11] As a result, humans evolved the ability to sweat: a process which was facilitated by the loss of body hair. She avers, the bipedalism of human ancestors led to the retention of hair on the scalp, where the absorption of solar radiation is greatest and the generation of heat from muscular activity is low. The bipedality hypothesis put forth by Wheeler (1984) argued that the reduction of body hair was made possible by the lower direct solar radiation fluxes incident upon a bipedal mammal **(Box 1.6)**.[8,9]

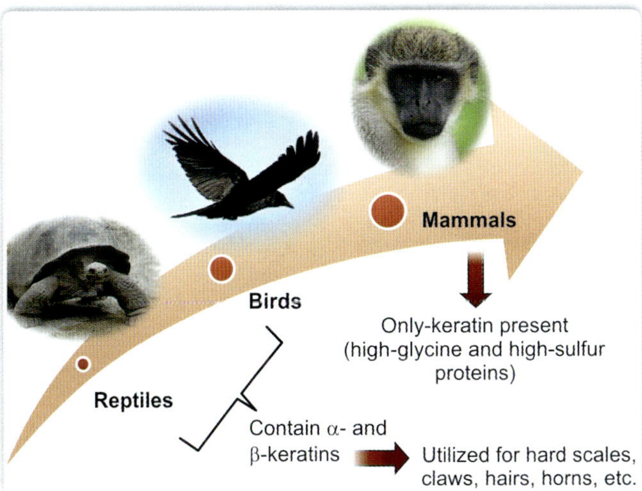

Fig. 1.3: Molecular evolution of alpha and beta keratins

> **Box 1.4: The cooling device hypothesis**
>
> The loss of hair was an adaptation to the less frequent sun exposure and colder temperatures to assist the body in absorbing UV rays from the sun

> **Box 1.5: Allometric theory and Diurnal hunter hypothesis**
>
> Increasing body size and intensified hunting during the day at the equator lead to sweating facilitated by loss of body hair

A few alternative theories have been proposed such as, sexual selection which played a significant role in the loss of human hair. This theory suggests that as humans had more choices in mating partners, those with less body hair (which according to this theory has historically been deemed unattractive—essentially in females) were chosen to mate with.[11] This theory accounts for the significant differences between the amount of hair in females and males (which for other mammals is typically equal).

The other theory proposed were the ancestral human beings having been through a semi aquatic stage, during which they lived on the sea shore, feeding on molluscs and other littoral animals. The fact that the animal morphology most like that of humans, the great apes, are all covered with thick hair and most aquatic mammals are hairless is important evidence for the aquatic ape theory supported by Sir Alister Hardy. This theory argues that many aspects of human anatomy resemble, not that of the great apes but, that of the aquatic mammals **(Box 1.7)**. Thus the idea that we once lived in water like dolphins is considered a reasonable interpretation.[12] The Adaptation against ectoparasite hypothesis putforth by Belt states that humans

> **Box 1.6: Bipedality hypothesis**
>
> Putforth by Wheeler (1984): Reduction of body hair was made possible by the lower direct solar radiation fluxes incident upon a bipedal mammal

> **Box 1.7: Aquatic ape theory**
>
> Putforth by Sir Alister Hardy: This theory argues that many aspects of human anatomy resemble, not that of the great apes but, that of the aquatic mammals

may have lost their body hair to reduce their vulnerability to fur-loving parasites and therefore attract the opposite sex.[13,14]

Thus several hypotheses have been proposed to explain the origins of humans devoid of hair may be summarized as follows, adaptations that facilitate heat exchange, conserve metabolic energy, reduce the incidence of ectoparasites, result from sexual selection or a combination of selective pressures. Hairlessness, combined with an efficient peripheral blood circulatory system and copious sweating may have been an adaption that, cooled the body when our ancestors first became predators.

The nakedness of the human species is extremely rare among the 3000 or so living mammal species. Other naked mammals include elephants, walruses, pigs, whales and the bizarre naked mole-rat.[11]

Conclusion

Evolution of human hair is an enigma that has long fascinated biologists and the phylogenetic origin of hair still remains speculative. The most common theory is that hair evolved from reptile scales as tiny projecting rods in the hinges between scales and served as tactile devices. This sensory protohair might have evolved into an insulative pelage as mammals became endothermic, thus forming hair. Humans seem to be hairless due to a predominance of vellus fibers that are thinner, shorter, and more transparent than terminal fibers rather than absence of follicles. Several such hypotheses have been proposed to explain the relative nakedness of skin but none have been completely accepted.

References

1. Cheng chang, Ping wu, Ruth e. baker, Philip k. maini, Lorenzo alibardi, Cheng-ming chuong. Reptile scale paradigm: Evo-Devo, pattern formation and regeneration. Int J Dev Biol. 2009;53:813-26.
2. Maderson PFA. When? Why? and How? Some speculations on the evolution of the vertebrate integument. Am. Zool. 1972;12:159-71.
3. Dhouailly D, Sun TT. The mammalian tongue filiform papillae: a theoretical model for primitive hairs. In: D van Neste, LaCapelle JM, Antoine JL (eds). Trends In Human Hair Growth and Alopecia Research. Kluwer Acad. Pub. Boston. 1989;pp. 29-34.
4. Alibardi L. Dermo-epidermal interactions in reptilian scales: speculations on the evolution of scales, feathers, and hairs. J. Exp. Zoolog. B. Mol. Dev. Evol. 2004a;302(4):365-83.
5. Eckhart L, Valle LD, Jaeger K, et al. Identification of reptilian genes encoding hair keratin-like proteins suggests a new scenario for the evolutionary origin of hair. Proceedings of the National Academy of Sciences of the United States of America. November 2008;105(47):18419–23. doi:10.1073/pnas.0805154105. PMC 2587626. PMID 19001262. http://www.pubmedcentral.nih.gov/articlerender.fcgi?tool=pmcentrez&artid=2587626.
6. Jerry Bergman. Why Mammal Body Hair Is an Evolutionary Enigma. Creation Research Society Quarterly. Mar 2004;40:240-3.
7. Nina G, Jablonski. The evolution of human skin and skin color. Annu. rev. anthropol. 2004;33:585-623.
8. Wheeler PE. The loss of functional body hair in man: the influence of thermal environment, body form and bipedality. Journal of Human Evolution. 1985;14:23. doi:10.1016/S0047-2484(85)80091-9.
9. Wheeler P. The evolution of bipedality and loss of functional body hair in hominids. Journal of Human Evolution. 1984;13:91. doi:10.1016/S0047-2484(84)80079-2.
10. Schwartz GG, Rosenblum LA. Allometry of primate hair density and the evolution of human hairlessness. American Journal of Physical Anthropology. 1981;55(1):9-12.
11. Rantala MJ. Evolution of nakedness in *Homo sapiens*. Journal of Zoology; 273.
12. Verhaegen MJB. The aquatic ape theory: evidence and possible scenario. Med. Hypothesis. 1985;16:17-32.
13. Pagel, Mark and Bodmer, Walter. A naked ape would have fewer parasites. Proceedings of the Royal Society B: Biological Sciences 2003;270(Suppl 1):S117-S119. doi:10.1098/rsbl.2003.0041. PMC 1698033. PMID 12952654. http://www.pubmedcentral.nih.gov/articlerender.fcgi?tool=pmcentrez&artid=1698033.
14. Rantala MJ. Human nakedness: adaptation against ectoparasites?. International journal for parasitology. 1999;29(12):1987-9. doi:10.1016/S0020-7519(99)00133-2. PMID 10961855. http://users.utu.fi/mjranta/reprints/1.%20Rantala1999.pdf.

2

Hair Anatomy

Shilpa K, S Sacchidanand

"The hair is the richest ornament of women."

—*Martin Luther*

Introduction

Hair has no vital function in humans, yet its psychological functions are extremely important, which brings one's self-image into focus. The human hair follicle (HF) is a sophisticated miniorgan, composed of multiple mesenchymal and epithelial cell layers, consisting of more than 20 different cell populations in total. Together with the arrector pili muscle and the sebaceous gland, the hair follicle forms the pilosebaceous unit **(Box 2.1)**. It has the extraordinary capability of self-renewal. Understanding the complex biology and function of the hair follicle requires familiarity with its anatomy, especially of the bulge region, the putative residence of the hair follicle stem cells, and the dermal papilla, which are believed to be responsible for the regulation of the hair cycle. Although the exact role of each part of the hair follicle has for long been a mystery, recent advances in hair follicle research have given us better insight on their function in maintaining hair follicle growth and cycle.[1]

Types of Hair (Box 2.2)

There are different types of hair on human body and different types of hair can be produced by any particular follicle under the influence of hormones or advancing age.[2] There are four different types of hair.

Box 2.1: Components of a pilosebaceous unit

- Hair follicles
- Arrector pili muscle
- Sebaceous gland

Lanugo Hairs (Latin: Lana-Wool) (Figure 2.1)

Lanugo hairs are the prenatal coat of hair consisting of fine, soft, unmedullated and usually unpigmented hair, which covers the entire body in humans in utero and is normally shed in the eighth to ninth month of gestation and are replaced by vellus hairs by 36–40 weeks. The presence of lanugo hairs at birth may indicate prematurity.[3] Lanugo

Box 2.2: Types of hair

- Prenatal—lanugo
- Postnatal—
  - Vellus
  - Terminal
  - Intermediate

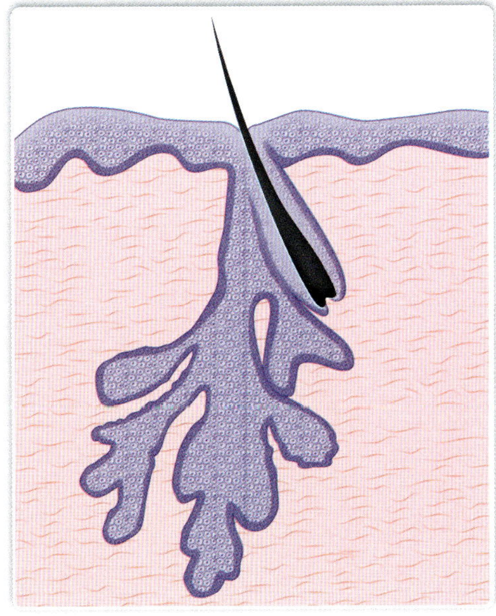

Fig. 2.1: Unmedullated lanugo hair

Box 2.3: Causes of persistent lanugo hairs

- Congenital hypertrichosis lanuginosa
- Acquired lanugo hair
  - Anorexia nervosa
  - Bulimia nervosa
  - Hypertrichosis lanuginosa acquisita—aero digestive tract malignancy

Box 2.4: Areas devoid of vellus hairs

- Lips
- Back of the ear
- Palms and soles
- Navel
- Some parts of external genitalia

hairs have been reported to occur in adults in psychiatric conditions like anorexia nervosa and bulimia nervosa and their occurrence in these conditions has been explained as an attempt to prevent heat loss from the body which can occur due to loss of subcutaneous fat in these patients.[4] In congenital hypertrichosis lanuginosa, the fetal pelage is not replaced by vellus and terminal hair but persists, grows excessively and is constantly renewed throughout life.[5] Hypertrichosis lanuginosa acquisita is a very rare condition characterized by the rapid growth of long, fine, lanugo-type hair particularly around the eyebrows, forehead, ears and nose seen with aero digestive tract malignancy as a cutaneous marker of internal malignancy **(Box 2.3)**.[6]

Postnatal hair may be divided into three kinds: Vellus, terminal, and intermediate hairs.

Vellus Hairs (Latin: Vellus-Fleece) (Figure 2.2)

The vellus hair is soft, unmedullated, occasionally pigmented and seldom grows more than 2 cms long and present over much of the body area, exceptions include lips, back of the ear, palm, sole, some external genital areas, the navel and scar tissue **(Box 2.4)**. After puberty, under the influence of androgen, vellus hairs are replaced by 'terminal' hairs in certain areas like beard, axilla, pubic area, etc.

Vellus hairs help in preventing heat loss from the body. An entity called eruptive vellus hair cyst has been reported in children.[7] Vellus hairs are resistant to laser hair reduction procedures.[8]

Terminal Hairs (Figure 2.3)

Terminal hair is the pigmented, longer, coarser hair and consistently possess a medulla. Till puberty, distribution of terminal hair is normally limited to the eyebrows, eyelashes and the scalp. After puberty they replace vellus hairs in areas like beard, axilla and pubic area, etc. Pubic and axillary hair will develop in both men and women, and they are considered as a secondary sex characteristics[9] although, males will develop terminal hair in more areas. This includes facial hair, chest hair, abdominal hair, leg and arm hair, and foot hair. Females, on the other hand retain more of the vellus hairs.[10]

Hypertrichosis is the term used for excessive hair growth on any part or whole body as compared to persons of the same age, sex and race.[11] Hypertrichosis must not be confused with hirsutism, which is defined as androgen-induced growth of terminal hair in women and children, in a male pattern distribution. Hirsutism is androgen-dependent while hypertrichosis is not.[12] In hirsute women, vellus follicles manufacture terminal hairs in certain areas of the body like cheeks, chin, chest, lower back and abdomen in response to increased circulating androgen levels.[13] Permanent reduction of pigmented terminal hairs can be done using laser **(Table 2.1)**.[14]

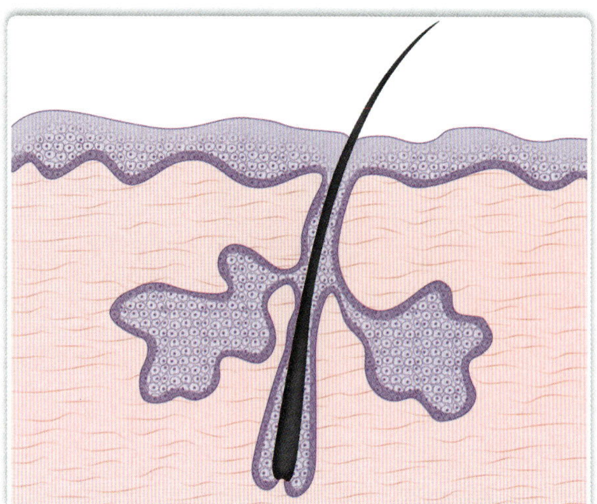

Fig. 2.2: Short unmedullated vellus hair

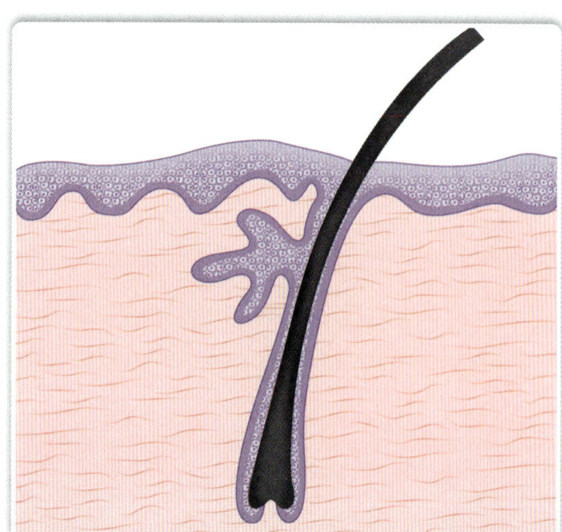

Fig. 2.3: Coarse thick medullated terminal hair

Table 2.1: Characteristics of hypertrichosis and hirsutism

	Hypertrichosis	*Hirsutism*
Definition	Excessive hair growth on any part or whole body in comparison to persons of same age, sex and race	Androgen induced growth of terminal hair
Sex predilection	No	Seen in women and children
Androgen dependency	Absent	Present
Areas affected	Generalized	Cheeks, chin, chest, lower back, abdomen

Intermediate Hairs

There is another variant of postnatal hair called as intermediate hair. It shows the characteristics of both vellus hairs and terminal hairs. Intermediate hairs have a medulla and contain a moderate amount of pigment, less than that found in the terminal hair type.

During the balding process terminal hair follicles and intermediate hair follicles change in such a way, that they no longer produce terminal hairs. In these areas, hair follicles grow vellus hairs rather than terminal hairs resulting in androgenic alopecia.[15]

Morphological Variants of Hair (Box 2.5)

Morphologically, hairs can be divided into four categories:

Spiral Hairs

Hairs in Blacks are spiral because the hair follicles are curved and the bases of their bulb are oriented somewhat horizontal to the skin surface. In addition, different rates of growth of matrical cells along the side of the bulbs may be responsible for the spirals. It is hypothesized that curly hair impedes the passage of UV light into the body relative to straight hair, thus curly or coiled hair would be particularly advantageous for dark-skinned hominids living at the equator.[16]

Straight Hairs

Hairs in Asians are straight because the follicles are straight and oriented vertically to thc skin surfacc. Straight hair would have been an adaptive liability as hominoids traveled farther from Africa or the equator. Straight hair may have (initially) evolved to aid the entry of UV light into the body during the transition from dark, UV-protected skin to pale-white skin.[16]

Box 2.5: Morphological variants of hair

- Spiral hair
- Straight hair
- Helical hair
- Wavy hair

Helical Hairs

It can be seen in Whites. Helical hair accompanying trichorrhexis invaginata and pili torti in an infant with Netherton's syndrome has been reported.[17]

Wavy Hairs

Hair in Whites may be any of these four types, but most are wavy or straight.

Woolly hair is the tightly coiled hair occurring over the entire scalp or part of it, in an individual of non-Negroid origin.[18]

Hair Thickness

Hair thickness can vary tremendously depending on race, continent, varies from person to person, day to day, year to year. It also depends on anatomical site-body hair or head hair and gender. Hair from a human head is normally between 0.04 and 0.25 mm, averaging normally 0.1 mm.[19] The term anisotrichosis has recently been proposed to describe diversity of hair shaft diameter. Anisotrichosis more than 20% on trichoscopy is diagnostic of female androgenetic alopecia (FAGA) **(Box 2.6)**.[20]

Hair Shape and Texture (Figure 2.4)

The shape of the hair strand when cut in cross-section varies depending on the race. It is round in shape in Asians, slightly less round in Caucasians and oval or elliptical in African hair.[21] However, nutritional status and intentional alteration (heat curling, "perms") can affect the physical appearance of hair.

Box 2.6: Anisotrichosis

- Refers to diversity in hair shaft diameter
- Average hair thickness 0.1 mm (0.04–0.25 mm)
- More than 20% anisotrichosis on trichoscopy implies FAGA

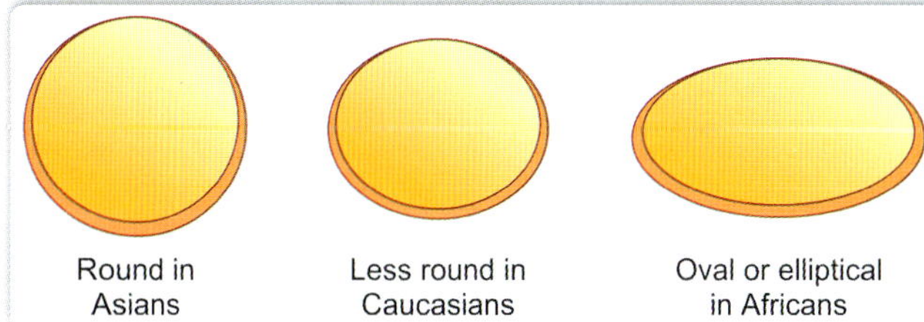

Fig. 2.4: Cross-section of terminal hair. It is round in shape in Asians, slightly less round in Caucasians and oval or elliptical in African hair

Hair shine is an optical phenomenon that depends on the light reflected by outer layers of the cuticle, higher the number of layers, the higher the ratio of the reflected light and the more intense is the luster. Luster may be affected by hair surface damage, hair color and their morphology. Other factors that influence luster include the presence of sebum, which eliminates this shine and renders the hair dull and unattractive by an interference mechanism.[22]

Composition of Hair

In terms of raw elements on an average hair is composed of 50% carbon, 20% oxygen, 17% nitrogen, 6% hydrogen and 5% sulfur. Hair also contains trace amounts of magnesium, arsenic, iron, chromium and other metals and minerals **(Table 2.2)**.[23]

Development of Hair Follicles

During embryonic development human hair follicles appear at about 9 weeks. First it emerges in the regions of the eyebrows, upper lip and chin, and by fourth month covers the entire body.[24] In humans, the full complement of hair follicles is probably established by the time of birth. New hair follicles are never formed after birth.

In many cases, areas on the human body that contain vellus hair will begin to produce darker, thicker body hair. An example of this is the growth of an adolescent's beard on a once smooth chin. Androgenic hair follows the same growth pattern as the hair that grows on the scalp, only the anagen phase is shorter, and the telogen phase is longer.

Follicle Density

There are approximately 100,000 hair follicles on the scalp.[25] It varies with the age, sex, race and area of the body. Follicle density is defined as number of hair follicles per unit area of skin. It is highest in the fetus, and is uniform across the skin surface because of the smaller body surface area. As the child grows there is a progressive reduction in follicle density, as skin surface area increases.

The forehead and cheeks have the highest hair follicle densities, which is approximately 800/cm^2 and in women on cheeks it is 400–450/cm^2.[26] Chest and back show lower hair densities of 50–100/cm^2,[26,27] and, follicle densities on the thigh and leg is around 50/cm^2.[28] Hair density on scalp varies between 250–320 hairs/cm^2.[29]

Density of scalp hair varies between various races, in Africans it is 187/cm^2,[30] in African Americans it is 171/cm^2,[31] and in Koreans 128/cm^2.[32]

On the scalp, and some other regions of the skin, hair follicles are arranged in groups of three or more follicles known as follicular units. The follicular unit is defined as a group of one to three hairs that grow naturally together, also includes one to two fine vellus hair, glands, muscle, nerves and blood vessels.[33] Several follicles within a follicular unit may coalesce so that hairs emerge through a common infundibulum **(Figure 2.5)**.

By keeping the transplanted micrografts to the size of a naturally occurring follicular unit, it is possible to provide hair restoration that is natural looking and undetectable.

Rate of Hair Growth

The rate of hair growth varies from species to species and within one species from region to region, as well as with sex and age. While there is some variation, human hair generally grows at a rate of 1 cm per month or 0.35 mm/day. According to a study done with graduated capillary tubes being fitted around the growing hairs, the average growth in males was as shown in **Box 2.7**.[34]

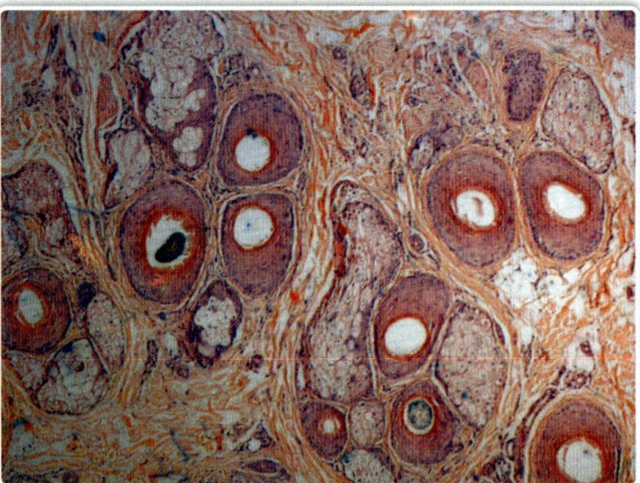

Fig. 2.5: Horizontal section of scalp specimen showing follicular unit

Table 2.2: Composition of hair

Carbon	50%
Oxygen	20%
Nitrogen	17%
Hydrogen	6%
Sulfur	5%
Traces of magnesium, arsenic, iron, chromium and other metals	

Box 2.7: Rate of hair growth

- 0.35 mm/day or 1 cm per month
- Vertex 0.44 mm/24 hours
- Temple 0.39 mm/24 hours
- Beard 0.27 mm/24 hours
- Chest 0.44 mm/24 hours in males

Hair Color

Hair color is determined by the melanocytes found in the matrix area of the follicle at the base of the cortex directly above the follicular papilla. Melanocytes transfer melanosomes to cortical cells during anagen. Eumelanin is the dominant global pigment and confers black or brown hair. Pheomelanin, a mutation of eumelanin, is the predominant pigment found in blond hair.[35] The proportions of eumelanin and pheomelanin and the total amount of melanin determine the hair color.[36] Graying of hair is a normal manifestation of ageing and illustrates progressive reduction in melanocyte function.

Just as epidermal keratinocytes incorporate melanosomes by clipping off the ends of melanocytic dendrites by apocopation, matrix cells of the follicle do the same to dendrites of melanocytes situated within the follicular bulb. The ratio of follicular cells to melanocytes in hair bulb is 1:1.[37] Cells of the cuticle of the hair do not contain melanosomes **(Table 2.3)**.

Black and dark brown are the prevalent natural hair colors of the people of all regions accounting for more than 90% of all human hair. Dark hair is characterized by very high levels of the dark pigment eumelanin. Blond hair is characterized by very low levels of the dark pigment eumelanin and very high levels of the pale pigment pheomelanin. Red hair (rutilism) is associated with the melanocortin-1 receptor gene anomaly, which is found on chromosome 16.[38] Red hair is an example of incomplete dominance **(Box 2.8)**. When only one copy of the red hair allele is present, red hair may blend with the other hair color, resulting in different types of red hair including strawberry blonde (red blonde) and auburn (red brown).

Anatomy of the Hair Follicle

Human hair is a filamentous outgrowth of the skin which grows from hair follicles deep in the skin dermis and projects out above the epidermis. The follicles are sloped in the dermis, and longer follicles extend into the subcutaneous layer. An oblique muscle, the arrector pili, runs from the mid-region of the follicle wall to a point in the papillary dermis close to the dermal epidermal junction. Above the muscle, one or more sebaceous glands and in some regions of the body an apocrine gland also, opens into the follicle.

Broadly, the structure of hair is divided into two components: the hair shaft and hair root.

The hair root may be divided anatomically into four parts from below upwards **(Figure 2.6)**.

1. The bulb consisting of the dermal papilla and matrix
2. The suprabulbar area from the matrix to the insertion of the arrector pili muscle
3. The isthmus that extends from the insertion of the arrector pili muscle to the sebaceous gland
4. The infundibulum that extends from the sebaceous gland to the follicular orifice.

Table 2.3: Factors determining the hair color

- ❑ Ratio of follicular cells to melanocytes in hair bulb (normal 1:1)
- ❑ Total amount of melanin in the follicular matrix at the base of cortex
- ❑ Dominant pigment : Eumelanin or pheomelanin
- ❑ Proportions of eumelanin and pheomelanin
- ❑ Melanosome transfer mechanisms in cortical cells
- ❑ Hair cycle stage: Anagen phase

Box 2.8: Rutilism

- Refers to presence of red hair
- Incomplete dominant pattern of inheritance
- Melanocortin 1 receptor gene anomaly found on chromosome 16
- Presence of one red allele copy may lead to strawberry blonde or Auburn hair

Hair Bulb (Figures 2.7 and 2.8)

The lowest part of a hair follicle is called the bulb because it resembles the bulb of a tulip or an onion. In large terminal follicles, the hair bulb is situated in the subcutaneous fat. The hair bulb encloses the dermal papilla which invaginates its base and is connected to the perifollicular dermal sheath by a narrow stalk.

The boundaries of a pear shaped follicular bulb are the base of a follicle below and the summit of the high arched curve of the "keratogenous zone" that ends at the distinct border known as Adamson's fringe **(Box 2.9)**.

The site at which Huxley's layer loses its trichohyalin granules and begins to cornify defines both Adamson's fringe and the upper boundary of the bulb. The epithelial

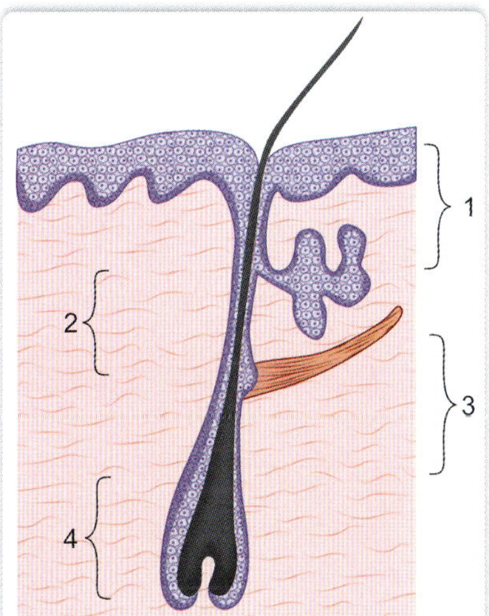

Fig. 2.6: Different parts of the hair bulb: 1. Infundibulum; 2. Isthmus; 3. Suprabulbar region; 4. Bulb

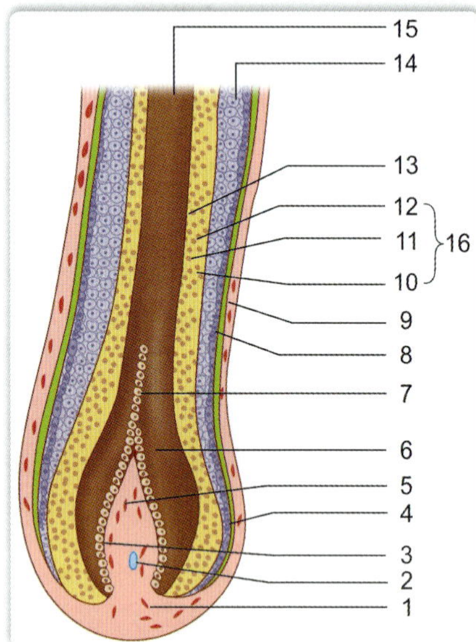

Fig. 2.7: Vertical section of the hair bulb: 1. Connective tissue of the cutis; 2. Blood vessel; 3. Glassy layer of the hair bulb; 4. Hair bulb; 5. Hair papilla; 6. Cortical substance of hair; 7. Medulla of the hair; 8. Basal cells of outer root sheath; 9. Glassy layer; 10. Henle's layer; 11. Huxley's layer; 12. Cuticle of inner root sheath; 13. Cuticle of the hair; 14. Stratum malphigii of outer root sheath; 15. The hair; 16. Inner root sheath

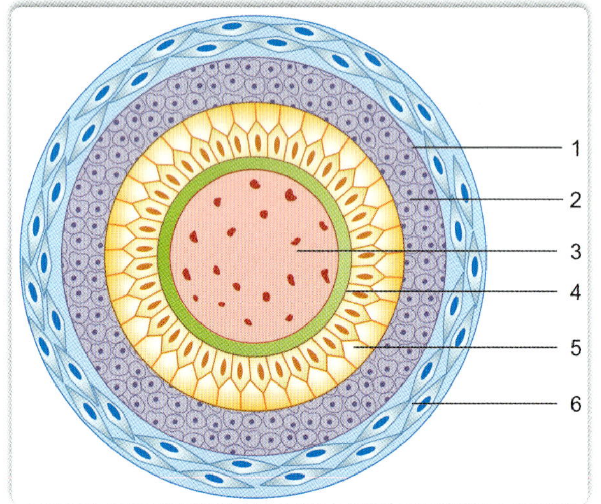

Fig. 2.8: Horizontal section of hair root: 1. Glassy layer; 2. Outer root sheath; 3. Cortex of the hair; 4. Cuticle of the inner root sheath; 5. Henle's layer; 6. Fibrous tissue sheath

Box 2.9: Adamson's fringe

- Imaginary border that marks the summit of keratogenous zone
- Huxley layer loses its trichohyalin granules and begins to cornify
- Layers lack complete cornification
- Keratinophilic dermatophytes fail to descend below this line

cells in the keratogenous zone are all nucleated, i.e. from the outside in, the pale and clear cells of the outer root sheath, trichohyalin granules containing cells of the inner root sheath, and the cells of the future hair. It is at Adamson's fringe that cornification of the viable keratinocytes can first be recognized, cells of the inner root sheath lose their trichohyalin granules and become bluish gray, and compactly arranged corneocytes and cells of maturing hairs lose their nuclei and come to resemble fully cornified hairs. The process of keratinization proceeds apace in pyriform bulb of a follicle, but complete cornification does not occur here. It is for this reason that dermatophytes, dependent on cornified cells to live never descend a follicle below Adamson's fringe.[39]

The hair bulb matrix or germinal epithelium constitutes epithelial cells surrounding the dermal papilla with a high mitotic rate and a rate of cell turnover similar to that in the bone marrow. The progeny of the dividing cells migrate upwards and differentiate in a highly ordered fashion to form the concentric layers of the inner root sheath and the hair shaft. The inner root sheath is derived from cells in the lower, more lateral part of the matrix, whereas the hair shaft is formed from the upper, centrally situated cells.

In pigmented hair follicles, highly melanized melanocytes are situated amongst cells destined to form the hair cortex.[34] Occasional Langerhans' cells may also be found in the matrix region.

The germinative (matrix) cells of follicular bulbs differentiate along seven separate pathways that, in part may be related to the distance of matricial cells from the center of the papilla. These morphological changes in follicular epithelium are discernable first near the base of the bulb where the outer root sheath, the three layers of the inner root sheath, and the three layers of the hair begin to be formed.

From outside, the seven components of the bulb are:

1. The outer root sheath filled with glycogen during anagen and therefore composed of pale and clear cells.
2. Henle's layer of the inner sheath, one cell thick with prominent trichohyalin granules and the first to cornify.
3. Huxley's layer of the inner sheath, two cells thick and characterized by numerous brightly eosinophilic trichohyalin granules.
4. Cuticle of the inner sheath, one cell thick.
5. Cuticle of the hair composed of a single layer of imbricated squames that wrap around the hair.
6. Cortex of the hair that constitutes the bulk of it.
7. The medulla of the hair, the last to cornify.

Dermal Papilla

The dermal papilla is a flask-shaped structure that invaginates the base of the hair follicle, derived from a condensation of mesenchymal cells. It is made up of specialized fibroblast-like cells embedded in an extracellular matrix rich in basement-membrane proteins and proteoglycans, and contains a loop of capillary blood vessels in large follicles. It is connected to the dermal sheath surrounding the follicle by a narrow stalk. The dermal papilla itself is not the source of the hair, the active germinal epithelium lying over it is. The presence and close proximity of the dermal papilla to the germinal matrix induces it to proliferate by sending chemical signals. When the signal is received, the germinal matrix proliferates and produces the hair and the inner root sheath. The triggering of hair growth by proximity of the dermal papilla is a classic example of the phenomenon of induction, the response of one cell population to signals from a second population.[40]

The bulbs and papillae in a given section of skin are not all the same size. In anagen, the growing phase, a well developed flask shaped dermal papilla is seen. In catagen phase, the dermal papilla shrinks and withdraws away from the bulb. This removes the necessary induction and the hair stops growing. The dermal papillae are smaller in hairs which are being shed (telogen hair).

The dermal papilla is the primary target of androgen action in the hair follicle. Androgen receptor expression in the lower part of the follicle is restricted to dermal papilla cells.[41,42] The size of the hair follicle is probably determined by the volume of the dermal papilla.[43] Dermal papillae express 5α-reductase type 2 whereas hair follicle epithelium expresses only 5α-reductase type 1 **(Box 2.10)**.[42]

Functions

1. Dermal papilla plays an essential part in the induction and maintenance of follicular epithelial differentiation.[40]
2. It is responsible for determining the follicle type.
3. The volume of the dermal papilla may also be responsible for controlling the size of the hair follicle, and that of the hair fiber.[44]

Suprabulbar Region

It is the longest section of terminal hair follicle in anagen. Isthmus and hair bulb form the upper and lower boundary of the suprabulbar region respectively. It is comprised of three layers from innermost to outermost: hair shaft, inner root sheath and outer root sheath. The outer root sheath is a multilayered epithelium enclosing the inner root sheath which, at this level, is a fully keratinized structure. Cells of the hair shaft, at the center of the follicle, undergo terminal differentiation within the keratogenous zone in the middle part of the suprabulbar region.

Isthmus

The isthmus extends from the opening of the sebaceous gland duct to the insertion of the arrector pili muscle. It consists of a multilayered outer root sheath that is continuous with the infundibulum but differs in its structure. The innermost cells undergo trichilemmal keratinization, a pattern of differentiation characterized by deposition of compact eosinophilic keratin without an intervening granular layer **(Box 2.11)**.[45] The keratinized inner root sheath, which lies within the outer root sheath, disintegrates at or about the level of the sebaceous duct. The bulge region below the isthmus, which allows insertion of arrector pili muscle also harbors a specialized compartment of outer root sheath, which form the niche for epithelial and neuroectodermal stem cells as well as various immature cell population including immature Langerhans cell and mast cell.

The stem cells were first described by Cotsarelis G [46] et al. These hair follicle stem cells are highly pluripotent which can proliferate and differentiate into various cell lines like neurons, muscles, etc.[47] In hair, these stem cells proliferate only during the onset of anagen. These dividing hair follicle stem cells, known as transient amplifying cells, migrate downwards and enter the hair bulb matrix where they proliferate and undergo terminal differentiation to form the hair shaft and inner root sheath. Not only the hair follicle, they also migrate distally to form the sebaceous gland and under certain circumstances such as wound healing, the epidermis **(Figure 2.9)**.[48]

The hair follicle stem cells may become the stem cells of choice in the future for regenerative medicine[47] since, (1) They are readily available from essentially anyone, (2) They are easily cultured and expanded, (3) They are highly pluripotent, (4) They have been demonstrated to be able to support the regrowth of nerves, (5) They do not carry the ethical issues that embryonic stem cells and fetal stem cells do. The near future should be an exciting time in stem cell.

Box 2.10: Dermal papillae

- Specialized fibroblast like cells embedded in extracellular matrix, mesenchymal in origin
- Rich in basement-membrane proteins and proteoglycans
- Contains a loop of capillary blood vessels
- Flask shaped in anagen while shrinks during catagen phase
- Primary target of androgen action in the hair follicle as they express 5α-reductase type 2
- Triggers hair growth by proximity of the dermal papilla (phenomenon of induction)

Box 2.11: Trichilemmal keratinization

- A pattern of differentiation characterized by deposition of compact eosinophilic keratin without an intervening granular layer
- The trichilemmal keratinization of ORS starts at the level of isthmus where the IRS disintegrates. At the level of the infundibulum, keratinization of the outer root sheath changes to normal epidermal keratinization
- Cysts arising from the isthmus portion of the hair follicle showing trichilemmal mode of keratinization termed as trichilemmal cysts/isthmus-catagen type of follicular cysts/pilar cysts

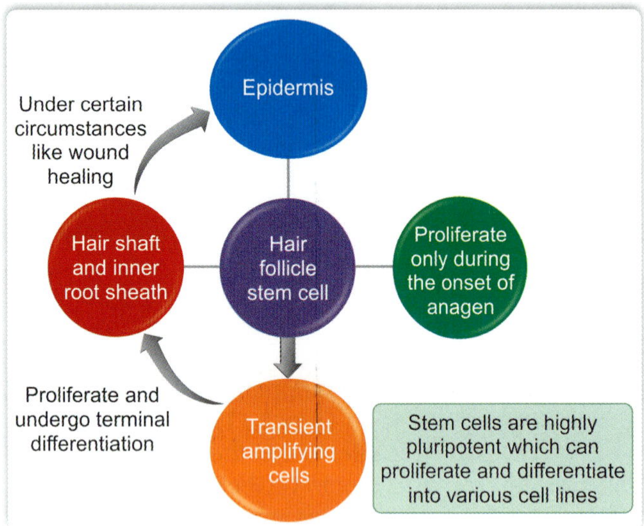

Figure 2.9: Schematic representation of hair follicle stem cell functions

Cysts arising from the isthmus portion of the hair follicle showing trichilemmal mode of keratinization termed as trichilemmal cysts or isthmus-catagen type of follicular cysts or pilar cysts has been reported.[49]

Arrector Pili Muscle (Box 2.12)

The arrector pili muscle associated with each follicle is a band of smooth muscle whose origin is in the fibrils of the dermis. It inserts onto the connective tissue investment of the follicle. Unlike the hair, which is ectodermal in origin, and part of the epidermis, the arrector pili is a true dermal structure and derived from embryonic mesoderm. Arrector pili muscle is absent in eye lashes.[20]

When the arrector pili contracts, it elevates the hair. This phenomenon of piloerection can occur in response to a number of stimuli. Piloerection is a common response to cold; lifting the hair increases the air spaces and hence the insulating value of the hair coat. It also occurs in response to anger or fear, because of the adrenaline surge that these emotions involve.[50]

Infundibulum (In Latin: Funnel) (Box 2.13)

The infundibulum extends from the skin surface, where it merges with the epidermis, to the opening of the sebaceous duct at the junction with the isthmus. The funnel shaped infundibulum eventually passes through the epidermis, where it is known as acrotrichium.

Box 2.12: Arrector pili muscle

- Band of smooth muscle ectodermal in origin
- Inserts onto the connective tissue investment of the follicle
- Absent in eyelashes
- It contracts to elevate the hair, i.e. piloerection in response to adrenaline surge.

Box 2.13: Infundibulum

- Extends from the skin surface, where it merges with the epidermis, to the opening of the sebaceous duct at the isthmus
- Epidermal surface opening referred to as acrotrichium
- Infundibular epithelium lacks rete ridges and is thinner
- Infrainfundibulum epithelium differs from that of an infundibulum by having walls that are parallel, a slightly thinner granular zone, and fewer corneocytes
- Harbor a variety of bacteria (e.g. *Staphylococcus epidermidis*, *Propionibacterium acnes*), yeasts (e.g. *Pityrosporum orbiculare* and *P. ovale*) and mite *Demodex folliculorum*

Infundibular epithelium is nearly identical morphologically to the epidermis with which it is continuous, and it cornifies in the same manner. The corneocyte of the epidermis and infundibulum are arranged in basket weave pattern. A granular zone with numerous keratohyalin granules is present beneath the cornified layer of the infundibulum, including infrainfundibulum. Infundibular epithelium differs slightly from epidermal epithelium because it generally lacks rete ridges and is thinner. The epithelium of infrainfundibulum differs from that of an infundibulum by having walls that are parallel, a slightly thinner granular zone, and fewer corneocytes.

Follicular infundibula, especially on the scalp, face and upper part of the trunk, normally harbor a variety of bacteria (e.g. *Staphylococcus epidermidis*, *Propionibacterium acnes*), yeasts (e.g. *Pityrosporum orbiculare* and *P. ovale*) and mite, *Demodex folliculorum*. They are normal non pathogenic commensals, and do not cause skin diseases in persons who are competent immunologically.

Sometimes a cyst occurring on the face and lined by epithelium like that of follicular infundibulum termed as infundibular cyst has been reported.[51] Infundibular carcinoma has also been reported as a separate entity with distinct histopathological and immunohistochemical markers.[52]

Dermal Sheath

The dermal or connective tissue sheath envelopes the lower part of the hair follicle. The dermal sheath becomes less distinct, both structurally and functionally, as it is traced upwards as it merges with the interfollicular dermis above the level of the arrector pili insertion. They contain progenitor cells which are specialized fibroblasts that maintain and regenerate the dermal papilla, a key component for hair growth. They can become wound healing fibroblasts and perform an important function in the repair of skin dermis after injury. In experimental animals, cultured peribulbar dermal sheath cells can induce hair follicle development and contribute to the dermal sheath and dermal papilla.[53]

Inner Root Sheath

The inner root sheath (IRS) of the hair follicle is located between the outer root sheath and the hair shaft. It is made of three layers: Henle's layer, Huxley's layer, and the cuticle **(Figure 2.10)**.

Henle's layer is the outermost layer of the inner root sheath, consisting of a single row of cubical transparent cells that do not contain nuclei. Huxley's layer is in the middle, made up of approximately two rows of flattened cells with granular protoplasm. The cuticle of the root sheath is in the center, continuous with the outermost layer of the hair fiber. Flugzellen (winged cells) are specialized cells of Huxley's layer in the supra-bulbous portion of the follicle, which shows elongated cytoplasmic pseudopods that traverse the rigid cornified impermeable Henle's layer and connect with the innermost cells of the outer root sheath **(Box 2.14)**.[54]

Henle's layer is the first to cornify followed by the cuticle while, the cells of Huxley's layer cornify last of all. The cornification occurs through the formation of bright pink trichohyalin granules (the trichological counterpart of the keratohyaline granules of the epidermis and the follicular infundibulum). As the cells transform and get fully keratinized, the cytoplasm appears homogenous with filaments in a dense matrix. The trichohyalin granules and the nucleus disappear with scattered remnants of cytoplasmic organelles and nuclear ghosts in fully developed cornified cells.[55]

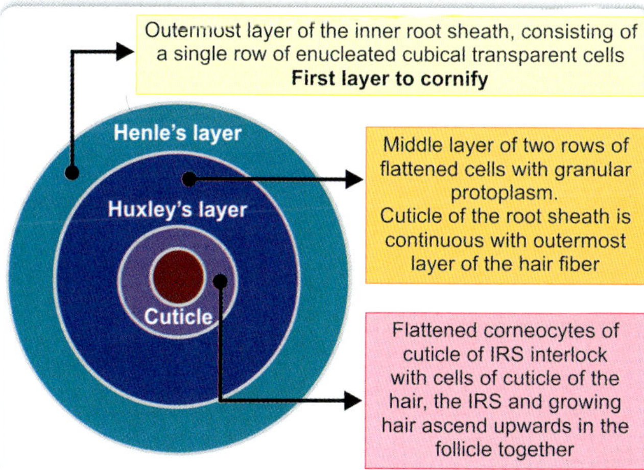

Fig. 2.10: Schematic representation of layers of inner root sheath

Box 2.14: Flugzellen cells (winged cells)

- Specialized cells of Huxley's layer in the supra-bulbous portion of the follicle, which shows elongated cytoplasmic pseudopod
- Cells traverse the rigid cornified impermeable Henle's layer and connect with innermost cells of ORS
- Function as nutritive canals between the not yet keratinized Huxley's layer and the ORS

Functionally, the inner root sheath serves as a rigid funnel-shaped protective covering around the hair and the flattened corneocytes of the cuticle of the inner root sheath overlap and interlock intimately with the cells of the cuticle of the hair ensuring that the inner root sheath and the growing hair that it protects, ascend upwards in the follicle together.[56] It is essential for the proper moulding, adherence, and keratinization of the growing hair. The Flugzellen of Huxley's layer are postulated to function as nutritive canals between the not yet keratinized Huxley's layer and the outer root sheath, bypassing the fully cornified and impermeable Henle's layer.[57] Premature keratinization of the inner root sheath has been implicated in the loss of the anchoring function and subsequent deformation of the hair shaft in loose anagen hair syndrome,[58] central centrifugal cicatricial alopecia (CCCA) and other cicatricial alopecia.[59]

Outer Root Sheath

The outer root sheath (ORS) is the outermost layer of hair follicle epithelium, enclosing the inner root sheath. Around the hair bulb it is a single layer of cuboidal cells, becomes multilayered in the region of the upper hair bulb. The outer root sheath cells appear as clear cells with routine histological stains as they are rich in glycogen.

The ORS does not consist of a homogeneous cell population. Ultrastructural studies have determined at least two distinct cell types in the ORS: (1) Multiple layers of cubical cells located at the outer surface, containing large quantities of glycogen, and (2) A single layer of flattened cells closely associated with the peripheral Henle's layer of the IRS. This single layer, referred by Ito as 'the innermost cell layer of the ORS,' was named by Orwin[60] as the 'companion layer' because of its close association with Henle's layer cells. At the level of the companion layer is the slippage plane at which the IRS-packaged hair shaft moves distally up to the skin surface. The companion layer can be followed from the hair bulb up to the isthmus, moving in conjunction with the IRS **(Box 2.15)**. At the end of terminal differentiation, at the upper isthmus level, both the cells

Box 2.15: Companion layer

- The innermost single cell layer of the ORS
- Named by Orwin because of its close association with Henle's layer cells
- Slippage plane at which the IRS-packaged hair shaft moves distally upto the skin surface
- Calretinin, calcium-binding protein is a marker of the companion cell layer
- At the upper isthmus level, both the cells of the IRS and companion layer cornify, degrade and slough in the follicular lumen while other ORS cells undergo trichilemmal keratinization

of the IRS and the companion layer cornify, degrade and slough in the follicular lumen, whereas the ORS cells undergo trichilemmal keratinization. The calcium-binding protein, calretinin is a marker of the companion cell layer of the human hair follicle.[61]

There appear to be two forms of melanocytes in the hair follicle: (1) An amelanotic melanocyte and (2) A dendritic DOPA-positive melanocyte. Distinctive cells believed to be non-functioning amelanotic melanocytes are present along the periphery of the outer root sheath of the human hair follicle.[62] It is believed that DOPA-negative melanocytes in the outer root sheath of the human hair follicle are activated, become identifiable by DOPA staining and migrate into the epidermis during the repigmenting phase of vitiligo. These cells are difficult to identify, however and otherwise have not been characterized. These cells are readily identified by immunofluorescence, immunohistochemistry and immunoelectron microscopy using the antibodies NKI/beteb and A4F11, which recognize premelanosome-related antigens.[63] Noncultured extracted hair follicle outer root sheath cell suspension has been tried in vitiligo.[64]

The trichilemmal keratinization of the outer root sheath starts at the level of isthmus where the inner root sheath disintegrates. At the level of the infundibulum, keratinization of the outer root sheath changes to normal epidermal keratinization.

Hair Shaft (Figure 2.11)

The hair shaft is made up of three cell layers:

1. An outer cuticle
2. The cortex
3. A variable central medulla.

Fig. 2.11: Hair (terminal) shaft under light microscope showing cortex and medulla

Cuticle (Figure 2.12)

Cuticle is the outermost layer of hair. It is made up of hard, transparent cells that overlap each other like the scales of a fish. It is formed initially as a single cell layer, but the cells become progressively imbricated (tile-like) as they move peripherally. The cells become flattened, and their outer edges point in an upward direction and interlock with the cuticle of the surrounding inner root sheath. In the fully formed hair shaft, the cuticle consists of 5–10 overlapping cell layers, each 350–450 nm thick. The cuticle cells may be elongated, acuminate (gradually tapering to a point), ovate (egg shaped), or flattened. Although the cuticle is the outermost layer of the hair, it does not give the hair its color because it has no melanin, which is found in the cortex.

Under electron microscopy, the mature cells of the cuticle consisting of compact cuticular keratin associated with ultra-high sulfur proteins show three distinct layers:

a. The outer a-layer, which is particularly rich in cysteine.
b. The exocuticle (also cysteine-rich). The exocuticle lies closer to the external surface and comprises of three parts; the b-layer, the a-layer and the epicuticle. The a- and b-layers are largely proteinaceous. The epicuticle is a hydrophobic lipid layer of 18-methyloctanoic acid on the surface of the fiber, or the f-layer **(Box 2.16)**.[51]
c. The inner endocuticle is virtually devoid of sulfur and has an irregular substructure of membrane-like elements which are probably the remnants of cytoplasmic structures.[65]

The cuticle has a smooth appearance and has important protective properties by limiting friction between the hair shafts, responsible for the luster, elasticity, resilience and

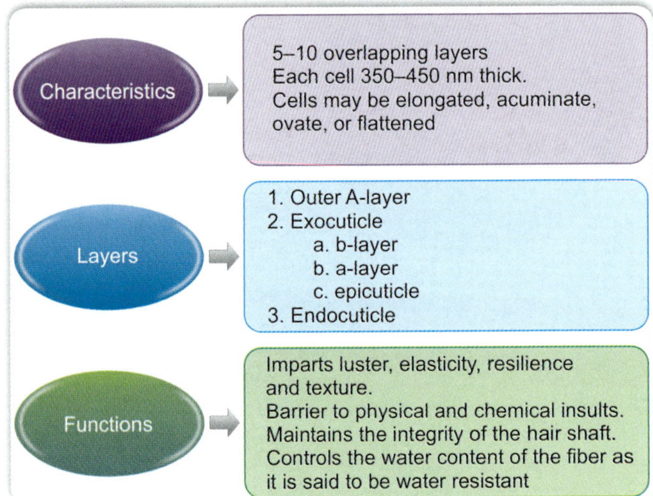

Fig. 2.12: Characteristics of cuticle of outer root sheath

Box 2.16: f- layer

- Epicuticle is a hydrophobic lipid layer of 18-methyloctanoic acid on the surface of the fiber, or the f-layer
- Chemical removal of the f-layer by oxidation eliminates the first hydrophobic defense and leaves hair more porous and vulnerable

texture, acts as a barrier to physical and chemical insults, also maintains the integrity of the hair shaft. The cuticle represents the structure that controls the water content of the fiber as it is said to be water resistant.

Brushing, using heat (like using curling irons) or chemical processing (like perms or texturizers), environmental factors such as the sun or wind can bring about wear and tear leading to gradual degradation of the cuticle which is called as' weathering', with breaking and lifting of the free margins of cuticular cells. Chemical removal of the f-layer particularly by oxidation eliminates the first hydrophobic defense and leaves the hair more porous and vulnerable. Cuticle disruption with alkaline chemicals is the first step in permanent hair styling.[22] This eventually leads to exposure of the cortex and fracture of the hair shaft resulting in dull lusterless hair.

Cortex (Figure 2.13)

Cortex forms the middle layer and makes for 90% of the hair's weight. The cortex is hydrophilic. As the cortical cells move upward they lose their nuclei and become more fusiform in shape. They develop a dense filamentous cytoskeleton in the upper hair bulb and become fully hyalinized in the suprabulbar region and they do not contain any keratohyaline or trichohyaline granules. The keratin of the cortex is hard in contrast to the soft keratin of IRS or epidermis. The cortex consists of closely packed spindle-shaped cortical cells rich in keratin filaments that are oriented parallel to the long axis of the hair shaft[66] and an amorphous matrix of high sulfur proteins. The intermediate filament hair keratin (40–60kDa), comprising 400–500 amino acid residues in heptad sequence repeats, form hard keratin polypeptide chains that pair together to form protofilaments, which make up a keratin chain.[22] The keratin chains have a large number of sulfur containing cysteine residues. Cysteine residues in the adjacent keratin filaments form covalent disulfide bonds, which create strong cross links between adjacent keratin filaments. The disulfide bonds confer shape, stability, and resilience to the hair shaft. Other weaker bonds such as van der Waals interactions, hydrogen bonds, and coulombic interactions known as salt links, link the keratin polypeptide chain.[67]

Recent genome analysis have increased the number of identified human keratins to 54; grouped into acidic type 1 and basic to neutral type 2 intermediate filaments, 11 of the 28 type 1 keratin and 6 of 26 type 2 keratin are hair keratin.[23] They are also classified into three major families: high sulfur, ultra-high sulfur and high glycine-tyrosine proteins.[68]

The cortex is responsible for providing hair its structure, strength, color, resistance, elasticity and texture. When the cuticle is damaged the cortex becomes weak and unraveled causing split-ends and damaged hair.

Medulla (Figure 2.14)

Medulla also called the marrow of the hair shaft is a variable structure, which may be continuous, discontinuous or absent. Lanugo and vellus hairs have no medulla. Large-diameter hairs are more likely to contain a medulla. The medulla develops quite abruptly around the upper pole

Characteristics → Cortex forms the middle layer and makes for 90% of the hairs weight. Consists of keratin rich spindle shaped cell oriented parallel to long axis of the hair shaft and an amorphous matrix of high sulfur proteins

Keratin of cortex → IF hair keratin (40–60kDa), comprising 400–500 amino acid residues in heptad sequence repeats, form hard keratin that pair to form protofilament. Sulfur containing cysteine residues form covalent disulphide bonds

Functions → Provides hair its structure, strength, color, resistance, elasticity and texture. When cuticle is damaged, cortex becomes weak and unraveled causing split-ends and damaged hair

Fig. 2.13: Characteristics of the hair cortex of outer root sheath. IF—Intermediate filaments

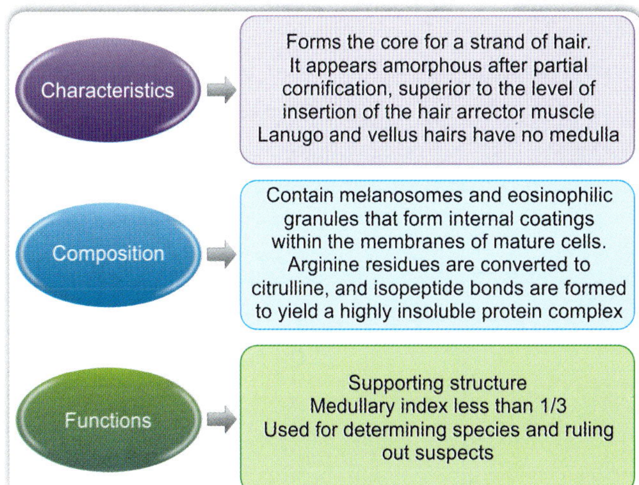

Fig. 2.14: Characteristics, composition and functions of medulla

of the dermal papilla, without any obvious precursor cell population.

When seen by electron microscopy, the medulla appears amorphous after partial cornification, superior to the level of insertion of the hair arrector muscle. The loosely aggregated cells of the medulla contain melanosomes and distinctive eosinophilic granules that eventually form internal coatings within the membranes of mature cells. As these cells develop, arginine residues are converted to citrulline, and isopeptide bonds are formed to yield a highly insoluble protein complex.[69]

It forms the core and is the supporting structure for a strand of hair. Human hairs are unique in that their medullary index (the fraction of the shaft's width that the medulla takes up) is small; generally less than 1/3. Other species will have ratios much larger, usually at least 1/2. Medulla patterns are not very good as individual evidence and are typically only used for determining species and ruling out suspects.[70]

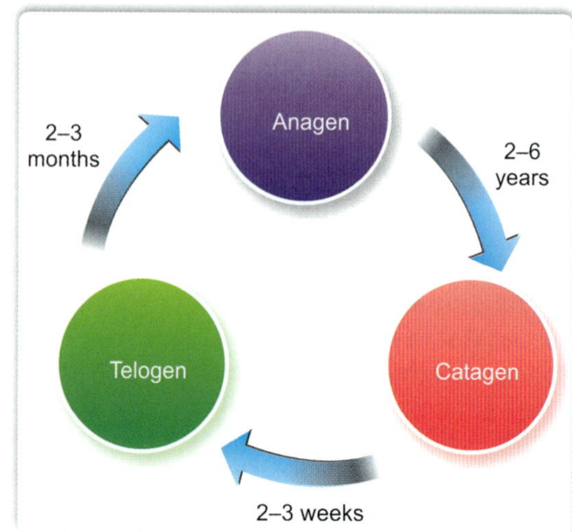

Fig. 2.15: Schematic representation of hair cycle

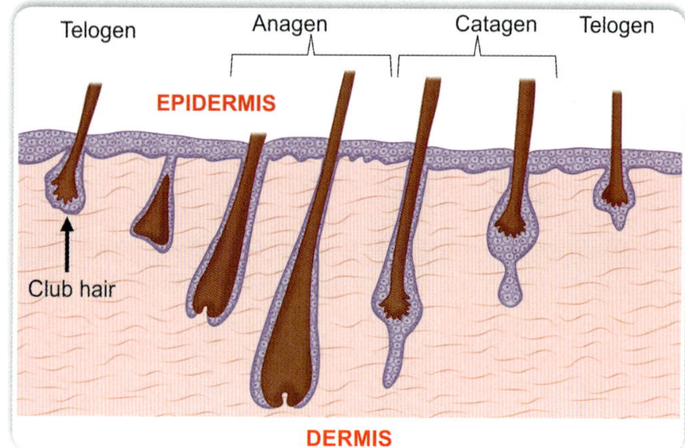

Fig. 2.16: Hair cycle-through anagen, catagen and telogen

Hair Follicle Innervations

There are two distinct neural networks that surround hair follicle. The first is located around the neck of the follicle just underneath the epidermis and contain sensory C fibers along with sympathetic fiber while the second is located around the permanent mid section of the hair follicle between the isthmus of sebaceous gland and insertion of arrector pili muscle and contain longitudinal A delta fiber and circular C fiber. Both the networks contain sensory nerve fiber, e.g. expressing calcitonin gene related peptide (CGRP) and autonomic nerves expressing choline acetyl transferase (ChAT).[23] Free nerve endings, pilo-Ruffini nerve endings and Merkel nerve endings are also found.[71] It has been postulated that Merkel cell secretions are involved in regulating the hair cycle.[72]

Hair Vasculature

During anagen phase rich vascular network surrounds lower end of the follicle. The network consists of parallel vessels connected by cross shunts extending between bulb and sebaceous gland. At the level of sebaceous gland the network terminate in loose network. The resting hair is supplied by palisade of capillaries connected by short transverse vessels. Vellus hair has very simple capillary system.[23]

Hair Cycle (Figures 2.15 and 2.16)

The hair follicle, a unique characteristic of mammals, represents a stem cell-rich, prototypic neuroectodermal-mesodermal interaction system. This factory for pigmented epithelial fibers is unique in that it is the only organ in the mammalian body which, for its entire lifetime, undergoes cyclic transformations from stages of rapid growth (anagen) to apoptosis-driven regression (catagen) and back to anagen, via an interspersed period of relative quiescence (telogen).[73]

Anagen

It is the period of active hair growth and the duration of this phase vary with age, sex and region. The duration of anagen phase determines the final length of the hair. In some hair follicles, such as those on human scalp, anagen may continue for several years, so that very long hairs are produced and in eyebrows and eye lashes, it is restricted to few days to month which explains their short length. At any one time normally 80–90% of hair follicles on the human scalp are in anagen phase.

When a resting hair follicle enters into early anagen phase, mitotic activity begins in the progenitor cells,

enveloping the dermal papilla, grows downwards into the skin and begins to differentiate into the inner root sheath and the hair shaft. The dermal papilla expands to form a flask-shaped structure. In the mid anagen, melanocytes located in the matrix begin to produce melanin and a new hair shaft emerges. Tightly packed cells of dermal papilla become separated due to deposition of extracellular matrix rich in proteoglycans and basement-membrane proteins. A network of capillary blood vessels develops around the growing follicle, sometimes extending into the dermal papilla in larger follicles. It correlates with the up regulation of the expression of vascular endothelial growth factor (VEGF) mRNA, a potent angiogenic growth factor, produced by keratinocytes of the outer root sheath. In transgenic mice over expressing VEGF, perifollicular vascularization was strongly induced, which resulted in accelerated hair growth and increased size of hair follicles and hair shafts.[74] In contrast, application of suppressors of angiogenesis leads to hair growth reduction.[75] Therefore, cutaneous vasculature may have a great impact on the hair shaft producing activity of hair follicle cells. The lower part of the follicle elongates downwards along the stele, a preformed dermal tract and in late anagen the hair fiber-producing unit is fully restored, characterized by the formation of the epithelial hair bulb surrounding the dermal papilla, located deep in the subcutaneous tissue, and the new hair shaft emerges from the skin surface.

Extensive remodeling of the follicle occurs during anagen. The transition of telogen follicles into anagen is associated with activation of Wnt/beta-catenin/Lef, [76] Sonic Hedgehog [77] (SHH) and STAT3 pathways, and down-regulation of BMP signaling. Other growth factors involved in promoting anagen include insulin-like growth factor 1 (IGF-1), hepatocyte growth factor, keratinocyte growth factor and vascular endothelial growth factor. Hair follicles also express tissue inhibitor of matrix metalloproteinase 3 (TIMP-3) in the outer root sheath during anagen, implying that remodeling involves a carefully controlled sequence of positive and negative influences **(Box 2.17)**.

Catagen

Catagen was first explained in detail by Kligman[78] and Straile.[79] Catagen phase is an involutionary phase in which the mitotic activity declines and ceases, during this phase, the proximal end of the hair shaft keratinizes to form a club-shaped structure and the lower part of the follicle involutes by apoptosis and thickens to form the 'glassy membrane'. During catagen, the dermal papilla is transformed into a cluster of quiescent cells that are closely adjacent to the regressing hair follicle epithelium and travel from the subcutis to the dermis to maintain contact with the distal portion of the hair follicle epithelium including the secondary hair germ and bulge. During the catagen phase the hair follicle shrinks in length by 70%.

Box 2.17: Growth factors involved in anagen phase

- Wnt/beta-catenin/Lef
- Sonic Hedgehog (SHH)
- STAT3 pathways
- Down-regulation of BMP signaling
- Insulin-like growth factor 1 (IGF-1), hepatocyte growth factor, keratinocyte growth factor and vascular endothelial growth factor

Catagen may be initiated as a passive process through exhaustion of the mitotic potential of transient amplifying cells in the hair bulb or the loss of action of growth promoting agents. Also, several growth factors and cytokines, including transforming growth factor-β (TGF-β), interleukin-1α (IL-1α) and tumor necrosis factor-α (TNF-α) have an inhibitory effect on hair growth and may be actively involved in triggering catagen. The ectodysplasin signaling pathway is involved in regulating apoptosis during catagen.[80] The expression levels of several proto-oncogenes associated with apoptosis, including c-*myc*, c-*jun* and c-*myb*, change immediately prior to or coincident with the onset of catagen.[81] The apoptosis-inhibitory proto-oncogene *bcl-2* is expressed in cycling follicular epithelium during anagen, disappears during catagen and is absent in telogen. One of the candidate molecules mediating apoptosis in hair matrix keratinocytes after growth factor withdrawal is p53. Mice lacking p53 showed significantly retarded catagen progression, compared with control mice confirming a pro-apoptotic role for p53 in the hair follicle.[82] The delicate proliferation-apoptosis balance, essential for follicle cyclic behavior, can also be controlled by survivin. Survivin, a member of the apoptosis inhibitor protein family, is implicated in the control of cell proliferation as well as the inhibition of apoptosis.[83] Survivin, expressed in the proliferating keratinocytes of the anagen hair matrix and outer root sheath, disappears with the progression of catagen.[84]

Towards the end of the first anagen phase, cells in the hair bulb undergo extensive premature apoptosis, and formation of the epithelial which is disrupted during catagen. The dermal papilla loses contact with the base of the hair follicle epithelium and the follicle is unable to re-enter anagen. Follicular remnants subsequently undergo cystic degeneration. Catagen is also initiated by several other molecules, such as endothelin-1, insulin-like growth factor binding proteins-3/4/5, interleukin-1, vitamin D receptor,[85] prolactin,[86] endocannabinoids,[87] or thrombospondin-1.[88]

Telogen

The period between the completion of follicular regression and the onset of the next anagen phase is termed telogen. The club hair lies within an epithelial sac to which it is attached by trichilemmal keratin. The club hair is eventually shed through an active process termed exogen.[89] Exogen hairs are passively retained within the follicles. In addition, exogen clubs do not retain remnants of the outer root sheath, in contrast to plucked telogen hairs.[90] Fifty to one-hundred club hairs are shed daily from a normal scalp. In human scalp, hair follicles may remain in a state of latency, also known as kenogen, for a prolonged period after the club hair is shed **(Box 2.18)**.[91]

The growth factor bone morphogenetic protein-4 (BMP-4)[92] produced by dermal papilla appears to play an important role in suppressing follicular growth and differentiation during telogen, by interacting with the receptor BMPR-IA, which is expressed by keratinocytes in the secondary epithelial germ.

Control of the Hair Cycle

It is thought that hair cycling is controlled primarily within individual hair follicles but that this intrinsic rhythmic behavior may be modulated by both local and systemic factors. The synchronous hair cycling seen during neonatal period is lost with the advancing age so that, hair follicles cycle independently of their neighbors. In these circumstances, hair cycling must be regulated by mechanisms intrinsic to the hair follicle. Although numerous systemic, metabolic, immunological, and nerve-derived factors (e.g. hormones, cytokines, neuropeptides, neurotransmitters, mast cells) can profoundly alter hair growth in vivo, neither vascular nor neural stimuli nor extrafollicular cells are essential for HF development or cycling. Rather, an intrafollicular "hair cycle clock" of as yet unknown nature drives the HF cycle. This elusive chronobiological timing device likely exploits secondary changes in the intra- and perifollicular signaling milieu for guiding the HF through its transformations. However, the supreme generator of cycling activity ("oscillator") that dictates any of these signaling switches is still as unknown as is its exact location. Since clinically, the control of catagen is of paramount importance (too early anagen termination: alopecia, effluvium; catagen too late: hirsutism, hypertrichosis), the controls of catagen-associated keratinocyte apoptosis and of dermal papilla secretory activities are discussed as crucial targets for future therapeutic manipulations **(Table 2.4)**.[93]

Box 2.18: Kenogen

A state of latency in which a hair follicle may remain for a prolonged period after the club hair is shed

Endocrine Factors

The type of hair produced is under endocrine control with androgens being key regulators of human hair growth; several other hormones are involved, particularly in other mammals, including melatonin, prolactin, melanocyte-stimulating hormone (MSH) and estrogens. Androgens have paradoxically different effects on human hair follicles depending on their body site. This ranges from stimulation, e.g. on the face, axilla, pubis and chest, though no effect on the eyelashes, to inhibition on parts of the scalp, causing balding in genetically susceptible individuals. All androgen effects require an intracellular androgen receptor in the hair follicle cells and most, except for pubic and axillary follicles, also require the intracellular enzyme 5α-reductase type 2 to metabolize testosterone to its more potent metabolite, 5α-dihydrotestosterone.

Exactly how androgens regulate hair follicles is not fully established, but most aspects appear to be coordinated via the mesenchyme-derived dermal papilla situated at the base of the follicle. In the current hypothesis androgens from the blood bind to androgen receptors in dermal papilla cells, altering their gene expression, particularly of paracrine signaling molecules, which influence the activity of the other follicular cells. Key signals identified so far include insulin-like growth factor-1 (IGF-1) in growth stimulation and transforming growth factor-β (TGF-β) in inhibition. IGF -1 plays an important role in many cell types as a survival factor to prevent cell death. This anti-apoptotic function of IGF-1 may be important to the development of follicle cells as follicles undergo a growth cycle where the regressive[94] TGF-β 2 suppresses proliferation of epithelial cells and stimulates synthesis of certain caspases. Then TGF-beta 2 triggers the intrinsic cascade network and subsequently epithelial cells are eliminated through apoptotic cell death. TGF-β antagonists are effective in preventing catagen-like morphological changes and in promoting elongation of hair follicles in vivo and in vitro.[95] It has been shown in animal

Table 2.4 : Intrinsic and extrinsic factors affecting hair cycle

1. **Endocrine factors:** Androgen, melatonin, prolactin, melanocyte-stimulating hormone (MSH) and estrogens
2. **Pregnancy**
3. **Seasonal hair growth:** Increases during spring while decreases in autumn
4. **Systemic factors:** Severe febrile illness (e.g. malaria), accidental trauma, major surgery, emotional stress, chronic systemic illness, large hemorrhage, and crash diet
5. **Intrinsic mechanisms within hair follicle**
6. **Neuronal influence:** Substance P, neurotrophic nerve growth factors (NGF)

models that estrogen has a role in hair cycle control in catagen induction via estrogen receptor alfa.[96]

Seasonal Hair Growth

Seasonal moulting is seen significantly in animals and is regulated by the endocrine system under the influence of environmental signals. Vestiges of seasonal variation in hair growth are present in humans, although it is insignificant. It has been shown in some studies that maximum number of anagen hairs (90%) on scalp are seen during spring, with falling down to 80% in autumn and also the number of follicle shed during autumn were more than double.[97]

Systemic Factors Affecting Hair Growth

Various systemic factors can regulate hair growth. The best example of a systemic influence on the human hair growth cycle is postpartum telogen effluvium.[98] During pregnancy there is prolongation of anagen phase and after parturition, there is precipitation of large numbers of follicles into telogen, leading to increased shedding from about 3 months postpartum. Telogen effluvium is also associated with iron deficiency anemia.[99] Other triggering events include severe febrile illness (e.g. malaria), accidental trauma, major surgery, emotional stress, chronic systemic illness, large hemorrhage, and crash diet.[100]

Intrinsic Control of the Hair Growth Cycle

The hair cycling is asynchronous, that is the follicles cycle independently of their neighbors. Hair follicles in different regions of the skin may also cycle differently. In humans, for example, the duration of anagen on the scalp may last several years, whereas on the eyebrows anagen is very brief. The telogen phase for body hair lasts close to a year.

The controls that underlie the hair cycle reside within the hair follicle itself, and are believed to result from changes in the intra and perifollicular expression of specific regulatory molecules and their receptors.[101] Much circumstantial evidence suggests that the dermal papilla which is composed of specialized fibroblasts located at the base of the follicle, determines hair follicle growth characteristics, especially the regulation of cell proliferation and differentiation of hair follicle matrix. Without papilla fibroblasts and an intimate contact with hair matrix keratinocytes, anagen cannot be sustained. Also, hair follicle morphogenesis can be induced by implanting dermal papilla cells under an appropriately receptive epithelium.[102] Interactions between two key cell populations in the hair follicle, epithelial stem cells in the outer root sheath and mesenchymal cells in the dermal papilla and dermal sheath, are thought to underlie intrinsic control of hair cycling, and a large number of molecules have been implicated in this process. However, the location and the nature of the 'switch' that initiates and terminates anagen growth are unknown. When scalp hair follicles are transplanted into other regions of the skin they retain the cyclical behavior of the donor site, supporting the fact that cycle control is determined within the follicle or its immediate tissue environment.

Neuronal Influences

Neuroimmune interaction and mediators are produced which fluctuate throughout the hair cycle affecting hair growth. Neuronal mediators such as sensory neuropeptide, substance P can turn on or terminate hair growth control mechanism such as keratinocyte proliferation or neurogenic inflammation associated with hair regression. At the same time growth factors secreted by HF such as the neurotrophic nerve growth factors (NGF), modulate the structure and function of their environment through perifollicular innervations, inter and perifollicular immune cell population and neuroimmune communication.[22]

Molecular Control of Hair Cycle (Figure 2.17)

A large number of molecular signals are involved in controlling the hair cycle. These include developmental genes, several families of growth factors and their receptors, transcription factors, nuclear receptors, neurotrophins, cytokines and intracellular signaling pathways. These factors interact to form signaling networks and their activity may also be modulated by interactions with extracellular matrix molecules that serve to increase or reduce the biological response.

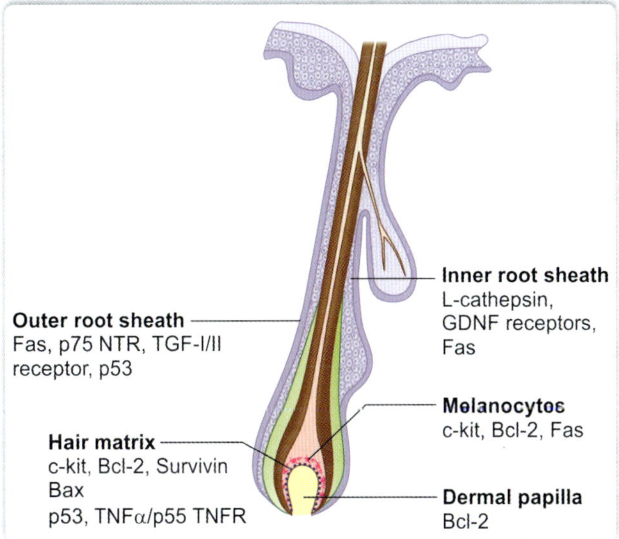

Fig. 2.17: Pro and antiapoptotic factors acting on different parts of the hair root

Catagen has been suggested to occur as a consequence of decreased expression of anagen maintaining factors, such as insulin-like growth factor 1 (IGF-1), basic fibroblast growth factor (bFGF), and vascular endothelial growth factor (VEGF), and increased expression of cytokines promoting apoptosis, such as transforming growth factor β 1 (TGF β 1), interleukin-1alpha (IL-1α), and tumor necrosis factor alpha (TNF alpha).[102] Since many extrinsic hair growth-modulatory factors, such as androgens, apparently operate at least in part via the dermal papilla, research is currently also focused on identifying androgen-regulated factors deriving from dermal papilla cells. Of the several factors that have been suggested to play a role in hair growth, stem cell factor (SCF) has been found to be produced in higher amounts by androgen-dependent beard cells than in control non-balding scalp cells, presumably also in response to androgens.[103] Since SCF is the ligand for the cell surface receptor c-kit on melanocytes, this may also play a role for hair pigmentation.

Role of the Immune System in Hair Cycle

The keratinocytes in healthy HF are protected from the attack by immune cells by their immune privilege characterized by low level of MHC class I and II antigens.[23] When there is breakdown of this putative immune privilege the disease states like alopecia areata results.

Androgen Receptor

The androgen receptor gene is located on the X chromosome.[104] The tissue effects of androgens are mediated through binding to the intracellular androgen receptor. Like all steroid hormones, androgens exert their effects by binding to an intracellular receptor, the androgen receptor (AR). Binding of androgens to their androgen receptor leads to conformational change of the AR-androgen complex (ARAC) which is then transported into the nucleus where it can bind to regions of DNA that have distinctive binding sites known as androgen-responsive elements (ARE). A wide variety of proteins have this ARE encoded in their DNA. In this way androgens are able to modulate the transcription of various genes, which may be activated or suppressed.[104]

Functions of Hair

1. It protects the scalp from sun rays.
2. Shields the eyelids from the droplets of sweat and sunlight.
3. It may also help to reduce friction in intertriginous area.
4. It is also a sexually attractive ornament.
5. In addition to its decorative value, hair screens the nasal passages from irritants.
6. As the isthmus of a follicle is surrounded by a network of myelinated sensory nerve fibers, hairs also contributes to the perception of tactile stimuli.
7. Hair is often interpreted as marker of age, healthy nutrition, fecundity, health, wealth and self esteem.
8. Hair examinations and comparisons, with the aid of a comparison microscope, and DNA examination can be valuable in an investigation of a crime.

References

1. Ramot Y. Basic hair anatomy. Int J Trichology. 2011;3(1):S1-S2.
2. Jakubovic HR, Ackeman AB. Structure and function of skin: Development, morphology, and physiology. In: Moschella LS, Hurley HJ, editors. Dermatology, 2nd edn. Philadelphia: WB Sounders Company. 1985.
3. Kligman AM. Pathologic dynamics of human hair loss. Arch Dermatol. 1961;83:175-98.
4. Walsh JME, Wheat ME, Freund K. Detection, evaluation, and treatment of eating disorders the role of the primary care physician. J Gen Intern Med. 2000;15(8):577-90.
5. Beighton P. Congenital hypertrichosis lanuginosa. Arch Dermatol. 1970;101:669-72.
6. Hensley GT, Glynn KP. Hypertrichosis lanuginosa as a sign of internal malignancy. Cancer. 1969;24:1051-6.
7. Esterly NB, Fretzin DF, Pinkus H. Eruptive vellus hair cysts. Arch Dermatol. 1977;113(4):500-3.
8. Goldberg DJ, Marmur ES, Hussain M. Treatment of terminal and vellus non-pigmented hairs with an optical/bipolar radiofrequency energy source—with and without pre-treatment using topical aminolevulinic acid. Journal of Cosmetic and Laser Therapy. 2005;7:25-8.
9. Heffner, Linda J. Human Reproduction at a Glance. Blackwell Publishing. 2001;p. 33.
10. Neal, Matthew, Lauren M. Sompayrac. How the Endocrine System Works. Blackwell Publishing. 2001;pp. 70,75.
11. Daniel S, Wendelin MD, David N. Hypertrichosis. Am J Acad Dermatol. 2003;48:161-79.
12. Valia RG. Hypertrichosis. Indian J Dermatol. 2005;50:119-24.
13. Redmond GP, Bergfeld WF. Diagnostic approach to androgen disorders in women: Acne, hirsutism, and alopecia. Cleve Clin J Med. 1990;57:423-7.
14. Ibrahimi OA, Avram MM, Hanke CW. Laser hair removal. Dermatologic Therapy. 2011;24:94-107.
15. Miranda BH, Tobin DJ, Sharpe DT, Randall VA. Intermediate hair follicles: A new more clinically relevant model for hair growth investigations. Br J of Dermat. 2010;163:287-95.
16. Jablonski NG. Skin: a natural history. Berkley, CA: University of California Press. 2006.
17. Lurie R, Garty BZ. Helical hairs: A new hair anomaly in a patient with Netherton's syndrome. Cutis. 1995;55(6):349-52.

18. Prasad GK. Familial woolly hair. Indian J Dermatol Venereol Leprol. 2002;68:157.
19. Rudnicka L,Olszewska M, Rakowska A, Oledjka EK, Slowniska M. Trichoscopy; A new method for diagnosis of hair loss. Journal of drugs in Dermatology. 2008;7(7).
20. Galliker NA, Trueb RM. Value of trichoscopy versus trichogram for diagnosis of female androgenic alopecia. Int J Trichol. 2012;4:19-22.
21. Dermatologic Therapy, Volume 17, Number 2, J pp. 164-176(13), 2004.
22. Gray J. Human hair. In: Mcmichael AJ, Hordinsky MK, editors. Hair and scalp diseases. 1st edn. New York: Informa health care. 2009;1-17.
23. Vogt A, McElwee KJ, Blume-Petavi U. Biology of hair follicle. In:Blume-Peytavi U, Tosti A, Whiting DA, Trueb R, editors, Hair growth and disorders. Velag Berlin Herdelberg: Springer. 2008;p.1-23.
24. Pinkus H. Embryology of hair. In: Montagna W, Ellis RA, eds. The Biology of Hair Growth. New York: Academic Press. 1958;1-32.
25. Venkataram M. Changing trends in hair restoration surgery. Indian J Dermatol Venereol Leprol. 2006;72:103-11.
26. Blume U, Ferracin J, Verschoore M, et al. Physiology of the vellus hair follicle: Hair growth and sebum excretion. Br J Dermatol. 1991;124:21-8.
27. Blume U, Verschoore M, Poncet M, et al. The vellus hair follicle in acne: Hair growth and sebum excretion. Br J Dermatol. 1993;129:23-7.
28. Szabo G. The Regional anatomy of the human integument with special reference to the distribution of hair follicles, sweat glands and melanocytes. Philos Trans R Soc Land B Biol sci. 1967;252:447-85.
29. Barman JM, Astore I, Pecoraro V. The normal trichogram of the adult. J Invest Dermatol. 1965;44:233-6.
30. Loussouarn G. African hair growth parameters. Br J Dermatol. 2001;145:294-7.
31. Sperling LC. Hair density in African Americans. Arch Dermatol. 1999;135:656-8.
32. Lee HJ, Ha SJ, Lee JH, et al. Hair counts from scalp biopsy specimens in Asians. J Am Acad Dermatol. 2002;46:218-21.
33. Poblet E, Ortega F, Jimenez F. The arrector pili muscle and the follicular unit of the scalp. 5A microscopic anatomy study. Dermatol Surg. September 2002;28:9:800-3.
34. Berker DAR, Messenger AG, Sinclair RD. Disorders of hair. In: Tony B, Breathnach S, Cox N, Griffiths C eds. Rook's Textbook of dermatology. 7th edn. Oxford: Blackwell Science. 2004;63:1-14.
35. Ha T, Rees JL. Red hair-a desirable mutation? J Cosmet Dermatol. 2002;1(2):62-5.
36. Dawber RPR, Gummer CL. The color of hair. In:Dawber, ed. Diseases of the Human hair and Scalp. Oxford: Blackwell Science.1997:408.
37. Tobin DJ. Pigmentation of human hair In. Hair in toxicology an important bio monitor. RSE publishing UK. 2005;p61.
38. Valverde P, Healy E, Jackson I, Rees JL, Thody AJ. "Variants of the melanocyte-stimulating hormone receptor gene are associated with red hair and fair skin in humans". Nat. Genet. 1995;11(3):328-30.
39. Joshi R. Adamson's Fringe, Horatio George Adamson, and Kligman's experiments and observations on Tinea capitis. Int J Trichol. 2011;3:14-9.
40. Hardy MH, Van Exan RJ, Sonstegard KS, Sweeny PR. Basal lamina changes during tissue interactions in hair follicles--an in vitro study of normal dermal papillae and vitamin A-induced glandular morphogenesis. J Invest Dermatol. 1983;80(1):27-34.
41. Elliott K, Stephenson TJ, Messenger AG. Differences in hair follicle dermal papilla volume are due to extracellular matrix volume and cell number: Implications for the control of hair follicle size and androgen responses. J Invest Dermatol. 1999;113:873-7.
42. Asada Y, Sonoda T, Ojiro M, et al. 5 alpha-reductase type 2 is constitutively expressed in the dermal papilla and connective tissue sheath of the hair follicle in vivo but not during culture in vitro. J Clin Endocrinol Metab. 2001;86:2875-80.
43. Van Scott EJ, Ekel TM. Geometric relationships between the matrix of the hair bulb and its dermal papilla in normal and alopecic scalp. J Invest Dermatol. 1958;31:281-7.
44. Ibrahim L, Wright EA. A quantitative study of hair growth using mouse and rat vibrissal follicles. I. Dermal papilla volume determines hair volume. J Embryol Exp Morphol. 1982;72:209-24.
45. Pinkus H, Iwasaki T, Mishima Y. Outer root sheath keratinization in anagen and catagen of the mammalian hair follicle. A seventh distinct type of keratinization in the hair follicle: Trichilemmal keratinization. J Anat. 1981;133(Pt 1):19-35.
46. Cotsarelis G, Cheng SZ, Dong G, Sun TT, Lavker RM. Existence of slow-cycling limbal epithelial basal cells that can be preferentially stimulated to proliferate: Implications on epithelial stem cells. Cell. 1989;57:201-9.
47. Robert M. Hoffman. The Pluripotency of Hair Follicle Stem Cells. Cell Cycle 5:3, 1 February 2006;232-3.
48. Ito M, Liu Y, Yang Z, Nguyen J, Liang F, Morris RJ, et al. Stem cells in the hairfollicle bulge contribute to wound repair but not to homeostasis of the epidermis. Nat Med. 2005;11:1351-4.
49. Freedberg, et al. Fitzpatrick's Dermatology in General Medicine, 6th edn. McGraw-Hill. 2003.
50. Poblet E, Ortega F, Jiménez F. The arrector pili muscle and the follicular unit of the scalp: A microscopic anatomy study. Dermatol Surg. 2002;28(9):800-3.
51. Klaus J. Busam, Dermatopathology: A Volume in the Foundations in Diagnostic Pathology Series, Chapter 9: Cysts and Sinuses.
52. Haykal S, Al Habeeb AS, Goldstein DP, Murray CA, Ghazarian D. Infundibular carcinoma of the skin: A distinct morphological and immunohistochemical entity, J Clin Pathol. 2010;63:455-62.
53. Mc Elwee KJ, Kissling S, Wenzel E, Huth A, Hoffma R. Cultured peribulbar dermal sheath cells can induce hair follicle development and contribute to the dermal sheath and dermal papilla. J Invest Dermatol. 2003;121:1267-75.
54. Joshi RS. The inner root sheath and the men associated with it eponymically. Int J Trichology. 2011;3(1):57-62.
55. Clemmensen OJ, Hainau B, Hanstead B. The ultrastructure of the transition zone between specialized cells (Flugelzellen) of

Huxley's layer of the inner root sheath and cells of the outer root sheath of the human hair follicle. Am J Dermatopathol. 1991;13:264-70.
56. Ackerman AB, Boer A, Bennin B, Gottlieb GJ. Embryonic, histologic, and anatomic aspects. In: Histologic Diagnosis of Inflammatory Skin Diseases. 3rd edn. New York: Ardor Scribendi. 2005;pp. 26-3.
57. Joshi RS. The inner root sheath and the men associated with it eponymically. Int J Trichology. 2011;3(1):57-62.
58. Hamn H, Traupe H. Loose anagen hair of childhood: The phenomenon of easily pluckable hair. J Am Acad Dermatol. 1989;20:242-8.
59. Horenstein MG, Simon J. Investigation of the hair follicle inner root sheath in scarring and non-scarring alopecia. J Cutan Pathol. 2007;34(10):762-8.
60. Orwin DFG. Cell differentiation in the lower outer sheath of the Romney wool follicle: A companion cell layer. Aust J Biol Sci. 1971;24:989-9.
61. Poblet E, Jimenez F, de Cabo C, Martin AP, Prieto RS. The calcium-binding protein calretinin is a marker of the companion cell layer of the human hair follicle. British Journal of Dermatology. 2005;152:1316-20.
62. Staricco RG. Amelanotic melanocytes in the outer sheath of the human hair follicle. The Journal of Investigative Dermatology. 1959;33:295-7.
63. Horikawa T, Norris DA, Johnson TW, Zekman T, Dunscomb N, Bennion SD, et al. DOPA-Negative Melanocytes in the Outer Root Sheath of Human Hair Follicles Express Premelanosomal Antigens But Not a Melanosomal Antigen or the Melanosome-Associated Glycoproteins Tyrosinase, TRP-1, and TRP-2. Journal of Investigative Dermatology. 1996;106:28-35.
64. Mohanty S, Kumar A, Dhawan J, Sreenivas V, Gupta S. Noncultured extracted hair follicle outer root sheath cell suspension for transplantation in vitiligo. British Journal of Dermatology. 2011;164:1241-6.
65. Jones LN. Hair structure anatomy and comparative anatomy. Clin Dermatol. 2001;19:95-103.
66. Dawber RPR, Messenger AG. Hair follicle structure, keratinisation and physical properties of hair. In: Dawber R, editor. Diseases of Human hair and scalp. Oxford, Blackwell Science. 1997;23-50.
67. Feughelman M, Lyman DJ, Willis BK.The parallel helices of intermediate filaments of alfa- keratin. Int J Biol Macroml. 2002;30(2):95-6.
68. Rogers GE, Powell BC. Organization and expression of hair follicle genes. J Invest Dermatol. 1993;101:50-5S.
69. Harding HW, Rogers GE. Epsilon-(gamma-glutamyl)lysine cross-linkage in citrulline-containing protein fractions from hair. Biochemistry. 1971;10:624-30.
70. Kshirsagar SV, Singh B, Fulari SP. Comparative study of human and animal hair in relation with diameter and medullary index. Indian Journal of Forensic Medicine and Pathology. 2009;2(3):59.
71. Hashimoto K, Ito M, Suzuki Y. Innervation and vasculature of the hair follicle. In: Orfanos CE, Happle R, eds. Hair and Hair Diseases. Berlin: Springer-Verlag. 1990;117-47.
72. Narisawa Y, Hashimoto K, Nakamura Y, et al. A high concentration of Merkel cells in the bulge prior to the attachment of the arrector pili muscle and the formation of the perifollicular nerve plexus in human fetal skin. Arch Dermatol Res. 1993;285:261-8.
73. Paus R, Foitzik K. In search of the "hair cycle clock": a guided tour. Differentiation. 2004;72(9-10):489-511.
74. Yano K, Brown LF, Detmar M. Control of hair growth and follicle size by VEGF-mediated angiogenesis. J Clin Invest. 2001;107:409-417.
75. Ahluwalia G, Styczynski P, Shander D. Inhibition of hair growth. USA, 2000, US6093748.
76. David Van Mater, Frank T Kolligs, Andrzej A Dlugosz, Eric R. Fearon Transient activation of β-catenin signaling in cutaneous keratinocytes is sufficient to trigger the active growth phase of the hair cycle in mice. http://genesdev.cshlp.org/content/17/10/1219.long#cited-by.
77. AE Oro, K. Higgins Hair cycle regulation of Hedgehog signal reception. Developmental Biology. 2003;255:238-48.
78. Kligman AG. The human hair cycle. J Invest Dermatol. 1959;33:307-16.
79. Straile WE, Chase HB, Arsenault C. Growth and differentiation of hair follicles between periods of activity and quiescence. J Exp Zoo. 1961;148:205-22.
80. Fessing MY, Sharova TY, Sharov AA, Atoyan R, Botchkarev VA. Involvement of the Edar signaling in the control of hair follicle involution (catagen). Am J Pathol. 2006;169(6):2075-84.
81. Seiberg M, Marthinuss J, Stenn KS. Changes in expression of apoptosis-associated genes in skin mark early catagen. J Invest Dermatol. 1995;104(1):78-82.
82. Botchkareva NV, Khlgatian M, Longley BJ, Botchkarev VA, Gilchrest BA. SCF/c-kit signaling is required for cyclic regeneration of the hair pigmentation unit. FASEB J. 2001;15:645-58.
83. Altieri DC. Survivin, versatile modulation of cell division and apoptosis in cancer. Oncogene. 2003;22:8581-9.
84. Botchkareva NV, Kahn M, Ahluwalia G, Shander D. Survivin in the human hair follicle. J Invest Dermatol. 2007;127:479-82.
85. Stenn KS, Paus R. Controls of hair follicle cycling. Physiol Rev. 2001;81:449-94.
86. Foitzik K, Krause K, Conrad F, Nakamura M, Funk W, Paus R. Human scalp hair follicles are both a target and a source of prolactin, which serves as an autocrine and/or paracrine promoter of apoptosis-driven hair follicle regression. Am J Pathol. 2006;168:748-56.
87. Telek A, Bir6 T, Bod6 E, T6th BI, Borbir6 I, Kunos G, et al. Inhibition of human hair follicle growth by endo- and exocannabinoids. FASEB J. 2007;21:3534-41.
88. Yano K, Brown LF, Lawler J, Miyakawa T, Detmar M. Thrombospondin-1 plays a critical role in the induction of hair follicle involution and vascular regression during the catagen phase. J Invest Dermatol. 2003;120:14-9.
89. Stenn KS, Parimoo S, Prouty SM. Growth of the hair follicle, a cycling and regenerating biological system. In: Chuong C-M, editor, Molecular Basis of Epithelial Appendage Morphogenesis. Austin, TX: RG Landes Co. 1998;pp. 111-30.

90. Van Neste D, Leroy T, Conil S. Exogen hair characterization in human scalp. Skin Res Techno1. 2007;13:43M43.
91. Rebora A, Guarrera M. Kenogen. A new phase of the hair cycle? Dermatology. 2002;205(2):108-10.
92. Botchkarev VA. Bone morphogenetic proteins and their antagonists in skin and hair follicle biology. J. Invest. Dermatol. 2003;120:36-47.
93. Paus R. Principles of hair cycle control. J Dermatol. 1998;25(12):793-802.
94. Su HY, Hickford JG, Bickerstaffe R, Palmer BR. Insulin-like growth factor 1 and hair growth. Dermatol online J. 1999;59(2):1.
95. Hibino T, Nishiyama T. Role of TGF-beta 2 in the human hair cycle. J Dermatol Sci. 2004;35(1):9-18.
96. Ohnemus U, Uenalan M, Conrad F, Handjiski B, Mecklenburg L, Nakamura M, et al. Hair Cycle Control by Estrogens: Catagen induction via estrogen receptor (ER): Is Checked by ER_ Signaling. Endocrinology. 2005;146(3):1214-25.
97. Randall VA, Ebling EJG. Seasonal changes in human hair growth. Br J Dermatol. 1991;124:146-51.
98. Millikan L. Hirsutism, postpartum telogen effluvium, and male pattern alopecia. Journal of Cosmetic Dermatology. 2006;5:81-6.
99. Obaidat NA, Rawashdeh BT, Razzac AA, Wreikat, Awamleh AA. A potential relation between telogen effluvium and iron difficiency in adult female.JRMS. 2005;12(1):62-6.
100. Shrivastava SB. Diffuse hair loss in an adult female: Approach to diagnosis and management. Indian J Dermatol Venereol Leprol. 2009;75:20-8.
101. Paus R, Rover MS, Botchkarev VA. Chronobiology of the hair follicle: Hunting the 'hair cycle clock.' J Invest Dermatol Symp Proc. 1999;4:338-45.
102. Trueb RM. Molecular mechanisms of androgenetic alopecia. Experimental Gerontology. 2002;37:981-90.
103. Hibberts NA, Messenger AG, Randall VA. Dermal papilla cells derived from beard hair follicles secrete more stem cell factor (SCF) in culture than scalp cells or dermal fibroblasts. Biochem. Biophys. Res. Commun. 1996;222:401-05.
104. Hoffmann R. Male androgenetic alopecia. Clinical and Experimental. Dermatology. 27:373-82.

3

An Approach to a Patient with Hair Disorder

S Sacchidanand, Archana L

"By three methods we may learn wisdom: First, by reflection, which is noblest; second, by imitation, which is easiest; and third by experience, which is the bitterest."

—*Confucius*

Introduction

Trichology is an integral part of dermatology as hair presents with a wide range of disorders including alopecias (cicatricial and non-cicatricial), hirsutism, hypertrichosis, infections (fungal), infestations (pediculosis), hair shaft anomalies and hair abnormalities as a component of genodermatoses.

The basic steps in the approach includes:

- An exhaustive history
- A thorough clinical examination
- Appropriate investigations.

History (Algorithm 3.1)

In a trichology OPD, patients usually come with the complaints of hair loss, bald patches, altered hair color, texture , increased hair fragility, itchy and scaly lesions over the scalp, pus filled lesions, associated matting of the hair, graying of the hair, increased facial hair to name a few. The details of the onset, duration and progression of the above complaints must be noted **(Boxes 3.1 and 3.2)**.

A few conditions presenting with acute onset include anagen effluvium, telogen effluvium, alopecia areata, infections and infestations. Conditions like androgenetic alopecia (AGA), female pattern hair loss (FPHL), chronic telogen effluvium (CTE), monilethrix, hair shaft anomalies can have an insidious onset and patient can present at a later stage of the disease due to the slow progression.

In case of alopecia being the presenting complaint of the patient one has to enquire if it is sudden in onset or a chronic condition and whether the hairloss is localized/diffuse/patterned. It is important to identify by history if it is a fallout or breakage as the latter would indicate shaft abnormalities. One has to ask if the hairloss was preceded by any inflammatory process and was it symptomatic or asymptomatic to rule out conditions leading to scarring alopecia.

History regarding presence of spontaneous hair regrowth and whether the hair grows to the normal length or not has to be elicited (helps to assess the disease activity and prognosis in cases of alopecia areata).

History of any illness/hospitalization/surgery in the preceding 2–6 months, drug intake in the recent past, prior radiation/chemotherapy, application of topical irritants has to be enquired in case of telogen effluvium.

When there is no positive history from the above set of questions it is essential to enquire regarding the habit of hair pulling, plucking, rubbing or cutting to rule out trichotillomania, trichoteiromania and trichotemnomania. It is wise to obtain the history from the patient's attender like parents especially in children as the patient denies the habit in majority of the cases. A behavioral history also should be obtained to detect presence of any underlying psychological disturbance.

History of itching or pain over the scalp has to be taken. History of boils or flakes is present in cases of seborrheic dermatitis or pityriasis capitis. Patient has to be asked about noticing lice or nits.

History of pain on combing indicates scalp dysesthesia or a sensitive scalp while a metallic sound on combing is indicative of piedra wherein hard concretions are present on the hair shaft.

In case of hirsutism, one has to enquire about the age at onset, sites of hair growth, regularity of menstrual cycles, drug intake, hoarseness of voice, pain or mass abdomen (in case of ovarian or adrenal tumors), history suggestive

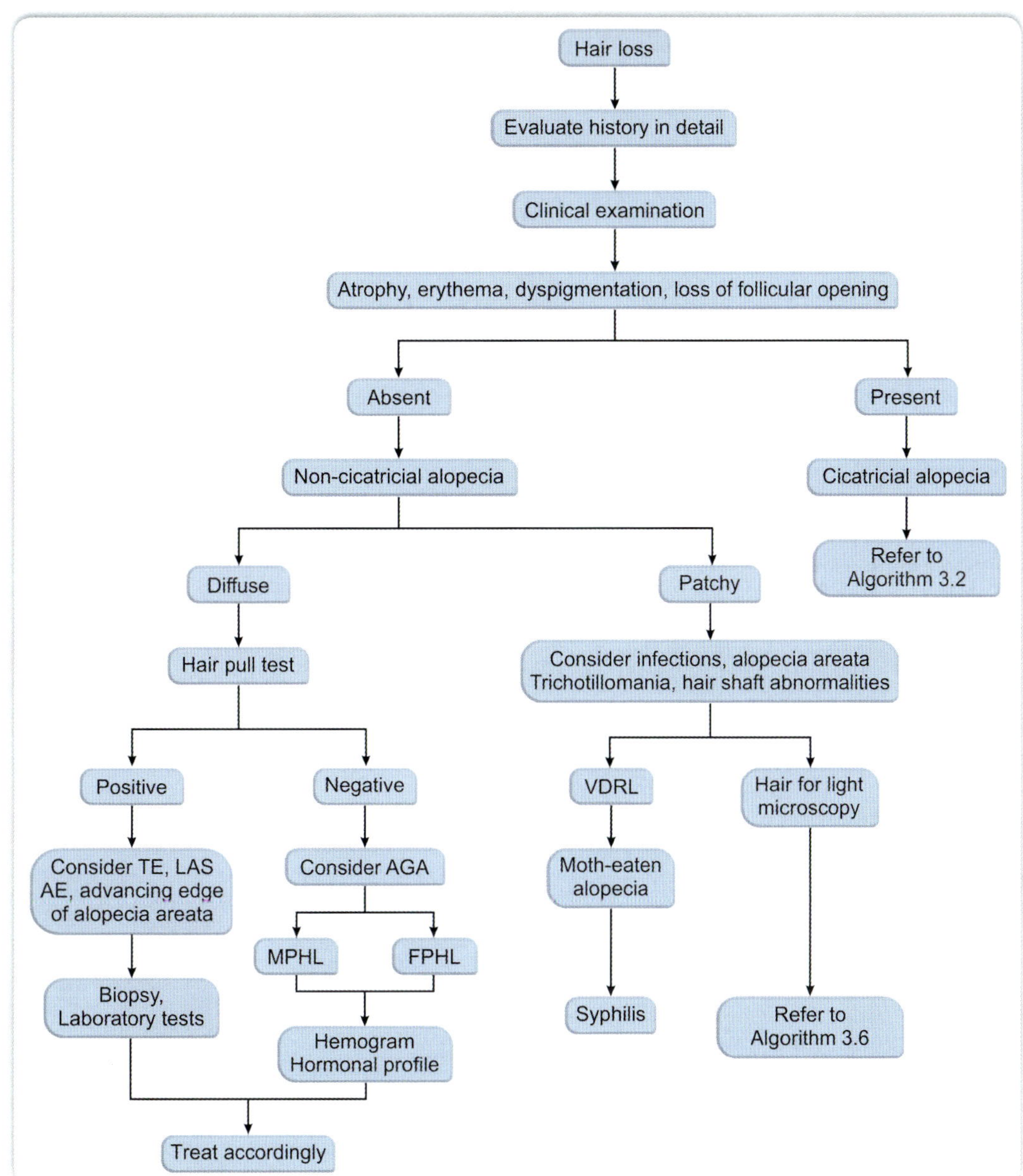

Algorithm 3.1: Algorithm showing approach to non-cicatricial alopecia

Box 3.1: OPD of a symptom

- O - Onset
- P - Progression
- D - Duration

of other endocrinopathies and family history of similar complaints (idiopathic familial hirsutism) **(Box 3.3)**.

In today's modern era, use of beauty care products is a rampant practice and multiple cosmetics and procedures find their place in the daily routine of women and men alike. Therefore, it becomes important to enquire regarding these as they can have deleterious effects on the hair **(Box 3.4)**.

Use of shampoos, conditioners, straightening serum, setting gels is asked for. Use of hairdryers or hot iron can

Box 3.2: History of hair loss

Things to remember:

- Onset: Sudden/Chronic
- Hairloss: Diffuse/Patterned/Localized
- Associated symptoms if any: Pruritus/Scaling
- Presence of spontaneous hair regrowth
- Other hair bearing areas involved esp axillary, pubic, beard region
- Preceding illness/hospitalization
- Drug intake
- Menstrual irregularities/Obstetric history
- Family history
- Behavioral history: habit of hair pulling, plucking, rubbing or cutting
- Hair care practices
- Diet history

Box 3.3: History of excessive hair growth

Things to remember:
- Age at onset
- Sites of hair growth
- Regularity of menstrual cycles
- Drug intake
- Hoarseness of voice
- Pain or mass abdomen (in case of ovarian or adrenal tumors)
- History suggestive of other endocrinopathies
- Family history of similar complaints (idiopathic familial hirsutism)

Box 3.4: History of hair care practices

- Use of shampoos, conditioners, straightening serum, setting gels
- Use of hairdryers or hot iron
- Tight braiding, high ponytails
- Straightening, perming, coloring and hair dyeing

cause weathering and hence increased fragility of the hair. One has to enquire about the cosmetic procedures patient has undergone like straightening, perming, coloring and hair dyeing. The hairstyle sported by the patient like tight braiding, high ponytails also contribute to hairloss by causing traction alopecia.

Hair disorders can be a part of a systemic pathological process or can be caused by any systemic assault. Hence a detailed history of any other skin disorders (lichen planopilaris, syphilis), history suggestive of thyroid dysfunction/anemia (telogen effluvium, alopecia areata), history suggestive of underlying malignancy, history suggestive of connective tissue disorders (lupus hair) should be taken. History suggestive of immunosuppressed state and genodermatoses should also be taken **(Box 3.5)**.

It is suggested that history of similar complaints in other family members and presence of early balding in relatives (AGA) has to be asked for. Family history of thyroid disorders or atopy gives a clue regarding a genetic predisposition to similar problems in the patient.

In a female patient, menstrual history is imperative which includes regularity of menstrual cycles (PCOS), presence of heavy bleeding (anemia causing telogen effluvium).

Obstetric history about pregnancy and postpartum period has to be enquired in case of telogen effluvium.

The dietary habits of the patient is also important to assess the nutritional status—whether the patient is on vegetarian or non-vegetarian diet, if he/she has adopted crash dieting and if there are any food fads. All these can play a role in causing diffuse hairloss in a patient.

Box 3.5: Hairloss and systemic association

- Other skin disorders (lichen planopilaris, syphilis)
- Thyroid dysfunction/anemia
- Connective tissue disorders
- Immunosuppressed state and genodermatoses
- Underlying malignancy

After a thorough history, we should proceed to a meticulous clinical evaluation which includes mucocutaneous and systemic examination.

In a **case of alopecia (Figure 3.1)** one has to look for the global appearance and assess the number of patches which indicates the extent and severity of the disease. The site of involvement has to be noted as it indicates the prognosis (like occipital involvement in alopecia areata indicates bad prognosis).

The pattern of hairloss has to be noted whether it is localized/patchy/diffuse/all over the scalp.

It is also important to look for involvement of other hairy areas like eyelash, eyebrows, trunk, axilla, pubic area to guage the severity of the disease.

An important step in the clinical examination is to assess whether the alopecia is of the scarring or non-scarring type. The below table enumerates the points to differentiate between the two **(Table 3.1) (Algorithm 3.2)**.

It is advised to examine for easy pluckability of the hairs to assess disease activity (along the periphery in case of alopecia areata patch) or to support the diagnosis (in tinea capitis).

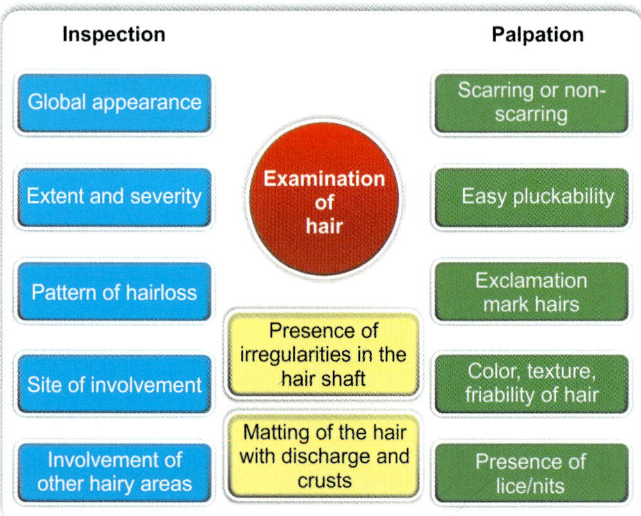

Fig. 3.1: Schematic representation of key points in examination of hair

Table 3.1: Pointers to differentiate cicatricial and non-cicatricial hairloss

Non-cicatricial	*Cicatricial*
Normal appearing skin	Erythema, dyspigmentation
Smooth patch of alopecia	Wrinkling of skin, depression- atrophy
Scaling, crusting present	Absent
Hair follicles retained	Absence of hair follicles

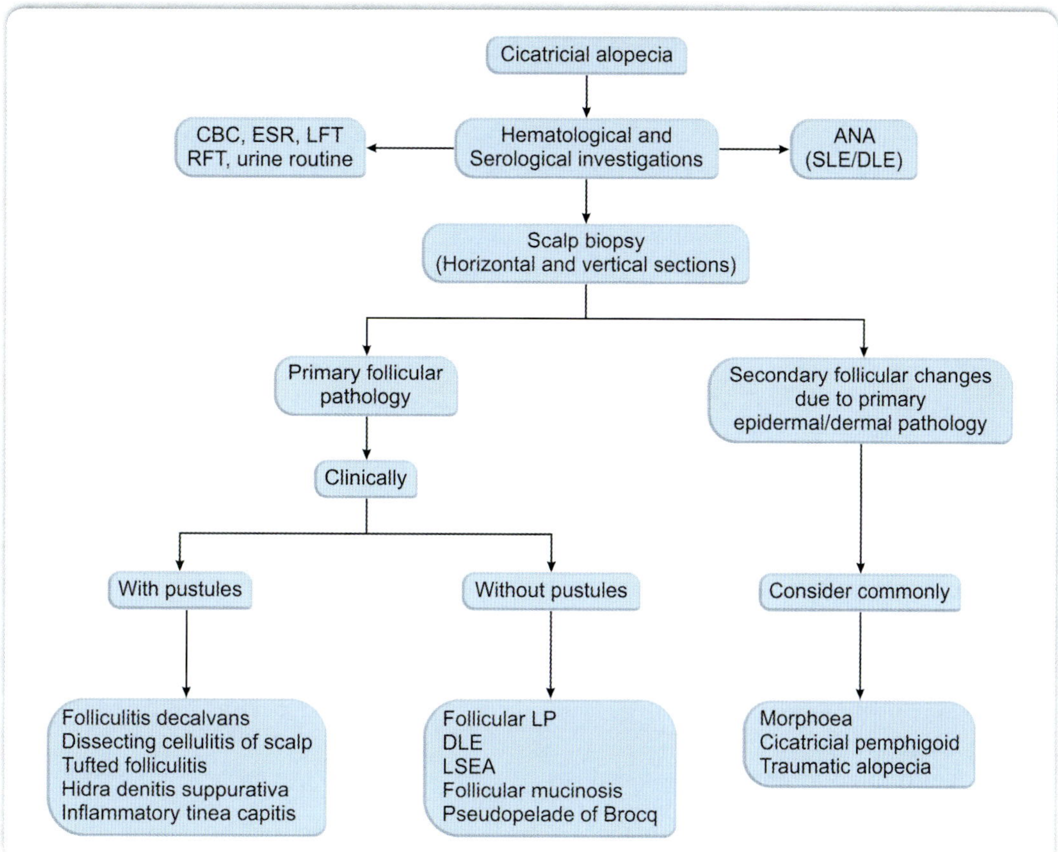

Algorithm 3.2: Approach to cicatricial alopecia

Abbreviations: Systemic lupus erythematosus (SLE); discoid lupus erythematosus (DLE); lichen planus (LP); lichen sclerosus et atrophicans (LSEA)

One has to examine for presence of exclamation mark hairs in case of alopecia areata.

Other points which have to be observed are color, texture, friability of hair in case of weathering effects, cosmetic induced hair damage and nutritional deficiency.

Presence of irregularities in the hair shaft point towards hair shaft anomalies or structural abnormalities. Presence of lice/nits (in the "louse pit"- occipital depression) has to be noted. Matting of the hair with discharge and crusts indicate secondary infection in severe cases of pediculosis neglected for a long time.

Scalp evaluation (Figure 3.2) is another important step as it may give a clue to the hair disorder. The various signs of inflammation like erythema, papules/pustules/plaques, crusting has to be noted as they may be seen in infections like simple folliculitis, folliculitis decalvans, early stages of scarring alopecia.

Scaling is another vital sign, therefore the nature and amount of scaling has to be examined for. In case of seborrheic dermatitis the scales are yellowish, greasy, adherent and limit themselves to the hairline, while in scalp psoriasis the scales are dry, gray to silvery white, loosely attached to the scalp and may cross the hairline (corona psoriatica). Thick asbestos like scales are seen in pityriasis amiantacea.

After a complete local examination, the next step is to look for **signs of other concomitant dermatological disease (which can involve hair/scalp as a part of the disease) (Box 3.6).**

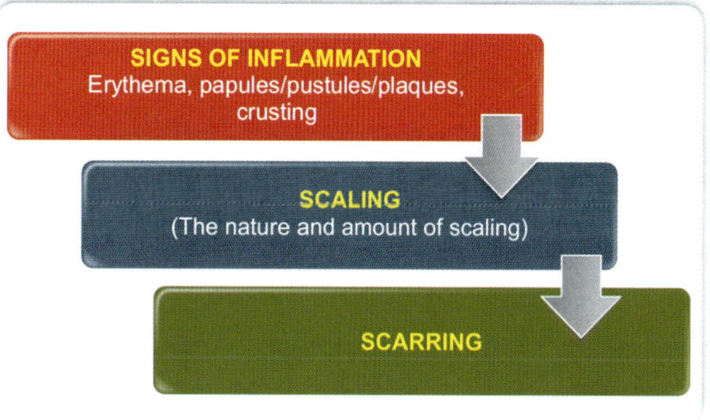

Fig. 3.2: Evaluation points in scalp examination

Box 3.6: Additive systems to be examined

- Concomitant dermatological disease
- Nail involvement
- Mucosal examination
- Genitalia

A few instances are presence of acne, pseudoacanthosis nigricans in hirsutism, female AGA; violaceous flat topped papules of lichen planus in lichen planopilaris or pseudopelade of Brocq; atrophic patches/plaques in the en coup de sabre variety of morphea; malar rash, discoid lesions in DLE, SLE ; genital ulcers, papulosquamous lesions, palms and soles involvement in syphilis.

Nail involvement can be seen in the form of geometric pitting, "Scotch plaid pattern", red lunula in alopecia areata, coarse nail pitting associated with scalp psoriasis.

Mucosal examination is needed to look for associated conditions like oral lichen planus, cheilitis/stomatitis in nutritional deficiency, snail track ulcers or patches in syphilis. One has to also examine the **genitalia** to look for evidence of active/healed syphilitic ulcers, look for pubic hair distribution, presence of clitoromegaly in case of hirsutism due to virilizing syndromes.

General physical examination is vital to the diagnosis as Subtle signs of underlying disorders can be picked up.

Pallor, tachycardia, feeble pulse, low blood pressure indicates a possibility of anemia which can cause telogen effluvium/diffuse hair loss. The BMI has to be calculated to assess the nutritional status. The presence of thyroid swelling if any should be examined. Signs of virilization are important in the evaluation of hirsutism. Signs of any syndromal involvement or genodermatoses should be picked up.

A complete examination of respiratory, cardiac, per abdomen and CNS has to be carried out to look for involvement of organs in endocrinopathies, collagen vascular diseases and malignancies.

After a complete history and examination one has to proceed to carry out a few investigations to assess the general state of the patient as well as few directed in particular to the hair and scalp.

Hematological Investigations include the Following (Figure 3.3)

Complete blood count with peripheral smear to confirm anemia and its type.

Serum iron, serum ferritin and TIBC also need to be done as they can contribute to telogen effluvium.

Thyroid function tests are done as it can be an etiology for diffuse hairloss or as a part of the autoimmune conditions like alopecia areata.

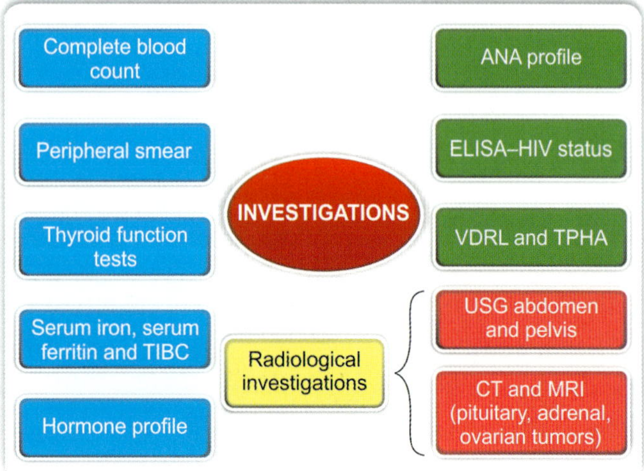

Fig. 3.3: Schematic representation of general investigations

Hormonal profile is indicated in cases of hirsutism to rule out conditions like PCOS, congenital adrenal hyperplasia, Cushing's syndrome, adrenal or ovarian tumors leading to aberrant secretion of hormones and pituitary disorders. The parameters measured include serum FSH, LH, FSH: LH ratio, prolactin, free testosterone, 17-hydroxy-progesterone, cortisol, ACTH, DHEAS, SHBG (the stepwise evaluation is shown in **Algorithms 3.3 to 3.5**).

Serological tests like ANA is done when there is scarring alopecia probably due to SLE or DLE.

VDRL and TPHA is advised in presence of a moth eaten appearance of hairloss seen in syphilitic alopecia.

Radiological Investigations

- USG abdomen and pelvis in PCOS where multiple follicles are seen arranged in a "string of pearls" like fashion in the periphery of the ovaries
- CT and MRI is peformed to detect pituitary, adrenal, ovarian tumors which can secrete abnormal levels of hormones
- After a general investigation, the next segment focuses on few investigations done specifically on the hair.

The various available modalities can be classified as:

Clinical Tests[1]

- Hair pull test
- Daily hair counts
- Wood's lamp examination
- Hair weight estimation
- Trichometry
- Trichotillometry.

Microscopic Examination of Hair

- Trichogram

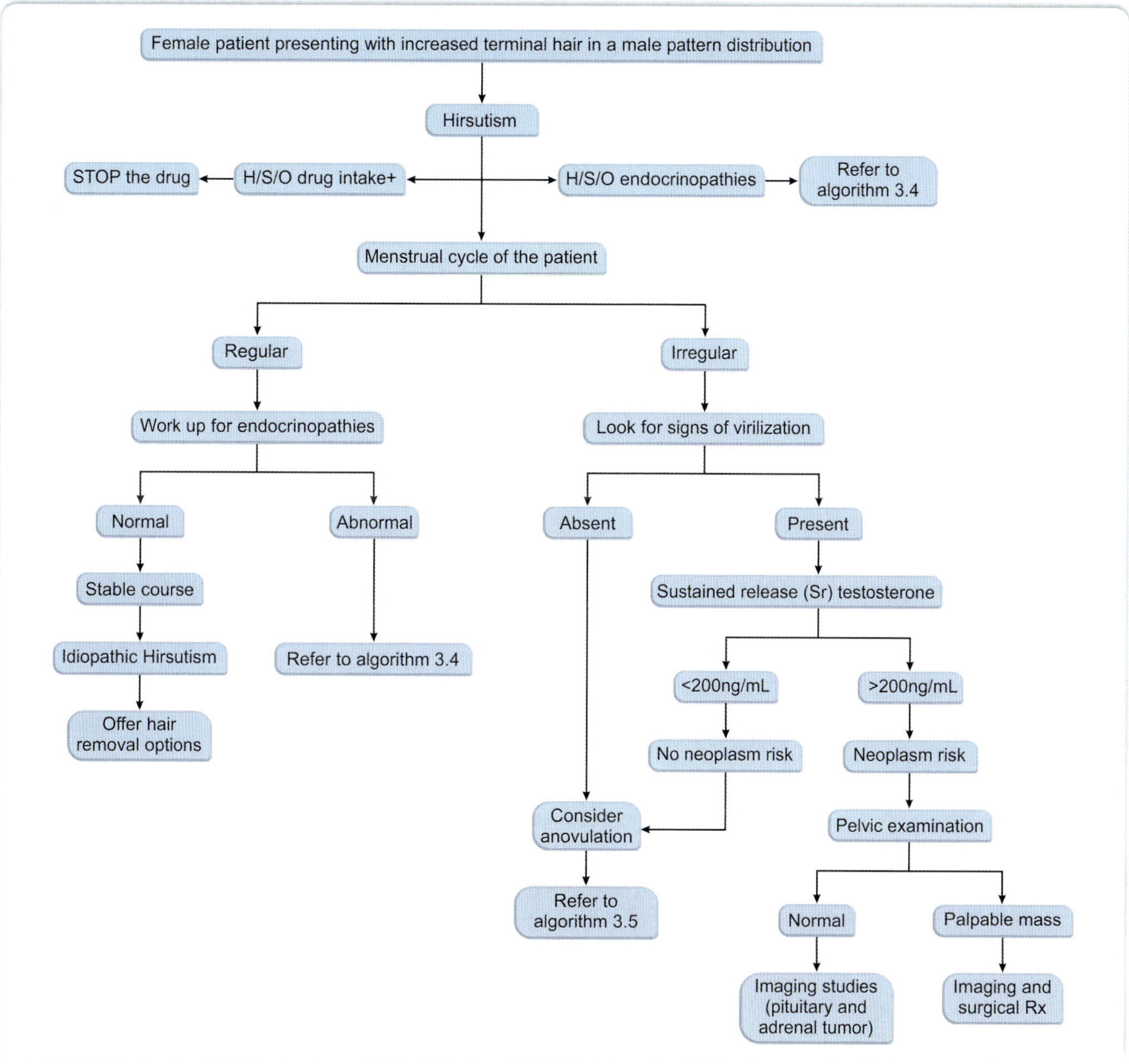

Algorithm 3.3: Hirsutism

- Photographic trichogram and its modifications
- Light microscopy
- Polarizing microscopy
- Electron microscopy
- Confocal microscopy

Hair Investigations in Systemic Diseases

- Hair bulb incubation (albinism)
- Zinc estimation
- Arsenic estimation
- Immunofluorescence in pemphigus

Scalp Biopsy

X-ray Diffraction Studies

It is used to study ultrastructural details of normal hair, effects of extraneous factors like hair dyes on the structure of hair and also used for the early diagnosis of breast and colon cancer.

Others

Dermoscopy, videodermoscopy.

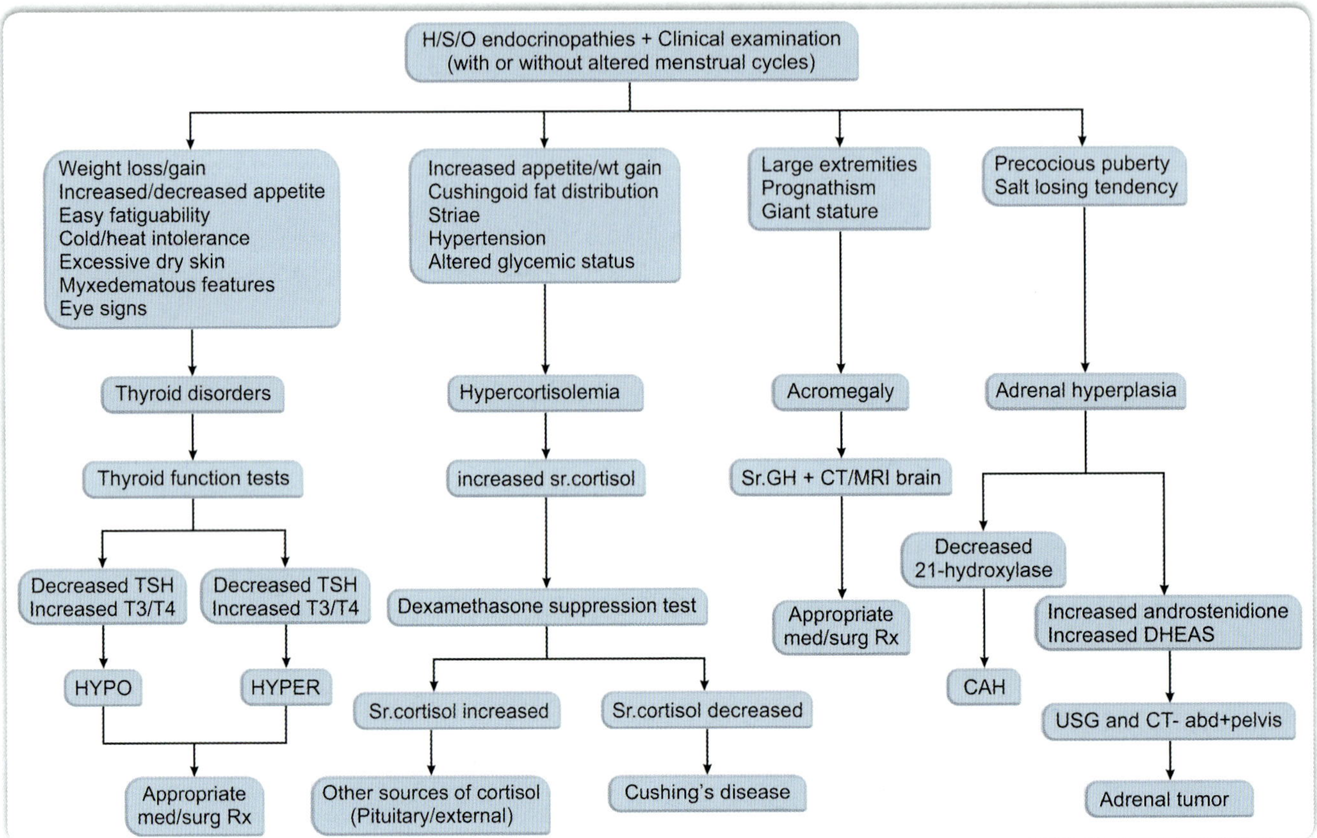

Algorithm 3.4: Approach to a patient with endocrinopathies

Abbreviations: History suggestive of (HSO); weight (WT); growth hormone (GH); congenital adrenal hypoplasia (CAH); dehydroepiandrosterone sulfate (DHEAS)

The above tests can also be grouped as non-invasive, semi-invasive and invasive methods.

These tests when interpreted with caution, are valuable tools for patient diagnosis and monitoring. Daily hair counts and wash test are good methods for primary evaluation of the patient and to get an approximate assessment of the amount of shedding. Some methods like global photography form an important part of any hair clinic. Analytical methods like phototrichogram are usually possible only in the setting of a clinical trial.

Daily Hair Count Test (Box 3.7)

This patient performed test is used to quantify the hair loss in order to rule out physiological hair loss (which amounts to <100 hairs/day).

Procedure

The patient is instructed to collect all shed hair in the bath, sink, during combing, in the brush, count them and place them in plastic bags on a day-to-day basis. This count is done for 7 days and reported to the dermatologist.

Box 3.7: Daily hair count test

- Subjective analysis of hair loss
- If more than 100 hairs are lost per day it is taken as pathological
- Anagen effluvium, telogen effluvium or alopecia areata

Inference

If more than 100 hairs are lost per day it is taken as pathological and one has to proceed to examine the hair root and the hair shaft for any changes. Based on the type of hair seen, the condition can be diagnosed as anagen effluvium, telogen effluvium or alopecia areata.

Drawbacks

- The procedure of collecting the hairs daily is cumbersome to the patient.
- There are no studies to confirm loss of <100 hairs/day as physiological.
- The assessment is very subjective.

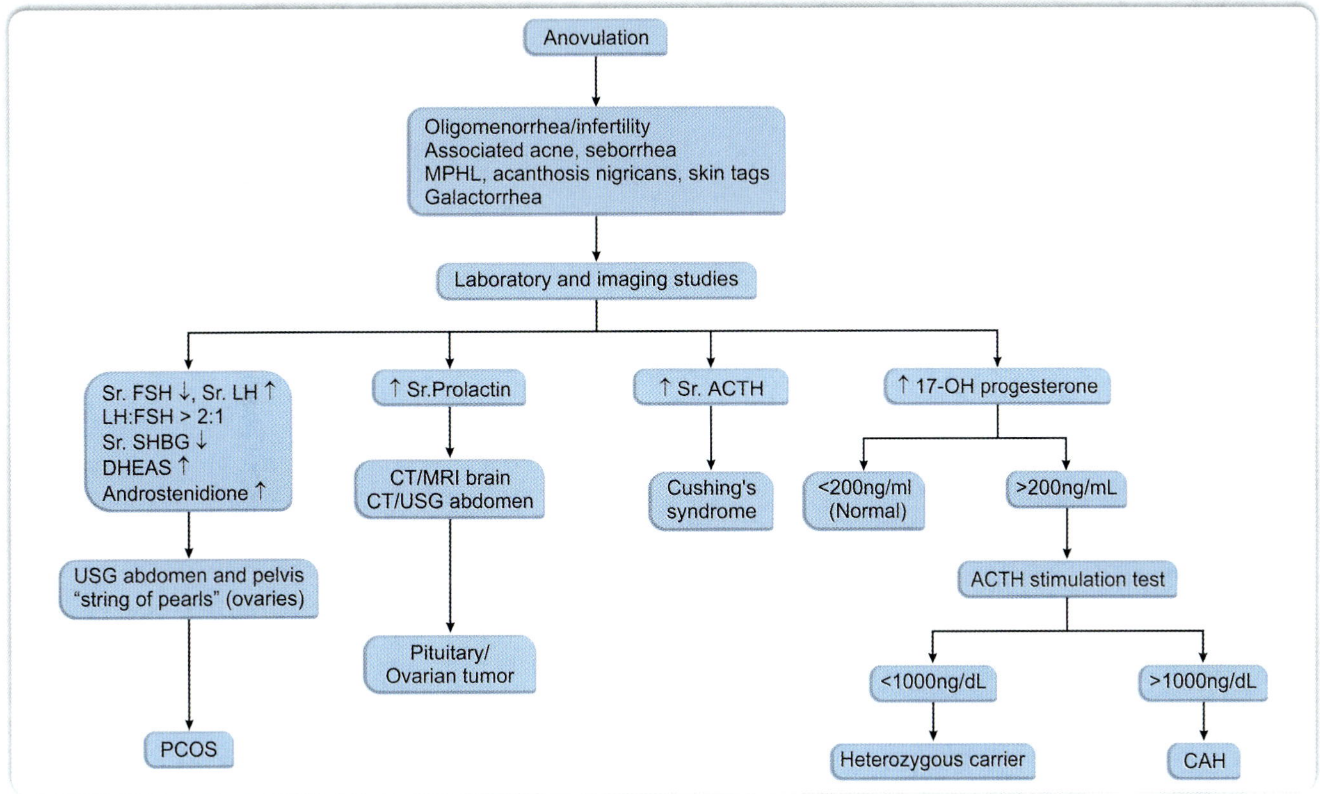

Algorithm 3.5: Anovulation

Abbreviations: Follicle stimulating hormone (FSH); leutinizing hormone (LH); steroid hormone binding globulin (SHBG); dehydroepiandrosterone sulfate (DHEAS); sr-serum; male pattern hair loss (MPHL); adrenocortical stimulating hormone (ACTH); congenital adrenal hypoplasia (CAH)

Standardized Wash Test (Box 3.8)

Aim

To differentiate FPHL from chronic telogen effluvium (CTE).

Procedure

Here the patient is asked to refrain from shampooing for 5 days and then wash the hair. They are instructed to rinse the hair in the basin with the outlet plugged, collect all the hair. They are then divided into hairs which are <3 cm (vellus) and >5 cm (terminal).

Inference

In female AGA 58.9% vellus hairs are found while only 3.5% vellus hairs are found in CTE.

Box 3.8: Standardized wash test

- Differentiates FPHL from chronic telogen effluvium
- AGA 58.9% vellus hairs, 3.5% vellus hairs are found in CTE

Drawbacks

To abstain from shampooing for 5 days may be difficult for the patients.

The tests and results are not standardized or diagnostic.

60 Second Hair Count Test

This is also a patient performed test to assess the amount of hairloss.

Procedure

Before shampooing, patient is advised to comb the hair for 60 s over a pillow or sheet of contrasting color, starting with the comb at the back top of the scalp and moving towards the front of the scalp. The procedure is repeated before three consecutive shampooing sessions using the same comb or brush. The number of hairs in the comb or brush and on the pillow after each hair count is recorded. The procedure is repeated monthly and results taken to the dermatologist.

Drawbacks

Falsely elevated number due to breakage while combing. Hairloss over lateral and posterior areas cannot be estimated.

Hair Pull Test

This is also known by the names Traction test/Saboraud's sign/Pull out sign **(Box 3.9)**.

Aim

To assess presence of active hair shedding, indicates severity and location of hairloss.

Procedure

Around 20–60 hairs are grasped between the thumb, index and middle fingers from the base of the hairs near the scalp and pulled away from it with a gentle but firm pressure.

Inference

If >10% of grasped hairs are pulled away it is taken as positive and it indicates active shedding.

Usually, telogen hairs are pulled out but the test is considered positive even if anagen hair is present along with thickened root sheath.

Conditions Where Test is Positive

- Telogen effluvium
- Anagen effluvium
- Loose anagen syndrome
- At advancing edge of alopecia areata.

Drawbacks

- The number of hairs grasped are difficult to count therefore results may be false
- The pulling force may vary from person to person making the test non-standardized.

Global Photography Technique (Box 3.10)

The procedure is also called Canfield technique which uses a stereotactic positioning device where the patient's chin and forehead are fixed.

Box 3.9: Traction test/Saboraud's sign/Pull out sign/Hair pull test

- If >10% of grasped hairs are pulled away, it is taken as positive and it indicates active shedding
- Indicates severity and location of hairloss

Box 3.10: Canfield technique/Global photography technique

- Four standard views (vertex, midline, frontal and temporal) are taken with standardized photographic techniques
- Paired photographs to assess hair growth
- A standardized seven-point rating scale used in assessment

The camera and flash device are mounted such that view, magnification and lighting are same at every exposure.

The patient is advised to maintain the same hairstyle and color at every follow up.

Four standard views (vertex, midline, frontal and temporal) are taken.

It is used to appreciate hair growth after drug therapy by taking paired photographs before and after treatment. A standardized seven-point rating scale (+3, +2, +1, 0, -1, -2, -3; greatly increased density to greatly decreased density) has been used in the assessment.

Dermoscopy and Videodermoscopy

These techniques take images upto 20X–40X and can also capture them digitally and store them for later use. Few of the clinical features can be appreciated better by this technique than the naked eye examination.

It has the advantage of diagnosing scalp disorders along with hair abnormalities.

The features examined are:

- Epidermal and perifollicular scale
- Follicular ostia
- Hair shaft diversity
- Exclamation mark hair.

Dermoscopic findings in few conditions are listed in **Table 3.2**.

Table 3.2: Table showing dermoscopic features in various conditions

Androgenetic alopecia	Hairs with a different caliber (miniaturized hair) Brown halo, about 1 mm in diameter, around the emergent hair shaft Small bald areas with numerous empty follicles and scalp pigmentation because of sun exposure
Cicatricial alopecia	Erythema, scaling, atrophy, dyspigmentation, hair tufting (doll's hair)
Alopecia areata	Yellow dots—represent degenerated follicular keratinocytes and sebum within the affected follicles. Exclamation mark hairs are also seen
Chronic cutaneous lupus erythmatosus (CCLE)	Red dots
Lichen planopilaris (LPP), folliculitis decalvans	White dots with honeycomb pattern—represent targeted follicular destruction
Tinea capitis	Comma shaped hairs are characteristic

Advantages

- It is a simple, non-invasive yet very informative procedure
- Best site for biopsy can be ascertained
- Both scalp and hair disorders can be diagnosed.

Hair Pluck Test/Trichogram (Figure 3.4)

This test is performed to ascertain the type of hair involved in the pathology.

Procedure

Around 60–80 hairs are held with hemostat covered with rubber and then plucked by a firm twisting action and lifting the hair shafts rapidly away from the scalp in the direction of its emergence. In most cases, two sites are investigated. The first site is 2 cm from the frontal hair line and 2 cm from the midline. The second site is in the occipital region, 2 cm lateral from the occipital protuberance. In alopecia areata, the first site would be in close proximity to a patch and the second in the contralateral, clinically uninvolved side.

The roots are cut off 1cm above root sheath, mounted on a slide side by side and fixed by adhesive tape.

The hair roots are then evaluated under light microscopy to determine the number of hair in the different phases of the hair cycle.

Findings

- *Anagen hair* (80–88%)—darkly pigmented, triangular/delta shaped bulb placed at an angle to hair shaft like a "hockey stick", intact inner root sheath.
- *Telogen hair* (10–20%)—less pigmented, club shaped bulb, absence of inner root sheath.
- *Catagen hair* (1–2%)—similar to telogen but the bulb is not smooth and it is covered by loose but thick outer and inner root sheath.
- *Dystrophic hair*—root is tapered severely to a point and root sheath is absent.

After identifying the hair types the percentage of individual types are calculated and the stage of hair cycle affected is assessed.

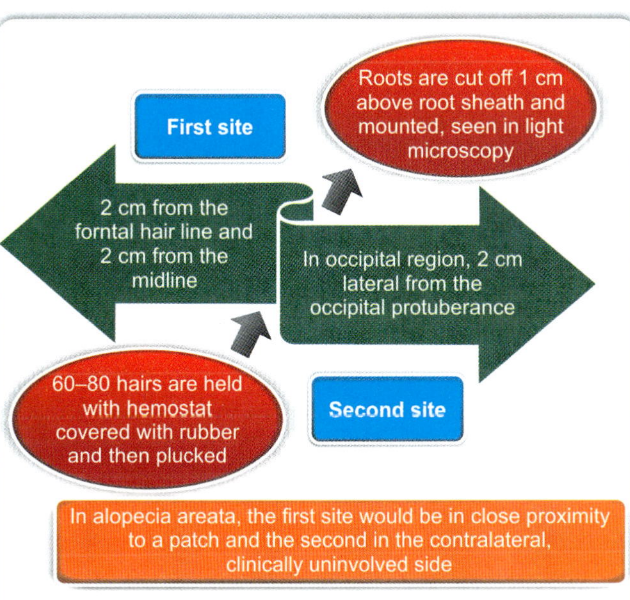

Fig. 3.4: Schematic representation of hair pluck test protocol

Inferences

- In acute telogen effluvium, the telogen hairs is double the normal upper limit
- In androgenetic alopecia, increased percentage of dystrophic hair and telogen hair with features of miniaturization are seen.

Unit Area Trichogram (UAT)

This is an improvised technique where a fixed area is marked on the scalp through a template with a uniform fiber tip pen. All hairs within and on the scribed line are epilated individually with forceps/tweezers in the direction of the hair growth to minimize damage to the hair bulb.

Unit area trichogram may be used for follow-up of scalp hair changes in clinical studies, for observing hair growth cycling and for monitoring topical or systemic drug and cosmetic effects **(Box 3.11)**.

Drawbacks

- The plucking of hair can be painful
- The procedure is laborious and time consuming
- Early anagen and vellus hairs are missed due to small size while plucking therefore results may not be accurate
- It is not a good indicator of disease severity or activity.

Phototrichogram (PTG)

It is a non-invasive in vivo study introduced by Saitoh in 1970.

Aim: This is used to study the physiology of the hair cycle and measure hair growth variables.

Principle: It is based on the observation that anagen hair grows about 1mm every 3 days; catagen hair shows moderate elongation while telogen hair does not grow at all.

Box 3.11: Unit area trichogram (UAT)

- Used for follow-up of scalp hair changes in clinical studies
- For observing hair growth cycling
- Monitoring topical or systemic drug and cosmetic effects

Procedures

- A selected area over the scalp is marked (1 sq cm^2) and the hairs are clipped
- Variables like hair density, thickness, length are measured
- The area is photographed, patient instructed not to wash hair for 48 hours
- A second photo is taken after 2 days and the same variables are measured.

Inferences

- Variables at D0—density, diameter, length (L1)
- Variables at D2—length (L2), number of anagen hairs, number of telogen hairs, anagen:telogen ratio
- Hair growth—(L2-L1)/2.

Modifications

Contrast enhanced PTG—black colored dye is used to color hairs (in case of thin and less pigmented hairs) to make them more visible.

Scalp immersion PTG—mineral oil is applied to improve visualization.

Trichoscan (standard epiluminescence microscopy combined with automatic digital image analysis) here the entire process is computerized where the serial photographs taken are stored and hence can be retrieved later for analysis **(Box 3.12)**.

Light Microscopy[2]

Light microscopy of the hair forms an important bedside clinical tool for the diagnosis of various disorders affecting the hair **(Figure 3.5)**.

Indications are grouped as the following:

1. Infections and infestations—tinea capitis, piedra, trichomycosis axillaris, pediculosis.
2. Hair shaft anomalies—structural defects, fractures, nodes, twists, bands, constrictions.
3. Assessment of hair loss—androgenetic alopecia, telogen effluvium.
4. Metabolic and nutritional disorders—kwashiorkor.
5. Genodermatoses—Chediak-Higashi syndrome, Griscelli syndrome, Netherton's syndrome, Menke's kinky hair disease.

Box 3.12: Trichoscan

- Standard epiluminescence microscopy combined with automatic digital image analysis
- The entire process is computerized where the serial photographs taken are stored and hence can be retrieved later for analysis

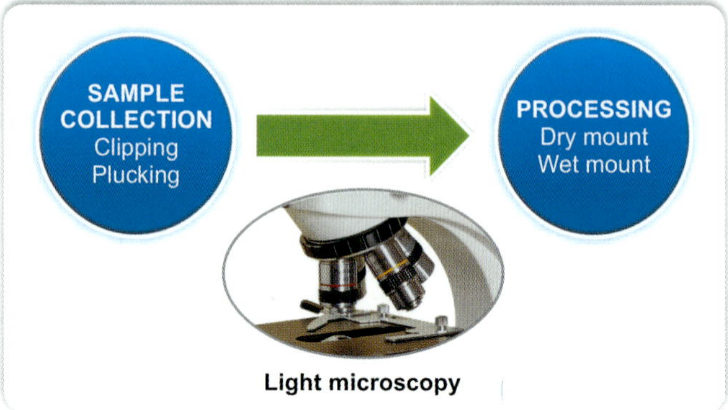

Fig. 3.5: Light microscopy sample collection and processing techniques

Procedures

Sample collection is done from the involved site by two methods namely:

- Clipping—where hair shaft has to be seen
- Plucking—where hair root needs to be visualized.

The collected samples are then processed in two methods namely:

- Dry mount—where the collected hairs are mounted on a slide and a cover slip is placed over.
- Wet mount—where fungal infection is suspected, KOH mount is prepared.

Findings on Light Microscopy

Normal Hair Shafts

These are cylindrical with a smooth surface, varying diameters and ovoid or round profiles on cross-section. Hair color is variable, but, in normal hair, the pigmentation within the shaft is usually uniform. The root of the hair in anagen is deeply pigmented and surrounded by a translucent inner sheath, whereas the bulbous tip of a hair in telogen is non-pigmented and whitish.

Tinea Capitis

- Endothrix—arthrospores and mycelia within the hair shaft
- Ectothrix—arthrospores are limited to only the outer aspect of the hair shaft
- Favus—longitudinally oriented fungal hyphae with degenerating tunnels
- Pediculosis—oval, transluscent, whitish nit attached to hair shaft
- Trichorrhexis nodosa—node formed by the frayed ends of the broken ends being thrust into each other

- Trichorrhexis invaginata—"bamboo" hairs caused by invagination of proximal concave end by the bulbous distal end
- Monilethrix—beaded appearance with swollen nodes and narrow internodal area
- Pili torti—flattened and twisted hair longitudinally at 180 degrees
- Pili annulati—hair looks banded and sandy with a spangled appearance
- Bubble hair—due to heating effects where hair appears spongy because of vacuolization
- Trichoclasis—transverse fracture of the cortex
- Peripilar cast—tubular amorphous structure completely encircling the hair
- Wooly hair—multiple grooves, twists, irregularity of the shaft
- Griscelli's syndrome—large clumps of melanosomes
- Chediak-Higashi syndrome—fine clumps of melanosomes

Polarizing Microscopy

- Trichothiodystrophy—"tiger tail" appearance
- Thallium poisoning

Electron Microscopy

- Loose anagen hair syndrome—"floppy sock" appearance
- Uncombable hair syndrome—triangular cross section
- Woolly hair—vacuolation of cortex
- Pili annulati—cobblestoning of cuticular cells
- Canities—melanosomal cytoplasmic vacuoles
- Trichothiodystrophy—abnormal microfibrils
- Marie-Unna syndrome—flattening and twisting of hairs; abnormal proliferation of hair sheath

Scalp Biopsy (Figure 3.6)

This is an invasive procedure carried out to identify the underlying pathological process.

Indications

1. All cases of cicatricial alopecia
2. Undiagnosed cases of non-cicatricial alopecia

Procedure

After adequate preparation of the scalp (clipping of hairs), under aseptic precautions, local anesthesia (lignocaine with 1:1,00,000 adrenaline) is given to the area to be biopsied.

A skin biopsy punch of at least 4 mm diameter is used, which gives an effective diameter of 12.6 mm^2.

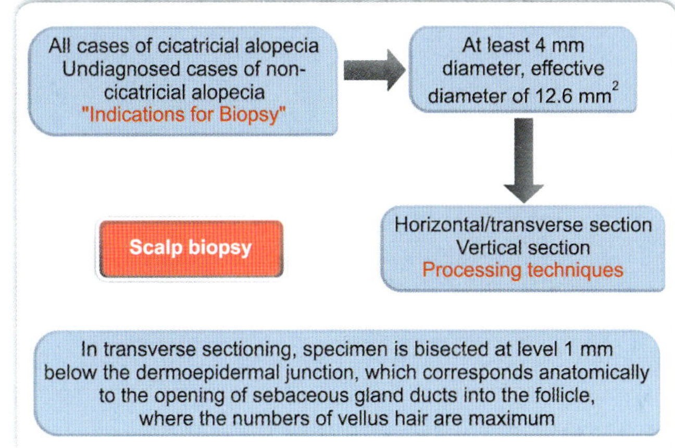

Fig. 3.6: Schematic representation of scalp biopsy—indications and processing techniques

The biopsy must be deep and should include the entire follicular unit, including some subcutaneous fat. Usually, this involves a depth of 4 mm.

While processing the sample two types of sections are preferred:

- **Horizontal/transverse section**—in cases of non-cicatricial alopecia, to count the number of hair follicles and also identify the type of follicle. In transverse sectioning, the biopsy specimen is bisected at a level 1 mm below the dermoepidermal junction, which corresponds anatomically to the opening of sebaceous gland ducts into the follicle, where the numbers of vellus hair are maximum.
- **Vertical section**—in cases of cicatricial alopecia, to identify the presence of infiltrates associated with the follicles and accompanying epidermal changes.

Normal scalp biopsy shows the following features:

- Upper level (papillary dermis)
  - Around 35-40 hairs are present
  - All type of hairs are seen
- Mid level (reticular dermis)
  - 35 hairs may be present
- Deeper level (subcutis)
  - Around 30 hairs are present
  - Only anagen hairs are seen at this level.

Appearance of Different Types of Hair in Hematoxylin and Eosin (H and E) Section (Figures 3.7 and 3.8):

- The **vellus** follicles are defined as follicles containing hairs in which the diameter of the hair shaft is equal to or less than the thickness of the inner sheath of the same follicle and the diameter is ≤0.03 mm.
- The **anagen** hairs are identified in transverse sections by the presence of a normal-appearing inner root sheath and the absence of individual cell necrosis.

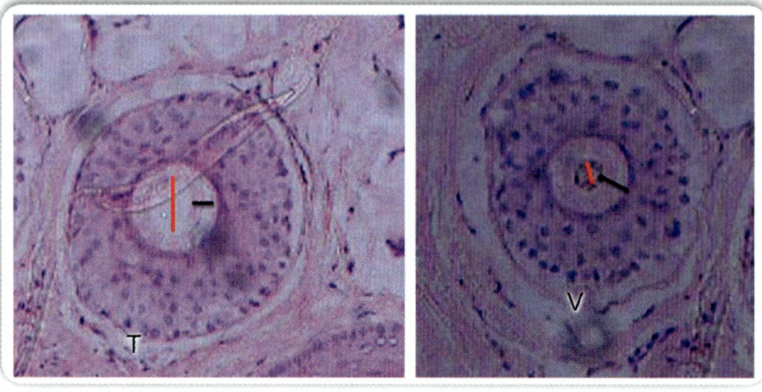

Fig. 3.7: Comparison between terminal and vellus hair. Red line- hair shaft, black line – inner root sheath. T- Terminal hair, V- Vellus hair

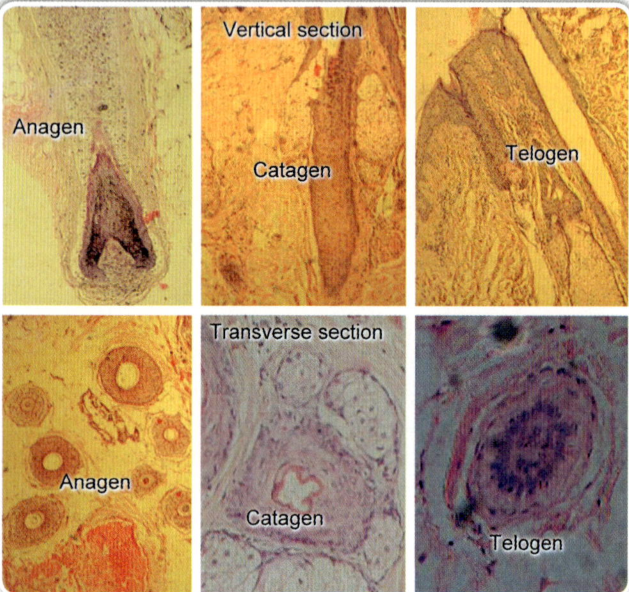

Fig. 3.8: Horizontal and transverse section of hair in various stages of hair cycle

- The **catagen** hair shows loss of matrix and thin epithelium of dermal papilla.
- The **telogen** hairs can be recognized below the level of the sebaceous duct by loss of inner root sheath. There is an irregular stellate configuration of the keratotic elements forming the remnants of the inner root sheath. Cornifying club having serrated rim, which interdigitates with surrounding outer root sheath, characterizes an early telogen hair bulb. Late telogen hair follicle shows completely cornified club.
- The end stage of telogen or **telogen germinal unit** is seen as an irregular basaloid star-shaped island of cells marked by a peripheral nuclear palisade.

Findings in few conditions:

Androgenetic Alopecia (AGA)

- In the transverse section, at the level of opening of sebaceous ducts into the hair follicle, the hairs shafts appear vastly different in diameter.
- Terminal hairs measure 06 mm and vellus hairs measure less than 0.03 mm, while the thickness of indeterminate hairs is between these two **(Refer Figure 13.10A)**.
- The original terminal follicle is replaced by a follicular streamer (stellae or fibrous tract) extending from the subcutaneous tissue up to the course of the follicle to the miniaturized hair. A streamer is characterized by a concentric arrangement of loose, fibrovascular tissue resembling a collapsed fibrous sheath. Streamers result from shortening of follicles, either from follicular miniaturization or an increased percentage of follicles in the resting (telogen) phase.
- Decreased terminal hairs and increased follicular streamers therefore characterize AGA. Sebaceous glands seem enlarged in relation to the miniaturized hair follicles.
- There is significant reduction in total follicular counts, measured by horizontal sectioning of scalp biopsy.
- The progressive reduction in the duration of anagen causes a relative increase in telogen hair. The terminal to vellus ratio is normally 7:1. In AGA, the ratio is < 4:1, which has been considered as diagnostic of AGA.

Telogen Effluvium

- The size of all the follicles is similar but there will be reduced number of terminal hairs when counted at the dermal-adipose tissue junction as compared with hairs counted at the upper dermis level.
- Total telogen hairs are counted and if the count is higher than 20%, it is suggestive of telogen effluvium **(Refer Figure 13.10B)**.
- The irregular island of basaloid epithelium represents a telogen germinal unit, an epithelial remnant of a telogen follicle. Such structures may be increased in telogen effluvium.

Alopecia Areata

- On vertical section, a dense lymphocytic infiltrate (swarm of bees) hugs the bulb of the terminal anagen follicle **(Refer Figure 10.8)**.
- Most of the hair show varying degrees of eosinophilic change of the hair shaft, indicating that they are in various stages of transition from catagen to telogen.

Trichotillomania

- At scanning magnification there is a normal number of hair follicles per cross section. There is a mild, predominantly superficial inflammatory infiltrate.
- Distortion of the hair follicle is seen, as manifested here by the twisted contour of the follicular canal, trichomalacia or follicular rupture.
- A characteristic finding in trichotillomania is the presence of pigment casts (clumps of pigment) that are present in the follicular canal and perifollicular hemorrhages.

Cicatricial Alopecia

- Early lesions are more suitable and multiple biopsies are preferred to study different stages of the disease
- Reduction in the size or absence of appendages like sebaceous and sweat glands
- Follicles are replaced by fibrotic tracts
- Dermal papillae are replaced by sclerotic whorls
- Based on the type of infiltrate they can be of neutrophilic, lymphocytic, mixed and non-specific types
- Infiltrate usually around upper two-thirds of the follicle
- Epidermal changes—atrophy, follicular plugging, lichenoid changes.

Other Tests

Contrasting Felt Examination (Box 3.13)

This test is used to see short, miniature hairs of the scalp.

Box 3.13: Contrasting felt examination

- Fine short hairs with broken or tapered distal tips project up along the edges of the felt
- Miniature hairs can be seen in the androgen-dependent areas
- In regrowing telogen effluvium, a classic short frontal fringe is seen

Procedure

An index card with black felt glued on one side and white felt on the opposite side is used. After making a parting in the hair, the index card is held along the scalp. Fine short hairs with broken or tapered distal tips project up along the edges of the felt.

Inference

These miniature hairs can be seen in the androgen-dependent areas of both men and women presenting with androgenetic alopecia.

In a regrowing telogen effluvium, a classic short frontal fringe is seen.

Trichometry

- It is the measurement of hair diameter
- The diameter is measured usually in the proximal 40 mm of the hair using dermoscopy or laser beam diffraction studies
- It is used in the objective assessment of patients with hirsutism, hypertrichosis or alopecia

Trichotillometry (Box 3.14)

- This procedure measures the mean force required for epilation of the hair using a trichotillometer
- The normal epilation force is around 36 g which is reduced to around 19 g in kwashiorkor

Box 3.14: Trichotillometry

- Measures the mean force required for epilation of the hair using a trichotillometer.
- Malnutrition and loose anagen hair syndrome, decrease in the force required to epilate the hair depicts the easy pluckability clinically

- There is decrease in the force required to epilate the hair in conditions like malnutrition and loose anagen hair syndrome, depicting the easy pluckability clinically.

Conclusion

In conclusion, diagnosis of hair disorders can be easily and accurately made with a systematic approach to the patient starting from history taking to the various investigative modalities.

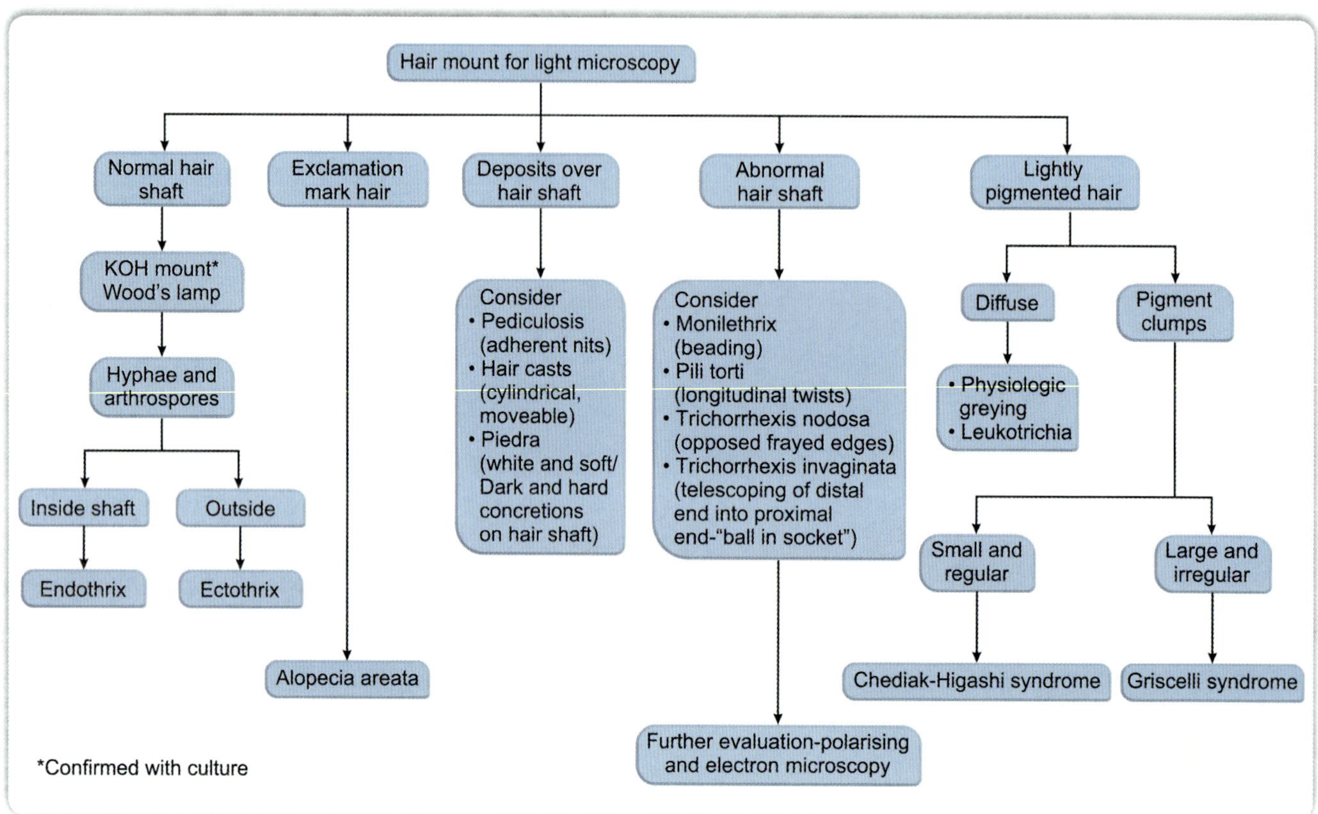

Algorithm 3.6: Hair microscopy

References

1. Dhurat R, Saraogi P. Hair evaluation methods: Merits and demerits. Int J Trichol. 2009;1:108-19.
2. Adya KA, Inamadar AC, Palit A, Shivanna R, Deshmukh NS. Light microscopy of the hair: A simple tool to "untangle" hair disorders. Int J Trichol. 2011;3:46-56.

4

Genetic Hair Disorders

Arun C Inamadar, Vishalakshi S Pandit, Aparna Palit

"My scientific labors have brought me a great deal of satisfaction, and I am convinced that before long the entire world will praise the result of these labors."

—*Gregor Mendel*

Introduction

Infant with sparse, lusterless, or broken - off hair suggest signs of genetic defect and may signal impending neurological and mental defects. These disorders are not very rare and molecular diagnostic methods are required for definitive diagnosis. Early recognition of genetic hair disorders can be done by simple hair microscopy. Hair mount **(Box 4.1)** is the basic procedure to differentiate between genetic hair disorders due to structural defect and otherwise.

Genetic hair disorders are grouped as given below:

1. Monilethrix
2. Pseudomonilethrix
3. Pili torti
4. Menkes disease
5. Netherton syndrome
6. Trichothiodystrophy
7. Ectodermal dysplasia.

Box 4.1: Hair mount

Hair mount is the basic procedure to differentiate between genetic hair disorders due to structural defect and otherwise

Monilethrix (Synonym: Beaded Hair)

Monilethrix is an autosomal dominant disorder characterized by periodic beading of hair shafts and pronounced hair fragility, leading to hair loss and eventual scarring alopecia.[1] This disorder was first described by Smith in 1879 as a rare nodose condition of the hair and the term "monilethrix" was later coined by Radcliff Crocker.[2]

Pathogenesis

It is an autosomal dominant transmitted disease with variable expressivity.

Around seven different types of mutations have been detected to be associated with monilethrix.[3] The three hair keratin genes proved to be causal for monilethrix encode the type II hair keratins Hb1, Hb3, and Hb6, **(Box 4.2)** and share a completely identical α-helical rod domain and, in line with the ultrastructurally observed disease symptoms, are all expressed in the hair cortex.[4] In these three keratins (hHb1, hHb3 and hHb6), the HTM was the most mutated region while a few HIM mutations occurred only in the hHb6 keratin.[3] There is conceivable evidence that mutation either in the cortex keratins, compromising the keratin-desmoplakin interaction, or in desmoglein 4 (DSG4), abrogating cell-cell adhesion, in cortex cells, entail a similar disease phenotype.[4] The mutation in transmembranous adhesion molecule desmoglein 4, a member of the two desmosomal cadherin subfamilies, desmocollins (DSCs) and desmogleins is implicated in the autosomal recessive pattern of monilethrix **(Figure 4.1)**.[5-7] Singh, et al.[8] have reported a case who showed higher acrocentric association using cytogenetic studies. This association could possibly indicate some predisposing factor between the satellite (acrocentric) chromosomes and mutation in the microsatellite DNA loci region on chromosome 12, containing the type II Keratin gene cluster.

Box 4.2: Genes involved in monilethrix

- hHb1, hHb3 and hHb6—autosomal dominant
- Mutations in desmoglein 4, desmocollins (DSCs)—autosomal recessive
- Mutation in the microsatellite DNA loci region on chromosome 12, containing the type II Keratin gene cluster

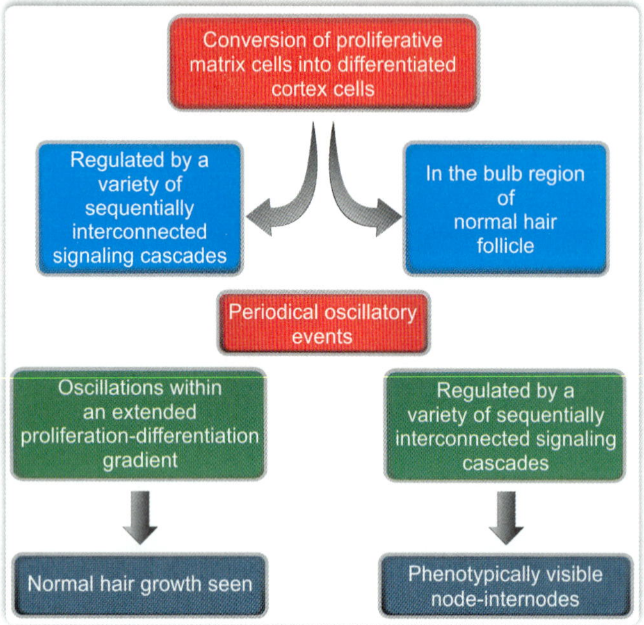

Fig. 4.1: Pathogenetic basis of formation of alternate node and internodes[4]

The beading or moniliform appearance of the hair shaft is caused by the nodes and internodal thinning of the shaft. The nodes seem to represent normal growth; the internodes are characterized by the wrinkling of corticle cells leading to fragility of the hair, with an absence of medulla. Ultrastructurally, vacuolation and alterations in the fibrillar structures of lower cortex cells have been described.[9]

Clinical Features (Box 4.3)

Affected individuals usually have normal appearing hair at birth but within the first few months of life, these fibers are replaced by short, fragile and brittle hair. Hairs rarely grow beyond 1 to 2 cm in length because of breakage, resulting in a stubbly appearance. In the mildest form, the disease involves only the occiput and nape of the neck, but in its severe form, the entire scalp, secondary hairs, eyebrows, and eyelashes may also be involved.[4] Alopecia is more severe in areas prone to friction. Perifollicular erythema and follicular hyperkeratosis are commonly observed in the occipital region **(Figure 4.2)**.

Box 4.3: Clinical clues in monilethrix

- *Mild form*—occiput and nape of the neck
- *Severe form*—entire scalp, secondary hairs, eyebrows, and eyelashes
- Perifollicular erythema and follicular hyperkeratosis in the occipital region
- Alopecia in pressure prone areas
- *Associated features*—keratosis pilaris, koilonychia, mental and physical retardation, syndactyly, cataract, teeth and nail anomalies

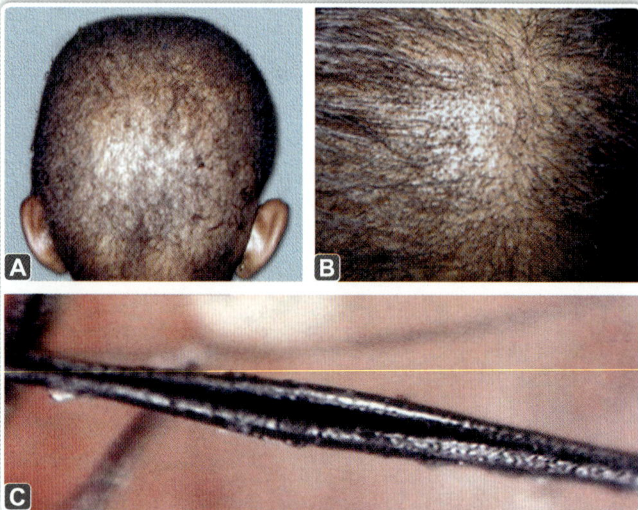

Figs 4.2A to C: (A) Sparse, fragile hair in monilethrix; (B) Follicular prominence on scalp; (C) Microscopic appearance of hair shaft showing fusiform nodes. (*Courtesy:* Department of Dermatology, STD and Leprosy, BMCRI, Bengaluru)

Lanugo hair is normal in the neonatal period. Clinical signs appear when terminal hair characteristics begin to form. Apart from short, sparse, fragile, non-growing hair, affected patients may have keratosis pilaris, koilonychia and rarely, systemic disturbances such as mental and physical retardation, syndactyly, cataract, teeth and nail anomalies.[10]

Investigations (Figure 4.3)

A diagnosis can be elucidated by examining hairs by light microscopy. It shows hair fibers with regularly spaced elliptical, fusiform or spindle-shaped nodes of normal thickness separated by intermittent abnormal constrictions that are the sites of fracture.[11] Infants with monilethrix may

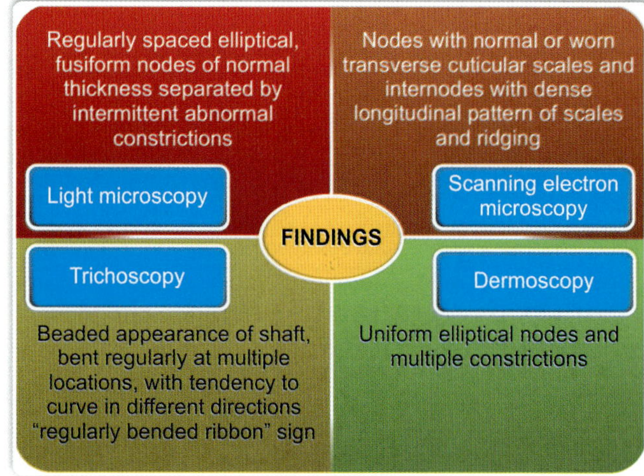

Fig. 4.3: Schematic representation of investigative findings in monilethrix

have a paucity of scalp hair, and it has been suggested that the examination of eyebrow hair may improve the likelihood of making the diagnosis in such settings.[12]

Advantages of simple microscopy: Inexpensive, rapid and non-invasive investigation.[12]

Scanning electron microscopy reveals nodes with normal or worn transverse cuticular scales and internodes with dense longitudinal pattern of scales and ridging. Trichoscopy reveals hair shafts with a beaded appearance, bent regularly at multiple locations, with a tendency to curve in different directions. These findings have been described as "regularly bended ribbon" sign by some authors.[11,13]

Dermoscopy (epiluminescence) of the papules reveals multiple stubs of broken hair arising from them with a similar beaded appearance.[14] Dermoscopy of hair reveals uniform elliptical nodes and multiple constrictions.[14]

Differential Diagnosis

The differential diagnosis between monilethrix and pseudomonilethrix can be made easily by trichoscopy.[15]

Treatment

There is no specific treatment for monilethrix although improvement has been reported with oral steroids, retinoids, griseofulvin and topical minoxidil.[16,17] Occasionally, regrowth of apparently normal hair may occur at the time of puberty or during pregnancy, suggesting some a hormonal influence.[17]

Pseudomonilethrix (Box 4.4)

In this condition, the hair shaft shows irregular flattened expanded areas that have an indented appearance. The beading is produced as an artifact of mounting hairs on glass slides and is of no significance.[18] On scanning electron microscopy, the widened beads can be seen to be an optical illusion. They merely represent artifactual indentations of the shaft viewed in cross section.[18] Although, some families with autosomal dominant transmission have also been described.[19]

Box 4.4: Pseudomonilethrix

Irregular flattened expanded areas on hair shaft with an indented appearance which is an artifact of mounting hairs on glass slides with no significance

Pili Torti (PT) (Synonym: Twisted hair, Corkscrew Hair[18])

In Latin, "pilus-hair", "torti-twisted".[20] It is characterized by hair shafts which are flattened and twisted at angles of about 180° with 4–5 twists at irregular intervals but in the same direction, giving it a spangled (glittering piece of metal) **(Box 4.5)** appearance in reflected light.[20] Fractures occur within the twists, which is the weakest point.[21] Occasional twists of less than 180 degrees do not qualify as true pili torti. These incomplete twists may occasionally occur in normal hair (seen in African hair and in the pubic/axillary hairs of other races).[18] Isolated twisted hairs are also seen in normal scalp, but in PT, the hairs appear in remarkably high number and density.[22]

Pili torti or 'twisting hair dystrophy' may be congenital, sporadic or acquired. Congenital pili torti may be seen as an isolated defect or in association with many different abnormalities and syndromes **(Table 4.1)**.[22]

Pathogenesis

The inheritance patterns can be autosomal dominant, autosomal recessive or sporadic in classic type. A limited number of cases have been reported and no gene defect has been elucidated. An autosomal dominant inheritance is seen in late-onset pili torti.[21] Bjornstad syndrome (congenital sensorineural deafness and PT) has been mapped to chromosome 2q34-36, with autosomal recessive inheritance pattern.[23] Genes encoding the major structural components of hair (cytokeratins and IFAPs) are particularly good candidate for mutations that account for the distinct manifestations of the disease.[23]

Box 4.5: Spangled appearance

- Hair shafts which are flattened and twisted at angles of about 180° with 4–5 twists at irregular intervals but in the same direction, giving it a glittering piece of metal appearance in reflected light
- Fractures occur within the twists, which is the weakest point

Table 4.1: Associations of pili torti

Associations with pili torti
❑ Inherited or congenital:
– Classic pili torti (Ronchese): Early onset
– Beare type: Late-onset PT
❑ Syndromal PT:
– Menke's kinky hair syndrome
– Bjornstad's syndrome
– Bazex syndrome
– Conradi-Hunermann syndrome
– Crandall's syndrome
– Citrullinemia
– Trichothiodystrophy
– Salti-Salem syndrome
– Laron syndrome
– Mitochondrial diseases
– Some ectodermal dysplasias
❑ Acquired:
– Cicatricial alopecia (due to distortion of the hair follicle caused by fibrosis by repeated trauma[21])
– Drugs: Isotretinoin, acitretin

Box 4.6: GRACILE

Growth retardation, aminoaciduria, cholestasis, iron overload, lactic acidosis and early death

Genetic mapping of the region 2q34-36 revealed a mutation in BCS1L, which encodes an ATPase required for the assembly of a mitochondrial complex.[24] The BCS1L protein plays a role in the assembly of mitochondrial complex III and in the electron-transport chain of energy production.[24] Patients with Bjornstad syndrome have mutations in BCS1L that alter protein-protein interactions, whereas patients with GRACILE **(Box 4.6)** syndrome, a multi-system lethal mitochondrial disorder, have altered adenosine triphosphate binding.[24]

Clinical Features and Types

In pili torti, hair is often normal at birth, but is gradually replaced by abnormal twisted hairs that may be detected as early as the third month. Affected hairs are brittle, fracture easily, and do not grow to any considerable length.[18] Patients present with a sparse and short coarse stubble over the entire scalp and may have a few circumscribed bald patches.

Classic pili torti: It is more common in females, primarily those with thin blond hair.[22] It may also be part of ectodermal dysplasia syndrome, associated with keratosis pilaris, widely spaced teeth, nail dystrophy, corneal opacities, cleft lip/palate and occasionally ichthyosis.[22]

Late-onset variant pili torti: It tends to manifest after puberty with patchy alopecia.[18] In some pedigrees of this type, an association with mental retardation has been reported.[25]

Pili Torti and Deafness

1. **Björnstad syndrome (Box 4.7)** is an autosomal recessive condition characterized by sensorineural hearing loss and pili torti.[24] The hearing loss in the Björnstad syndrome is congenital and of variable severity. Pili torti is recognized early in childhood.[24]
2. **Crandall syndrome** is similar with findings of hypogonadism.[26]

Box 4.7: Bjornstad syndrome

- Autosomal recessive
- Mutation in BCS1L, which encodes an ATPase required for the assembly of a mitochondrial complex (chromosome 2q34-36)
- Congenital sensorineural deafness and PT

Mental retardation is rarely associated with either.[27] The severity of hair shaft abnormality has been shown to correlate with the severity of hearing loss.[27]

Investigations (Figure 4.4)

On light microscopy, groups of three or four (up to 20) regularly spaced twists, each 0.4-0.9 mm in width, may be seen at irregular intervals along the shaft in some hairs within a sample.[28] Light microscopy remains a more flexible tool in terms of adapting the method to allow use of cross-polarized light sources and histological mountant to enhance light penetration and detection of detail within the hair shaft. It also has a greater resolution for smaller or more subtle abnormalities, including fractures (to examine milder forms of monilethrix or pili torti).[29]

Trichoscopy in pili torti shows typical, regular twists of the hair shaft along the long axis, which is best visible at 70-fold and higher magnifications. The 20-fold magnification demonstrates hair shafts with sharp bending at irregular intervals.[15]

Treatment

The twisting hair dystrophies are a diverse group and prognosis is variable. Its frequent association with sensorineural hearing loss (as in Björnstad syndrome and Crandall syndrome) emphasizes the importance of early auditory testing in children with this hair defect. Minimizing trauma is the key aim. There are several cases reports of PT which have improved after an episode of alopecia areata.[20] Patients with true pili torti can be reassured that most will improve at puberty.[18]

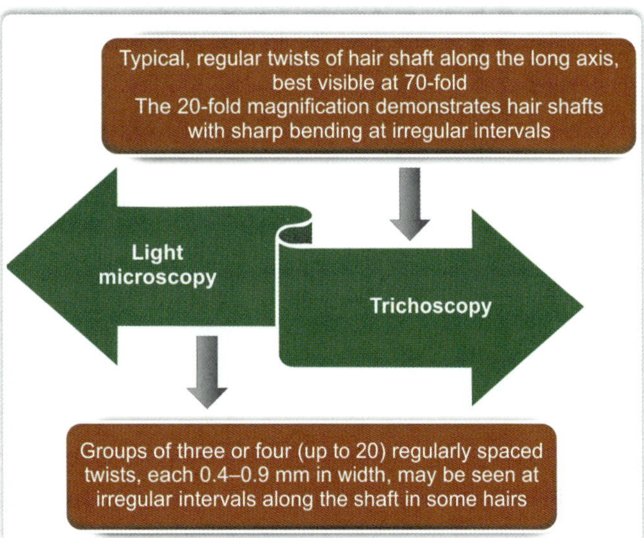

Fig. 4.4: Schematic represention of findings in pili torti

Differential Diagnosis (Figures 4.5A and B shows Algorithm to Diagnose Disease Associated with Pili Torti)

1. Monilethrix: It is often confused with PT, since irregular torsions along the hair shaft resemble the moniliform appearance.[22] Examination of hair with light microscopy or trichoscopy differentiates these two conditions.
2. Spun glass hair or uncombable hair **(Box 4.8)**: Children with this disorder have pili trianguli et canaliculi, which may be confused with the PT.[21] Characteristic findings are triangular or kidney-shaped hairs seen in cross-sections and longitudinal grooves which are responsible for the frizzy, stand-away appearance of uncombable hair.[22] Hair shafts are not twisted as in PT. The hair cannot be combed flat.

Box 4.8: Spun glass hair

- Uncombable hair
- Characterized by pili trianguli et canaliculi-triangular or kidney-shaped hairs seen in cross-sections and longitudinal grooves which are responsible for the frizzy, stand-away appearance

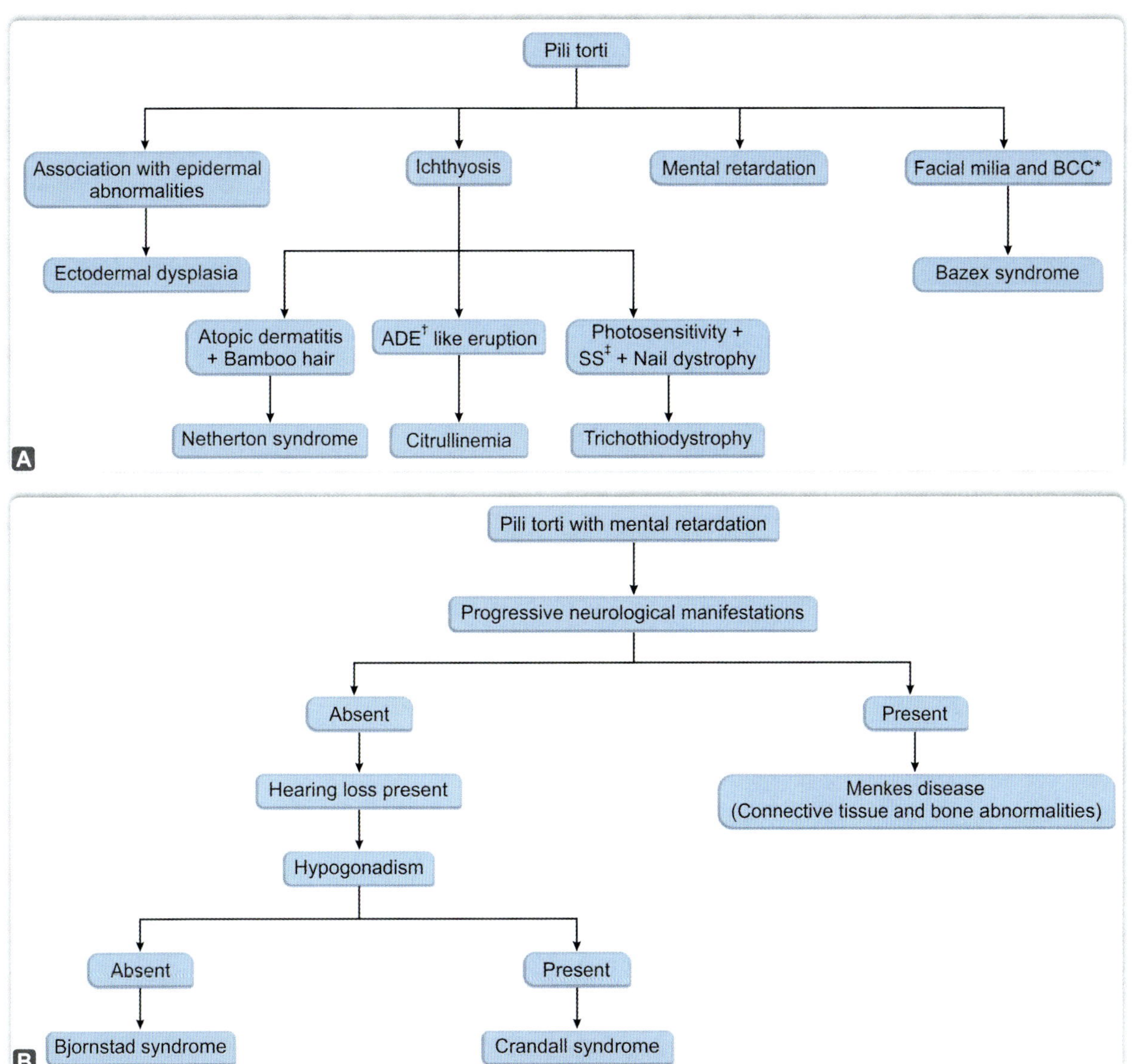

Figs 4.5A and B: Shows the algorithm to diagnose diseases associated with pili torti
*BCC- Basal cell carcinoma, †ADE- Acrodermatitis enteropathica, ‡SS- Short stature

Menkes Disease (Synonyms: Kinky Hair Disease, Trichopoliodystrophy, Steely Hair Disease)

Menkes disease (MD) is a lethal multisystemic disorder of copper metabolism.[30] This is an X-linked recessive condition characterized by skin and hair hypopigmentation, progressive neurologic degeneration with mental retardation, bone and connective tissue alterations with soft doughy skin and joint laxity, and vascular abnormalities, including aneurysms and bladder diverticula.[21]

Pathogenesis

Pili torti with copper deficiency was first described by Menkes, who listed cuproenzymes which may account for features of the disoder **(Table 4.2)**.[22] It is caused by mutations in the ATP7A gene encoding a copper-translocating P-type ATPase, which contains six N-terminal copper-binding sites (CBS1–CBS6).[31] The vast majority of ATP7A mutations are intragenic mutations or partial gene deletions.[30]

ATP7A is an energy-dependent, transmembrane protein, which is expressed in almost all organs except liver where ATP7B is predominantly expressed.[30] ATP7A is involved in the delivery of copper to the secreted copper enzymes, in presence of normal intracellular copper levels and in the export of surplus copper from cells, in the presence of increased copper levels **(Table 4.2 and Figure 4.6)**.[32] Mutations in the MNK gene lead to accumulation of intracellular copper and prevent copper transport to copper dependent enzymes such as lysyl oxidase. With excess intracellular copper, RNA synthesis of metallothionine is triggered, which chelates the accumulated copper to prevent cellular toxicity, but further reducing the transfer of copper to enzymes.[21]

There is no obvious correlation between the mutations and the clinical course of MD. In general patients with a milder phenotype [like occipital horn syndrome (OHS)]

Table 4.2: Cuproenzymes and consequences in their deficiencies

Enzyme	*Function*	*Manifestations in deficiency*
1. Lysyl oxidase	Cross-linking of collagen/elastin	Connective tissue abnormalities, laxity of skin/joints, vascular abnormalities, bony abnormalities, and bladder diverticula
2. Tyrosinase	Melanin formation	Depigmentation of hair and skin pallor
3. Cytochrome C oxidase	Electron transport chain	Hypothermia, CNS degeneration, muscle weakness, ataxia and energy deficiency
4. Peptidylglycine α-amidating monooxygenase (PAM)	Neuropeptide processing	Unknown, possible neurodegeneration
5. Superoxide dismutase	Free radial scavenger	Low tolerance of oxidative stress, demyelination
6. Cross-linkase	Cross-linkage of keratin	Coarse, brittle hair
7. Dopamine B hydroxylase	Catecholamine production	Hypothalamic imbalance, hypothermia, hypotension

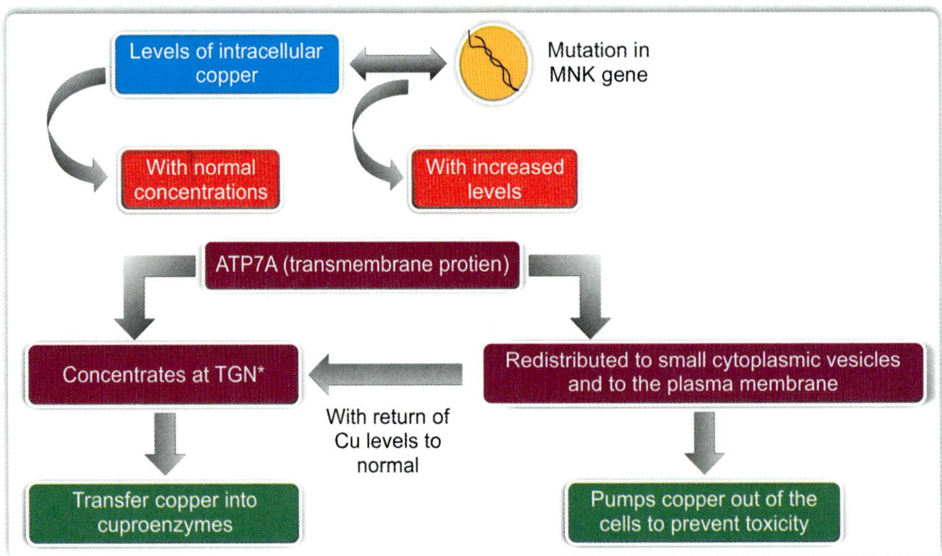

Fig 4.6: Activity of ATP7A in varying intracellular copper levels
*TGN: Trans-Golgi network

have a higher proportion of mutations, which lead to a partially functional protein or result in reduced amounts of an otherwise normal protein.[33]

Clinical Features

MD shows considerable variability in its severity. Classical MD is the most severe form, while OHS is the mildest recognized form.[34]

Classical MS

Affected infants may develop normally until the onset of symptoms, usually between age of 5 weeks and 5 months.[22]

Pregnancy is usually uncomplicated or there may be premature labor and delivery.[30] Cephalohematomas and spontaneous fractures are occasionally observed at birth. In the early neonatal period, patients may present with prolonged jaundice, hypothermia, hypoglycemia and feeding difficulties.[30] Umbilical and inguinal hernias have also been reported.[35]

Affected males have pili torti, growth retardation and progressive psychomotor retardation. Female carriers may have more limited features due to random X inactivation. Affected females demonstrate patchy areas of short, broken, and twisted hairs, along Blaschko's lines on their scalp.[18] As copper is a cofactor for tyrosinase, affected hairs have characteristically hypopigmented "kinky hair" appearance.[35]

The first sign of MD may be unusual sparse and lusterless scalp hair that becomes tangled on the top of the head at the age of 1–2 months. At this time the appearance may be described as being odd, with pale skin, frontal or occipital bossing, micrognathia, pudgy cheeks, and a rather expressionless appearance. However, these changes are often too subtle to attract attention. Initial psychomotor development is usually unremarkable, with normal babbling and smiling up to about 2–4 months of age. The baby then ceases to develop further and gradually loses some of the previously developed skills. The developmental regression becomes obvious around 5-6 months of age.[30]

Subsequently, hypotonia, seizures, failure to thrive, poor eating, vomiting, and diarrhea develop.[36] As the motor dysfunction progresses, spontaneous movements become limited and drowsiness and lethargy emerge. The patients are typically diagnosed at 3-6 months of age, often due to the abnormal hair that is a striking feature of the disease. The hypopigmented or depigmented hair resembles and feels like steel wool; it is lusterless and friable, especially in the areas of the scalp subjected to friction.[30]

Epilepsy is a major feature of Menkes disease; seizure types include focal or multifocal tonic-clonic, myoclonic, infantile spasms, and status epilepticus.[36]

Vascular, urogenital and skeletal abnormalities are numerous.

Urological complications include

1. Congenital—bladder diverticula, hydronephrosis, vesicoureteral reflux, rupture of the bladder diverticulum, hydroureter, obstruction of bladder outflow and rupture of the kidney
2. Acquired—urinary tract infection and bladder calculi.[37]

Skeletal abnormalities include pectus excavatum or pectus carrinatum, and spontaneous fractures due to generalized osteoporosis. The joints are hyperextensive, and loose and dry skin may be observed very early. Thick, scaly seborrheic dermatitis is also a frequent feature.[30] Routine ophthalmoscopy is usually normal, but in later stages patients frequently fail to follow visual stimulus.

Late manifestations of the disease are blindness (secondary to optic atrophy), subdural hematoma, and respiratory failure. Most patients die within the third year of life due to infection, vascular complications (such as sudden and massive cerebral hemorrhage due to vascular rupture), or from the neurological degeneration itself.[30]

Occipital Horn Syndrome (OHS)

The mildest form is primarily characterized by pronounced connective tissue symptoms such as soft doughy lax skin and diverticula, and little neurologic aberration.[31]

It is called OHS because of bony projections (exostoses) which occur on the occipital bone of the skull. These are symmetric exostoses (occipital horns - **Box 4.9**) protruding from the occipital bone and pointing down.[21] These are formed as a result of the calcification in the trapezius and sternocleidomastoid muscles at their attachments to the occipital bone.[38]

The skin may appear wrinkled and loose at birth. The extent of skin laxity is variable and may increase with age, resulting in droopy wrinkles around the trunk. Within days similar to classic MS, neonatal problems such hypothermia, jaundice, hypotonia, and feeding difficulties may develop.[30] Facial appearance gradually becomes distinctive. Unusual features include long, thin face, often with a high forehead, down-slanting eyes, hooked or prominent nose, long philtrum, high arched palate, and prominent large ears (**Box 4.10**).[30]

Box 4.9: Occipital horns

- Symmetric exostoses protruding from the occipital bone and pointing down
- Result of the calcification in the trapezius and sternocleidomastoid muscles at their attachments to the occipital bone

Box 4.10: Dysmorphic facies of OHS

Long, thin face, often with a high forehead, down-slanting eyes, hooked or prominent nose, long philtrum, high arched palate, and prominent large ears

Motor development is delayed due to muscular hypotonia and is associated with unusual clumsiness. Height is usually normal, while mild disproportion with long trunk, narrow chest and shoulders, thoracolumbar kyphosis or scoliosis, and pectus deformity are common. The joints are hypermobile.[30] Childhood-onset seizures, dysarthric speech, elbow deformities and dislocations, bladder diverticula, recurrence of the inguinal hernia and tortuous vessels are the features of OHS.[38]

Hair is usually not conspicuously abnormal, although some patients may have lusterless and unusually coarse hair. Vascular anomalies, such as varicose veins are common, and arterial aneurysms have also been described. A particular problem is orthostatic hypotension. The intellectual capacity is described as low to borderline normal. Pubertal development is normal.[30]

Central nervous system similarities shared by classic Menkes' syndrome and occipital horn syndrome include generalized cerebral and cerebellar atrophy, cerebellar and cortical neuronal loss, depletion of the central nervous system white matter, and cerebellar heterotopias (reduplication of the cerebral vasculature).[38]

Clinical problems become gradually obvious, and the first signs that bring the child to medical attention may be intractable diarrhea or recurrent urinary tract infections. In spite of these problems, diagnosis of OHS is usually made only around 5-10 years of age.[30]

Investigations

Initial diagnosis of MD is suggested by clinical features (especially typical hair changes) and supported by demonstration of reduced levels of serum copper and ceruloplasmin.[30]

Box 4.11: Rapid diagnostic test of MD in neonatal period

Plasma catecholamine analysis (ratio of DOPA to dihydroxyphenylglycol) indicative of dopamine β-hydroxylase deficiency

The recognition of MD in early neonatal period is difficult and these markers should be interpreted with caution, as their levels may be within the range of normal infants in the first week; they are higher than normal in the cord blood of affected infants and fall gradually after 4 weeks of age.[22] In this period, plasma catecholamine analysis (ratio of DOPA to dihydroxyphenylglycol) indicative of dopamine β-hydroxylase deficiency may be the choice as a rapid diagnostic test **(Box 4.11)**.[39]

Hair Examination (Figure 4.7)

Light microscopy of either eyebrow/scalp hair shows classic short, pale "kinky hairs" with twists, which are completely rotated through 180° around their long axis at irregular intervals in the shaft.[12] Other hair changes include varying hair shaft diameter (monilethrix) and fragmentation at regular intervals (trichorrhexis nodosa).[30] It is important to examine as many strands of hair as possible because not every hair may demonstrate morphological abnormalities in the lengths examined. This may not always be easy, because many infants often have sparse, fine, wispy, blond hair. So, examination of eyebrow hair may improve the likelihood of diagnosis.[12]

Examination of scalp hair using dermoscopy shows twisted hair with greater clarity than with the light microscopic examination.[29]

Different clinical features of MD are detected by using other laboratory investigations like cystourethrography,

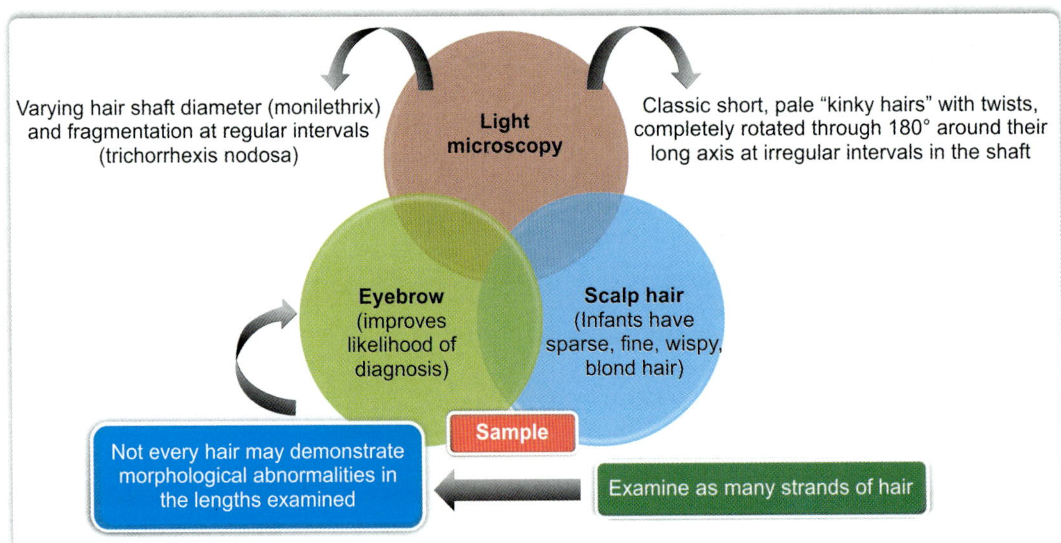

Fig. 4.7: Schematic representation of light microscopic features of menkes disease

arteriography, radiography, computed tomography, and magnetic resonance imaging.

Radiographic features of patient with classical MD includes generalized osteoporosis, metaphyseal flaring and spurs in the long bones, diaphyseal periosteal reaction and thickening, and Wormian bones in the cranial sutures.[30] Other skeletal abnormalities include loss of curvature of the cervical spine, pectus excavatum, short ribs, short and widened clavicles, deformed radii with radial head dislocations and bilateral ulnar deformities.[38] In OHS, multiple horns protruding down from occipital bones and short and broad clavicles are seen.[38]

The CT and MR imaging reports on Menkes disease have shown severe neuronal loss that is manifested by diffuse cerebellar and cortical atrophy, white matter lesions and subdural hematoma or effusions.[35] Magnetic resonance angiography shows tortuosity of cerebral vessels.

EEG findings in MD include absence of age-appropriate features, background slowing and disorganization, polymorphic slow waves, focal or diffuse spike and waves, status epilepticus, and hypsarrhythmia.[36]

The specific diagnostic test for MD is the demonstration of the molecular defect in ATP7A. Detection of the genetic defect in a given family may take time, because of the large size of the gene and the variety of the mutations observed in different families.[30]

Carrier Identification and Prenatal Diagnosis (Table 4.3)

In at-risk families only male fetuses need to be evaluated, and rapid sex determination can be made using Y-chromosome-specific DNA sequences. Carrier determination by measuring radioactive copper accumulation in cultured fibroblasts is not reliable due to random X-inactivation, and mutation analysis should be performed. In informative families, the intragenic polymorphic markers may also be used for carrier detection.[30]

Table 4.3: Carrier detection and prenatal diagnosis

	Diagnostic tests
Carrier detection	Measuring radioactive copper accumulation in cultured fibroblasts, intragenic polymorphic markers
At-risk families	Only male fetuses need to be evaluated, and rapid sex determination made using Y-chromosome-specific DNA sequences
First trimester	The total copper content in chorionic villi can be measured directly by neutron activation analysis and atomic absorption
Second trimester	Copper accumulation is measured in cultured amniotic fluid cells

In at-risk pregnancies where the mutation of the family is unknown, biochemical analysis remains a possibility as identification of the genetic defect may be challenging in limited time. In the first trimester the total copper content in chorionic villi can be measured directly by sensitive and accurate methods like neutron activation analysis and atomic absorption, and in the second trimester copper accumulation is measured in cultured amniotic fluid cells. Although there are potential pitfalls for these analyses, they have been performed routinely at the Kennedy Center in Denmark since 1975.[40]

Differential Diagnosis

The diagnosis of Menkes disease may present problems in early neonatal period. Pili torti may develop later, as the primary fetal hair is usually normal.[22]

The roentenographic signs may not be evident until after 6 weeks of age. Menkes disease should be included in the differential diagnosis of unexplained rib and metaphyseal fractures, sub-dural hematomas, and neurological impairment in infants where the diagnosis of non-accidental injury such as in shaken baby syndrome is considered.[22]

Treatment

MD is a progressive disorder with poor prognosis and most of the patients die within 3 years of life in its severe form.[22] Treatment in major cases is mainly symptomatic. However, careful medical care, and possibly copper administration, may extend life span up to 13 years or even more.[30]

The specific treatment for MD is infusion of copper-histidine **(Box 4.12)**.[21] Objective of this treatment is to provide extra copper to the tissues and copper-dependent enzymes.[30] The full function of copper histidine and how it works is not well characterized. It must be administered early in life, because it may prevent but not reverse permanent neurologic damage.[41,42] Copper-histidine therapy has limited effects on connective tissue abnormalities and many patients subsequently die of these complications.[21]

Box 4.12: Copper histidine

- Specific treatment of MD
- To be administered early in life
- May prevent but not reverse permanent neurologic damage

Netherton Syndrome (Box 4.12) (Synonyms: Netherton's Disease, Bamboo Hair)

Netherton syndrome (NS) is an autosomal recessive inherited disorder characterized by congenital ichthyosis

Box 4.13: Triad of Netherton syndrome

- Trichorrhexis nodosa
- Ichthyosis linearis circumflexa
- Atopic diathesis

(ichthyosis linearis circumflexa ILC), trichorrhexis invaginata, and features of atopic dermatitis (AD) with high serum IgE levels[43] **(Box 4.13)**. Ichthyosis linearis circumflexa (ILC) was first described by Dr Comel in 1949. It consists of migratory polycyclic erythematous patches surrounded by a serpiginous overlying double-edged scale.[44] In 1958, Netherton[45] described a young girl with generalized scaly dermatitis and fragile nodular hair shaft deformities that he termed trichorrhexis nodosa (bamboo hair). Later, this was more appropriately renamed as trichorrhexis invaginata. In 1974, the clinical relationship between ichthyosis linearis circumflexa and Netherton's syndrome was established by Mevorah, et al.[46]

Pathogenesis

The syndrome is caused by the mutation in SPINK 5 gene, which is located on long arm of Chromosome 5. This gene codes for production of a protein LEKT1 (lympho-epithelial Kazal-type related inhibitor), which inhibits the enzyme serine proteinase in the outermost layer of the skin **(Figure 4.8)**.[47] LEKTI is expressed in the stratum granulosum of the epidermis, and it was shown that bioactive LEKTI fragments inhibit 3 major proteases involved in stratum corneum desquamation, kallikreins (KLK) 5, 7, and 14.[48] Lack of LEKTI led to kallikrein 5 (KLK5) and KLK7 proteolytic hyperactivity, resulting in desmoglein-1 degradation and, in turn, to abnormal corneodesmosome cleavage below the stratum corneum.[49] ELA2 is a new epidermal protease which is hyperactive in LEKTI-deficient epidermis.[50] ELA2 directly degrades (pro) filaggrin, promoting skin barrier impairment.

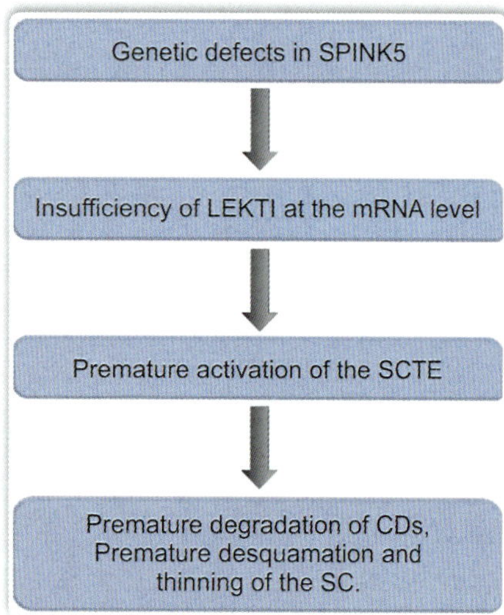

Fig. 4.8: Sequence involved in the pathogenesis of the skin lesions in NS
Abbreviation: SCTE—Stratum corneum tryptic enzyme, CDs—corneodesmosomes, SC—stratum corneum

Clinical Features (Figure 4.9)

At birth, infants exhibit generalized erythroderma and scaling, which is similar to other types of infantile erythroderma.[51] Continuous peeling of the skin can persist in NS similarly to peeling skin syndrome.[52,53] The congenital ichthyosiform erythroderma-like features can persist throughout life in the most severe cases or evolve into a unique milder condition known as ichthyosis linearis circumflexa, consisting of migratory, serpiginous, and erythematous plaques, which are bordered by a peculiar double-edged scale.[54]

Like ichthyosis linearis circumflexa, trichorrhexis invaginata (bamboo hair) is pathognomonic for NS.[47] Trichorrhexis invaginata causes patchy hair thinning, but rarely complete alopecia.[44] Trichorrhexis invaginata is a focal defect of the hair shaft that produces development of torsion nodules and invaginated nodules **(Box 4.14)**. The proximal element of the node overlaps the distal portion, causing an intussusception.[44] Other hair shaft abnormalities manifested as pili torti (twisted hair), helical hair and trichorrhexis nodosa. This may not be detected

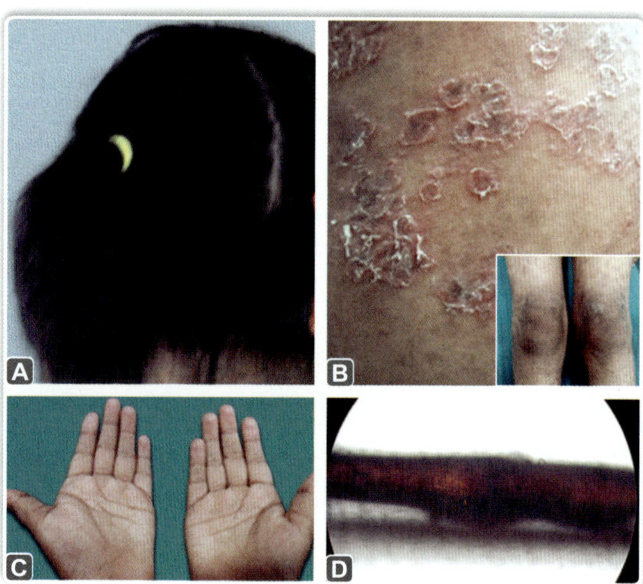

Figs 4.9A to D: (A) Sparse brittle hair; (B) Ichthyosis linearis circumflexa- double edge scales (Inset showing scaly lesions over knees; (C) Hyperlinearity of palm noted as a component of atopic diathesis, child also had atopy; (D) Microscopic appearance of bamboo hair. (*Courtesy:* Department of Dematology, STD and Leprosy, BMCRI, Bengaluru)

Box 4.14: Trichorrhexis invaginata ('bamboo hair')

- Pathognomonic for NS
- A focal defect of hair shaft that produces development of torsion nodules and invaginated nodules
- The proximal element of the node overlaps the distal portion, causing an intussusception
- Causes patchy hair thinning, but rarely complete alopecia

at birth and may disappear with age.[55] These hair defects can be found in scalp, eyebrow or eyelash hairs. Ito, et al.[56] have reported the hair shaft abnormality to be secondary to intermittent incomplete formation of disulfide bonds in the keratogenous zone.

Affected individuals have a broad range of atopic manifestations, including eczema-like rashes, hay fever, angioedema, allergic rhinitis, asthma, food allergy, heat intolerance, eosinophilia and high levels of IgE in the serum.[47]

Other associated manifestations include aminoaciduria, recurrent infections, mental and neurological retardation, seizures or spastic diplegia, hyper/hypogammaglobulinemia and impaired cellular immunity.[47] Gastrointestinal involvement in the form of dermopathic enteropathy with villous atrophy and diarrhea may lead to poor weight gaining in early childhood.[55] NS patients with ichthyosis linearis circumflexa have a normal general development, whereas those presenting with generalized exfoliative erythroderma display life-threatening complications such as hypernatremic dehydration, electrolyte imbalances, hypothermia, failure to thrive, and recurrent infections resulting in high postnatal mortality. These complications might be attributed to the severe alteration of the epidermal barrier function.[54]

Investigations

Hair microscopy is crucial for diagnosis of NS and shows **(Box 4.15)**:

1. 'Ball and socket' or 'pencil in cup' configuration with various patterns.
2. Bamboo hair: A shallow invagination of the distal shaft into the proximal part of the shaft.
3. Tulip-like form: A deeper invagination and long sides of the 'cup'.
4. Circumferential strictures: These represent the earliest stage of the invagination.[57]

Box 4.15: Hair findings in NS

- 'Ball and socket' or 'pencil in cup' configuration
- Bamboo hair
- Tulip-like form
- Circumferential strictures

Trichorrhexis nodosa and pili torti also occur. Often only 20–50% of hair is affected; therefore hairs should be cut (not plucked) from multiple areas of the head to be examined. Hairs can also be examined from axillary, pubic, and eyebrow regions for abnormalities.[44]

Histopathologic examination of NS skin reveals a 'psoriasiform' epidermis, hyperplasia of the subcorneal epithelium (acanthosis) with varying degrees of epidermal invaginations into the dermis (papillomatosis).[54]

Electron microscopic examination of skin lesions of NS reveals abnormalities including premature secretion of lamellar bodies, and a less cohesive stratum corneum with loosely packed parakeratotic corneocytes which are often separated by elongated clefts with fewer or greatly reduced numbers of desmosomes and the presence of electron-dense material in the interstices of the stratum corneum.[58]

Peripheral eosinophilia is commonly found.[44] The serum IgE level is often elevated, sometimes to extreme levels. Positive skin tests or RAST responses to environmental and/or food allergens are commonly observed.[59]

Differential Diagnosis

The diagnostic features of NS are helpful in making a differential diagnosis of other causes of neonatal and infantile erythroderma.

Petechiae and purpura due to thrombocytopenia are typical signs in Wiskott-Aldrich syndrome; diarrhea and vesiculobulbous lesions distributed in a periorificial and acral pattern on the face, scalp, hands, feet and the anogenital areas are typical signs in acrodermatitis enteropathica; diarrhea and periorificial eczematous eruption are typical signs in biotinidase deficiency.[60]

Treatment

Many treatments have been attempted in patients with Netherton syndrome. Patients with Netherton syndrome are likely more susceptible to systemic absorption of medication, and are therefore at increased risk to experience adverse reactions to topical therapies.[55]

A crucial point in topical therapy is an intensive skin care by application of hydrophobic creams without additives or with a low dose of urea, for treating only specific parts of the body surface daily.[22]

The cutaneous manifestations of NS are frequently resistant to conventional therapy (emollients and topical corticosteroids).[61] Topical calcineurin inhibitors - tacrolimus and pimecrolimus have been demonstrated to improve the skin findings and quality of life in patients with several chronic dermatoses, including atopic dermatitis. The use of topical tacrolimus has been associated with significant systemic absorption in children with NS. Use of tacrolimus ointment should be reserved for the short-term management of flares and should be considered only when the benefits outweigh the risks.[22] The absorption of pimecrolimus through the skin in patients with NS is, by contrast, considerably diminished.[61]

Various treatments have been attempted, including low-dose oral corticosteroids, etretinate, and psoralen ultraviolet A therapy.[44] The use of oral retinoids has yielded mixed results.[21]

Trichothiodystrophy (Acronyms: PIBIDS, IBIDS and BIDS)

(From Greek: tricho- meaning hair; thio- sulfur; dys-faulty; trophy- nourishment).

Trichothiodystrophy (TTD) is a heterogeneous group of autosomal recessive disorders characterized by brittle sulfur-deficient hairs.[18] In 1979, Price coined the term "trichothiodystrophy," which encompasses a wide spectrum of neuro-cutaneous findings, to describe the unifying feature.[62]

TTD can be associated with a spectrum of symptoms affecting organs of ectodermal and neuroectodermal origin. These include nail dystrophy, mental and growth retardation, ichthyosis, decreased fertility, and cutaneous photosensitivity, but not cancer.[63] Many terms have been proposed to subcategorize patients by groups of clinical features, which are variable (up to 100). Eight subgroups have been categorized by Itin, et al.[64] and include **(Figure 4.10)**:

1. BIDS - Brittle hair, intellectual impairment, decreased fertility, and short stature
2. IBIDS - BIDS + Ichthyosis
3. PIBIDS - IBIDS +Photosensitivity
4. SIBIDS - Otosclerosis + IBIDS
5. ONMR - Onychotrichodysplasia, chronic neutropenia, and mentral retardation
6. Tay - Brittle hair, intellectual impairment, short stature, Non-bullous congenital ichthyosiform erythroderma
7. Sabinas – Brittle hair, ichthyosis, decreased fertility, ocular abnormalities
8. Pollitt syndromes - Brittle hair, intellectual impairment short stature.

Pathogenesis

TTD is a member of a group of nucleotide excision repair disorders which includes xeroderma pigmentosum (XP).[65] Cells from many TTD patients have defects in nucleotide excision repair (NER) as well as in transcription, which eliminates ultraviolet light induced cyclobutane pyrimidine dimers, pyrimidine pyrimodone photoproducts (6-4PP), and intrastrand crosslinks in the DNA.[66] NER comprises a complex-overlapping network of enzymatic pathways for DNA repair with approximately 30 gene products involved.[21]

TTD patients have abnormal production of transcription factor II H (TFIIH), a general transcription factor active in basal transcription and nucleotide excision repair, due to mutations in genes encoding 3 subunits of TFIIH— ERCC2 (XPD), ERCC3 (XPB), and GTF2H5 (TTDA) - most with mutations of XPD. Photosensitive TTD patients with (~50%) have defective nucleotide excision repair mechanisms

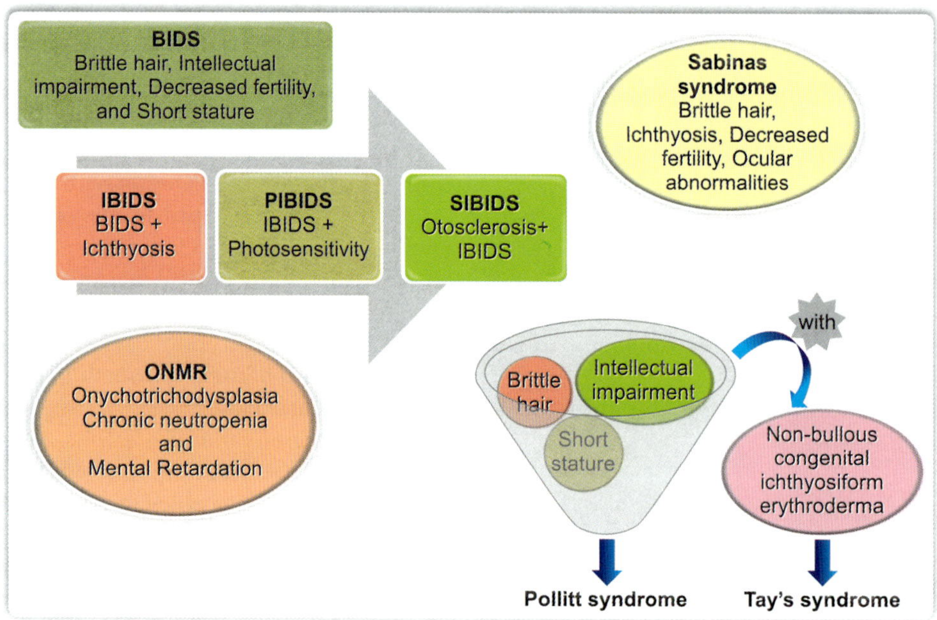

Fig. 4.10: Schematic representation of syndromes associated with trichothiodystrophy

due to reduced amounts of TFIIH, without the increased incidence of skin cancer seen in xeroderma pigmentosum, another autosomal recessive disorder of DNA repair demonstrating mutations in XPB and XPD.[67] The severity of symptoms ranges widely and correlates with the amount of damaged TFIIH and abnormal transcription product.[67]

Nakabayashi K, et al.[68] have identified gene C7orf11 as mutated in patients with non-photosensitive TTD. The protein of this gene demonstrates a nuclear localization, and C7orf11 may have a role in transcriptional processes but have no role in DNA repair.[68]

Clinical Features

The clinical features in different patients are remarkably varied ranging from only hair involvement to severe neurological and somatic developmental abnormalities.

Pregnancy is usually uncomplicated. Many TTD patients were born prematurely or were small for gestational dates.[69]

TTD is associated with several disorders such as mental and physical retardation, low-set and posteriorly rotated ears, nail abnormalities, follicular keratosis, erythroderma, hypohidrosis, ocular dysplasia, dental caries and hypoplasia and cryptorchidism.[70]

Cutaneous Manifestations

Common skin finding is lamellar ichthyosis; many of the patients are born with the collodion membrane. Ichthyosis may be seen in almost all age groups.[62] Crovato and Rebora underlined that if ichthyosis developed in late infancy, patients are affected by IBIDS, and if congenital ichthyosis is present, Tay syndrome must be considered.[71] Follicular keratosis as a sign of ichthyosis, pruritus, eczema, freckles, telangiectasias, and actinic cheilitis have also been found.[70]

Photosensitivity is the second most common skin finding reported with TTD.[62] Photosensitivity may be extreme in patients affected by PIBIDS; in particular photosensitivity to ultraviolet (UV) B and for UVA is impressive.[70] Interestingly, photosensitivity seems to diminish with age, and it does not affect patients with congenital ichthyosis, but only those with ichthyosis that develops later in infancy.[71]

TTD patients, while sun sensitive, do not develop the pigmentary abnormalities of XP and do not have an increased frequency of skin cancer.[69]

Hair Abnormalities

The most frequent hair findings are brittle hair or hair shaft abnormalities. Patients with TTD share the distinctive feature of short, brittle hair. Persistent alopecia is often found; eyebrows, eyelashes and body hair may also be affected.[22] Trichoschisis is characteristically seen on light microscopy. Under polarized light, the characteristic "tiger tail" pattern of alternating bright and dark diagonal bands is seen in most TTD patients and is rarely found in normal individuals (**Box 4.16**).[21] The underlying cause of the tiger tail pattern is unknown, but it is hypothesized to be secondary to the irregular sulfur content of the hair shaft.[72] This pattern can be seen in utero, but its absence does not exclude the diagnosis. The sulfur and cystine content of the hair is reduced to approximately 50% in both the cuticle and the cortex, with a marked absence of high sulfur content proteins and an increase in low sulfur content proteins in the hair shaft.[21]

Box 4.16: Tiger tail appearance in TTD

- It is a polarized light microscopy feature of hair shaft
- Refers to alternating bright and dark diagonal bands
- Hypothesized to be secondary to the irregular sulfur content of the hair shaft
- Absence does not exclude the diagnosis

Central Nervous System Manifestations

These include microcephaly, spasticity, ataxia, and altered reflexes.[67] Generalized dysmyelination is the most common neuroimaging abnormality in TTD.[67] While TTD patients may have intellectual impairment, they usually are very social and have an outgoing, engaging, friendly personality. Typically, standard intelligence tests appear to underestimate their capability for social interactions. The MRI shows predominantly hypomyelination of the white matter of the cerebrum. Atrophy of the brain is not a major feature. Some patients may have calcification of the basal ganglia.[69] Impaired transcription of structural components of myelin and of high-sulfur content molecules important in central nervous system (CNS) development, such as neurocan and phosphacan, has been implicated in the dysmyelination present in TTD.[67]

Genitourinary System

Hypogonadism, cryptorchidism, delayed pubertal development, poor sexual maturation and partial panhypopituitarism have been reported in few patients of TTD.[62]

Cardiovascular System

Cardiac defects in the form of cardiomyopathy, pulmonic stenosis and ventricular septal defect have been reported in some patients of TTD.[73] Toelle, et al.[73] suggests to monitor TTD patients for developing severe cardiomyopathy using echocardiography.

Nail Abnormalities (Box 4.17)[62]

Box 4.17: Nail changes in TTD

Onychodystrophy, brittle nails, hypoplasia, koilonychia, splitting (onychoschizia), peeling, ridging

Skeletal System

They may have skeletal abnormalities including delayed bone age, peripheral osteopenia and central osteosclerosis.[69] Joint abnormalities including contractures and joint dislocation/subluxation, clinodactyly of 5th finger, short limbs, tapering fingers, syndactyly and joint hypermobility have been noted.[62]

Others

Ophthalmic findings include cicatricial ectropion with bilateral corneal opacities, superficial punctate keratitis and a high frequency of congenital cataracts.[74]

Immunodeficiency with history of multiple infections has also been noted.[69]

Investigations (Figure 4.11)

Light microscopy of scalp hair reveals numerous clean-cut transverse fractures (trichoschisis), trichorrhexis nodosa-like fractures, ribboning and alterations of the cuticle.[75] Higher magnification reveals ridging of the cuticle layer and a cribiform-like shaft surface.[66] Some cases may show spherical hair shaft and abrupt narrowing.[66]

Cross-polarizing microscopy shows the alternating dark and light bands that give the shaft "tiger tail pattern".[75]

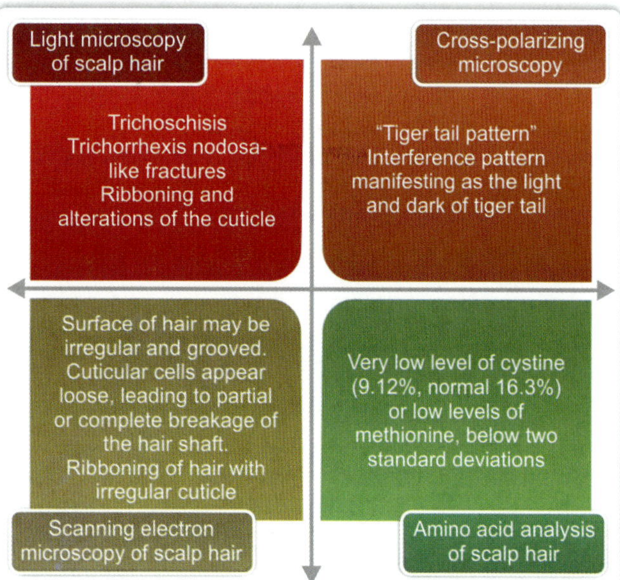

Fig. 4.11: Schematic representation of investigative findings in trichothiodystrophy

This pattern arises through sinusoidal distortion of the weakened cortical keratin fibrils. As they flow through the sine wave morphology they act as polarizing filters in their own right giving rise to the interference pattern manifesting as the light and dark of the tiger tail.[76]

Scanning electron microscopy allows detailed examination of hair shaft abnormalities. The surface of the hair may be irregular and grooved. The cuticular cells appear to be coming loose, leading to partial or complete breakage of the hair shaft. Ribboning of the hair with an intact yet irregular cuticle may also be noted.[66]

Amino acid analysis of scalp hair reveals a very low level of cystine (9.12%; normal value 16.3%)[75] or low levels of methionine, below two standard deviations.[76]

MRI Findings

Magnetic resonance imaging (MRI) discloses diffuse signal hyperintensity throughout the cerebral white matter on T2-weighted images. In normal brain, the signal intensity of white matter on T2-weighted images is dark compared with the cerebral cortex due to myelin sheaths. This finding is compatible with a diffuse hypomyelination of cerebral white matter. The lateral ventricles are moderately dilated, indicating a loss of periventricular tissue, probably as a consequence of hypomyelination.[75]

Other nonspecific structural abnormalities observed in TTD include cortical heterotopias, partial agenesis of the corpus callosum, perimedullary fibrosis of the spinal cord, and intracranial calcifications.[67]

Differential Diagnosis

1. It is important to distinguish tiger tail banding from non-specific banding that occurs without abnormalities or undulation of the hair shaft. All TTD hairs display tiger tail banding with polarizing microscopy and with rotation of the microscope stage.[66]
2. Conditions such as anorexia nervosa and acrodermatitis enteropathica, where malnutrition or malabsorption leads to secondary hair changes share features with TTD. However, with improvement in bowel function, assessment demonstrates normalization of the hair. These diseases are correctable with diet. In acrodermatitis enteropathica, the distinction between the primary disease (e.g. Argininosuccinic aciduria) and the hair features of TTD is important as specific management is required for the primary diagnosis. Urinary amino acids analyses helps in such cases.[76]
3. Differential diagnosis for diffuse dysmyelination **(Box 4.18)** in the absence of gray matter abnormalities in children include Pelizaeus-Merzbacher disease, 18q-syndrome, and Salla disease.[67] Although inborn

Box 4.18: Diffuse dysmyelination

- TTD
- Pelizaeus-Merzbacher disease
- 18q-syndrome
- Salla disease

errors of metabolism may result in delayed myelination mimicking the diffuse dysmyelination present in TTD, atrophy and distinct clinical syndromes generally allow differentiation.[67]

Treatment

There is no specific treatment for TTD and there is no trend towards spontaneous resolution.[18] Associated abnormalities require attention, particularly minimizing sun-related skin damage.[22] Dietary cytosine supplementation has been suggested, but its value is unproven.

Ectodermal dysplasia

Ectodermal dysplasia (ED) defines a family of congenital, developmental disorders with primary defects in at least two ectoderm-derived structures.[77] The main tissues of ectodermal origin affected in EDs are hair, teeth, nails and eccrine glands. Hair shaft abnormalities are found in various ectodermal dysplasias. In general, hair may be sparse, curly, and fair. Alopecia may be due to hair shaft anomaly with increased fragility, or to hypotrichosis.[22]

Several classifications have already been proposed on the basis of clinical point of view;[78] molecular genetic data and clinical findings,[79] and the recent one by Lamartine[80] on the basis of functions of genes.

Pathogenesis

Ectodermal dysplasias are the result of molecular causative defects involving, for instance, widely expressed proteins with essential roles in control of cell cycle progression, in replication and/or DNA repair.[79] Embryogenesis is regulated by a number of complex signaling cascades that are critical for normal development.[22] One of the best investigated pathways is the sonic hedgehog, leading to interactions with transcription factors within the Gli family. Dysregulation of this pathway lead to different diseases including some from the spectrum of EDs.[79]

Clinical Features

The spectrum of primary hair shaft abnormalities reported in ectodermal dysplasia ranges from flattened hair, twisted hair, longitudinal impressions to a combination of both twisting and impressions of the hair shaft in pili torti et canaliculi and corkscrew hairs.[77]

These abnormalities often present as alopecia, one of the features of subtypes in EDs.[22] Hair is generally fair, curly and scanty, sometimes brittle and uncombable. Body hair is often diminished or absent. Eyebrows and eyelashes may be lacking.[22]

The different shaft abnormalities may be detected in various ectodermal dysplasias, sometimes in the same patient. Whereas longitudinal grooves are a frequent finding; pili torti et canaliculi appears to be a characteristic finding in ectodermal dysplasias combined with clefting of lip/palate **(Box 4.19)**.[77] There thus seems to be a crescendo in structural abnormalities, with increasing shaft defects associated with the degree of clinical dysmorphology, with corkscrew hairs as an exaggeration of pili torti et canaliculi.[81]

Secondary unspecific changes, such as trichorrhexis nodosa and loss of cuticle, are due to the increased fragility often seen in these hair shaft abnormalities.[77] Differences in the calibre of the hair and cuticular irregularities are other findings previously reported.[82]

Box 4.19: Pili torti et canaliculi

- Longitudinal grooves along hair shaft
- Characteristic finding in ectodermal dysplasias combined with clefting of lip/palate
- Increasing shaft defects associated with degree of clinical dysmorphology in ED, with corkscrew hairs as an exaggeration of pili torti et canaliculi

Treatment

The prognosis and treatment depend on underlying defects, which are heterogenous as the group of EDs itself. In general, maintenance of a cool, ambient temperature is vital in management of these patients. Air-conditioned environments reduce the chances of sudden hyperpyrexia.[83] Light clothing, repeated cold water spray and avoidance of hot food or exertion can help the patient to combat the daily heat stresses of life.

Approach to patient with genetic hair disorder

Given the extensive list of genetic hair disorders, it is imperative that the clinician have an organized approach to the diagnosis of these conditions. It should cover the history, physical examination and laboratory evaluation.

History

Prenatal history: Family history, history of problems during pregnancy like – bleeding, medications and gestational age are important. Postnatal history of heat intolerance (ectodermal dysplasia), photosensitivity (PIBIDS), skin eruptions (Netherton syndrome), and delayed developmental milestones (Menkes disease) are essential.

Physical examination: Examination of all body part hairs (eyebrow, eyelash and scalp hair), determination of deafness by ENT examination (Bjornstad's syndrome), examination of eye (trichothiodystrophy), teeth (ectodermal dysplasia), nail (trichothiodystrophy) and skin (Netherton syndrome) will throw light on the probable cause of genetic hair disorder.

Investigations

Simple hair microscopy (to see structural hair defect as in monilethrix, pili torti), scanning EM (to see cuticular abnormality in monilethrix, TTD), polarized microscopy ('tiger tail' appearance in TTD), X-ray (Menkes disease), and mutation analysis (as in Netherton syndrome, Bjornstad's syndrome) will add to the diagnostic assay of the genetic hair diseases.

References

1. van Steensel MAM, Steijlen PM, Bladergroen RS, Vermeer M, van Geel M. A missense mutation in the type II hair keratin hHb3 is associated with monilethrix. J Med Genet. 2005;42:e19.
2. Messenger AG, de Barker DAR, Sinclair RD. Disorders of hair. In: Burns T, Breathnach S, Cox N, Griffith C, (eds). Rook's textbook of dermatology, 8th edition. Wiley-Blackwell Publications. 2010;66:1-100.
3. Zhang Shi-de, Meng J, Zhao Jing-jun, Tian W. Mutation E402K of the hHb6 in a Chinese Han family with monilethrix. Euro Jr Derm. 2009;19:508-9.
4. Schweizer J. More than One Gene Involved in Monilethrix: Intracellular but also Extracellular Players. J Invest Dermatol. 2006;126:1216-20.
5. Schaffer JV, Bazzi H, Vitebsky A, Witkiewicz A, Kovich OI, Kamino H, et al. Mutations in the desmoglein 4 gene underlie localized autosomal recessive hypotrichosis with monilethrix hairs and congenital scalp erosions. J Invest Dermatol. 2006;126:1286-91.
6. Shimomura Y, Sakamoto F, Kariya N, Matsunaga K, Ito M. Mutations in the desmoglein 4 gene are associated with monilethrix-like congenital hypotrichosis. J Invest Dermatol. 2006;126:1281-5.
7. Zlotogorski A, Marek D, Horev L, Abu A, Ben-Amitai D, Gerad L, et al. An autosomal recessive form of monilethrix is caused by mutations in DSG4: clinical overlap with localized autosomal recessive hypotrichosis. J Invest Dermatol. 2006;126:1292-6.
8. Singh A, Ambujam S, Srikanth S, Uma AN. Monilethrix: One Step More on the Ladder of Cytogenetics. Int J Trichology. 2010 Jan-Jun;2(1):18-9.
9. Langbein L, Schweizer J. Keratins of the human hair follicle. Int Rev Cytol. 2005;243:1-78.
10. Karincaoglu Y, Basak KC, Muammer ES, Nalan B. Monilethrix Improvement with Acitretin. Am J Clin Dermatol. 2005;6:407-10.
11. Rakowska A, Slowinska M, Czuwara J, Olszewska M, Rudnicka L. Dermoscopy as a tool for rapid diagnosis of monilethrix. J Drugs Dermatol. 2007;6:222-4.
12. Smith VV, Anderson G, Malone M, Sebire NJ. Light microscopic examination of scalp hair samples as an aid in the diagnosis of paediatric disorders: retrospective review of more than 300 cases from a single centre. J Clin Pathol. 2005;58:1294-8.
13. Tosti A. Hair shaft disorders. In: Tosti A, editor. Dermoscopy of hair and scalp: Pathological and clinical correlation, illustrated edition. USA: CRC press; 2007;pp. 51-3.
14. Jain N, Khopkar U. Monilethrix in Pattern Distribution in Siblings: Diagnosis by Trichoscopy. Int J Trichology. 2010 Jan-Jun;2(1):56-9.
15. Rakowska A, Slowinska M, Kowalska-Oledzka E, Rudnicka L. Trichoscopy in genetic hair shaft abnormalities. J Dermatol Case Rep. 2008 July 7;2(2):14-20.
16. Ito M, Hashimoto K, Katsuumi K, Sato Y. Pathogenesis of monilethrix: Computer stereography and electron microscopy. J Invest Dermatol. 1990;95:186-94.
17. Sandhu K, Handa S, Kanwar AJ. Monilethrix. Indian J Dermatol. 2002;47:169-70.
18. Dinh HV, Sinclair RD, Green J. Hair and Scalp Diseases Medical, Surgical, and Cosmetic Treatments. Informa Healthcare USA, Inc. p.149-62.
19. Bentley-Phillips B, Bayles MAH. A previously undescribed hereditary hair anomaly (pseudomonilethrix). Br J Dermatol. 1973;89:688-90.
20. Valia RG, Valia AR. IADVL textbook of Dermatology. Bhalani Publishing House. 3rd edition. 2008.
21. Cheng AS, Bayliss SJ, Louis S. The genetics of hair shaft disorders. J Am Acad Dermatol. 2008;59:1-22.
22. Blume-Peytavi U, Tosti A, Whitling DA, Trüeb R. Hair growth and disorders. Springer International Edition. 2010.
23. Lubianca Neto JF, Lu L, Eavey RD, Flores MA, Caldera RM, Sangwatanaroj S, et al. The Bjornstad syndrome (sensorineural hearing loss and pili torti) disease gene maps to chromosome 2q34-36. Am J Hum Genet. 1998;62:1107-12.
24. Hinson J, Fantin V, Schonberger J, Breivik N, Siem G, McDonough B, et al. Missense mutations in the BCS1L gene as a cause of the Bjornstad syndrome. N Engl J Med. 2007;356:809-19.
25. Beare JM. Congenital pilar defect showing features of pili torti. Br J Dermatol. 1952;64:366-72.
26. Crandall BF, Samec L, Sparkes RS, Wright SW. A familial syndrome of deafness, alopecia, and hypogonadism. J Pediatr. 1973;82:460-5.
27. Voigtlander V. Pili torti with deafness (Bjornstad syndrome). Report of a family. Dermatologica. 1979;159:50-4.
28. de Berker D, Sinclair RD. The hair shaft: normality, abnormality, and genetics. Clin Dermatol. 2001;19:129-34.
29. Wallace MP, de Berker D. Hair diagnoses and signs: the use of dermatoscopy. Clinical and Experimental Dermatology. 2009;35:41-6.

30. Tümer Z, Møller LB. Menkes disease. Eur J Hum Genet. 2010;18(5):511-8.
31. Paulsen M, Lund C, Akram Z, Winther JR, Horn N, Mølle LB. Evidence That Translation Reinitiation Leads to a Partially Functional Menkes Protein Containing Two Copper-Binding Sites. Am. J. Hum. Genet. 2006;79:214-29.
32. Camakaris J, Petris MJ, Bailey L, et al. Gene amplification of the Menkes (MNK; ATP7A) P-type ATPase gene of CHO cells is associated with copper resistance and enhanced copper efflux. Hum Mol Genet. 1995;4:2117-23.
33. Møller LB, Bukrinsky JT, Mølgaard A, et al. Identification and analysis of 21 novel disease-causing amino acid substitutions in the conserved part of ATP7A. Hum Mutat. 2005;26:84-93.
34. Horn N, Tümer Z. Menkes disease and the occipital horn syndromein Royce PM, Steinmann B (eds): Connecitive Tissue and its Heritable Disorders: Molecular, Genetic, and Medical Aspects New York: John Wiley and Sons Inc. 2002. 2nd edn 651-85.685.
35. Lee ES, Ryoo JW, Choi DS, Cho JM, Kwon SH, Shin HS. Diffusion-Weighted MR Imaging of Unusual White Matter Lesion in a Patient with Menkes Disease. Korean J Radiol. 2007 Jan-Feb;8(1):82-5.
36. Kaler SG, Clarissa J. Liew CJ, Donsante A, Hicks JD, Sato S, et al. Molecular correlates of epilepsy in early diagnosed and treated Menkes disease. J Inherit Metab Dis. 2010;33(5):583-9.
37. Zaffanello M, Maffeis C, Fanos V, Franchini M, Zamboni G. Urological complications and copper replacement therapy in childhood Menkes syndrome.
38. Palmer CA. Neuropathology of Occipital Horn Syndrome. Journal of Child Neurology. 2001;16:764-66.
39. Kaler SG. Menkes disease. Adv Ped. 1994;41:263-304.
40. Tümer Z, Horn N. Menkes disease: recent advances and new aspects. J Med Genet. 1997;34:265-74.
41. George DH, Casey RE. Menkes disease after copper histidine replacement therapy: case report. Pediatr Dev Pathol. 2001;4:281-8.
42. Kirodian BG, Gogtay NJ, Udani VP, Kshirsagar NA. Treatment of Menkes disease with parenteral copper histidine. Indian Pediatr. 2002;39:183-5.
43. Hosomi N, Ukai KF, Nakanishi T, Unaki SF, Shii MI. Caspase-1 activity of stratum corneum and serum interleukin-18 level is increased in patients with Netherton syndrome. Br J Dermatol. 2008;159:733-72.
44. Sun JD, Linden KG. Netherton syndrome: a case report and review of the literature. Int J Dermatol. 2006;45:693-7.
45. Netherton EW. A unique case of trichorrhexis nodosa; bamboo hairs. AMA Arch Derm. 1958;78:483.
46. Mevorah B, Frenk E, Brooke EM. Ichthyosis linearis circumflexa comèl. A clinico-statistical approach to its relationship with Netherton's syndrome. Dermatologica. 1974;149:201-9.
47. Salodkar AD, Choudary SV, Jadwani G, Singh A. Int J Trichology. 2009;1:143-4.
48. Deraison C, et al. LEKTI fragments specifically inhibit KLK5, KLK7, and KLK14 and control desquamation through a pH-dependent interaction. Mol Biol Cell. 2007;18(90):3607-19.
49. Descargues P, Deraison C, Bonnart C, Kreft M, Kishibe M, Ishida-Yamamoto A, et al. Spink5-deficient mice mimic Netherton syndrome through degradation of desmoglein 1 by epidermal protease hyperactivity. Nat Genet. 2005;37(1):56-65.
50. Bonnart C, Deraison C, Lacroix M, Uchida Y, Besson C, Robin A et al. Elastase 2 is expressed in human and mouse epidermis and impairs skin barrier function in Netherton syndrome through filaggrin and lipid misprocessing. J Clin Invest. 2010;120(3):871-82.
51. Chavanas S, Garner C, Bodemer C, Ali M, Hamel- Teillac D, Wilkinson J. Localization of the Netherton Syndrome Gene to Chromosome 5q32, by Linkage Analysis and Homozygosity Mapping. Am J Hum Genet. 2000 March;66(3):914-21.
52. Sardy M, Fay A, Karpati S, Horvath A. Comel–Netherton syndrome and peeling skin syndrome type B: overlapping syndromes or one entity? Int J Dermatol. 2002;41:264-8.
53. Schneider I, Sebok B, Kosztolanyi G, Szekeres G. Comel–Netherton syndrome: evolution of manifestation in a 20-year follow-up and phenotypic overlap with peeling skin syndrome type B. Acta Dermatol Venereol. 2000;80:209-10.
54. Descargues P, Deraison C, Prost C, Fraitag S, Mazereeuw-Hautier J, D'Alessio M et al. Corneodesmosomal Cadherins Are Preferential Targets of Stratum Corneum Trypsin- and Chymotrypsin-like Hyperactivity in Netherton Syndrome. J Invest Dermatol. 2006;126:1622-32.
55. Dey VK. Netherton syndrome: A rare genodermatosis. Ind Dermatol Online J. 2011;2:38-9.
56. Ito M, Ito K, Hashimoto K. Pathogenesis in trichorrhexis invaginata (bamboo hair). J Inv Dermatol. 1984;83:1-6.
57. Rogers M. Hair shaft abnormalities: Part II. Australas J Dermatol. 1996;37:1-11.
58. Chao SC, Richard G, Lee J Y-Y. Netherton syndrome: report of two Taiwanese siblings with staphylococcal scalded skin syndrome and mutation of SPINK5. Br J Dermatol. 2005;152:159-65.
59. Smith DL, Smith JG, Wong SW, deShazo RD. Netherton's syndrome: a syndrome of elevated IgE and characteristic skin and hair findings. J Allergy Clin Immunol. 1995;95(1 Part 1):116-23.
60. Kilic G, Guler N, Ones U, Tamay Z, Guzel P. Netherton syndrome: report of identical twins presenting with severe atopic dermatitis. Eur J Pediatr. 2006;165:594-7.
61. Yan AC, Honig PJ, Ming ME, Weber J, Shah KN. The Safety and Efficacy of Pimecrolimus, 1%, Cream for the Treatment of Netherton Syndrome.
62. Faghri S, Tamura D, Kraemer KH, DiGiovanna JJ. Trichothiodystrophy: a systematic review of 112 published cases characterizes a wide spectrum of clinical manifestations. J Med Genet. 2008;45:609-21.
63. Bergmann E, Egly JM. Trichothiodystrophy, a transcription syndrome. Trends Genet. 2001;17:279-86.
64. Itin P, Sarasin A, Pittelkow M. Trichothiodystrophy: update on the sulfur- deficient brittle hair syndromes. J Am Acad Dermatol. 2001;44:891-920.
65. Bootsma D, Kraemer KH, Cleaver JE, Hoeijmakers JHJ. Nucleotide excision repair syndromes: xeroderma pigmentosum, Cockayne syndrome, and trichothiodystrophy. In: The Genetic Basis of Human Cancer, 2002 second edition. (Vogelstein B, Kinzler KW, eds) New York: McGraw-Hill, 211-37.

66. Liang C, Morris A, Schlücker S, Imoto K, Price VH, Menefee E, et al. Structural and Molecular Hair Abnormalities in Trichothiodystrophy. J Invest Dermatol. 2006;126:2210-6.
67. Harreld JH, Smith EC, Prose NS, Puri PK, Barboriak DP. Trichothiodystrophy with Dysmyelination and Central Osteosclerosis. Am J Neuroradiol. 2010;31:129-30.
68. Nakabayashi K, Amann D, Ren Y, Saarialho-Kere U, Avidan N, Gentles S. Identification of C7orf11 (TTDN1) Gene Mutations and Genetic Heterogeneity in Non photosensitive Trichothiodystrophy. Am J Hum Genet. 2005;76:510-6.
69. Kraemer KH, Patronas NJ, Schiffmann R, Brooks BP, Tamura D, DiGiovanna JJ. Xeroderma pigmentosum, Tricchothiodystrophy and Cockayne syndrome: A complex genotype-phenotype relationship. Neuroscience. 2007;145:1388-96.
70. Richetta A, Giustini S, Rossi A, Calvieri S. What's new in trichothiodystrophy. J Eur Acad Dermatol Venereol. 2001;15:1-4.
71. Crovato F, Rebora A. PIBI(D)S syndrome: a new entity with defect of the deoxyribonucleic acid excision repair. J Am Acad Dermatol. 1985;13:683-5.
72. Calvieri S, Zampetti M, Corbo A. Preliminary results using a microanalysis system on the hair of patients affected by trichothiodystrophy. Clin Exp Dermatol. 1989;14:404.
73. Toelle SP, Valsangiacomo E, Bolthauser E. Trichothiodystrophy with severe cardiac and neurological involvement in two sisters. Eur J Pediatr. 2001;160:728-31.
74. Dahbi-Skali H, Benamar L, Benchikhi H, Lakhdar H, Pinel N. PIBID S syndrome (trichothiodys trophy type F) and skin cancer: an exceptional association. Photodermatol Photoimmunol Photomed. 2004;20:157-8.
75. Fortina AB, Alaibac M, Piaserico S, Peserico A. PIBI(D)S: clinical and molecular characterization of a new case. J Eur Acad Dermatol Venereol. 2001;15:65-9.
76. Cheng S, Stone J, de Berker D. Trichothiodystrophy and fragile hair: the distinction between diagnostic signs and diagnostic labels in childhood hair disease. Br J Dermatol. 2009;161:379-1383.
77. Selvaag E, Aas AM, Heide S. Structural hair shaft abnormalities in hypomelanosis of Ito and other ectodermal dysplasias. Acta Pñdiatr. 2000;89:610-2.
78. Pinheiro M, Freire-Maia N. Hair-nail dysplasia—a new pure autosomal dominant ectodermal dysplasia. Clin Genet. 1992;41:296-8.
79. Priolo M, Silengo M, Lerone M, Ravazzolo R. Ectodermal dysplasias: not only 'skin' deep. Clin Genet. 2000;58:415-30. © Munksgaard, 2000.
80. Lamartine J. Towards a new classification of ectodermal dysplasias. Clin Exp Dermatol. 2003;28:351-5.
81. TruÈ eb RM, Bruckner-TudermanL, WyssM,WuÈ thrich B, Burg G. Scalp dermatitis, distinctive hair abnormalities and atopic disease in the ectrodactyly-ectodermal dysplasia-clefting syn-drome. Br J Dermatol. 1995;132:621-5.
82. TruÈ eb RM, Spycher MA, Schumacher F, Burg G. Pili torti et canaliculi beiektodermaler Dysplasie. Hautarzt. 1994;45: 372-7.
83. Itin PH, Burgdorf WHC, H app le R et al. G enoderma-toses. In: Schachner LA, Hansen RC, eds. Pediatric der-matology, 3rd e d. Edinburgh: Mosby. 2003;263-383.

5

Hair Shaft Disorders

Savitha AS, S Sacchidanand

"Supposing is good, but finding out is better."
—*Mark Twain*

Introduction

The function of scalp hair is mainly cosmetic, though in other regions of the body, it has a variety of functions. The part of the hair above the hair bulb is hair shaft. Hair shaft defects may give the hair an unusual appearance, make it fragile or act as a marker for a syndrome **(Box 5.1)**. Hair shaft disorders may occur as localized or generalized disorders. They may be primary and hereditary or secondary to external factors.

Classification of Hair Shaft Disorders (Box 5.1)

Price classified hair shaft anomalies into those with increased fragility and those that are not **(Table 5.1)**.[1]

Hair shaft disorders can also be classified according to the morphological appearance (**Table 5.2**).[2]

Monilethrix (Beaded Hair, Nodose Hair, Moniliform Hair)

'Monilethrix' is derived from 'monile' (Latin), which means necklace, and 'thrix' (Greek), which means hair. This term indicates the resemblance of the hair to a string of beads

Box 5.1: Presentation of hair shaft defects

- Unusual appearance
- Fragile hair
- Abnormal color
- Abnormal length
- Abnormal density

Table 5.1: Price classification of hair shaft defects

Structural defects with increased fragility	*Structural defects without increased fragility*
Monilethrix	Trichoptilosis
Pseudomonilethrix	Trichoclasis
Pili torti	Circle hair
Netherton syndrome	Bubble hair
Trichorrhexis nodosa	Trichonodosis
Trichothiodystrophy (TTD)	Hair casts
	Pili multigemini
	Trichostasis spinulosa
	Pohl Pinkus constriction
	Tapered hair
	Loose anagen hair syndrome
	Uncombable hair
	Woolly hair
	Pili annulati/ringed hair

Table 5.2: Classification of hair shaft defects according to morphology[2]

Fractures ❑ Trichoclasis ❑ Trichoptilosis ❑ Trichoschisis ❑ Trichorrhexis nodosa	**Multiple hairs** ❑ Pili bigeminy ❑ Pili multigemini ❑ Trichostasis spinulosa
Nodes ❑ Pseudomonilethrix ❑ Trichorrhexis nodosa ❑ Trichorrhexis invaginata ❑ Trichonodosis ❑ Infective–Nits, piedra ❑ Bayonet hair ❑ Hair casts	**Nodes** ❑ Monilethrix ❑ Pohl-Pinkus mark ❑ Tapered hair ❑ Exclamation mark hair ❑ Hypoplasia
Twists and curls ❑ Pili torti ❑ Woolly hair ❑ Circle hair ❑ Corkscrew hair ❑ Trichomalacia	**Grooves** ❑ Spun glass hair ❑ Pili bifurcati ❑ Trichothiodystrophy
Unruly hair	**Bands** ❑ Pili annulati ❑ Trichothiodystrophy

or a necklace. It is an autosomal dominant (AD) disorder. Abnormalities are attributed to mutations in human keratin type II genes hHb1 and hHb6 on chromosome 12q31.[3] The hair shaft is beaded and breaks easily **(Figure 5.1)**. The normal hair is succeeded by horny follicular papules from the summit of which emerge fragile beaded hairs (Refer Chapter 4).

Pseudomonilethrix

Bentley-Phillips and Bayles described a condition termed as pseudomonilethrix in South Africans of European or Indian descent. The shaft abnormality diagnosis is uncertain and may be artifactual. Patients present with alopecia starting in childhood. The hair readily breaks with trauma of combing or brushing. Microscopy shows irregular nodes, twists without flattening of hair, breaks with brush like ends on normal shaft.[1] Keratosis pilaris is absent. Similar changes can be produced in normal hair by tweezers or forceps or by compression. Hair lacquer and gel also causes beading visible under light microscope.[4]

Pili Torti (Trichokinesis, Corkscrew Hair, Twisted Hair)

In pili torti the affected hair is flattened and twisted through 180° along their long axis at irregular intervals **(Figure 5.2)**. Autosomal dominant mode of inheritance is seen in those cases in which pili torti of early onset appears to have occurred as an isolated defect (Refer to chapter 4).[5]

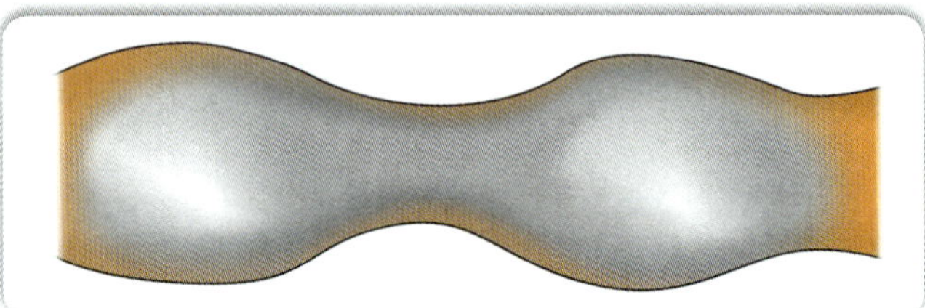

Fig. 5.1: Diagram of Monilethrix

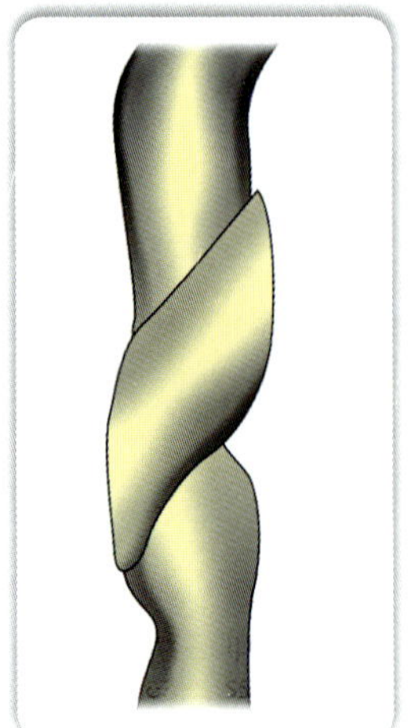

Fig. 5.2 : Diagram of pili torti

Netherton Syndrome (Trichorrhexis Invaginata, Comel-Netherton Syndrome, Bamboo Hair)

Netherton syndrome has a triad of atopic dermatitis, ichthyosis linearis circumflexa and bamboo hair/ Trichorrhexis invaginata. The defect has been located to a gene on chromosome 5q32 known as SPINK 5 acronym for serum protease inhibitor.[6] Finding a single trichorrhexis invaginata node in a single hair is conclusive of Netherton syndrome. Characteristic "bamboo" shape under light microscopic examination is due to invagination of the distal part of the hair shaft to its proximal part **(Figure 5.3)**. The proximal remnant of the invaginate node may resemble a golf tee and can allow diagnosis where a classic node is absent **(Refer to Chapter 4)**.[7]

Trichorrhexis Nodosa

One of the most common hair shaft defects, a dermatologist encounters is trichorrhexis nodosa (TN).

History

In 1852, Samuel Wilks of Guy's Hospital first described the condition, although the term trichorrhexis nodosa was not proposed until 1876 by M Kaposi.[8]

Etiology

Trichorrhexis nodosa (TN) is a distinctive response of hair shaft to injury. If the degree and frequency of injury is sufficient, it can be induced in normal hair also.[9] The

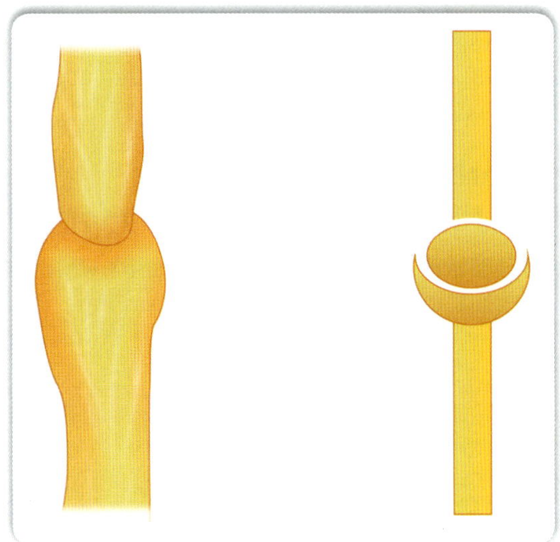

Fig. 5.3: Diagram of Bamboo hair

cuticular cells become disrupted allowing the cortical cells to splay out to form nodes. The trauma of hair dressing procedures has been frequently incriminated. Scratching may produce identical changes in pubic hair. The cumulative effect of shampooing, brushing, sea bathing and sunlight has led to seasonal recurrences.[2]

A primary congenital form of TN is inherited as an autosomal dominant trait in some families.

Trichorrhexis nodosa is a manifestation of rare metabolic defect argininosuccinic aciduria in which it is associated with mental retardation.[10] A case of TN isolated in beard has been reported.[11]

The TN has also been described in a case of hypothyroidism. The accumulation of mucin in the outer root sheath is postulated to press on the IHS, causing the hair-shaft defect (**Box 5.2**).[12]

Pathology

The shaft may appear normal with light or electron microscope. However, in isolated spots along the length of a fiber swelling and/or fraying can be seen **(Figures 5.4 and 5.5)**. These focal defects develop where there is an absence of cuticle. At the nodes the cuticle bulges and is split by longitudinal fissures.[9]

Clinical Features

Congenital trichorrhexis nodosa is very rare and it often develops at a very young age. TN appears as minute grayish nodes along the shaft where the cuticle is lost. The number of these nodes along a single hair shaft varies from one to several depending upon the length. The frayed cortical fibers project out giving the appearance of two paint brushes thrust into one another.

In trichorrhexis nodosa complicating congenital defect of hair shaft, the hair breaks so easily that large or small portions of scalp show only broken stumps and alopecia may be gross. However the common situation is where trauma plays a major role. In this setting there are three principal clinical presentations.[1]

- Distal trichorrhexis nodosa: Affects primarily Asians and white patients, and occurs several inches from the scalp, and is associated with trichoptilosis. Clinically hair is dry, dull or brittle.
- Generalized variant seen in Afro-Caribbean women called proximal TN. Hair is universally short and brittle demonstrating severe weathering of the hair in those who traumatize their hair with styling or chemicals.
- Sabouraud described a rare form in which localized area of scalp, moustache and beard show one to five nodules.[13]

Box 5.2: Etiology of trichorrhexis nodosa

- Primary congenital form- AD
- Hair dressing procedures
- Sunlight
- Arginosuccinic aciduria
- Hypothyroidism

Differential Diagnosis

The congenital forms must be differentiated from other shaft defects. The distal acquired form simulates dandruff or even pediculosis.

Treatment

Regardless of the presence or the absence of an underlying defect of the hair shaft, TN is ultimately the result of trauma. Therefore, treatment is aimed at minimizing physical or chemical trauma. Excessive brushing, hot combing, permanent waving, and other harsh hair treatments should be avoided.

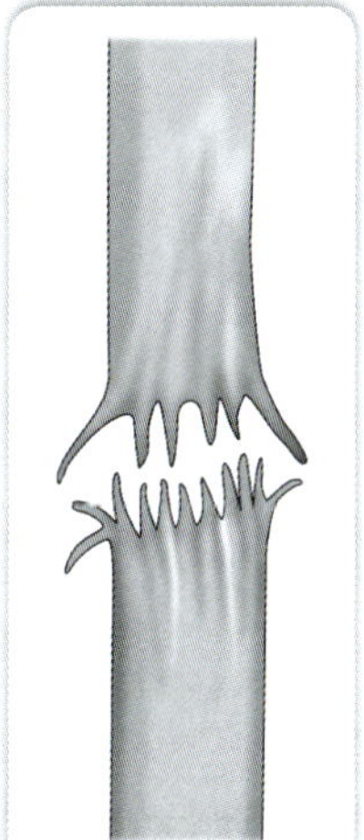

Fig. 5.4: Diagram of trichorrhexis nodosa

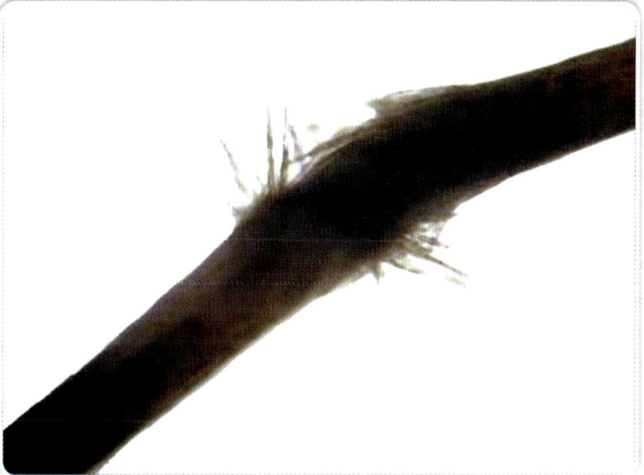

Fig. 5.5: Trichorrhexis nodosa under light microscope

Trichothiodystrophy

The term trichothiodystrophy (TTD) was used to describe brittle hair with abnormally low sulfur content. Approximately 50% are photosensitive and in this group there is phenotypic and genetic crossover with xeroderma pigmentosa (XDP). The common genetic defect in XDP and photosensitive TTD is within excision repair cross complementation 2 (ERCC2) gene on chromosome 19q. (Refer to chapter 4).[14]

Trichoschisis

Trichoschisis is a clean transverse fracture across the hair shaft through the cuticle and cortex **(Figure 5.6)**. At the site of fracture, there is localized absence of cuticular cells. Trichoschisis is a common association with syndromes associated with trichothiodystrophy. Electron-probe X-ray microanalysis of the defective hair shaft revealed a marked deficiency of sulfur in a few cases.[15]

Trichoptilosis (Fragilitis Crinium, Split Ends, Schizotrichia)

The term comes from the Greek root "tricho" meaning hair and "ptilosis" meaning "falling out of the eyelashes."

Etiology

Trichoptilosis is the most common macroscopic response of the hair shaft to trauma. It is a component of weathering process especially in those with long hair.[2] Thermal, chemical or mechanical stress can cause split ends. Excessive application of hair products such as perms and hair coloring may strip protective layering off the outside of the hair's shaft and weaken the hair, making the hair prone to split ends. Mechanical stresses include pulling a comb forcefully through tangled hair and repeated combing. Split ends can be seen as a symptom of copper transport disorders such as Menkes disease and occipital horn syndrome.

Pathology

The distal end of the shaft is split longitudinally into two or several divisions. Other microscopic evidence of hair damage may be present. The split commences from the distal tip thus distinguishing the problem from pili bifurcati or multigemini.

Clinical Features

Trichoptilosis is asymptomatic and usually an incidental finding. The common complaint is brittle hair. Trichoptilosis may be central or distal **(Figures 5.7 and 5.8)**. Central trichoptilosis is longitudinal splitting of hair shaft in the center without involving the tip, sometimes occurs particularly in knotted hair (trichonodosis). Trichorrhexis nodosa and trichoptilosis are often present in the same patient.[16]

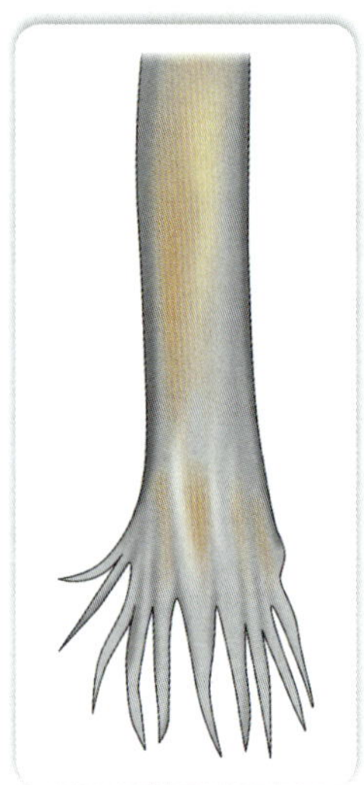

Fig. 5.7: Diagram of trichoptilosis

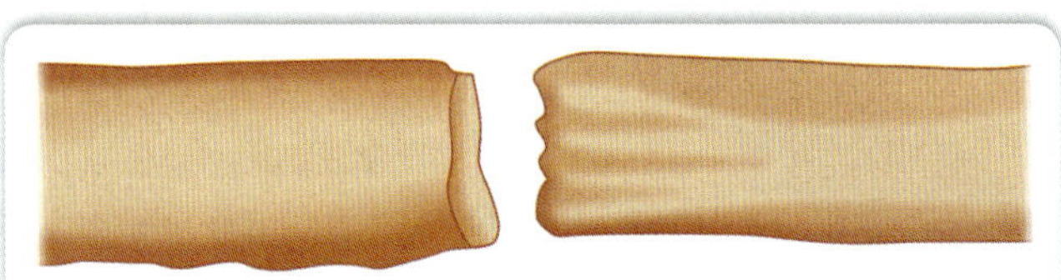

Fig. 5.6: Diagram of trichoschisis

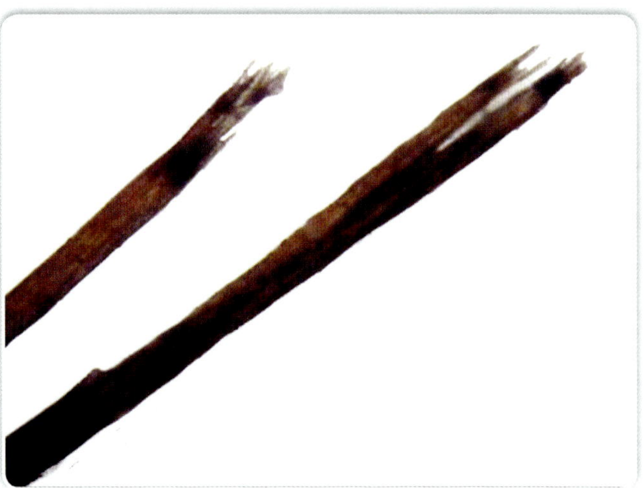

Fig. 5.8: Light microscopy of distal trichoptilosis

Treatment

Careful explanation to the patient is necessary to avoid further hair trauma, otherwise the condition will definitely recur. Short hair and frequent trimming solves the problem.

Trichoclasis

Trichoclasis is the common greenstick fracture of hair shaft. The transverse fracture is partly splinted by the cuticle, unlike in trichoschisis. It is seen in a variety of congenital and acquired fragile hair states **(Figure 5.9)**.[17] It can also be seen in normal hair where vigorous grooming stresses the fiber to such an extent that the hair suddenly snaps and breaks off. It is common to see some trichoclasis as a result of trichotillomania (obsessive hair plucking). Treatment for trichoclasis involves reducing the physical manipulation of hair and the recommendation of gentle handling of hair.

Idiopathic trichoclasis was first described by Jackson. Sabouraud, in a descriptive article on the subject, distinguished three forms of the disease:

1. A rare form of trichorrhexis that is localized in and involves the entire moustache, the hairs presenting five or six pearls or nodules from 3 to 5 mm apart, and in which relapses continue in spite of the avoidance of trauma.
2. A trichoclasis involving circumscribed rounded or oval patches on the scalp in which hairs are broken off from 6 to 8 mm from the skin, and in which the skin appears normal, the plaques healing spontaneously, but new areas appearing on other parts of the scalp.
3. A trichoclasis occurring in patches on the scalp, the skin of the plaque being dry, thickened, rough and bound down.[18]

Circle Hair

Circle hair and spiral hair occur in middle aged men on back, abdomen and thighs as small dark circles next to hair follicles. They are an unusual form of ingrown hair lying in a coiled track just below stratum corneum and can be easily extracted.[19]

Bubble Hair

History

Brown et al. published the first report of bubble hair in 1986.[20]

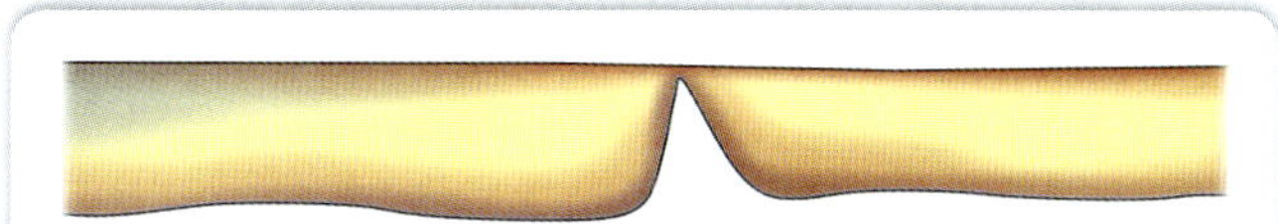

Fig. 5.9: Diagram of trichoclasis

Etiology

Bubble hair is a sign of thermal injury. Hair dryers operating at 175°C or more can cause bubble hair. The use of hair curling tongs operating at 125°C and applied to the hair for one minute can also induce bubbles in hair fiber.[21]

Pathology

Bubble hair is full of bubbles. All hair fibers contain minute air filled spaces called vacuoles. These spaces can also become filled with water when the hair is wet. Too much heat may make the water in the hair fiber spaces vaporize into steam. This vaporization of the water may force the spaces in the hair to expand eventually turning the hair into a sponge-like structure. These damaged hairs are weak and brittle as the bubbles destroy the integrity of the fiber.[20] Chemical treatment may also precipitate the onset of bubble hair and any already weak hair, whatever the cause, may be more susceptible to bubble development **(Figure 5.10)**.[22]

Clinical Features[22]

The hair may be kinked, break off, and over time the condition may develop into a localized alopecia. The hair appears to "come out in clumps," and the overall texture of the hair changing from soft and naturally curly to straight and stiff has been reported.[23]

Electron microscopic studies of previously reported cases revealed a loss of cortical cells and medulla at these sites. Cross-section images showed either a single large cavity or a reticulated, "Swiss cheese-like" loss of cells.[24]

Under dermatoscopy, dysmorphia of distal hair shaft was observed in bubble hair. In large hair samples

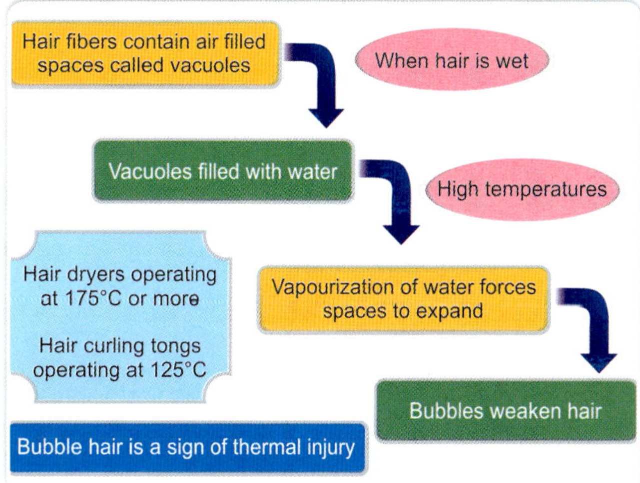

Fig. 5.10: Pathogenesis of bubble hair

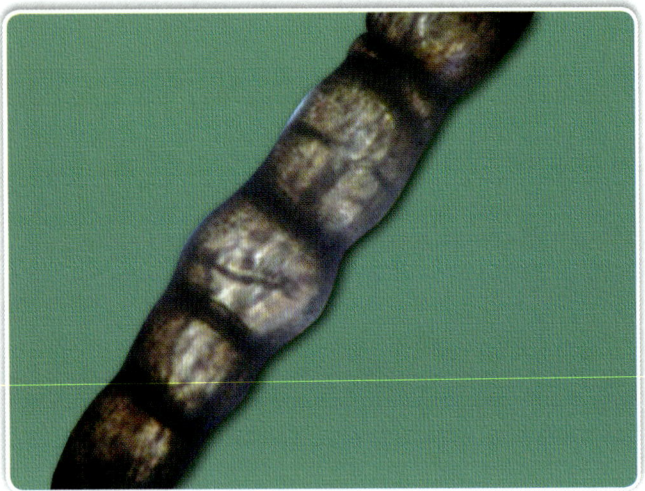

Fig. 5.11: Light microscopy of bubble hair

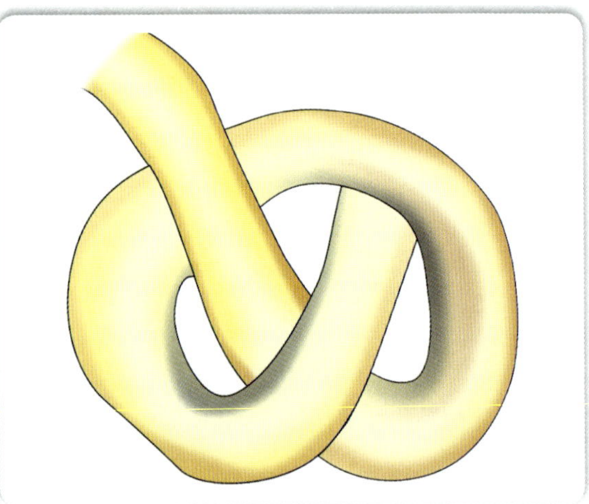

Fig. 5.12: Diagram of trichonodosis

dermatoscopy can be used to highlight hair that warrants closer examination under light microscopy **(Figure 5.11)**.[25]

Treatment

Stop using heat and chemicals on the hair and cut off the old damaged hair.

Trichonodosis (Knotted Hair)

History

Michelson first proposed the term noduli laqueati for knotted hair and noted that naturally curly hair was most frequently affected.[26]

Etiology

Trichonodosis may be caused by trauma, head rests, hats and pillows.

Clinical Features

Incidental clinical finding of trauma induced knotting of the naturally curly/wavy hair-shaft is seen frequently over lower occipital regions **(Figure 5.12)**. Microscopic examination may be needed to differentiate from piedra and the pediculosis capitis ova.

Hair Casts (Pseudonits, Peripilar Keratin Cysts)

History

Grindon in 1897 described hair casts under the heading of "Ecbolic folliculitis" which was named as "Hair casts" by Kligman.[27]

Etiology

There are two types of hair casts:

- The common type is found frequently in association with parakeratotic scalp disorders like psoriasis, lichen planus, seborrheic dermatitis or trichotillomania and hair styles requiring traction. They occur in children and adults of either sex. It is suggested they be called parakeratotic hair casts, as this name reflects the cause and composition of the casts.
- The uncommon type is not usually associated with diseases of the scalp and has only been reported in female subjects. It is suggested they be called peripilar keratin casts, as this is the name frequently used for them.[28]

Pathology

Electron microscopy studies showed that the true peripilar hair casts are usually compounds of the outer root sheath and are rarely composed of the internal root sheath, and often some are made up of both the sheaths, internal and external.[29]

Scalp histology shows follicular openings packed with parakeratotic squames which break off at intervals to form casts.[30]

Clinical Features

Hair casts often occur in great numbers and may mimic nits in scalp. They are 2–5 mm, firm, and tubular movable structures around the hair shafts **(Figure 5.13)**. While nits are firmly cemented to hair shaft, hair casts slide freely along the shaft **(Table 5.3)**.[27]

Differential Diagnosis

Pediculosis capitis, piedra, trichomycosis, trichonodosis and trichorrhexis nodosa.

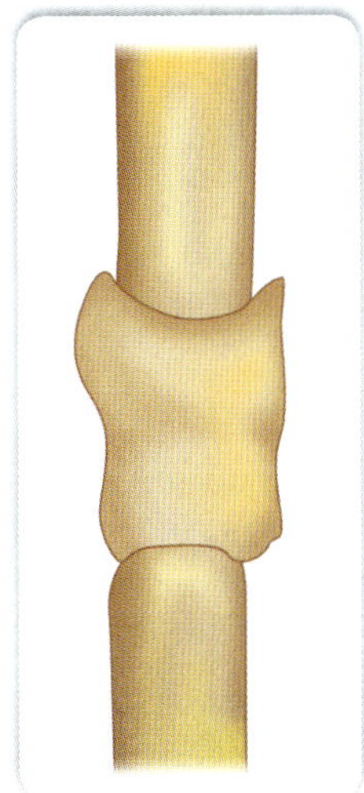

Fig. 5.13: Diagram of peripilar hair cast

Table 5.3 : Differences between nits and pseudonits[31]

True nits	*Pseudonits*
Tiny yellow, brown or tan dots attached to the hair shaft near the scalp	Firm, shiny , white, freely movable tubular accretions that encircle the hair shafts of the scalp
Caused by pediculus humanus capitis, female lays eggs at the base of the follicle	Etiology unknown
Common in childhood	Seen in all age groups
Contagious	Non contagious
Causes an itchy scalp	Usually asymptomatic

Treatment

Any causative disease must be treated. Prolonged brushing and combing is needed to slide off cast.

Pili Multigemini (Compound Hairs)

History

Pili multigemini was first described by Flemming (1883).[32]

Etiopathogenesis

Pili multigemini is a rare developmental anomaly where several dermal papillae are closely situated, with each producing a fiber, but these separate hair follicle bulbs combine together into one hair canal towards the skin surface. Each hair has its own inner root sheath and the hairs are surrounded by a common outer root sheath.[33]

Clinical Features

Several separate hair fibers bunch together and emerge from the skin through a single hair canal **(Figure 5.14)**. The hair looks like a bunch of flower stalks in a vase. Hairs are often flattened, ovoid, grooved or triangular in configuration.[33] Common site affected is face along the lines of jaw. Patient may complain of recurrent inflammatory nodules, leaving scars.

Treatment

There is very little information published on the treatment of pili multigemini. Plucking the hair seems to be very difficult as the hair fibers are deep rooted and it does not stop the hair growth. Shaving the hair may stop any associated folliculitis. Permanent hair reduction techniques like electrolysis, ablative lasers and cryosurgery may be tried.

Trichostasis Spinulosa

Etiology

Trichostasis spinulosa (TS) is a normal age related phenomenon, which results from successive production and retention of vellus telogen club hairs from a single hair matrix in a follicle. Hyperkeratosis plugs the follicle and results in the retention of the vellus hairs.[34] The precise cause of this phenomenon remains undetermined. Widespread trichostasis spinulosus has been reported with renal failure. External mechanisms include the use of irritating soaps or paraffin-containing creams and prolonged exposure to dust, hydrocarbons, or industrial oils. Trichostasis spinulosa has also been associated with prolonged use of clobetasol.[35]

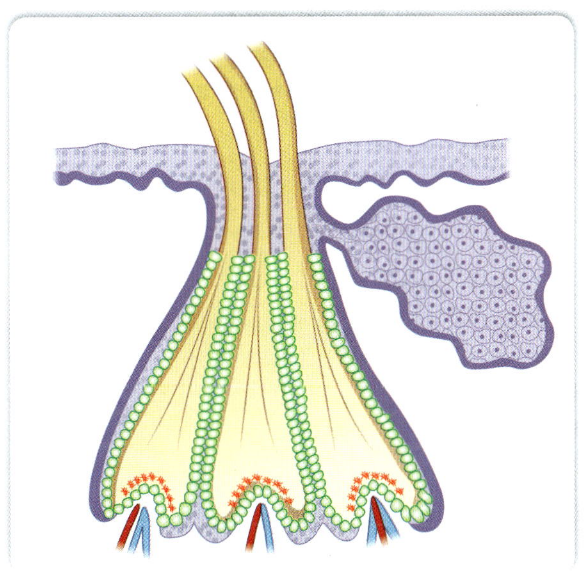

Fig. 5.14: Diagram of pili multigemini

Pathology

Histopathological examination reveals a dilated hair follicle with hyperkeratosis and acanthosis of the follicular epithelium. Inflammatory changes are not a characteristic feature of TS.

Clinical Features

The lesions are elevated, dark, spiny papules resembling comedones occurring predominantly on nose, forehead and cheeks. TS frequently are discovered as an incidental finding, and often it is confused with keratosis pilaris or acne comedones.[36] Pruritus is occasionally present, as is roughness of the skin. Pruritus may be more common when lesions are present on the trunk and arms of young adults.[37] A case of trichostasis spinulosa on the vertex is reported.[38] On examination with hand lens, comedones are prominent with a tuft of hair projecting through the horny plug.

Differential Diagnosis

Acne vulgaris, keratosis pilaris, lichen spinulosa, comedones.

Treatment

The individual plugs of impacted hairs may be removed by following means and topical retinoic acids can be used to help prevent future lesions

- Tweezing with forceps
- Pressure expression with a comedone extractor
- Use of depilatory wax, adhesive strips[39]
- Laser treatment with a 755-nm long-pulsed Alexandrite laser may also be considered[40]
  Emollients and keratolytics may also be helpful.

Pohl Pinkus Constriction

History

This was first described by Pohl in 1894, and he later changed his name to Pinkus.

Etiology and Pathogenesis

In some individuals, a zone of decreased shaft diameter coincides with a surgical operation, illness, administration of folic acid antagonists or any other drugs which inhibit mitosis.[41] The proportion of hair affected is variable and it seems probable that hairs in early anagen are easily susceptible to periods of hypoproteinemia or disturbed protein synthesis. These constrictions of hair shaft have been analogous to Beau's lines in nails which also coincide with periods of ill health.[42]

Tapered Hair

Etiology and Pathogenesis

Tapered hair may occur in association with many other structural abnormalities of hair shaft. They can arise in any process which inhibits the cell division in the hair matrix.[43]

Clinical Features

The distal end of hair shaft resembles the tip of javelin. Fracture of the shaft could occur if there is severe narrowing. If the inhibitory factors are temporary then the shaft would widen again giving a local dumb -bell -like appearance.[41] Another type of tapered hair is the young anagen hair or 'embryonic hair' with tapered points seen particularly in trichotillomania, alopecia areata and acquired progressive kinking of hair.[43] If many such young anagen hairs are seen, this usually represents a phase post-dating a period of acute hair shedding.

Treatment

Diffuse alopecia involving tapered hairs can only be remedied by removing the precipitating factor. For example, stopping chemotherapy will allow cell proliferation in the hair follicles to recover and fiber production should resume.

Loose Anagen Hair (LAH) Syndrome

History

Loose anagen syndrome was first reported in 1986 by Nodl and later by Zaun under the name of 'syndrome of loosely attached hair in childhood'.[44]

Etiopathogenesis

The precise pathogenesis of loose anagen syndrome is not known, but theories postulating an abnormality in the anagen hair's anchoring mechanism predominate. The inner root sheath (IRS) is thought to play an integral role in anchoring the hair shaft within the follicle and first layer to keratinize playing a key role in the differentiation of the layers. Most authors believe that LAH results from a premature keratinization of the IRS that produces an impaired adhesion between the cuticle of the IRS and the cuticle of the hair shaft.[45] Mutations in genes coding for cytokeratins have been identified in some cases and are thought to result in abnormal keratinization of the inner root sheath. This faulty keratinization leads to impaired adherence of the deformed hair shafts to their follicles.[46] Reports of autosomal dominant and sporadic occurrences are there.[47]

Clinical Features

This condition features anagen hair that are loosely anchored and easily, painlessly plucked from the scalp. Hair is thin, fine, sparse, lusterless and short. This is usually seen in young fair haired females between 2 and 6 years. There is patchy alopecia leading to a misdiagnosis of alopecia areata. The repeated rubbing of the occipital region of the head against the pillow at night pulls out more hair and this explains why the occiput is affected most.[48] The hair shaft may show twists and grooves.

Three phenotypes have been identified, with each having in common the finding of easily and painlessly extracted LAH on gentle hair pull. These phenotypes are:

1. Type A LAS, characterized by decreased hair density
2. Type B LAS, characterized by mainly unruly hair
3. Type C LAS, characterized by normal appearing hair with excessive shedding of LAH

The above phenotypes appear to be age-dependent, with types A and B occurring in children, possibly evolving into the type C phenotype around the age of eight years and occurring in adults.[49] The hair becomes more normal with age.

Trichograms show 98–100% anagen hair devoid of outer and inner hair root sheaths. The proximal segment of hair shaft closest to the root appears distorted and twisted with the characteristic ruffling of the cuticle seen. This has been described as the 'floppy sock appearance', which is characteristic. Some of the hair bulbs are positioned at an acute angle to the shaft resembling mouse tails.[43] On histopathology, the characteristic findings are clefting between IRS, IRS and ORS, ORS and fibrous sheath and lack of inflammation.[50]

Associated Conditions[45] (Box 5.3)

Box 5.3: Associated conditions in loose anagen hair syndrome

- Coloboma
- Noonan syndrome
- Hypohidrotic ectodermal dysplasia
- EEC (ectrodactyly–ectodermal dysplasia–clefting) syndrome
- Trichorhinophalangeal syndrome
- Nail-patella syndrome
- Neurofibromatosis
- Trichotillomania
- Woolly hair

Electron Microscopy

The epilated anagen hair shows rippling of the hair cuticle of the proximal hair shaft. Triangular or flattened shapes and longitudinal grooves and torsions are also occasionally present. The only characteristic finding is a premature keratinization of the cells of the Henle and Huxley layers of the IRS. Such premature keratinization could interfere with the normal interdigitation of the IRS cuticle and the hair shaft cuticle and disturb anchorage of anagen hairs.[48]

Diagnostic Criteria[52]

Tosti, et al. proposed diagnostic criteria for LAS on the basis of hair pull test and trichogram:

1. Positive pull test results with painless extraction of at least 10 LAHs.
2. The presence of more than 80% LAH on trichogram.

However, these criteria are too strict and only permit the severely affected to be diagnosed. Therefore, Tosti et al revised these criteria and suggested that the diagnosis of LAS should not be made if the trichogram does not show at least 70% LAH.[51]

Differential Diagnosis

Alopecia areata, trichotillomania, telogen effluvium, anagen effluvium.

Treatment and Prognosis

Most cases of LAS resolve spontaneously with age. The successful use of minoxidil is encouraging and may be a reasonable first-line therapy for patients with disease at the severe end of the LAH syndrome spectrum.[2]

Uncombable Hair Syndrome (Spun Glass Hair; Cheveux Incoiffables, Pili Trianguli et Canaliculi)

History

This condition was first described by Dupre et al in 1973 although the German fairy tale has a character "Struwwelpeter" whose hair was a mess.[53]

Etiology

Spun glass hair has both inherited (autosomal dominant and recessive) and sporadic modes of inheritance.[54] The early keratinization of the sheaths forms a straight, strong tube through which the hair fiber must pass. This inflexible tube forces the shape of the fiber to be straight and inflexible.[55]

Pathology

Light microscopy features are triangular to reniform to heart shaped in cross section and longitudinal grooving in at least 50 percent of hair. On histological examination of scalp hair, cross sectional characteristics are more easily seen. The pili canaliculi are seen in all cases and pili trianguli in majority with pili torti in a few. The misshapen dermal papilla alters the shape of internal root sheath, which hardens in a triangular cross sectional shape.[55]

Clinical Features

The abnormality may first become obvious from 3 months to 12 years of age.

The names "spun glass hair" literally describes the hair fiber. The hair looks like spun glass strands growing in any and all directions and are difficult to control and maintain a hairstyle. Diffuse alopecia is possible because the hair is not always anchored in the hair follicle and also due to the brittle nature of the hair. The eyebrows and eyelashes are normal.[51] Diagnosis is best made by scanning electron microscopy of hair fibers.

Light microscopy does not always show up the abnormalities in the hair fibers although polarized light is helpful.

No treatment is known although oral biotin therapy is suggested.[53]

Associated conditions of uncombable hair are given in **Box 5.4**.

Differential Diagnosis

Syndromes with hair abnormalities which may mimic uncombable hair syndrome clinically are given in **Box 5.5**. Unlike other conditions with an uncombable hair component, uncombable hair syndrome alone (cheveux incoiffables, pili trianguli et canaliculi) is not associated with physical, neurologic, or mental abnormalities.[56]

Box 5.4: Conditions associated with uncombable hair

- Ectodermal dysplasia
- Retinal dysplasia/pigmentary dystrophy, juvenile cataract
- Digit abnormalities
- Tooth enamel anomalies, oligodontia
- Phalango epiphyseal dysplasia

Box 5.5: Syndromes mimicking uncombable hair

- Rapp-Hodgkin ectodermal dysplasia
- Loose anagen hair syndrome
- Ectodermal dysplasia
- Ectrodactyly
- Cleft lip/palate (EEC) syndrome
- Familial tricho-odonto-onchyial ectodermal dysplasia with syndactyly.

Grooved Hair

Grooved hair has one or more grooves running for part or all of the hair fiber length. The hair fiber is structurally sound and strong with a normal cuticle. With just one groove the hair has a quarter moon cross section shape. With two grooves it may have an hour glass cross section shape, and with three or more grooves the cross section is star shaped. A few grooved fibers can be found in almost all individuals with healthy hair. However, an increased number of grooved hairs are found in conditions such as trichothiodystrophy, pili torti, woolly hair, uncombable hair syndrome, argininosuccinase deficiency, and ectodermal dysplasias.[57]

Woolly Hair

History

Woolly hair syndrome was first observed in a European family in 1907 by Gossage.

Definition

Woolly hair syndrome is a condition affecting a small percentage of persons of Caucasian and Asian heritage. It is characterized by extremely frizzy and wiry hair that looks almost woolly in appearance **(Figure 5.15)**.[25]

Classification[2]

1. Dominant woolly hair: Some families have woolly hair inherited as an autosomal dominant trait
2. Recessive woolly hairs
3. Acquired woolly hair also termed as progressive kinking of hair
4. Woolly hair nevus.

Pathology

The soft, woolly, Afro-textured hair lies typically separate and is tightly coiled or spiraled while the curls of the woolly

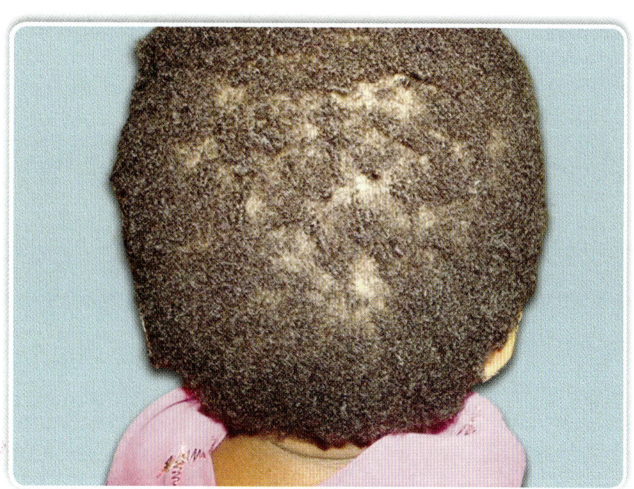

Fig. 5.15: Wooly hair

hair syndrome tend to merge. Hair of persons afflicted with this syndrome covers only portions of the scalp. Hair microscopy reveals nonspecific features. Usual associations are grooves, twists, irregularity of bore and sometimes trauma.[58] The changes are subtle and better appreciated on assessment of at least 20 to 50 hairs or more.

Acquired Woolly Hair

May develop as a part of ageing or may be attributable to trauma and drugs.

An irregular band of coarse whisker like hair extends around the edge of the scalp from above the ears towards the occipital area.[59] The hair shaft features are similar to congenital woolly hair.

Retinoids are the most commonly cited drugs.[43]

Woolly Hair Nevus

Hair in a circumscribed area of scalp is woolly and contrasts in color and coarseness with surrounding hair.

Naxos Disease

Naxos disease is a rare autosomal recessive inherited association of right ventricular dysplasia/dilated cardiomyopathy, palmoplantar keratoderma with woolly hair which appears from birth.[60]

Acquired Progressive Kinking of Hair[61]

Acquired progressive kinking of hair is also called pubeshaarnaevus because it resembles pubic hair. In this rare disorder, scalp hair becomes progressively curly, frizzy, dry and difficult to comb. It usually affects the vertex or frontotemporal area of young men and may progress to male pattern balding (androgenetic alopecia). Acquired progressive kinking of hair may also be a side effect of retinoid therapy.

Pili Annulati (Ringed Hair)

Etiology

Most common mode of inheritance is autosomal dominant, few reports of autosomal recessive and sporadic cases are seen. A gene for pili annulati maps to the telomeric region of chromosome 12q.[62]

Pathology

With the polarizing microscope the abnormal dark bands alternating with the light bands is reversed. The bright appearance of abnormal bands is due to the reflected light caused by air spaces in the cortex. The pathogenesis remains uncertain.[63]

Clinical Features

Pili annulati is normally diagnosed as a coincidental finding or as part of pursuance of unusual but attractive spangled appearance. The hair appears banded and sandy in reflected light. Axillary hair may occasionally be affected.

Prognosis is good and the severity does not progress with age.

Weathering of Hair

While "weathering" is a term very familiar in association with skin, hair is also subject to cosmetic and structural damage that some experts call "weathering". In the normal hair growth cycle, a hair tends to become shaggier in appearance as it ages; this is due to gradual breakdown of the structural proteins in the hair shaft. The normal structural breakdown can be hastened by hair-damaging environmental factors and cosmetic procedures that contribute to "weathering".

If the cuticle is absent, then the cortex underneath is directly exposed. The cortex is less resistant to the physical and chemical factors in the environment compared to the cuticle, and it forms ridges, fissures and nodules. This focal disruption of the hair fiber is a prime area for hair shaft breakage. As we comb, brush, and generally manipulate our hair, these defective nodes in the hair fiber may break. Hair that has lost its structure is a common cause of frizzy, hard-to-manage hair.

Excessive UV radiation exposure, excessive wetting especially in salt water, vigorous combing or brushing, chemical and physical damage caused by long-term permanent waving, hair curling and hair straightening, bleaching, dyeing, and the use of degreasing shampoos can cause significant damage to the hair shaft.

Body hair can be similarly damaged by environmental factors and by hard scratching with fingernails.

Because so many environmental and cosmetic factors may be at work in the life of any one person, it may be difficult to point to one factor as "**The cause**" of hair weathering. In rare instances, a genetic condition may contribute to breakage and frizzing of the hair shaft.

Weathering damage can occur to hair without one's knowledge. Hair has no nerve connections and thus cannot give one a feeling of pain when it is damaged.

Cosmetic and environmental factors that contribute to hair weathering should be avoided.[8]

Infections

Nits

The average nit (egg) of lice is 0.8 mm long, oval, translucent and whitish. The nit attaches to the base of the hair shaft or to fibers of clothing with strong, highly insoluble cement.

Children aged 3–11 years are most likely to become infested with head lice because of close contact in classrooms and daycare facilities. Pruritus is the major symptom, and parents may note the lice and nits in the hair of the child. The nits are laid close to the scalp and they grow along with the hair; their distance from the scalp gives an indication of duration of infestation.

Diagnosis

Close inspection of the scalp in affected patients may reveal the nits, live lice, and small dark specks of insect feces. Wood's lamp examination reveals yellow and/or green fluorescence of the lice and their nits **(Refer to Chapter 8)**.

Tinea Capitis

Tinea capitis is superficial fungal infection of the skin of the scalp, eyebrows, and eyelashes, with a propensity for attacking hair shafts and follicles. Tinea capitis is caused by keratinophilic fungi of species of genera *Trichophyton* and *Microsporum*.

Three types of in vivo hair invasion are recognized.

a. Ectothrix invasion is characterized by the development of arthroconidia on the exterior of the hair shaft **(Figure 5.16)**. The cuticle of the hair is destroyed, and infected hairs usually fluoresce a bright greenish-yellow color under a Wood's lamp examination. Common agents include *Microsporum canis, M. gypseum, Trichophyton equinum*, and *Trichophyton verrucosum*.
b. Endothrix hair invasion is characterized by the development of arthroconidia within the hair shaft only. The cuticle of the hair remains intact and infected hairs do not fluoresce under a Wood's lamp ultraviolet light. All endothrix-producing agents are anthropophilic (e.g. *Trichophyton tonsurans, Trichophyton violaceum*). Infected hairs break off sharply at the follicular orifice, leaving a conidia-filled stub or black dot **(Figure 5.17)**.
c. Favus, usually caused by *Trichophyton schoenleinii*, produces scutula and corresponding hair loss.

Spread of infection is the result of person-to-person transmission. The organism remains viable on combs, brushes, couches, and sheets for long periods.

Diagnosis

Fungus identification by KOH mount and culture.

Treatment

The mainstay of treatment is griseofulvin or other antifungals like itraconazole.

Topical therapy has little role in the management **(Refer to Chapter 7)**.

Piedra

Piedra means stone in Spanish. Piedra is superficial fungal infection, which affects exclusively the hair. It occurs in two varieties:

- The black variety called piedra hortae is common in South India. It is seen as 1–2 mm hard dark nodes along the shaft of the hair that are difficult to scrape off. Combing with a metal comb produces characteristic sound.
- White piedra, caused by *Trichosporon cutaneum*, is recognized as a common infection of genital hair. It is seen as whitish, soft, spongy nodular concretions that may be discrete or may coalesce to form a sheath along the scalp, beard, and axillary or perigenital hair.[64]

Plica Polonica (Plica Neuropathica, Hair Matting, Polish Plait, Elflock)[65]

History

The most notable person in history said to be afflicted with plica polonica was King Christian IV of Denmark (1577–1648).[66] The term "Plica neuropathica" was first

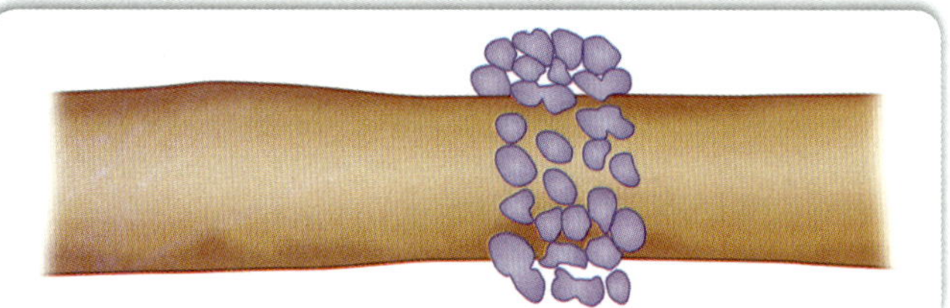

Fig. 5.16: Diagram of ectothrix infection

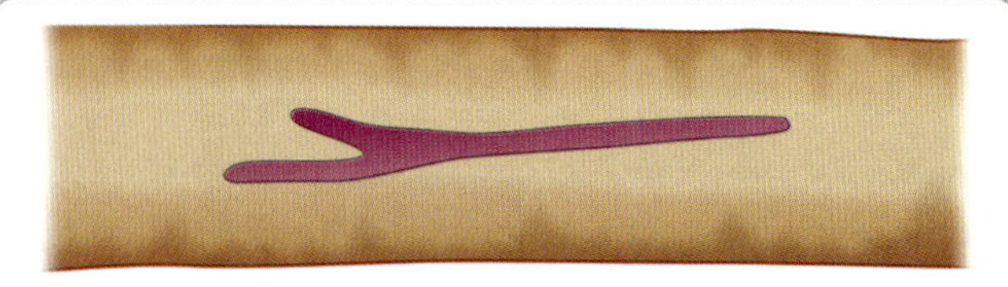

Fig. 5.17: Diagram of endothrix infection

used by Le Page in 1884 to describe a case of sudden onset entangled hair in a patient with hysteria.[67]

Etiopathogenesis

Plica polonica results from deficient hair care and use of shampoos containing cationic detergents. Uncombed hair becomes irreversibly entangled, forming a matted, malodorous and encrusted or sticky moist mass. It may be caused or accompanied with lice infestation.

It has been suggested that plica polonica may be associated with damage to sections of the cuticle thereby exposing the moist sticky cortex to which other similarly affected hair shafts adhere **(Figure 5.18)**.

Plica polonica is made of a hard impenetrable mass of keratin fibers permanently cemented together with dried pus, blood, old lice egg-casings and dirt.[68] Plica neuropathica has also been reported in two cases with pancytopenia following azathioprine use and it was attributed to cuticular damage of hair shaft in absence of poor hair care practices.[69]

Treatment

The disease may be easily prevented by washing and combing of the hair. Treatment involves cutting the affected hair.

Diagnosis of Hair Shaft Disorders

To establish an exact diagnosis of dysplastic hair shafts, a structured history and physical examination are needed which emphasizes on other skin appendages such as the nails, sweat and sebaceous glands. Hair microscopy including polarizing microscopy can be a useful part of clinical assessment in some situations, including a range of hereditary or acquired metabolic disorders where the hair shaft can sometimes provide clues to diagnosis.[70]

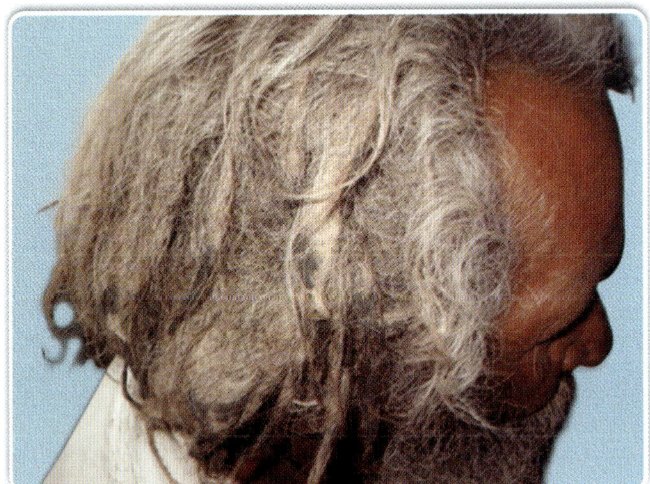

Fig. 5.18: Plica polonica

Examination of hair for structural defects is facilitated by a method devised by Shely wherein putting a piece of double stick tape on a microscope slide and aligning 5 cm segments of hair in parallel on it.[71]

Polarizing Microscopy

- Polarized light is transverse wave light whose vibration possesses direction.
- A polarizing microscope is a special microscope that uses polarized light for investigating the optical properties of specimens.
- Polariscopic examination of the hair in trichothiodystrophy shows characteristic alternate dark and white bands of hair shaft called as 'tiger tail' appearance which is not visualized on light microscopic examination.[72]

Applications of Wood's Lamp in Hair Shaft Disorders

Tinea Capitis

Some dermatophyte species produce characteristic fluorescence under UV light. The chemical responsible for the fluorescence is pteridine. Wood's lamp is helpful in the diagnosis and treatment of an individual patient as well as for mass screening and control of epidemics in schools. Dermatophytes that cause fluorescence are generally members of the *Microsporum* genus.[73]

Conclusion

Therapy of hair shaft disorders should focus on the cause. In addition, minimizing traumatic influences to hair shafts, such as drying hair with an electric dryer or permanent waves and coloring dyes, is important. A short hairstyle is more suitable for patients with hair shaft disorders

References

1. De Berker DAR, Messenger AG, Sinclair RD. Disorders of hair. In: Tony Burns, Stephen Breathnach, Neil Cox, Christopher Griffiths, editors. Rook's Textbook of Dermatology. 7th edn. Massachusetts: Blackwell Publishing. 2004;pp.63.72-120.
2. Wadhwa SL, Uday Khopkar, Vandhana Mhaske. Hair and scalp disorders. In: Valia RG, Valia AR, editors. IADVL Textbook and Atlas of Dermatology. 2nd edn. Mumbai: Bhalani Publishing House. 2001;pp.744-51.
3. Cheng AS, Bayliss SJ. The genetics of hair shaft disorders. J Am Acad Dermatol. 2008;59(1):1-22.
4. Itin PH, Schiller P, Mathys D, Guggenheim RJ. Cosmetically induced hair beads. J Am Acad Dermatol. 1997;36:260-1.

5. Rief PH, Patrizi A, Piraccini BM. Autosomal dominant pili torti. Eur J Dermatol. 1996;6:385-7.
6. Emmanuelle Bitoun, Stephane Chavanas, Alan D Irvine. Netherton syndrome: Disease expression and spectrum of SPINK5 mutations in 21 families. J Invest Dermatol. 2002;118:352-61.
7. Powell J. Increasing the likelihood of early diagnosis of Netherton syndrome by simple examination of eyebrow hairs. Arch Dermatol 2000;136(3):423-4.
8. Robert A Schwartz, Bryan D Seiff. Trichorrhexis Nodosa. [Online]. 2008 [cited 2013 Aug 21];Available from: URL:http://www.emedicine.com/derm/topic896.htm.
9. Whiting DA. Structural abnormalities of the hair shaft. J Am Acad Dermatol. 1987;16:1-25.
10. Fichtel JC, Richards JA, Davis LS. Trichorrhexis nodosa secondary to argininosuccinic aciduria. Pediatr Dermatol. 2007;24(1):25-7.
11. Bhushan Kumar, Kumar Vinod Sharma, Surrinder Kaur. Trichorrhexis nodosa confined to the beard hairs. Indian J Dermatol Venereol Leprol [serial online] 1984 [cited 2013 Aug 29];50:113-14. Available from: URL:http://www.ijdvl.com/article.asp?issn=0378-6323/ 1984/50/2/113 =114.
12. Lurie R, Hodak E, Ginzburg A, David M. Trichorrhexis nodosa: A manifestation of hypothyroidism. Cutis. 1996;57(5):358-9.
13. Camacho-Martinez. Localized trichorrhexis nodosa. J Am Acad Dermatol. 1989;20(4):696-7.
14. Christine Liang, Andrea Morris, Sebastian Schlücker, Kyoko Imoto, Vera H Price, Emory Menefee, et al. Structural and molecular hair abnormalities in trichothiodystrophy. J Invest Dermatol. 2006;26:2210-6.
15. Brown AC, Belser RB, Crounse RG, Wehr RF. J Invest Dermatol. A congenital hair defect: Trichoschisis with alternating birefringence and low sulfur content.1970;54(6):496-509.
16. Pasricha JS, Jain GL. Scanning electron microscopy of terminal parts of hair in Indian girls. Indian J Dermatol Venereol Leprol. 1989;55:44-6.
17. Kippax John. A Handbook of Diseases of skin. Delhi: B. Jain Publishers. 2002;p.227.
18. Chris R Halloran. Idiopathic trichoclasis report of a case. Arch Derm Syphilol. 1932;25(2):317-20.
19. Levit F, Scott MJ. Circle hair. J Am Acad Dermatol. 1983;8:423-7.
20. Gummer CL. Bubble hair: A cosmetic abnormality caused by brief, focal heating of damp hair fibres. Br J Dermatol. 1994;131(6):901-3.
21. Detwiler SP, Carson JL, Woosley JT, Gambling TM, Briggaman RA. Bubble hair: A case caused by an overheating hair dryer and reproducibility in normal hair with heat. J Am Acad Dermatol. 1994;30(1):54-60.
22. Krasnoff J, Glusac E, Bolognia JL. Bubblse hair-a possible explanation for its distribution. Int J Dermatol. 1998;37(5):380-2.
23. Savitha AF. Sacchidanad G, Revathy Tn.Lat
24. Elston DM, Bergfeld WF, Whiting DA, McMahon JT, Dawson DM, Quint KL, et al. Bubble hair. J Cutan Pathol. 1992;19(5):439-44.
25. Wallace MP, De Berker DA. Hair diagnoses and signs: the use of dermatoscopy. Clinical and Experimental Dermatology. 2010;35(1):41-6.
26. Khumalo NP, Doe PT, Dawber RP, Ferguson DJ. What is normal black African hair? A light and scanning electron-microscopic study. J Am Acad Dermatol. 2000;43:814-20.
27. Thappa DM, Kumar V, Sharma RC, Lal S. Hair casts. Indian J Dermatol Venereol Leprol. 1993;59:201-2.
28. Keipert JA. Hair casts: Review and suggestion regarding nomenclature. Arch Dermatol. 1986;122(8)927-30.
29. Taïeb A, Surlève-Bazeille JE, Maleville J. Hair casts: A clinical and morphological study. Arch Dermatol. 1985;121:1009-13.
30. Fabbri P, Difonozo EM, Palleschi GM, Pacini P. Hair casts. Int J Dermatol. 1988;27:319-21.
31. França K, Villa RT, Silva IR, de Carvalho CA, Bedin V. Hair casts or pseudonits. Int J Trichol. 2011;3:121-2.
32. Joong Sun Lee, You Chan Kim, Hee Young Kang. The nevoid pili multigemini over the back. Eur J Dermatol. 2005;15(2):99-101.
33. Pili multigemini. [online]. 2007 Aug [cited 20013 sep 8]; Available from: URL:http://en.wikipedia.org/wiki/Pili_multigemini.
34. Janjua SA, McKoy KC, Iftikhar N. Trichostasis spinulosa: Possible association with prolonged topical application of clobetasol propionate 0.05% cream. Int J Dermatol. 2007;46(9):982-5.
35. Sidwell RU, Francis N, Bunker CB. Diffuse trichostasis spinulosa in chronic renal failure. Clin Exp Dermatol. 2006;31(1):86-8.
36. Harford RR, Cobb MW, Miller ML. Trichostasis spinulosa: A clinical simulant of acne open comedones. Pediatr Dermatol. 1996;13(6):490-2.
37. Krivda SJ, Elston DM. Trichostasis spinulosa.[online]. 2012 [cited 2013Aug 21]. Available from :URL:http://emedicine.medscape.com/article/1071782-overview.
38. Bhargava RK, Mukul. Trichostasis spinulosa. Indian J Dermatol Venereol Leprol [serial online] 1987 [cited 2013 15];53:183-184. Available from: URL:http://www.ijdvl.com/searchresult.asp?search/trichostasis+spinulosa&author&journal/.
39. Elston DM, White LC. Treatment of trichostasis spinulosa with a hydroactive adhesive pad. Cutis. 2000;66(1):77-8.
40. Toosi S, Ehsani AH, Noormohammadpoor P, Esmaili N, Mirshams-Shahshahani M, Moineddin F. Treatment of trichostasis spinulosa with a 755-nm long-pulsed alexandrite laser. J Eur Acad Dermatol Venereol. 2009;23.
41. Willimson PJ, de Berker. Pohl-Pinkus constrictions of hair following chemotherapy for Hodgkin's disease. Br J Haematology. 2005;128(5):582.
42. Raymond Bonnett, Rodney PR, Dawber, Dominique Van Neste. Hair and Scalp Disorders: Common Presenting Signs, Differential Diagnosis and Treatment. 2nd edn. USA: Informa Health Care. 2004;pp.68-9.
43. Stroud JD. Hair-shaft anomalies. Dermatol Clin. 1987;5(3):581-94.
44. Zaun H. Differential diagnosis of alopecia in children. In: Happle R, Grosshans E, editors. Pediatric dermatology. New York NY: Springer-Verlag NY Inc. 1987;pp.157-66.
45. Dhurat RP, Deshpande DJ. Loose Anagen hair syndrome. Int J Trichology. 2012;2(2):96-100.

46. Piraccini BM, Tosti A. Loose anagen hair syndrome and loose anagen hair. Arch Dermatol. 2002;38:521-2.
47. Hamm H, Traupe H. Loose anagen hair in childhood: The phenomenon of easily pluckable hair. J Am Acad Dermatol. 1989;20:242-8.
48. Abdel-Raouf H, El-Din WH, Awad SS, Esmat A, Al-Khiat M, Abdel-Wahab H, et al. Loose anagen hair syndrome in children of upper Egypt. J Cosmet Dermatol. 2009;8:103-7.
49. Chong AH, Sinclair R. Loose anagen syndrome: A prospective study of three families. Aust J Dermatol. 2002;43:120-4.
50. Sperling LC. Loose Anagen Hair syndrome. In An Atlas of Hair Pathology with Clinical Correlations. 1st edn. USA: Parthenon Publishing Group. 2005;pp.155-62.
51. Tosti A, Piraccini BM. Loose anagen hair syndrome and loose anagen hair. Arch Dermatol. 2002;138:521-2.
52. Tosti A, Peluso AM, Misciali C, Venturo N, Patrizi A, Fanti PA. Loose anagen hair. Arch Dermatol. 1997;133:1089-93.
53. Mallon E, Dawber RP, De Berker D, Ferguson DJ. Cheveux incoiffables-diagnostic, clinical and hair microscopic findings, and pathogenic studies. Br J Dermatol. 1994;131(5):608-14.
54. Hicks J, Metry DW, Barrish J, Levy M. Uncombable hair (cheveux incoiffables, pili trianguli et canaliculi) syndrome: brief review and role of scanning electron microscopy in diagnosis. Ultrastruct Pathol. 2001;25(2):99-103.
55. Itin PH, Buhler U, Buchner SA, Guggenheim R. Pili trianguli et canaliculi: a distinctive hair shaft defect leading to uncombable hair. Dermatology. 1993;187(4):296-8.
56. Hicks J, Metry DW, Barrish J, Levy M. Uncombable hair (cheveux incoiffables, pili trianguli et canaliculi) syndrome: brief review and role of scanning electron microscopy in diagnosis. Ultrastruct Pathol. 2001;25(2):99-103.
57. Kevin. Grooved hair. [Online]. [Cited 2008 Sep 15];Available from: URL:http://www.keratin.com/ag/ag004.shtml.
58. Prasad GK. Familial woolly hair. Indian J Dermatol Venereol Leprol. 2002;68:157.
59. Mortimer PS, Gummer C, English J, Dawber RP. Acquired progressive kinking of hair. Report of six cases and review of literature. Arch Dermatol. 1985;121(8):1031-3.
60. Rai R, Ramachandran B, Sundaram VS, Rajendren G, Srinivas CR. Naxos disease: A rare occurrence of cardiomyopathy with woolly hair and palmoplantar keratoderma. Indian J Dermatol Venereol Leprol. 2008;74:50-2.
61. http://dermnetnz.org/hair-nails-sweat/hair-shaft-defects.html.
62. Jack Green, Elizabeth Fitzpatrick, David de Berker, Susan Forrest M, Rodney Sinclair D. A gene for pili annulati maos to the telomeric region of chromosome 12q. J Invest Dermatol. 2004;123(6):1070-2.
63. Feldmann KA, Dawber RP, Pittelkow MR, Ferguson DJ. Newly described weathering pattern in pili annulati hair shafts: A scanning electron microscopic study. J Am Acad Dermatol. 2001;45(4):625-7.
64. Pasricha JS, Nigam PK, Banerjee U. White piedra in Delhi. Indian J Dermatol Venereol Leprol. 1990;56:56-7.
65. Morewitz H. A Brief History of Plica Polonica. [Online]. 2008 [cited 2008 Aug 28]; [6]. Available from: URL:http://nuvoforheadlice.com/Plica.htm.
66. Pavithran K. Plica neuropathica causing traction alopecia. Indian J Dermatol Venereol Leprol. 1990;56:141-2.
67. Le Page JE. Neuropathica plica. Br Med J. 1884;1:160.
68. Pushpa Gnanaraj, Venugopal V, Pandurangan CN. Plica polonica in association with pediculosis capitis and scabies—A case report. Int J Dermatol. 2007;46(2):151-2.
69. Kwinter J, Weinstein M. Plica neuropathica: Novel presentation of a rare disease. Clin Exp Dermatol. 2006;31:790-2.
70. Smith VV, Anderson G, Malone M, Sebire NJ. Light microscopic examination of scalp hair samples as an aid in the diagnosis of paediatric disorders: Retrospective review of more than 300 cases from a single centre. J Clin Pathol. 2005;58(12): 1294-8.
71. Jones LN. Hair structure anatomy and comparative anatomy. Clin Dermatol. 2001;19:95-103.
72. Dongre A, Bhisey P, Khopkar U. Polarized light microscopy. Indian J Dermatol Venereol Leprol. 2007;73:206-8.
73. Gupta LK, Singhi MK. Wood's lamp. Indian J Dermatol Venereol Leprol. 2004;70:131-5.

6

Bacterial Infections of Hair and Scalp

Leelavathy B, Eswari L

"The appearance of a disease is swift as an arrow; its disappearance slow, like a thread".

—*Chinese proverb*

Introduction

Bacterial infections of hair and scalp are very common, varying from folliculitis, furuncles, carbuncles to secondary infections. They are easily treatable but recurrence is a problem.

Scalp anatomy has an important bearing in understanding the outcome of scalp infections **(Box 6.1)**. Of the five layers of scalp (skin, connective tissue, galea aponeurotica, loose connective tissue and pericranium), the first three layers move as a single unit. Access to the subgaleal space may permit extensive spread of infection. Scalp is richly vascular, conferring a natural resistance to infection and also providing a potential route for hematogenous spread from other locations. The extensive anastomosis of vessels of the scalp, face and neck allow retrograde extension of scalp infections. Lymphatics form a rich network in the neighborhood of the vertex, and enlarged, tender lymph nodes may indicate an occult scalp infection.

Box 6.1: Scalp en route to infection

- Five layers: Skin, connective tissue, galea aponeurotica, loose connective tissue, and pericranium
- Break in subgaleal space permits extensive spread of infection
- Rich vascularity: Potential route for hematogenous spread
- Extensive anastomosis: Retrograde extension of scalp infections

Classification

Bacterial infections of the hair and scalp can be classified as given in **Table 6.1**.

Table 6.1: Classification of bacterial infections

Primary bacterial infections
1. Folliculitis
2. Furuncle
3. Carbuncle
4. Sycosis and lupoid sycosis
5. Erysipelas and scalp cellulitis
6. Trichomycosis axillaris and pubis

Secondary bacterial infections
1. Secondary bacterial infections following fungal and arthropod diseases of scalp
2. Infections following operative procedures of scalp
3. Scalp infections in neonates following intrauterine fetal monitoring devices

Diseases of the scalp due to presumed bacterial etiology
1. Folliculitis keloidalis
2. Acne necrotica miliaris
3. Acne necrotica varioliformis
4. Folliculitis decalvans
5. Tufted folliculitis
6. Dissecting cellulitis of scalp

Miscellaneous bacterial infections
1. Syphilis
2. Mycobacterial infections

Folliculitis

Folliculitis is the inflammation of one or more hair follicles and can occur on any hair bearing areas of the skin. Causes can be fungal, bacterial or viral. Folliculitis can be superficial or deep, depending on the depth of infection **(Table 6.2)**. Bacterial folliculitis can be classified as:

1. *Staphylococcus aureus* folliculitis
   - Superficial folliculitis (follicular impetigo or Bockhart's impetigo)
2. Deep folliculitis (sycosis)
3. *Pseudomonas aeruginosa* folliculitis (hot tub folliculitis)
4. Gram negative folliculitis
5. Syphilitic folliculitis.

Superficial Folliculitis (Figure 6.1) (Box 6.2)

These are usually small follicular papules or pinhead sized pustules. Here the inflammatory changes are confined to the ostium of the pilosebaceous canal or extend slightly below. They heal without scarring. Isolated lesions of folliculitis may occur on the scalp, beard, neck, buttocks, and thighs which go unnoticed usually. Culture of these lesions yield coagulase negative *Staphylococcus*.

Staphylococcus aureus superficial folliculitis, also called as Bockhart's impetigo **(Figure 6.2) (Box 6.3)** is an infection of the ostium/infundibulum of hair follicles. Application of potent topical steroids for a long time is a predisposing factor. It is common in childhood, occurs on scalp and scalp margins, also in beard area, axilla, extremities and buttocks. They are dome shaped yellow pustules with surrounding erythema, occurring in crops and heal within 7 to 10 days. Some lesions may become deep and chronic and some may merge imperceptibly with folliculitis decalvans and other related processes.

Chronic folliculitis of legs is seen in the middle aged males in India. The lesions are profuse in number, may be superficial or deep, common on thighs and legs. *Staphylococcus aureus* is the organism mostly isolated.

The pustular dermatitis atrophicans of the legs,[1] described as accounting for 0.5% of skin diseases in Lagos

Table 6.2: Comparison between superficial and deep folliculitis

Superficial folliculitis	*Deep folliculitis*
Involves upper portion of hair follicles	Involves entire or deep portion of the hair follicles
Small tender/nontender pruritic papules and pustules which heal without scarring	Erythematous, tender papules, pustules, and nodules, may heal with scarring
Example: Staphylococcal folliculitis	Example: Furuncle, carbuncle, sycosis barbae, scalp sycosis, gram-negative folliculitis, pseudomonas folliculitis

Box 6.2: Variants of superficial folliculitis

- Bockhart's impetigo
- Chronic folliculitis of legs
- Pustular dermatitis atrophicans of the legs
- Community-acquired methicillin resistant staphylococcal infections

Box 6.3: Bockhart's impetigo

- Infection of the ostium/infundibulum of hair follicles
- Application of potent topical steroids for a long time is a predisposing factor
- Common in childhood
- Crops of dome shaped yellow pustules with surrounding erythema, heal within 7 to 10 days on scalp, beard area, axillae, extremities and buttocks

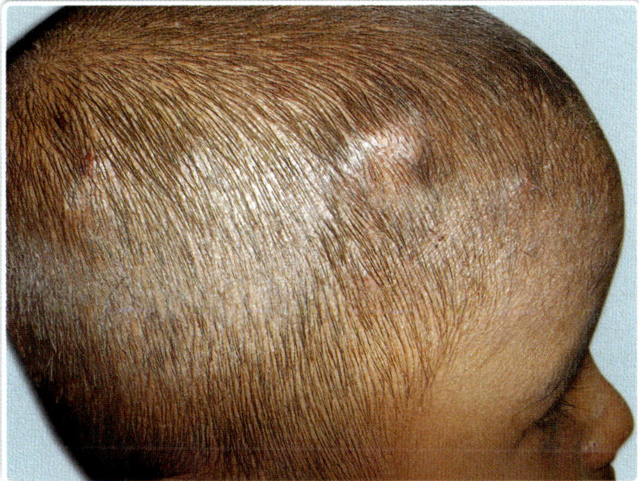

Fig. 6.1: Superficial folliculitis of scalp

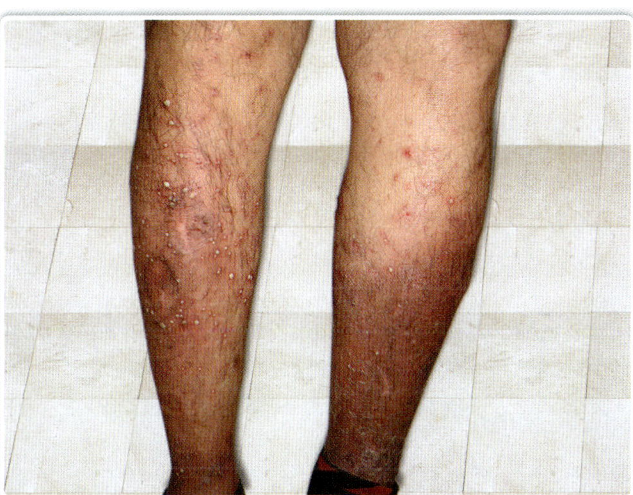

Fig. 6.2: Bockhart's impetigo

in West Africa, appears to be a similar condition. It is predominantly seen on the anterior tibial surface of the legs in males. The pustules usually heal with atrophic scars.

Community-acquired methicillin resistant staphylococcal infections (CAMRSA) may present with folliculitis or an abscess. They are common in athletes, military personnel and prisoners.

Histopathology

It is a subcorneal pustule, situated at the opening of the hair follicle. The upper portion of the hair follicle is surrounded by considerable inflammatory infiltrate composed predominantly of neutrophils.

Diagnosis

Follicular pustules are cultured, not by deroofing the pustule and taking swab, but by scraping off the entire pustule with a No. 15 blade and depositing the material onto the cotton swab of a transport medium kit.

Differential Diagnosis

Pustular miliaria, subcorneal pustular dermatoses.

Treatment

Mild folliculitis usually subsides by cleansing or topical antibiotics. Sometimes they may be self limiting. More severe infections are treated with topical or systemic antibiotics. In chronic conditions, carrier state must be sought for and managed. Hand washing and avoiding sharing of personal clothing will go in a long way in preventing such infections. Daily application of 6.25% aluminum chloride hexahydrate in completely anhydrous ethyl alcohol was reported to be very effective treatment for chronic folliculitis of unspecified type (except for scalp lesions).[2]

Deep Folliculitis

In deep folliculitis the entire hair follicle or the deeper portion of the hair follicle is affected.

Sycosis Barbae

[Greek: Sycosis - ripe fig]. This is a sub acute or chronic pyogenic deep folliculitis with perifollicular inflammation occurring in the beard and upper lip area. They present as deep seated pustules **(Box 6.4)**.

Box 6.4: Sycosis barbae

- Sub-acute or chronic pyogenic deep folliculitis with perifollicular inflammation
- Causative agent: *Staphylococcus aureus*
- Seborrheic diathesis and greasy skin are the predisposing factors
- Groups of papules studded on an elevated plaque which resembles a ripe fig
- Can be recurrent and chronic

Etiopathogenesis

Commonly affects males after puberty. *Staphylococcus aureus* is the causative organism. Seborrheic diathesis and greasy skin are the predisposing factors. Clerical and indoor workers who work in an environment with no fresh open air are commonly affected.

Clinical Features **(Figure 6.3)**

Follicular oriented papules and/or pustules are seen. There is perifollicular edema. They may be discrete or groups of papules studded on an elevated plaque which resembles a ripe fig, and hence the name. Scaling and crusting can occur but scar formation is rare. The lesions can be recurrent and chronic, sometimes persisting for as long as 20 years.

Histopathology

There is perifollicular infiltrate composed largely of neutrophils. Lymphoid cells, histiocytes and plasma cells may also be seen. Later perifollicular abscess forms and destroys the hair and hair follicles. Older lesions show chronic granulation tissue, usually heal with fibrosis.

Lupoid Sycosis

In this condition, the follicular papules and pustules heal with severe scarring. Multiple active infected follicles are seen in the advancing margin of the atrophic scar. The papules show granulomatous inflammatory change and hence the name 'lupoid'. Sites involved commonly are the front of ears, chin, scalp, axillary and pubic area, lower legs,

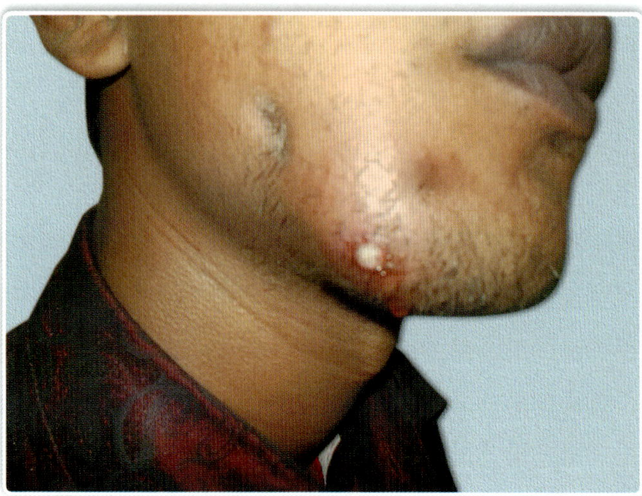

Fig. 6.3: Sycosis barbae

Box 6.5: Lupoid sycosis

- Follicular papules and pustules heal with severe scarring
- Histologically granulomatous inflammatory change (lupoid)
- Sites: Front of ears, chin, scalp, axillary and pubic area, lower legs, thighs and arms
- Chronic forms, treat with topical antibiotics and steroids
- Resistant cases, systemic antibiotics can be given for 10 to 14 days
- Nasopharyngeal sepsis to be managed to prevent the chronicity of infection

thighs and arms. Scalp can be extensively involved. This condition tends to persist indefinitely **(Box 6.5)**.

Differential Diagnosis

Pseudofolliculitis barbae, mycotic sycosis, lupus vulgaris.

Treatment

Subacute forms usually are treated with topical antibiotic creams. Chronic forms are treated with a combination of topical antibiotics and steroids for a long time. In resistant cases, systemic antibiotics can be given for 10 to 14 days. Chronic carrier state and chronic nasopharyngeal sepsis must be managed to prevent the chronicity of infection.

Furuncle

[Latin: furuncle-boil]. It is a deep seated inflammatory nodule around a hair follicle developing usually from a preceding superficial folliculitis and may evolve into an abscess.

Etiopathogenesis

Caused by *Staphylococcus aureus*, usually occurs on hair bearing sites such as nape of neck, axilla, face and buttocks. Mostly affects males, in adolescence or early adulthood. Local predisposing factors are pre-existing dermatoses like atopic dermatitis, abrasions, excoriations, scabies or pediculosis. Systemic host factors like obesity, blood dyscrasias, diabetes, defective neutrophil function, immunoglobulin deficiency states and treatment with glucocorticoids and cytotoxic agents may all play a role. Malnutrition can be an important predisposing factor, and is also common in patients infected with HIV.

Recent epidemics of furunculosis, attributable to specific strains of staphylococci have occurred. Many of these have been associated with community-acquired staphylococcal infections. In a French study, patients with furunculosis showed staphylococci in the majority of swabs, and 42% of the isolates had Panton-Valentine leukocidin (PVL) genes present **(Box 6.6)**. These were associated with epidemic furunculosis. Nasal carrier state of staphylococci is responsible for chronicity and recurrence of furunculosis. The observation of families over a period of years showed that the same phage type may be responsible for irregular episodes of infection between long intervals of clinical quiescence.[3]

Box 6.6: Panton-Valentine leukocidin (PVL)

- Predominant Genes in staphylocci found to be responsible for furunculosis
- Associated with epidemic furunculosis
- May be responsible for irregular episodes of infection between long intervals of clinical quiescence

Histopathology

Furuncles usually affect vellus hair. There is an area of perifollicular necrosis containing fibrinoid material and many neutrophils. At the deep end of necrotic plug, in the subcutis, there is an abscess. Gram stain of pus from the center of the abscess shows clusters of staphylococci.

Clinical Features

There is a hard tender folliculocentric inflammatory nodule which later develops into a painful abscess. Abscess becomes fluctuant and ruptures, discharging pus and the necrotic core, leaving a permanent scar. The entire process may take 2 days to 2 weeks. The lesions may be single or multiple, associated with mild constitutional symptoms like fever. Furuncles occurring on the upper lip region and cheek may lead to cavernous sinus thrombosis, which is a dangerous and rare complication. There can be recurrent and chronic attacks at irregular intervals. In HIV disease, furuncles may coalesce into violaceous plaques **(Figure 6.4)**.[4]

Differential Diagnosis

Disseminated herpes simplex, halogen eruptions, cystic acne, kerion, hidradenitis suppurativa, ruptured epidermal inclusion cyst, furuncular myiasis.

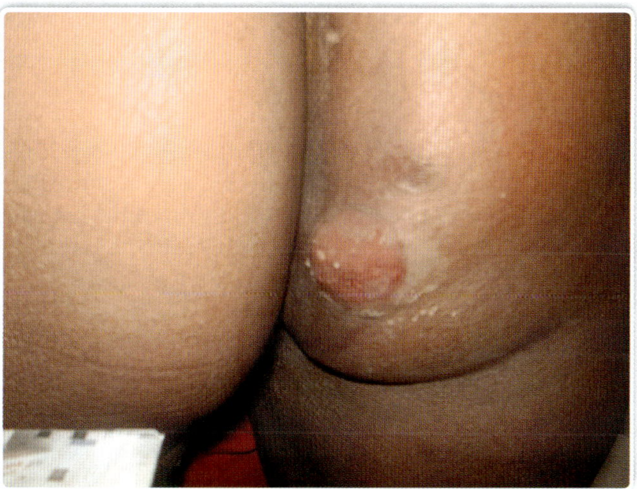

Fig. 6.4: Furuncle

Prognosis

The course can be recurrent and chronic if left untreated. Where CAMRSA is prevalent, systemic infections such as bacterial endocarditis can occur.

Treatment

Simple furunculosis may be aided by local application of moist heat. Each episode must be treated systematically with oral antibiotics like dicloxacillin, cotrimoxazole, ciprofloxacin or minocycline. Topical antibiotic will take care of the surrounding contamination. Nasal and perineal carriage of *Staphylococcal aureus* must be sought for and managed. Addition of rifampicin[5] or intravenous gammaglobulin to neutralize the toxin may be helpful.[6] Antimicrobial therapy should be continued until all signs of inflammation regress.

Management of Recurrent Furunculosis

1. Underlying predisposing factors must be managed.
2. General skin care measures must be undertaken.
3. Sharing of personal clothing should be avoided.
4. General measures like stress free life and living in a cool dry climate may help a long way.
5. Nasal carriage of *Staphylococcus aureus* must be eliminated by topical application of antibiotics in the nasal vestibule. Intranasal application of 2% mupirocin calcium ointment for 5 days can eliminate *S.aureus* nasal carriage in 70% of healthy individuals for 3 months.
6. In patients where all measures have failed oral antibiotics like Rifampicin, 600 mg daily for 10 days have been effective in eradicating *S.aureus* from most nasal carriers for almost 12 weeks.
7. Adding other oral antibiotics can prevent emergence of Rifampicin resistance and to treat recurrent furunculosis.

Carbuncle

[Latin: carbuncle- small fiery coal]. It is a deep extensive infection of contiguous hair follicles accompanied by intense inflammatory reaction of the surrounding and underlying connective tissues including subcutaneous fat. It occurs when multiple closely set furuncles coalesce.

Etiopathogenesis

Affects men above middle age. Commonly seen in the presence of diabetes, malnutrition, cardiac failure, drug addiction or severe generalized dermatoses, such as exfoliative dermatitis or pemphigus and during prolonged steroid therapy.

Clinical Features

Usually starts of as a single smooth dome shaped nodule, which is tender and inflamed. Later, enlarges in size and suppurates with discharge from multiple follicular orifices. The intervening skin undergoes necrosis and a yellow gray crateriform nodule is formed. After the discharge of the central core a deep ulcer is left behind with a purulent floor. The resulting scar is very deep and evident. Nape of the neck, back, thighs are the most common sites of occurrence.

Constitutional symptoms like fever, malaise may occur. Sometimes death may occur due to toxemia or metastatic infection **(Figure 6.5)**.

Differential diagnosis: Anthrax.

Treatment: Systemic antibiotics like flucloxacillin and other penicillinase resistant antibiotics must be given. Underlying conditions like diabetes has to be treated.

Gram Negative Folliculitis **(Figure 6.6)**

First reported in 1968 by Fulton, et al. in a group of patients with acne vulgaris, resistant to conventional treatments. Gram-negative folliculitis (GNF) is a hair follicle infection by Gram-negative organism; can occur as a complication in patients receiving broad spectrum antibiotics for prolonged periods, as in the treatment of acne vulgaris and rosacea.

Etiopathogenesis: Prolonged treatment with broad-spectrum antibiotics alters the normal bacterial flora of the nasal mucosa and adjacent skin with reduced gram-positive bacteria and coagulase positive aerobic diphtheroids, with an increase in gram-negative bacilli mainly enteric bacteria. It is well known that tetracyclines, the most commonly used systemic antibiotic in acne and rosacea, impair protein synthesis and function of

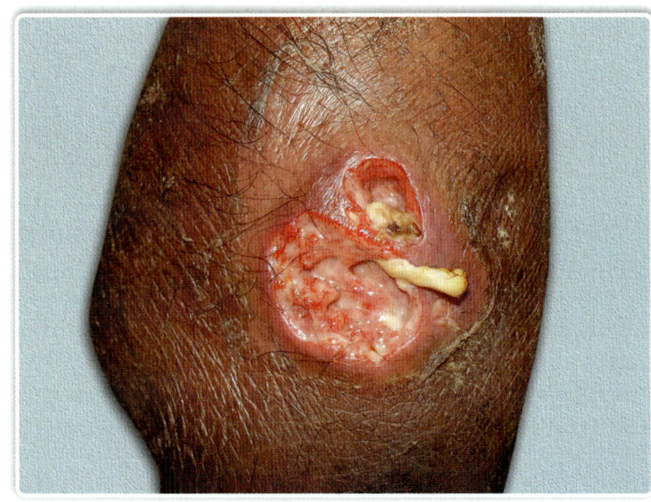

Fig. 6.5: Carbuncle

lymphocytes and neutrophil chemotaxis, thus increasing the risk of bacterial infections.

Clinical features: Characteristic features include:

- Predominance in males
- Severe seborrhea
- Papules, pustules and perinasal and/or perioral involvement
- Recurrent folliculitis of the scalp
- Prolonged antibacterial pre-treatment
- Shortened asymptomatic intervals
- Gram-negative bacteria isolated in cultures.

Leyden, et al.[7] clinically differentiated two types of GNF. The type I, superficial or pustular form, is the most common (80–90%), with presence of multiple papules and pustules in the middle of the face, 3 to 6 mm in diameter with an erythematous halo, mainly caused by *E.coli, Klebsiella* sp., *Enterobacter* species and *P. aeruginosa*. The type II, deep or nodular (10–20%), is characterized by deep and painful inflammatory nodules or cysts, on the face, neck and/or chest, caused by *Proteus mirabilis* **(Box 6.7)**. Sebaceous follicles are colonized with these bacteria, mainly in the perioral and perinasal zone, with subsequent follicular and perifollicular inflammation with formation of papules and pustules.

Diagnosis: Confirmed with a smear from pustules. The lesions (pustules) and the anterior nasal mucosa should be sampled for bacteriological studies.

Box 6.7: Common organisms causing GNF

- *E.coli* (Type 1)
- *Klebsiella sp* (Type 1)
- *Enterobacter species* (Type 1)
- *P. aeruginosa* (Type 1)
- *Proteus mirabilis (Type 2)*

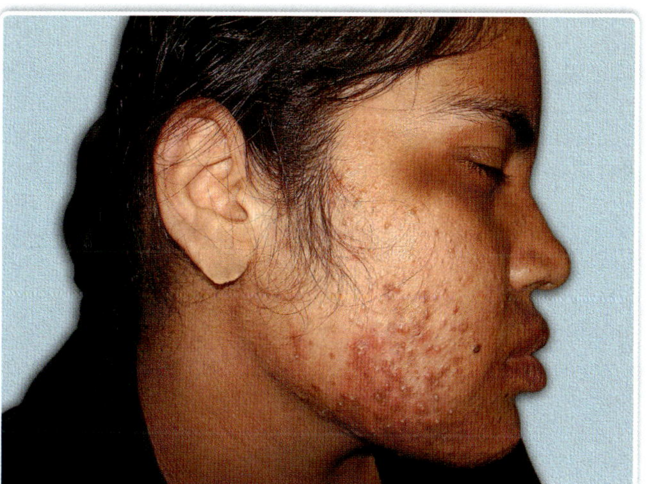

Fig. 6.6: Gram negative folliculitis

Treatment: Conventional broad spectrum antibiotics must be withdrawn. Oral isotretinoin is the treatment of choice—0.5 to 1mg/kg/day for a period of 4–5 months. The therapeutic success of isotretinoin is due to decreased secretion of the sebaceous glands and reduction of the follicular space size and anti-inflammatory effect, making it non-conducive for the growth of gram-negative bacteria. The most effective dose with a lower recurrence rate is 1mg/kg/day. Systemic antibiotics such as cephalosporins combined with oral isotretinoin for 2 weeks are often useful in patients with frequent relapses.[8] Ampicillin and trimethoprim-sulfamethoxazole can also be given. The clinical course determines the time of withdrawal of the antibiotics.

Pseudomonas Aeruginosa Folliculitis/ Hot Tub Folliculitis

Folliculitis caused by *Pseudomonas aeruginosa* is a rare, adverse effect of therapeutic or recreational use of hot tubs, whirlpools (Jacuzzis), spa pools, saunas, and occasionally swimming pools, water slides and physiotherapy pools. *P. aeruginosa* thrives in warm and moist areas and is commonly found in soil, sinks and drains, shower-floors, carpets and even tap water. *Pseudomonas aeruginosa* is able to withstand relatively high temperatures and high chlorine levels. The organism colonizes the overhydrated stratum corneum of the follicular ostia **(Figure 6.7)**.

Clinical features: Symptoms usually appear 8–48 hours after exposure, quite often with multiple members of a family being affected. The rash is usually itchy and polymorphous, with erythematous macules, papules, vesicles and pustules. The areas most affected are those covered by the bathing suit. The head and neck are rarely affected. There may be associated conjunctivitis, pharyngitis and, occasionally, swollen and painful breasts, abdominal symptoms and lymphadenopathy.

Differential diagnosis: Acne, bromide sensitivity, staphylococcal folliculitis, gram-negative folliculitis.

Diagnosis: *Pseudomonas aeruginosa* can often be cultured from papules and pustules on the skin.

Treatment: Mild cases of hot tub folliculitis are typically self-limiting, resolving in a few days, and do not require treatment. Severe cases may require treatment with topical or systemic antibiotics specific for gram-negative organism, including gentamicin cream, polymyxin B spray, and oral ciprofloxacin. Proper maintenance and control of the pH and disinfectant levels in the water pools will prevent the growth of *Pseudomonas aeruginosa*.

Erysipelas and Scalp Cellulitis

Erysipelas is an infection of the upper dermis usually caused by Group A Streptococci. The scalp can be involved

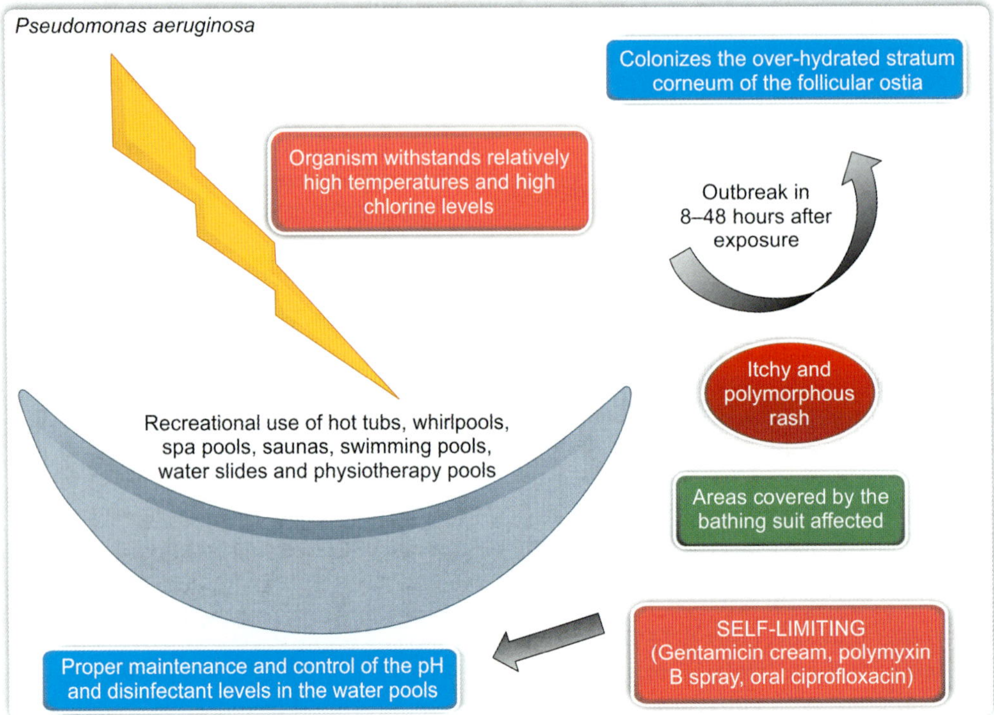

Fig. 6.7: Schematic representation of hot tub folliculitis: Etiopathogenesis, clinical features and management

due to extension of infection from the face or pinna or due to a scalp wound or a chronic skin condition. Clinically, a well-demarcated erythematous plaque is seen, associated with fever. Lymphadenopathy can be associated. An acute telogen effluvium can follow. Lymphedema predisposes to this infection.

Cellulitis or infection involving the deep dermis and subcutaneous fat can be caused by *Streptococcus pyogenes* and/or *Staphylcoccus aureus* or MRSA. Entry for the bacteria can be a scalp wound, scalp surgery, or a chronic skin condition. Diffuse, poorly demarcated erythema, heat, swelling, and pain are the hallmarks of cellulitis **(Box 6.8)**. Systemic symptoms and lymphadenopathy can also be associated. Laboratory investigations of cellulitis rarely identify a specific causative organism.

Diagnosis is clinical, with possible identification of the infecting agent on skin swabs and cultures. Blood cultures are recommended in elderly patients with fever and leukocytosis as well as in immunocompromised patients.

For both erysipelas and cellulitis, treatment with systemic antibiotics is required.

Box 6.8: Clinical hallmark of cellulitis

- Diffuse
- Poorly demarcated erythema
- Heat/warm
- Swelling
- Pain/tender

Necrotizing Fasciitis of Scalp

It is a rapidly progressive, highly destructive, fatal bacterial invasion of the subcutaneous and subgaleal spaces. Spread is limited by the scalp attachments: The supra orbital ridges anteriorly, and the occipital protuberance posteriorly. It commonly occurs spontaneously, following minor trauma, and may present following craniotomy. Neonatal necrotizing fasciitis of the scalp has been reported in association with intrapartum fetal scalp electrode monitoring.

There is a diffuse patch of erythema which progresses and rapidly undermines the scalp with widespread necrosis. It is associated with severe toxemia. There is sloughing and ulceration due to vascular thrombosis in the subcutaneous tissue and deep dermis. The entire calvaria may be denuded as the pericranium becomes incorporated into a layer of thick fibrous tissue. Bacteriology shows multiple organisms, often *Staphylococcus epidermidis, Staphylococcus aureus,* and *Streptococcus* species. Immediate generous debridement, with copious antibiotic irrigation of the subgaleal space is advocated. Multiple postoperative inspections and debridement are usually necessary with a planned second-look operation after the first 24 hours. Split skin grafting can then be applied after 2 weeks. Systemic toxicity must be treated aggressively. Mortality may be from multiple organ failure but commonly there is septic shock, cardiac failure and respiratory failure. Hyperbaric oxygen may help in the treatment of necrotizing fasciitis.

Trichomycosis Axillaris and Pubis

It is also known as trichomycosis nodosa. The term trichomycosis is a misnomer because the causative agent of this condition is not a fungus. This is a superficial bacterial infection of axillary and pubic hair with yellow, black or red adherent granular nodules on the hair shaft. These nodules contain tightly packed bacteria. They grow between and within cuticular cells of hair shaft and may invade the cortex.

Etiology

It is common in hot, damp and tropical climate. As a rule, it disappears spontaneously once a person returns to temperate environment. It can occur in any sex or race. Hyperhidrosis is a predisposing factor. The causative agent is aerobic corynebacteria with no particular species like *Corynebacterium tenuis*, which was once believed to be the causative agent. The changes in the chemical environment of the organism are responsible for the pigment production, imparting different colors to the nodules like yellow black or red.

Clinical Features

Patients are usually unaware of its presence as it is asymptomatic. Yellow, black or red waxy concretions are present, adherent to the hair shaft imparting same color to the sweat as the concretions and thus staining clothes. Yellow type is the most common. Hair is usually brittle, breaks easily and the underlying skin is normal. Pubic hair is less commonly affected. Corynebacterial infections like erythrasma and pitted keratolysis may coexist in some patients **(Figure 6.8)**.

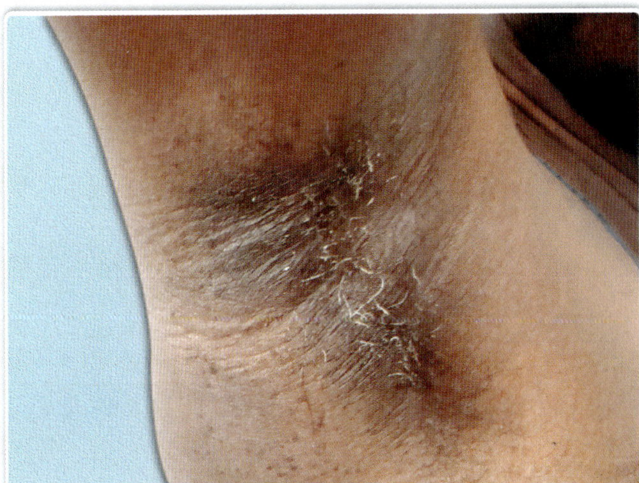

Fig. 6.8: Trichomycosis axillaris

Differential Diagnosis

Pediculosis pubis, piedra.

Laboratory Diagnosis

These are gram-positive organisms. For culture, the hair sample must be surface sterilized by immersing in 70% alcohol. Incubation at 37°C in blood agar is recommended. Light microscopy and ultrastructural studies, together with various stains, have shown that a variety of coryneforms adhere to the hair shaft and some are encapsulated in an extracellular encasing. This was analogous to glucan, synthesized by streptococci, which is responsible for the adhesion.[9]

Treatment

Affected hair should be removed by shaving. Benzoyl peroxide washes and gel are used for treating and also preventing recurrences. Benzoic acid compound ointment or 1% aqueous formalin, are also effective. Antiperspirants such as anhydrous aluminium chloride are also helpful. Erythromycin can also be used.

Postoperative Scalp Infections

Postoperative scalp infections usually occur following post-hair transplant procedures and neurosurgeries.

Though infections are rare after hair transplantation, localized folliculitis can occur occasionally at the graft site. This usually presents as small red pustules several days or weeks following transplant procedure. Treatment consists of de-roofing the pustule and probing the site for any ingrown hair. Patients should be reassured that folliculitis is a simple condition and will not affect the graft. Topical or systemic antibiotics should be prescribed for a prolonged period.

The scalp is a common site for infections in neurosurgery procedures. Preoperative evaluation of a craniotomy patient should include scalp examination. Any evidence of infection should be treated prior to the interventional procedures. Elderly males with a postoperative cerebrospinal fluid (CSF) leak were found to be at risk for scalp infections following neurosurgical procedures.

Propionibacterium acnes is increasingly recognized as a causative organism in post-neurosurgical infections. It is part of the normal skin flora, especially of the scalp, and is therefore a common contaminant of scalp wound swabs. Methicillin-resistant *Staphylococcus aureus* (MRSA) is a well known nosocomial pathogen that can cause soft tissue infections such as abscesses and cellulitis and should always be considered as a potential pathogen in scalp infections. The rate of community-acquired MRSA (CA-MRSA) infections is also on the rise. Culture and antimicrobial sensitivity should be obtained and appropriate antibiotic therapy initiated. Intravenous vancomycin or linezolid, is a highly effective treatment option for MRSA-positive wounds.

Infection in Scalp Lacerations

Most scalp wounds heal satisfactorily, including those that are grossly contaminated at the time of closure. Any delay in debridement increases the risk of infection. Unfortunately, minor scalp wounds are usually ignored, and these may result in serious infections. Principles to be followed in managing scalp lacerations are:

- The entire scalp must be inspected thoroughly and cleansed to remove debris
- The depth of the wound must be assessed for penetrating wounds
- Any CSF leak—a skull fracture with dural tear to be suspected
- The wound must be thoroughly cleansed with a sterile solution and foreign material and devitalized tissue removed. Tetanus prophylaxis should be administered.

Scalp Infections in Neonates

Since head is the common presenting part of the baby during parturition, the scalp is prone to trauma and infections. Secondary bacterial infections are usually caused by injuries inflicted by instrumentation, especially the use of scalp electrodes for monitoring fetal heart rate. Infections following placement of intrauterine fetal monitoring (IFM) devices is between 0.1% to 5.2%. Gonococcal scalp infections have also occurred via such portal of entry. Trauma from forceps and aplasia cutis may also be responsible. Other predisposing factors include prolonged duration of monitoring, prolonged rupture of membranes, vaginal contamination by feces, puerperal infections. Scalp abscess has been noted among infants delivered by vacuum extraction.

Clinical infection varies from a solitary pustule to abscess, cellulitis, necrotising fasciitis and osteomyelitis. Most bacterial infections are evident within few days after birth, whereas anaerobic infections may take several days or weeks to present. Sensitive culture techniques have revealed a polymicrobial etiology like *S.aureus, S.epidermidis,* β Hemolytic streptococci, *Hemophilus influenza* type B, *Neisseria gonorrhea, Pseudomonas, Klebsiella* and many anaerobes.

Many bacterial infections of the fetal scalp resolve spontaneously, if not, incision and drainage is necessary; extensive debridement should not be performed. However, if surrounding cellulitis is present, a 5- to 7-day course of parenteral antibiotic therapy is usually sufficient, with culture results guiding antibiotic choice. If insufficiently treated, osteomyelitis of the occipital bone, meningitis, and sepsis may all occur as sequelae. IFM devices should be avoided in fetuses of mothers infected with gonorrhea, amnionitis, endometritis and the ones who have undergone repeated per vaginal examinations.

Diseases of the Scalp Due to Presumed Bacterial Etiology

Folliculitis Keloidalis [Synonym: Acne Keloidalis] (Figure 6.9)

It is a chronic inflammatory process involving the hair follicles of the nape of the neck, presenting as papules and plaques with hypertrophic scarring. Although, infection is not the primary etiology, *Staphylococcus aureus* is frequently isolated from the lesions. Black pubertal males are usually affected.

Clinical Features

Multiple follicular oriented papules or pustules are seen on the nape of the neck sometimes extending on to the scalp and hence called acne keloidalis nuchae. These lesions may undergo hypertrophy forming keloidal papules or plaques. Mild burning or itching may be present. They are usually chronic with underlying abscess and sinus formation. New crops of lesions keep occurring at irregular intervals.

Histopathology

There is chronic perifollicular inflammation, with follicular destruction, lamellar fibrosis and acute inflammatory infiltrate around degenerating follicles. Foreign body

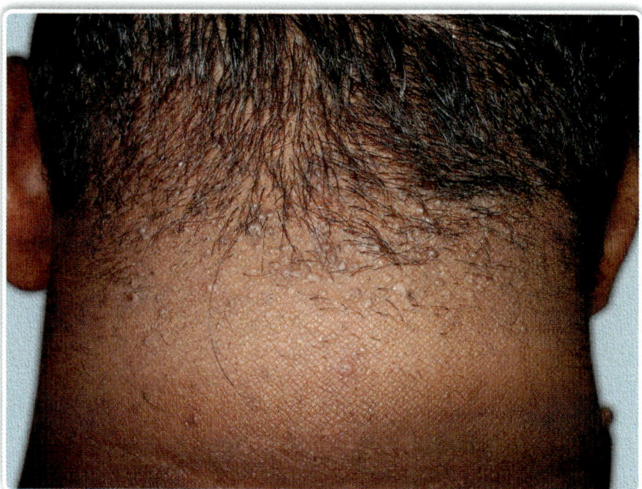

Fig. 6.9: Acne keloidalis

reaction to hair and follicular remnants occurs. All these suggest that follicular antigens like bacteria and skin flora stimulate inflammatory reaction destroying sebaceous glands and follicles, resulting in scarring.

Differential Diagnosis

Folliculitis decalvans; acne necrotica; dissecting folliculitis; bacterial, fungal, or viral folliculitis.

Treatment

A bacterial etiology has never been proven but acne keloidalis usually responds to short or long term courses of oral antibiotics. Different classes of antibiotics may have to be tried for long periods before control is achieved. Cephalosporins, trimethoprim-sulfamethoxazole, dicloxacillin, and amoxicillin-clavulanate potassium have been successful in individual cases. Frequent haircuts, and shaving too close to skin must be avoided. Intralesional steroids reduces scarring and inflammation. If medical management is unsatisfactory, then excision of the affected area with grafting can be done or allow it to it heal by secondary intention.

Acne Necrotica

It is a chronic necrotizing folliculitis mainly involving the scalp margins, which evolves into small round scars. This is called acne necrotica varioliformis. Similar kinds of lesions occurring on entire scalp but with not much of a scarring is called acne necrotica miliaris **(Figures 6.10A and B)**.

Etiopathogenesis

Commonly affects people with seborrheic diathesis. Men between 30 to 40 years of age are commonly affected. Widely suggested pathogens are *Staphylococcus aureus* and *Propionibacterium acnes*. But the disease is mainly due to the host response mechanisms. *Staphylococcus aureus* is frequently isolated from the surface swabs which may be a contaminant or secondary pathogen because, treatment with antibiotics is often disappointing. Emotional disturbances have been a frequent finding in some studies; it has been suggested that repeated excoriation of lesions of a primary folliculitis leads to more destructive changes.[10] *Propionibacterium acnes* play a major role in acne necrotica miliaris **(Box 6.9)**.

Clinical Features

Initially, occur as tiny red papules later heal with hemorrhagic crusts. When this adherent crust separates a deep permanent scar is formed, which is varioliform. Subjective symptoms like burning and pruritus can be severe. Lesions may be few or multiple. They usually occur on the temples and anterior scalp margins. They also occur on the cheek, nose and midline of chest. Recurrent attacks at the same site can be severely disfiguring.

Histopathology

There is follicular lymphocytic infiltration with extensive individual cell necrosis of keratinocytes in the outer root sheath and surrounding epidermis. Subepidermal edema is present. Later confluent necrosis occurs.

Box 6.9: Acne necrotica varioliformis

- Chronic necrotising folliculitis mainly involving the scalp margins which evolves into small round scars
- If, not much of a scarring is present, its termed acne necrotica miliaris

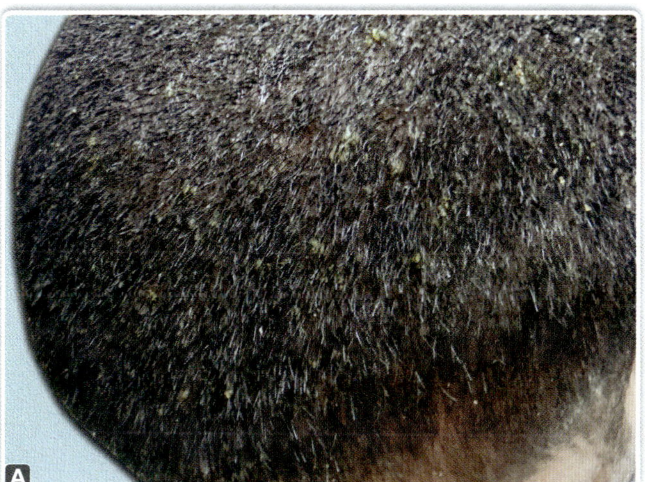

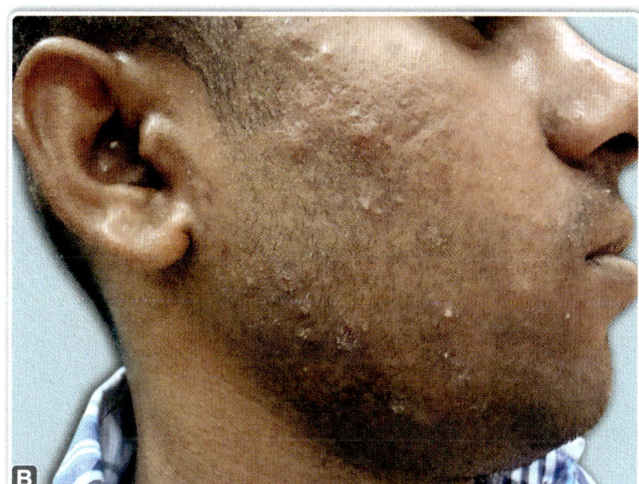

Figs 6.10A and B: (A) Acne necrotica miliaris of scalp; (B) Acne necrotica miliaris of face

Differential Diagnosis

Papulonecrotic tuberculids, tertiary syphilis.

Treatment

If *Staphylococcus aureus* is isolated, appropriate antibiotics must be given. If no response, then prolonged treatment with tetracyclines and topical clindamycin should be tried. Doxepin is given to manage the emotional disturbances and also the associated intense pruritus. In severe chronic cases, isotretinoin can be tried.

Perifolliculitis Capitis (Abscedens et Suffodiens) [Latin: suffodio-dig under]

[Synonym: Dissecting cellulitis of the scalp]

Perifolliculitis capitis abscedens et suffodiens (PCAS) is a therapeutically challenging chronic suppurative scalp disease of unknown etiology. Spitzer first described the disease in 1903, and Hoffman named it descriptively in 1907.[11]

Etiopathogenesis

It affects black males of African origin between 2nd to 4th decade of life. It commonly occurs in association with acne conglobata and hidradenitis suppurativa where the basic pathogenesis is follicular occlusion. Other associations are pilonidal sinus and spondylo arthropathy **(Figure 6.11)**. Keratin and organisms from the ruptured hair follicles initiate a neutrophilic and granulomatous response. Bacterial infection appears to be a secondary event, not an etiologic factor in the pathogenesis.

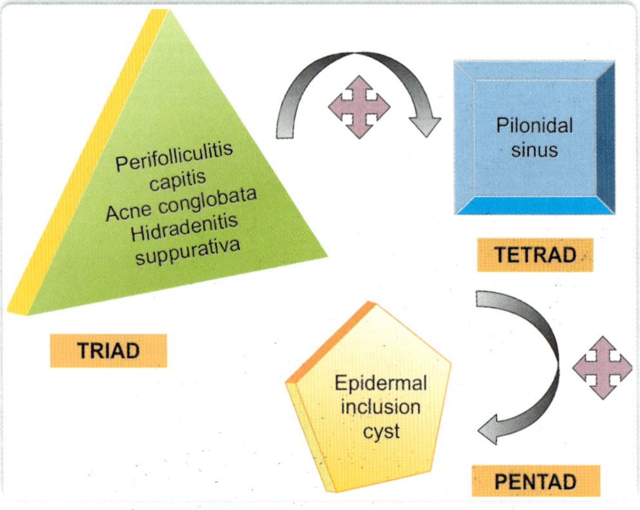

Fig. 6.11: Associations of perifolliculitis capitis

Clinical Features

Usually starts as simple folliculitis on the vertex and occiput. Later inflammatory nodules occur which develop rapidly into abscesses and sinuses with seropurulent discharge. There is scarring alopecia on the summit of the nodules with sparing of hair in between the nodules. Eventually nodules occur on entire scalp and persist for years. Regional lymphadenopathy is rarely seen. Fatal squamous carcinoma has been reported.

Histopathology

Early lesions show follicular hyperkeratosis with plugging and dilatation of the follicle. Eventually perifolliculitis develops with extensive infiltration of neutrophils, lymphocytes and histiocytes. Abscess formation destroys the pilosebaceous structures and other cutaneous appendages. When they extend deeper into subcutaneous tissues, sinus tracts are formed which later heal by extensive fibrosis.

Differential Diagnosis

Kerion, tufted folliculitis.

Treatment

Bacterial pathogens must be sought for and treated. Treatment with isotretinoin gives temporary remissions. Zinc sulfate 400 mg three times a day for 12 weeks, followed by half that dose for 10 more weeks, resulted in complete healing with satisfactory hair regrowth in one patient with no relapse in 5 years.[12] Oral steroids relieve inflammation. Carbon dioxide and ruby laser therapy has been reported to be successful.[13] In recalcitrant cases, widespread excision and grafting may be considered.

Folliculitis Decalvans and Tufted Folliculitis

Folliculitis decalvans (FD) is a type of chronic folliculitis leading to progressive cicatricial alopecia. This entity was first described by Quainquad (1889). Various terminologies like Lupoid sycosis (Brocq 1888), Ulerythema sycosiforme (Unna 1889), Epilating folliculitis of the glabrous skin (Arnozan 1892 and Dubreuilh 1894), essentially imply the same process. Similar lesions involving the hairy regions of the lower limbs are termed as folliculitis depilans, Folliculitis cruris et atrophicans.[14] It is believed that all these entities are variants of a single syndrome.

Etiopathogenesis

Affects men during their adolescence. Females are affected after 3rd decade. The cause of folliculitis decalvans is still unknown. Staphylococcal infection has been found in the majority of cases. Local defect in immune response or leukocyte function is considered to be an important etiological factor. The superantigens theory,[15] with an abnormal host defense mechanism is widely accepted. Some times folliculitis when not treated properly may become persistent and may spread to neighboring follicles, later on resulting in scarring alopecia. The protective barrier of inner root sheath is destroyed by the bacterial proteases and thus there is failure to confine the *Staphylococcus aureus* at the infundibulum. No consistent defect in cell-mediated immunity or inner root sheath keratinization has been identified in patients with folliculitis decalvans.

Clinical Features

Initially starts of as pustular folliculitis of the scalp. Successive crops of pustules occur destroying the follicles which later form areas of cicatricial alopecia with further pustules at the periphery. There are areas of "corn stalking", grouped hairs arising within the area of alopecia **(Box 6.10)**. They usually occur on the scalp margins in a coronal pattern. This is a chronic condition.

Histopathology

There is follicular abscess with dense perifollicular infiltration of neutrophils, eosinophils and plasma cells. Foreign body reaction with granuloma formation may occur when there is follicular disruption. This is followed by scarring and extensive fibrosis.

Tufted Hair Folliculitis

Is a variant of folliculitis decalvans.

Etiopathogenesis

The precise role of *Staphylococcus aureus* in this condition is also unclear. *S. aureus* frequently, but not invariably, is cultured from lesions of tufted hair folliculitis. It is likely that the organism is a secondary invader, but still may contribute to the progression of the disease. However, some authors postulate that infection is the primary process; toxins elaborated by *S. aureus* trigger an inflammatory process in the superior dermis, leading to scarring.

Clinical Features

The most prominent feature of this disorder is the presence of tufts of 8–15 hairs that appear to emerge from a single follicular orifice in a "doll's hair" pattern **(Box 6.11)**. Adjacent to and intermingled with the tufts are areas of scarring alopecia, with complete loss of follicles. The area of tufts and scarring is somewhat well circumscribed and may be accompanied by varying degrees of edema, erythema, and tenderness. Boggy plaques have been described. There may be crusts adherent to the scalp or hair, often in a collarette, around the most proximal portion of the hair. Pustules are not common, but pus may be expressed from the follicular openings. Several reports have noted that a high percentage of telogen hairs are obtained when tufts of hair are forcibly extracted.[16]

Case reports describe tufted folliculitis in association with medication use, specifically with cyclosporine[17] and lapatinib.[18]

Histopathology

The epidermis shows hyperkeratosis, parakeratosis, overlying a hyperplastic epidermis. Follicular plugging may be observed. In the papillary and upper reticular dermis, a perifollicular, mixed inflammatory cell infiltrate seen, including lymphocytes, plasma cells, and neutrophils. In areas of follicular rupture, giant cells that may contain fragments of hair shafts are present. In areas of tufting, the outer root sheath in the infundibular section of the follicle is thinned. The normal spacing of the hairs is disrupted, resulting in convergence of the upper portion of the follicles. Multiple hairs are seen emerging from a single follicular

Box 6.10: Corn stalking

- Grouped hairs arising within the area of alopecia
- Occur on the scalp margins in a coronal pattern

Box 6.11: Doll's hair

- Tufts of 8–15 hairs that appear to emerge from a single follicular orifice
- Seen in tufted hair folliculitis
- Areas of circumscribed scarring alopecia intermingled with the tufts seen

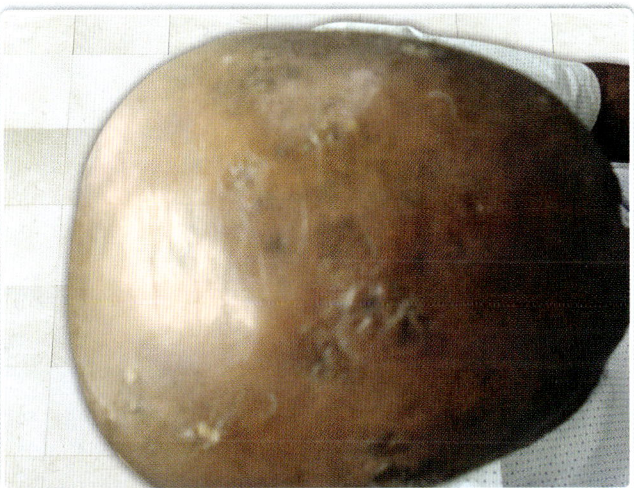

Fig. 6.12: Lepromatous lesions on the scalp

opening. Large numbers of telogen hairs may be identified in the tufts.

Diagnosis

- A scalp biopsy to confirm the diagnosis.
- Bacterial culture of purulent exudate, biopsy specimen, or plucked hair, including antibiotic sensitivity, may be helpful in guiding treatment.
- Fungal cultures are not positive. If a fungal organism is identified, consideration should be given to an alternate diagnosis.

Differential Diagnosis

Kerion.

Treatment

Eradication of *Staphylococcus aureus* from the scalp with prolonged oral antibiotics like flucloxacillin, tetracyclines along with topical clindamycin is helpful. But prolonged remission is seen when Rifampicin is given 300 mg BD along with other antibiotics in order to prevent emergence of Rifampicin resistance.

Tufting may be reduced by measures directed at reducing the scale, such as the use of tar shampoos and topical keratolytics.

Disorders of the scalp in other bacterial infections

Syphilis

Alopecia syphilitica is an uncommon manifestation of secondary syphilis. It is non-inflammatory and non-cicatricial hair loss that can present in a diffuse pattern, a moth-eaten pattern, or a combination of both **(Box 6.11)**. The scalp is the most commonly affected area. However, eyebrows, eyelashes, axilla, pubis, chest and legs can also be affected. Diffuse shedding of telogen hair (telogen effluvium) may occur 3 to 5 months after infection. Other hairy areas may also be affected. Hair growth resumes spontaneously after a few months. In Jarisch-Herxheimer reaction, acceleration of hair loss can occur as a rare feature.

Trichogram shows a decrease in anagen hair and an increase in catagen hair in both primary and secondary stages of syphilis.

Less commonly, small closely set, non-coalescing groups of papules occur on scalp or beard. Nodulo ulcerative lesions can also occur in secondary syphilis. The serpiginous nodulo-squamous syphilid of tertiary syphilis may affect the scalp. Syphilitic gumma on scalp can cause scarring alopecia.

Diagnosis of syphilis is based on serological tests. Spirochetes can be visualized on dark field microscopy of the smear from the lesions. Scalp biopsy is also helpful for active scalp lesions, and in the noduloulcerative forms, spirochetes may be seen with the Warthin-Starry stain. *Treponema pallidum* can also be identified in the peribulbar region in biopsy specimen from the nonscarring alopecia patch.

Mycobacterial Infections

Cutaneous mycobacterial infection can cause scalp hair loss. *Mycobacterium neoaurum* has been shown to cause an indurated plaque of scarring alopecia in an immunocompetent host.[19] Histology showed granulomatous inflammation and PCR was positive on scalp biopsy for *Mycobacterium neoaurum;* however, culture was negative. Supportive of the causative origin of this alopecia, antimycobacterial treatment was initiated and the plaque improved and flattened; however there was no hair regrowth.

Other nontuberculous mycobacterial species can also infect the scalp, causing soft tissue infections and skin ulcers. Large crusted, exudative and verrucous plaques affecting the forehead and scalp producing patchy alopecia and cervical lymphadenopathy caused by *M.kansasii* in a black woman has been described. Treatment with rifampicin and ethambutol produced complete resolution with normal regrowth of hair.

M.leprae rarely infects the scalp **(Figure 6.12)** because it prefers the cooler regions of the body compared to scalp which has higher surface temperature due to abundant blood supply. However in one study[20] lepra bacilli were found in 100% of apparently normal scalp of patients with lepromatous leprosy and 75% of those with borderline leprosy.

Biopsy, culture, and PCR should be done on any suspected, atypical infection. Treatment is guided by the *Mycobacterium* species identified on culture or PCR.

Box 6.12: Alopecia syphilitica

- Non-inflammatory and non-cicatricial hair loss that can present in a diffuse pattern, a moth-eaten pattern, or a combination of both
- Uncommon manifestation of secondary syphilis
- Sites: Scalp, eyebrows, eyelashes, axilla, pubis, chest and legs

References

1. Clarke GHV. Note on dermatitis cruris pustulosa et atrophicans. Trans R Soc TropMed Hyg. 1952;46:558-9.
2. Shelley WB, Hurley HJ. Anhydrous formulation of aluminium chloride for chronic folliculitis. JAMA. 1980;244:1956-7.
3. Roodyn L. Epidemiology of staphylococcal infections. J Hyg. 1960;58:1-10.

4. Becker BA, Frieden IJ, Odom R, et al. Atypical plaquelike staphylococcal folliculitis in human immunodeficiency virus-infected persons. J Am Acad Dermatol. 1989;21:1024-6.
5. Hoss DM, Feder HM. Addition of rifampicin to conventional treatment for recurrent furunculosis. Arch Dermatol. 1995;131:647-8.
6. Gauduchon V, Cozon G, Vandenesch F, et al. Stapylococcus aureus leukocidin: a new virulence factor in cutaneous infections? An epidemiological and experimental study. J Infect Dis. 2004;189:346-53.
7. Leyden JJ, Marples RR, Mills OH Jr, Kligman AM. Gram-negative folliculitis-a complication of antibiotic therapy in acne vulgaris. Br J Dermatol. 1973;88:533-8.
8. Böni R, Nehrhoff B: Treatment of gram-negative folliculitis in patients with acne. Am J Clin Dermatol. 2003;4:273-6.
9. Shelley WB, Miller MA. Electron microscopy, histochemistry and microbiology of bacterial adhesion in trichomycosis axillaris. J Am Acad Dermatol. 1984;10:1005-14.
10. Fisher DA. Acne necroticans (varioliformis) and Staphylococcus aureus. J Am Acad Dermatol. 1988;18:1136-7.
11. Hoffman E. Perifolliculitis capitis abscedens et suffodiens: Case Presentation. Dermat Ztschr. 1908;16:122-3.
12. Kobayashi H, Aiba S, Tagami H. Successful treatment of dissecting cellulitis and acne conglobata with oral zinc. Br J Dermatol. 1999;141(6):1137-8.
13. Glass LF, Berman B, Laub D. Treatment of perifolliculitis capitis abscedens et suffodiens with the carbon dioxide laser. J Dermatol Surg Oncol. 1989;15(6):673-6.
14. Sri KV, Garg BR, Ratnakar C. Folliculitis decalvans. Indian J Dermatol Venereol Leprol. 1995;61:233-4.
15. Chandrawansa PH, Giam YC. Folliculitis decalvans: A Retrospective Study in a Tertiary Referred Centre, Over Five Years. Singapore Med J. 2003;44(2):084-7.
16. Dalziel KL, Telfer NR, Wilson CL, Dawber RP. Tufted folliculitis: a specific bacterial disease?. Am J Dermatopathol. 1990;12(1):37-41.
17. Farhi D, Buffard V, Ortonne N, Revuz J. Tufted folliculitis of the scalp and treatment with cyclosporine. Arch Dermatol. 2006;142(2):251-2.
18. Ena P, Fadda GM, Ena L, Farris A, Santeufemia DA. Tufted hair folliculitis in a woman treated with lapatinib for breast cancer. Clin Exp Dermatol. 2008;33(6):790-1.
19. Martin LK, Lawrence R, Kossard S, Murrell DF. Cutaneous Mycobacterium neoaurum infection causing scarring alopecia in an immunocompetent host. Br J Dermatol. 2007;157(1):204-6.
20. Vaishnavi C, Kaur S, Kumar B, Thakur M, Ganguly NK. Indian J Lepr. 1985;57:519.

7

Fungal Infections of Hair and Scalp

R Madhu, C Janaki, G Sentamil Selvi

"He who cures a disease may be the skill fullest, but he who prevents it is the safest physician."

—*Thomas Fuller*

Introduction

Trichomycoses, the fungal infections of the hair and scalp include tinea capitis, piedra, Majocchi's granuloma, pityrosporum or malassezia folliculitis and pityriasis capitis simplex/seborrheic dermatitis. Dermatophytes and organisms causing piedra cause infection by direct hair invasion, whereas *Malassezia*, play an important role in the etiopathogenesis of pityriasis capitis/seborrheic dermatitis along with other factors like sebum and individual susceptibility. Majocchi's granuloma caused by dermatophytes is the result of a foreign body granulomatous reaction. Majocchi's granuloma, Piedra and Malassezia or pityrosporum folliculitis are relatively uncommon. While the diagnosis of trichomycoses caused by dermatophytes and those that cause piedra is by KOH wet mount examination, pityriasis capitis is essentially a clinical diagnosis. Infections of the hair assume increasing significance in this modern era, due to the prevailing cosmetic concern and mental trauma associated with visually obvious impact of the fungal infections of the hair and hence warrant early diagnosis and effective management of these conditions.

Trichomycoses Caused by Dermatophytes

Dermatophytes causing infection of hair may be anthropophilic (human), zoophilic (animal) or geophilic (soil). Infection can involve the scalp (tinea capitis), eye brows, eye lashes (tinea faciei), beard, moustache area (tinea barbae) and for that matter, any hair bearing area on the body surface. Clinical presentation depends on the virulence of the organism, type of hair invasion namely endothrix, ectothrix or favic, host resistance and immunological response of the various sites involved **(Box 7.1)**.

Tinea Capitis

Tinea capitis is dermatophytosis of the scalp and scalp hair caused by dermatophytes belonging to the genera *Trichophyton* and *Microsporum*.[1] It is also referred to as ring worm of the scalp or tinea tonsurans.[2] Tinea capitis is the most common dermatophytosis of children in the prepubertal age group.[1] History reveals that during the 1830s, Gruby described all the major types of hair invasion known today, but his clinical description was imprecise. In 1894, Sabouraud unaware of Gruby's contribution had described the main types of tinea capitis and culture methods, which were soon adopted worldwide.[3]

Among the dermatophytes causing tinea capitis, the anthropophilic species predominate. Amidst the various species of dermatophytes causing hair infection, *Microsporum audouinii, Trichophyton violaceum* and *T. schoenleinii* have a specific predilection for hair. It is known that *Epidermophyton floccosum, T. concentricum* and *T. mentagrophytes var interdigitale* apparently never cause tinea capitis. All dermatophytes causing tinea capitis can invade glabrous skin and many may cause nail infection

Box 7.1: Factors affecting clinical presentation of trichomycoses

- Source of organism: Zoophilic/anthropophilic/geophilic
- Virulence of the organism
- Type of hair invasion namely endothrix, ectothrix or favic
- Host resistance
- Immunological response of the various sites involved

too.[2] Predominant organisms vary with geographic area and from time to time. For instance, in North America, initially *Microsporum canis* and later *M. audouinii* were the dominant organisms, which have now been replaced by *T. tonsurans*. Both *M.canis* and *M. audouinii*, ectothrix causing organisms produce brilliant green fluorescence under the Wood's lamp, whereas organisms that cause endothrix type of hair invasion such as *T. tonsurans, T.violaceum* do not fluoresce. *Trichophyton schoenleinii* produces a pale green fluorescence. With the transition from *M.canis* and *M. audouinii* to *T. tonsurans,* the utility of Wood's lamp as a screening tool has greatly reduced. *Microsporum canis* is the most common causative organism in most parts of Europe. In the urban areas of United kingdom, a rise in the prevalence of *T.tonsurans* has been recorded. [4] In India, the various organisms causing tinea capitis are *T.violaceum, T.tonsurans, T.simii, T. rubrum* and *T. mentagraphytes*, with *T.violaceum* being the most common agent **(Table 7.1 and Figure 7.1)**.[5]

Table 7.1: Organisms causing tinea capitis [2,3]

Species	Type
Trichophyton violaceum	Anthropophilic
T. tonsurans	Anthropophilic
T.mentagrophytes	Anthropophilic/zoophilic
T.schoenleinii	Anthropophilic
T. verrucosum	Zoophilic
T. simii	Zoophilic
T. rubrum	Anthropophilic
T.megninii	Anthropophilic
T. soudanense	Anthropophilic
T. yaoundei	Anthropophilic
Microsporum audouinii	Anthropophilic
M. canis	Zoophilic
M. ferrugineum	Anthropophilic
M. nanum	Zoophilic/geophilic
M. gypseum	Geophilic
M. fulvum	Geophilic
M.distortum	Zoophilic

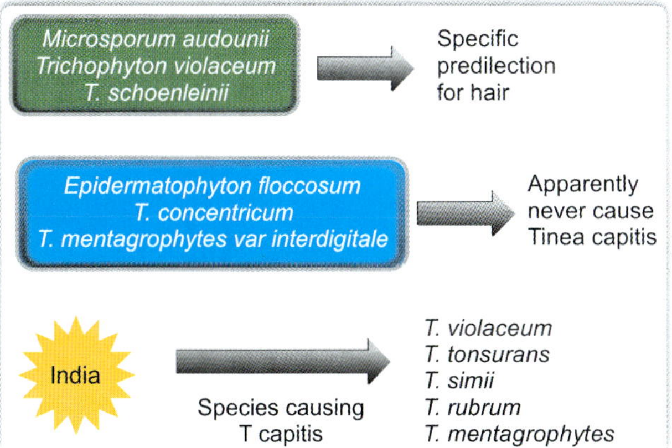

Fig. 7.1: Schematic representation of species causing trichomycoses

Tinea capitis occurs predominantly in prepubertal children in the age group of 4 and 14 years.[1] The fungistatic properties of fatty acids of short and medium chains in post pubertal sebum and the lipolytic activity of pityrosporum species are known to have an inhibitory effect on the dermatophytes. However, infection can occur in all age groups. Tinea capitis has been reported in neonates and in infants.[6,7] Ratio of sexual predilection may vary with the causative organism. With the *Microsporum* species, infection rate is higher in boys, while in infection with *Trichophyton* species, boys and girls are equally infected.[3] Incidence is more in adult females who fondle children.[8] Tinea capitis is transmitted via infected persons, select animal vectors and fomites such as contaminated barber shop instruments, combs, hair brush, caps, towels, pillow covers, theatre seats, etc.[3,9] It is most often seen in children who have undergone tonsure in pilgrimage places.[10] Intrafamilial infection has been reported **(Figure 7. 2)**.[11] Poor personal hygiene, overcrowding and low socioeconomic status act as predisposing factors for this infection.[3] Studies have shown that this infection is endemic in south India and that it is more common in the residential schools.[12-15] Asymptomatic carrier is defined as a person, from whom positive scalp cultures have been isolated in the absence of symptoms and signs of tinea capitis. Carriers who are usually the adults in the family, siblings, care takers and playmates act as a major reservoir for transmission of the organisms causing tinea capitis. Asymptomatic carrier state is most common with the anthropophilic organisms **(Box 7.2)**. Hair care practices

Box 7.2: Asymptomatic carrier

- Defined as a person, from whom positive scalp cultures have been isolated in the absence of symptoms and signs of tinea capitis
- Adults in the family, siblings, care takers and playmates act as a major reservoir for transmission. Asymptomatic carrier state is most common with the anthropophilic organisms

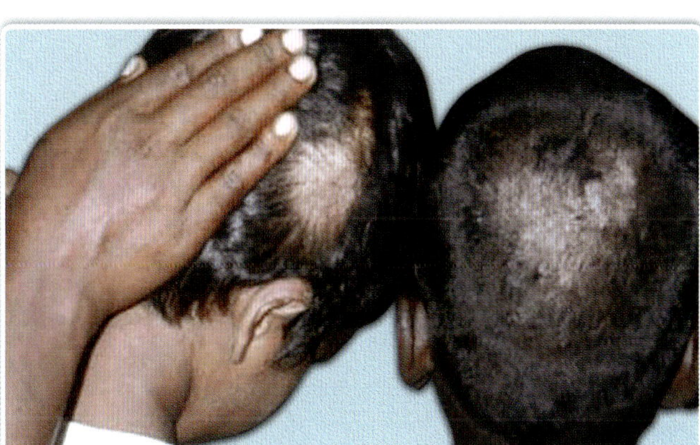

Fig. 7.2: Two siblings with tinea capitis

(use of oils or greases, frequency of hair wash, styling of hair, etc.) do not appear to play a major role in the acquisition of infection.[16]

Pathogenesis

The pathogenesis of tinea capitis has been studied by Kligman and by Frieden and Howard.[1] Hair appears to be susceptible to dermatophytes during mid to late anagen phase. Trauma assists inoculation which is followed approximately after 3 weeks by clinical evidence of hair shaft infection. Kligman describes the initial phase as follicular phase wherein fungal spores enter into follicle and germinate into extrapilary hyphae which entwine around the hair forming parallel chains along its long axis. During the second phase named as pilar phase, the hyphae penetrate under the cuticle, proliferate in the subcuticular cortex and descend until they reach the upper limit of keratigenous zone (Adamson's fringe) by about the 12th day after inoculation **(Figure 7.3)**. External branches of the intrapilar hyphae produce short chains of ectothrix spores. The hyphae never enter the nucleated zone. Kligman postulated that a biochemical substance produced by the cornifying cells may function as inhibitor of the fungus and also said that there is a unique dynamic relationship between the host and the parasite at the Adamson's fringe **(Box 7.3)**. It is said that as long as the fungus maintains the same rate of growth as the hair shaft, the infection persists.[17]

There are three types of hair invasion namely endothrix, ectothrix and favic. In the ectothrix type, secondary extrapilary hyphae burst out and grow over the surface of the hair shaft, which further segment to produce arthroconidia. In the endothrix type of invasion, intrapilary hyphae proliferate and divide into arthroconidia that fill the hair shaft and are transported upward. Hair thus affected is fragile and breaks off close to the surface of the scalp. In the favic type caused by *T. schoenleinii*, broad, regularly septate hyphae run parallel to the long axis of the hair shaft. Degeneration of the hyphae results in tunnels seen as air spaces within the hair shaft in wet mount **(Table 7.2)**.[2]

Histologically, rounded and box like arthrospores may be found within the hair shaft in endothrix infection and around in ectothrix infection, which are better visualized with special stains such as periodic acid schiff (PAS) (purple) and gomori's methenamine stains (GMS) (black). In the non-inflammatory type, there is mononuclear inflammatory infiltrate around the follicles. Follicular disruption may result in foreign body giant cell reaction. In kerion, there is follicular pustule formation and a dense

Box 7.3: Adamson's fringe

- Imaginary line that marks non-keratogenous zone of hair shaft
- A biochemical substance produced by the cornifying cells may function as inhibitor of the fungus preventing spread beyond fringe

Table 7.2: Types of hair invasion[2]

Ectothrix causing organisms	*Endothrix causing organisms*
Small spore ectothrix	*T. tonsurans*
M. audouinii	*T. violaceum*
M. canis	*T. soudanense*
M. canis var *distortum*	*T. yaoundei*
M. equinum	*T. gourvilii*
M. ferrugineum	*T. rubrum* (rare)
Large spore ectothrix	**Favic type**
M. gypseum	*T.schoenleinii*
M. fulvum	*T.violaceum* } less
M. nanum	*M.gypseum* } frequently
M. vanbreuseghemii	
T. verrucosum	
T. mentagrophytes var. *mentagrophytes*	
T. mentagrophytes var. *erinacei*	
T. megninii	
T. rubrum (rare)	

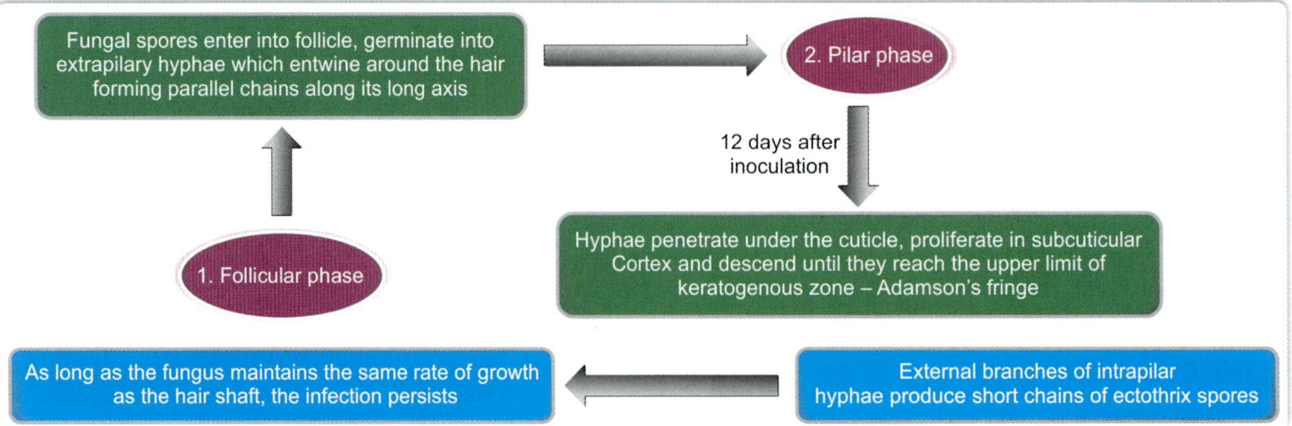

Fig. 7.3: Schematic representation of pathophysiology of tinea capitis

perifollicular neutrophilic inflammatory infiltrate in the dermis.[1,18]

Clinical Features

The clinical presentation depends on the type of hair invasion, virulence of the organism, host resistance and degree of the inflammatory response. Hence this infection may range from an asymptomatic carrier state/chronic non-inflammatory to acute inflammatory type **(Box 7.4)**. Non-inflammatory types are the gray patch, black dot, seborrheic type, smooth patch of baldness and the glabrous (adult) type. Inflammatory types are kerion, abscess, favus, pustular and agminate folliculitis. Mixed type comprising of non-inflammatory and inflammatory types or different types of non-inflammatory or inflammatory may present depending on the immunological response of the various sites of the scalp and immunity of the patient.[19] Chronicity of the non-inflammatory types plays an important role in increasing the prevalence of the infection. Non-inflammatory types are more often caused by anthropophilic organisms. Grey patch or epidemic type is characterized by patches of partial hair loss with scales. Broken off hairs are dull grey and lusterless in appearance due to the overcoating by arthrospores **(Figure 7.4A)**. Black dot pattern is caused by endothrix organisms such as *T. violaceum* and *T. tonsurans*. Infected fragile hair breaks at the level of scalp leaving the remnant of hair in the infected follicle which appears as a black dot **(Figure 7.4B)**. Seborrheic type characterized by diffuse scaling may occur with or without discrete patches of hair loss **(Figure 7.5A)**. Smooth patch of baldness mimics alopecia areata but there is minimal scaling **(Figure 7.5B)**. Hence it becomes important to have a wet mount examination done in all children with patchy loss of hair. In the glabrous type, lesions extend from the less hairy area to the scalp and this is the common type seen in adults **(Figure 7.6)**. Among the inflammatory types, kerion is a painful inflammatory boggy swelling studded with broken hairs and follicular pustules on its surface, associated with regional lymphadenopathy **(Figure 7.7A)**. Untreated kerion may result in scarring. Abscess is characterized by the presence of smooth, boggy swelling without follicular pustules on the surface **(Figure 7.7B) (Box 7.5)**. Id reaction, which presents as papules over the trunk, is associated more often with inflammatory types like kerion and abscess. Follicular pustules may present in a

Box 7.4: Types of tinea capitis

Non-inflammatory types:
- Gray patch, black dot, seborrhoeic type, smooth patch of baldness and the glabrous (adult) type

Inflammatory types:
- Kerion, abscess, favus, pustular and agminate folliculitis

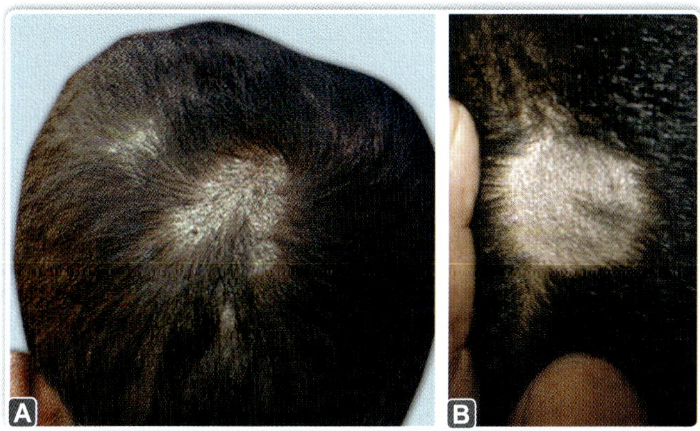

Figs 7.4A and B: (A) Gray patch; (B) Black dot

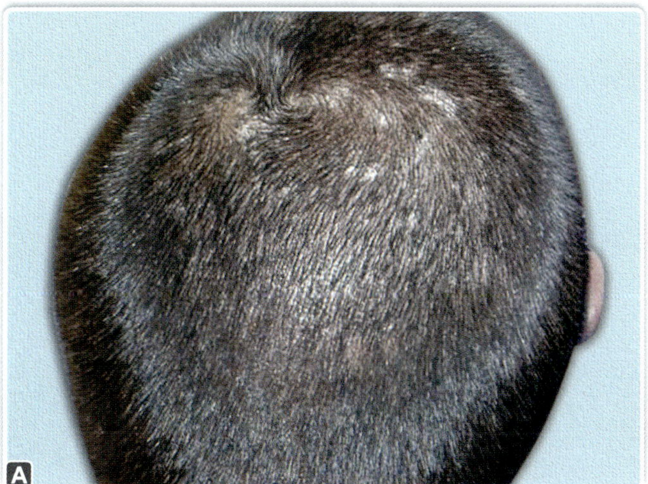

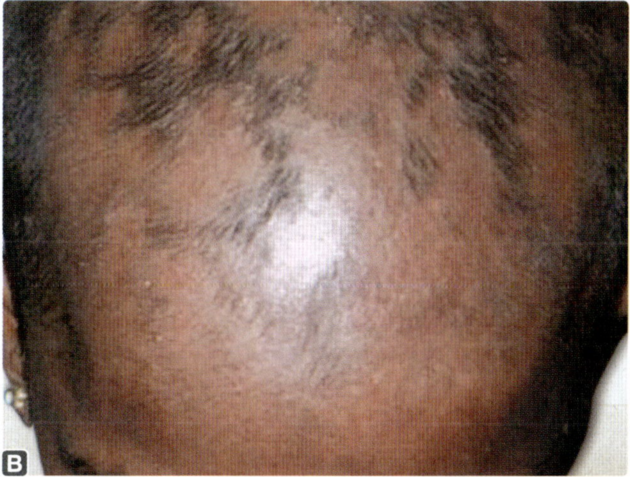

Figs 7.5A and B: (A) Seborrheic type; (B) Smooth patch of baldness

discrete pattern (pustular type) **(Figure 7.7C)** or as grouped pustules studded on a erythematous plaque (agminate type). Favus caused by *T.schoenleinii* and at times by *T.violaceum* and *M.gypseum* is characterized by presence of yellow shaped crust known as scutula pierced by a long hair. This condition always heals with scarring. Mixed type of tinea capitis may comprise of combinations of different types of non-inflammatory/inflammatory or different types of non- inflammatory and inflammatory types **(Figure 7.7D)**. Cervical or occipital lymphadenopathy occurs in all types of tinea capitis and is due to the antigen antibody reaction **(Figure 7.8)**.[2,3]

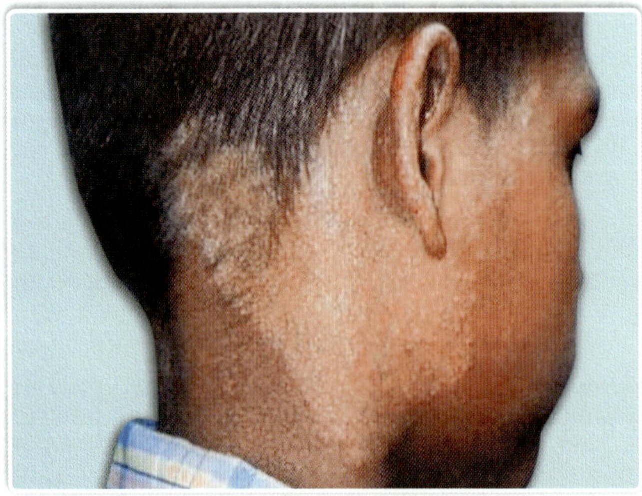

Fig. 7.6: Glabrous type

Differential Diagnosis

When there is scaling and minimal inflammation, differential diagnosis will include seborrheic dermatitis and scalp

Box 7.5: Kerion vs abscess

- Kerion is a painful inflammatory boggy swelling studded with broken hairs and follicular pustules on its surface, associated with regional lymphadenopathy with/without scarring
- Abscess is characterized by the presence of smooth, boggy swelling without follicular pustules on the surface

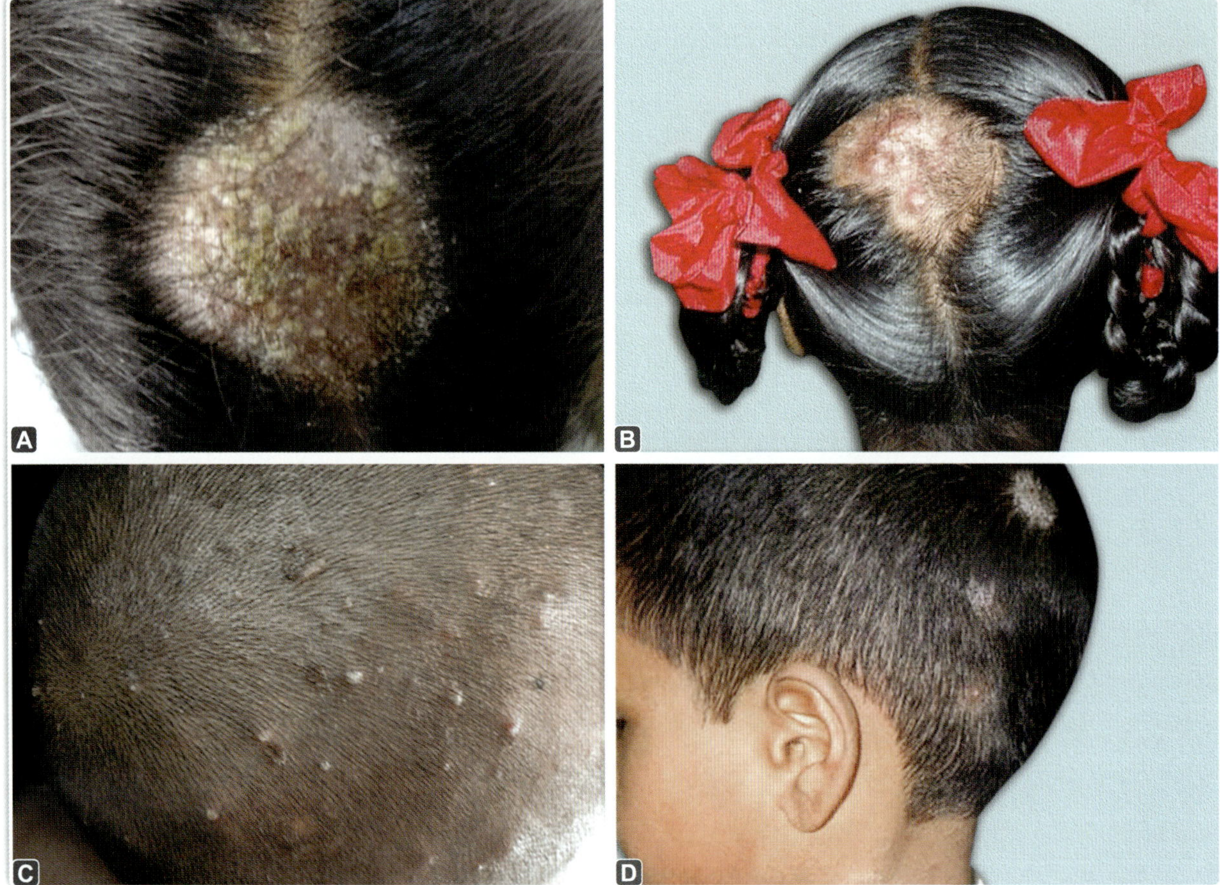

Figs 7.7A to D: (A) Kerion; (B) Abscess; (C) Pustules; (D) Mixed type of tinea capitis showing gray patch, black dot and pustules

psoriasis. In both these conditions, there is no patchy loss of hair. Alopecia areata, trichotillomania are to be considered when the clinical lesion appears as smooth patch of baldness. **(Figure 7.9)** In alopecia areata, scaling is absent while one can look for the presence of exclamation mark hair. In trichotillomania, which usually occurs in easily accessible sites of the scalp, hairs are of varying length. Bacterial pyoderma (impetigo, folliculitis) form a close differential diagnosis for the inflammatory types. However, there is no loosening of hair in these conditions. In the presence of scarring, conditions like lichen planopilaris, pseudopelade, discoid lupus erythematosus and radiation dermatitis need to be considered **(Box 7.6)**.

Tinea Barbae and Tinea Faciei

Tinea barbae denotes the dermatophyte infection of the beard and moustache areas of the face with invasion of coarse hairs. Zoophilic organisms such as *T. verrucosum*, *T. mentagrophytes var. mentagrophytes* are the most common causative organisms while, anthropophilic organisms like *T. violaceum, T.schoenleinii, T.rubrum, T.simii, T. megninii* may be occasionally involved. There are three forms namely superficial, inflammatory and circinate types, with the inflammatory type being analogous to kerion in tinea capitis. Clinical features include erythematous perifollicular papules and pustules with oozing and crusting. Hair is brittle, lusterless and easily pluckable. Loss of hair may be seen **(Figure 7.10A)**. Infection of the area around the eyes in tinea faciei may result in invasion of the hair in eyelashes and eye brows **(Figure 7.10B)**. Pathogenesis of hair invasion is essentially the same as in tinea capitis. Tinea barbae mus be differentiated from bacterial folliculitis (sycosis barbae) severe herpes simplex, herpes zoster contact dermatitis, acne, rosaceae and pseudofolliculitis.

Box 7.6: Differentials in the presence of scarring

- Lichen planopilaris
- Pseudopelade
- Discoid lupus erythematosus
- Radiation dermatitis

Majocchi's Granuloma

Majocchi's granuloma or Granuloma trichophyticum was first described by Domenico Majocchi in 1883, which he referred to as Granuloma trichofitico.[20] It is a deep folliculitis usually caused by *T.rubrum* that may occur in any hair bearing area on the body surface. It starts as a suppurative folliculitis and results in a foreign body granulomatous reaction. Usual sites of involvement are the scalp, face, forearms, hands and legs. Women with the habit of repeated shaving of legs may develop multiple perifollicular papulopustules and nodules with or without erythema. Tinea pedis due to *T.rubrum* has been observed in these women.[1,20] Histologically, perifollicular and dermal granulomas with chronic inflammatory infiltrate consisting of lymphoid cells, epitheloid cells, macrophages and multinucleated giant cells are present. Fungal hyphae and spores are seen within the hair follicles and in the inflammatory infiltrate in the dermis, which are better visualized with special stains.[21] Sometimes, Splendore Hoeppli material (eosiniphilic mantle) may be seen around the fungal hyphae which will mimick a

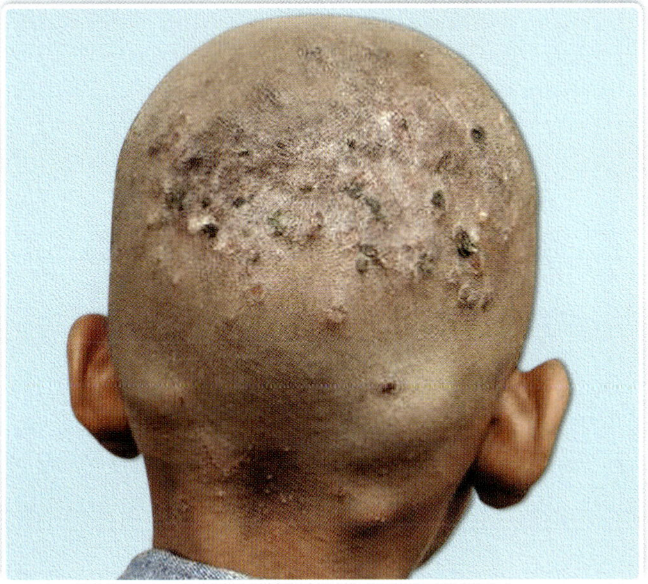

Fig. 7.8: Posterior cervical and occipital lymphadenopathy

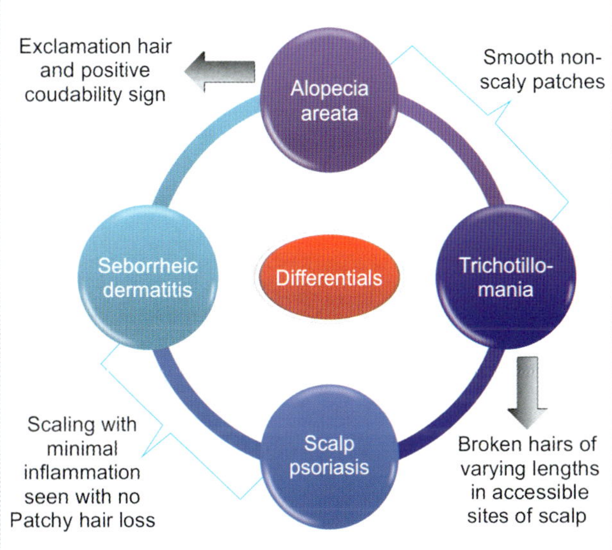

Fig. 7.9: Schematic representation of differentials of tinea capitis

mycetoma grain, resulting in this condition being also termed as dermatophyte pseudomycetoma.[22] Differential diagnosis includes bacterial folliculitis, nodular vasculitis, eosinophilic pustular folliculitis, lymphocytoma cutis, Kaposi sarcoma and acne keloidalis nuchae.

Box 7.7: Majocchi's granuloma/Granuloma trichophyticum/ Granuloma trichofitico

- A suppurative form of deep folliculitis usually caused by *T.rubrum* with a foreign body granulomatous reaction
- Sites: Scalp, face, forearms, hands and legs
- Seen in women with habit of repeated shaving of legs
- Splendore Hoeppli material (eosiniphilic mantle) may be seen around fungal elements with perifollicular dermal granulomas

Diagnosis (Figure 7.11)

Clinical diagnosis of dermatophyte infections of hair may be confirmed by a wet mount examination. It is important to examine the hair root and not a cut portion of hair in the case of dermatophytosis, whereas in piedra, the latter would suffice. Samples to be examined include skin scrapings and hair root, which may be collected using a blunt scalpel. Other methods of collecting samples are by using sterile tooth brush, hair brush, moistened gauze and cotton swabs.[2,23,24] Microscopic examination of the scales in 10% KOH and hair in 40% KOH solution will show arthroconidia within the hair shaft (endothrix) **(Figure 7.12)** or outside the hair shaft (ectothrix) or both within and outside the

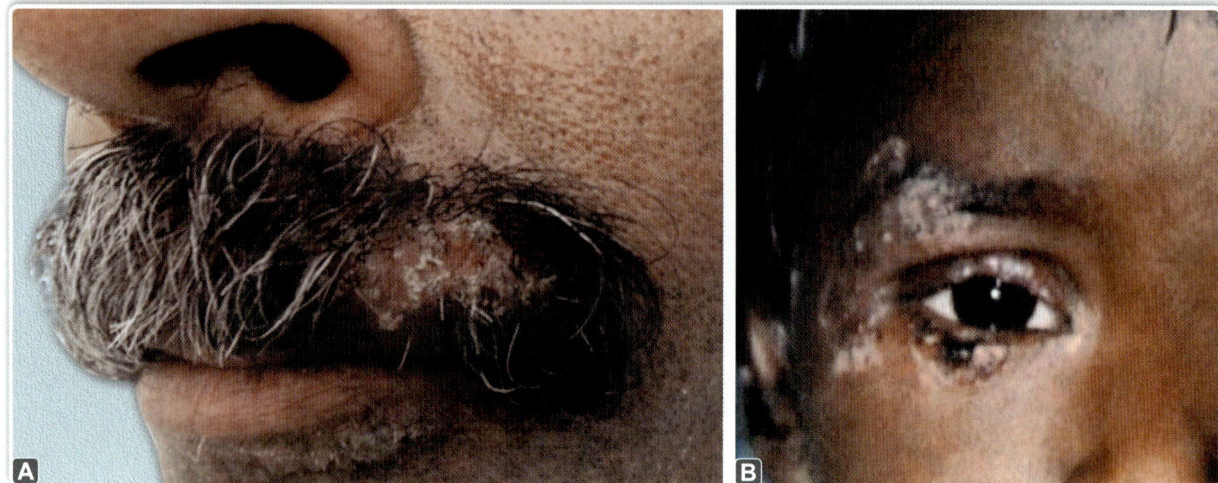

Figs 7.10A and B: (A) Tinea barbae; (B) Tinea faciei

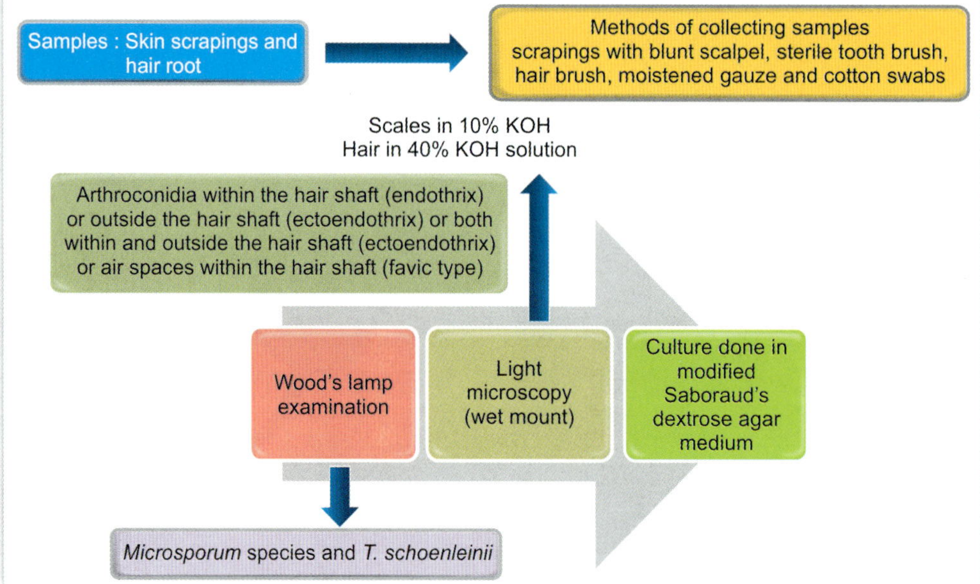

Fig. 7.11: Schematic representation of investigative findings in tinea capitis

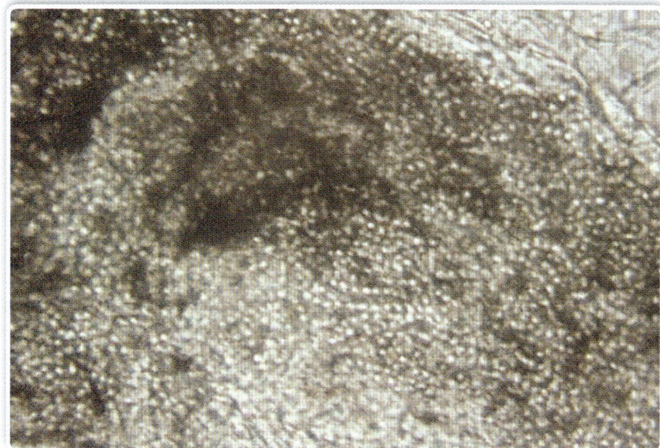

Fig. 7.12: Endothrix spores in wet mount

hair shaft (ectoendothrix) or air spaces within the hair shaft (favic type). Wood's lamp examination is useful as a screening tool in infections due to *Microsporum* species and *T. schoenleinii*. Culture done in modified Saboraud's dextrose agar medium to isolate the organism, is mainly of academic interest and for epidemiological studies.

Treatment

Systemic antifungal agents are the mainstay of treatment of tinea capitis, with the topical antifungals being used as adjuncts to reduce the spore load in patients and asymptomatic carriers because, the topical agents do not penetrate the infected hair shaft. Among the systemic antifungal agents used, griseofulvin is the only FDA approved drug that has been the gold standard treatment for more than 50 years. Griseofulvin microsize formulation is given in the dosage of 20 to 25 mg/kg, whereas ultramicrosize formulation dosage is 10 to 15 mg/kg for a period of 12 weeks. It is to be taken after a fatty meal. The main disadvantages of this drug are the long duration of treatment and poor compliance. Newer antifungals like fluconazole, itraconazole and especially terbinafine with its fungicidal activity, though not approved by FDA for use in tinea capitis have benefits like short duration of treatment, good compliance and less side effects, but are more costly than griseofulvin. Liquid formulations are available for griseofulvin, fluconazole and itraconazole though not in our country. Daily dosage of fluconazole and itraconazole is 5 mg/kg, given for a period of 30 days and 4 weeks respectively. Weekly once dose of fluconazole 8 mg/kg given for a period of 8–12 weeks has also been found to be effective. Itraconazole pulse regimen with capsules (5 mg/kg/day for 1 week given 3 weeks apart for 3 pulses), and itraconazole pulse regimen with oral solution (3 mg/kg/day for 1 week given 3 weeks apart for 3 pulses) have been tried. Itraconazole should be taken with food or a cola beverage to enhance absorption. With terbinafine tablets, the continuous regimen (>40 kg body weight, 250 mg/day; 20–40 kg, 125 mg/day; and <20 kg, 62.5 mg/day) is given for 4 weeks **(Table 7.3)**.[25-27] In case of pulse therapy, terbinafine is given in the dosage as in the continuous regimen for 1 week with 2 weeks off period between the first two pulses and 3 weeks off period between the second and third pulses of treatment.[28] Currently, oral terbinafine is approved for the treatment of tinea capitis in many countries.[29] Itraconazole may also be given in a pulse regimen similar to that of terbinafine **(Table 7.4)**.[26] Pulse therapy with terbinafine and itraconazole has been found to be very effective due to the reservoir effect of these drugs. The treatment may be stopped when hair regrowth is clinically evident. Thus, the duration of treatment may be individualized according to the response. Treatment of tinea barbae is with systemic antifungal agents given for appropriate duration, as in tinea capitis. Duration of treatment of tinea faciei is 2–4 weeks with terbinafine/itraconazole and 6–8 weeks with griseofulvin. In children with tinea capitis, adjunctive therapy with 1%–2% ketoconazole or 2.5% selenium sulfide shampoo or zinc pyrithione shampoo helps to reduce the spore load and shedding of infected hairs and thus minimizes the spread of infection. Close contacts of infected children should be advised to use these topical agents. Antifungal shampoo should be applied to the scalp and hair weekly twice or thrice until there is clinical cure and when investigated, mycological cure.[26] Sharing of fomites such as combs, brushes, toys, etc. should be discouraged. In case of zoophilic infections, infected animal must be treated. Infected children can be allowed to attend school. Children with tinea capitis undergo mental turmoil as they are bullied by their friends. Hence, it is imperative to provide psychological support to these children.

Table 7.3: Dosage schedule of various systemic antifungal agents in tinea capitis[25-27]

Drug	Dosage/Day	Duration
Tab Griseofulvin 125 mg	Microsize 20 to 25 mg/kg Ultramicrosize 10 to 15 mg/kg after food in 2 divided doses	12 weeks
Tab Fluconazole 150 mg	5 mg/kg/od	30 days
Cap Itraconazole 100 mg Itraconazole solution	5 mg/kg/od 3 mg/kg/od	4 weeks 4 weeks
Tab Terbinafine 250 mg	< 20 kg 62.5 mg od 20–40 kg 125 mg od > 40 kg 250 mg od	4 weeks

Table 7.4: Pulse therapy in tinea capitis[26-28]

Drug	Dosage	Pulse regimen
Terbinafine	10–20 kg: 62.5 mg/day 20–40 kg: 125 mg/day >40 kg: 250 mg/day or 4–5 mg/kg/day	1 week with 2 weeks off between the first 2 pulses and 3 weeks off between the 2nd and 3rd pulse 2–3 pulses
Itraconazole	Capsules: 5 mg/kg/day Oral solution:3 mg/kg/day	1 week with 2 weeks off between the first 2 pulses and 3 weeks off between the 2nd and 3rd pulse 2–3 pulses (range: 1–5) OR 1 week with 3 weeks apart, i.e monthly once 2–3 pulses
Fluconazole	8 mg/kg once weekly	8–12 weeks

Majocchi's granuloma is treated with a combination of topical and systemic antifungal agents. Topical azole creams along with itraconazole given in a dosage of 200 mg twice a day for 1 week has been found to be effective. In some patients, a second pulse after a period of 3 weeks may be given depending on the clinical response. Terbinafine 250 mg/day given for a period of 2-4 weeks has been reported to be effective.[27]

Piedra

Piedra also known as trichomycosis nodularis, is an asymptomatic superficial fungal infection of the hair shaft. In 1865, Biegel described Piedra and later in 1911, Horta classified this condition into two types namely black piedra and white piedra. The word, "Piedra" means stone in Spanish. Black piedra is caused by *Piedraia hortae,* whereas white piedra is caused by yeast like fungus, *Trichosporon beigelii* which is now considered to include a complex of different species such as *T.asahii, T.inkin, T.ovoides, T. asteroides, T.mucoides* and *T.cutaneum.*[30] High humidity, abundant rainfall, straight hairs and use of hair oils may be predisposing factors **(Box 7.7)**. In addition, individuals who swim or wash their hair in stagnant water may develop this infection.[31]

Black piedra is seen in the tropical regions such as South America, Pacific islands and far East and less commonly in Asia. *Piedraia hortae* is present in the soil, stagnant water and crops. Among the human pathogenic fungi, *P.hortae* is unique as it produces sexual spores in the parasitic phase. As the fungus grows, cuticle ruptures followed by its growth on the outer surface of the cuticle, completely surrounding the entire hair shaft. Black piedra typically involves the scalp hair and less frequently the beard, moustache or pubic area. It is characterized by the presence of multiple, firmly adherent, oval, black, brown, hard gritty nodules on the hair shaft **(Figure 7.13)**. As the nodules are gritty to feel, a metallic sound may be heard when hair is combed.[30]

Box 7.7: Predisposing factors for piedra

- High humidity
- Abundant rainfall
- Straight hairs and use of hair oils
- Swimming or washing hairs in stagnant water

White piedra is seen in the temperate and sub-tropical regions. *Trichosporon asahii* is generally found in the soil, but may also be present in air, rivers, lakes, sewage, bird droppings, sputum and body surfaces. This yeast like fungus occasionally constitutes substantial proportion of normal flora of human skin. Trichosporon ovoides and T. inkin are associated with infection of the scalp hair and pubic hair respectively. Sexual transmission acts as a predisposing factor in patients with pubic white piedra. Cutaneous lesions are caused by T.cutaneum and T.asteroides. Systemic infection is seen to be associated with T.asahii and T.mucoides. While T.asahii causes hematogenous dissemination, T.mucoides affects the central nervous system. It has been postulated that a bacteria, Brevibacterium mcbrellneri may have a synergistic role in the causation of infection, as the strong proteolytic activity of the bacterium facilitates hair shaft invasion by both yeasts and bacterium, while the fungal by products stimulate the bacterial growth. HIV patients have been reported to have an increased carriage of T.beigelii in the perianal area. Infection involves the hairs of the beard, moustache, axilla and genital areas and less commonly scalp, eyebrow and eyelashes. It is characterized by the presence of soft, white to light brown gelatinous nodules that are less adherent and easily detachable from the hair **(Figure 7.14)**. As the hair shaft becomes weak, broken hairs are seen in both the types. Cutaneous manifestations occur in the form of purpura or papulovasicular lesions. Clinically piedra may be confused with nits, hair casts, trichomycosis axillaris, monilethrix and trichorrhexis nodosa. In white piedra, nodules are easily pulled off unlike the nits.[1,2,30,32]

Laboratory Diagnosis

In potassium hydroxide mount, the nodules of black piedra are seen to be comprised of closely packed demetiaceous

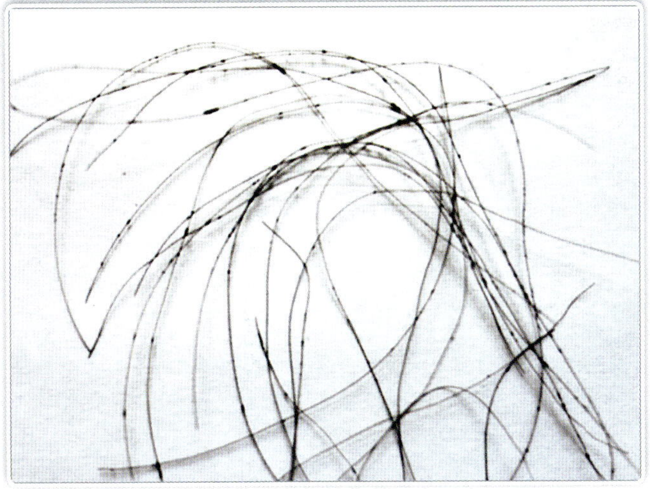

Fig. 7.13: Scalp hairs showing black nodules attached to the hair shaft

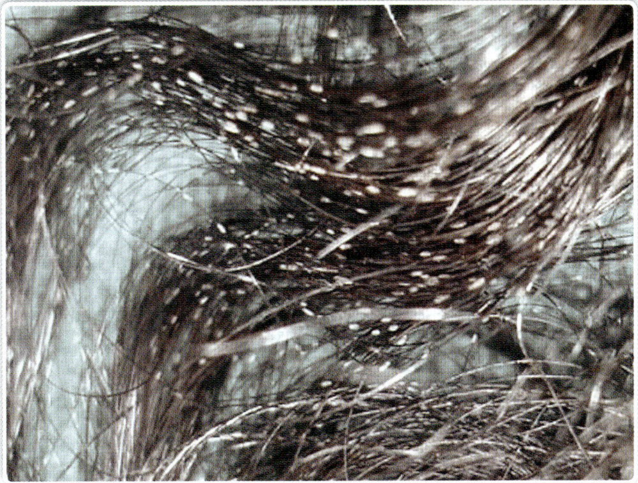

Fig. 7.14: Scalp hairs showing white nodules attached to the hair shaft

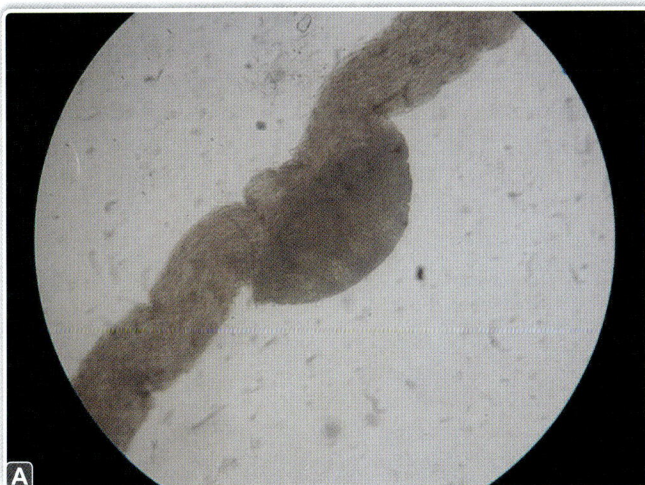

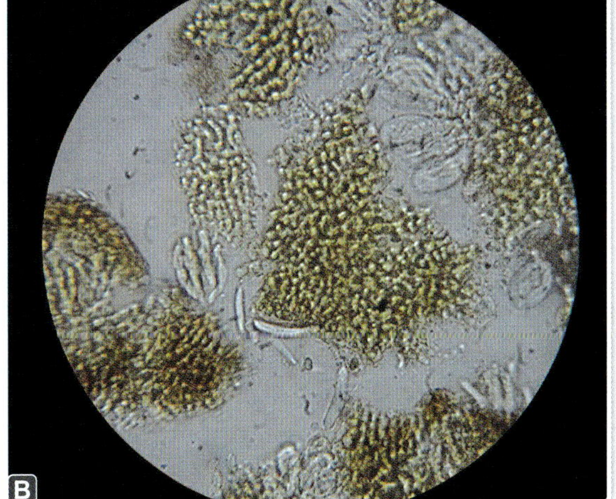

Figs 7.15A and B: (A) Photomicrograph of a black nodule in KOH; (B) Black piedra—closely packed spores and ascospores are seen

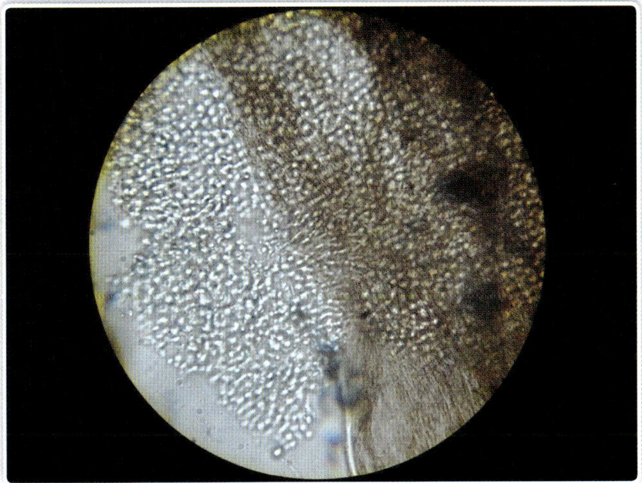

Fig. 7.16: White piedra—blastospores and arthrospores are seen

hyphae. Mature nodules will show asci containing eight ascospores which have a flagellum at the tip, better seen when they are crushed **(Figures 7.15A and B)**. In white piedra, grouped, polygonal, hyaline spores are seen **(Figure 7.16)**.[2]

Treatment

Preventive measures in both types of piedra, consists of avoidance of moisture and application of plant oil on wet hair. Treatment comprises of shaving of hair followed by application of high concentrations of topical terbinafine, azoles, benzoic acid ointment compound, tolnaftate and 1 in 2000 mercury perchloride solution after shampooing. These topical antifungal agents are to be applied for a period of two to six weeks or until remission. Oral terbinafine has been used to treat black piedra while itraconazole has been found to be effective in the treatment of white piedra. Relapse is known to occur. However shaving of hair followed by topical and systemic antifungal therapy reduces the recurrences.[1,2,33]

Pityriasis Capitis Simplex/Seborrheic Dermatitis

Pityriasis capitis simplex or dandruff present in about 15–20% population, refers to the mild form of the seborrheic dermatitis of the scalp, wherein the inflammation is minimal and remains subclinical. Seborrheic dermatitis is a common, chronic, inflammatory papulosquamous disorder characterized by the presence of erythema covered with greasy scales in the sebaceous glands rich areas namely, the scalp, face, chest, back and flexural areas. Lipophilic yeasts, *Malassezia* have been implicated in the etiopathogenesis of dandruff, seborrheic dermatitis, pityrosporum folliculitis and pityriasis versicolor. Malassez in 1874 isolated the yeast forms of the fungi from dandruff scales. In 1904, Saboraud considered *Pityrosporum malassezia* as the causative organism of dandruff. Subsequently, it was renamed as *Pityrosporum orbiculare* and *Pityrosporum ovale* and finally, this organism regained its original name, "Malassez" in1984. Initially, only *Malassezia furfur* and the non-lipid dependent species, *Malassezia pachydermatis* were known. At present, the genus consists of 12 distinct species **(Box 7.8)**.[34] *M. restricta* and *M. globosa* are the most prevalent organisms in dandruff affected population. Etiology of seborrheic dermatitis depends on 3 main factors namely sebum, microfloral metabolism, and individual susceptibility. The *Malassezia* yeasts are most common on sebum-rich areas of the body and they degrade sebum. Specifically, the organisms contain lipases that hydrolyze triglycerides, resulting in specific saturated fatty acids that the yeast requires to proliferate and unsaturated fatty acids that cause scalp irritation. It has been shown that fatty acid metabolites like oleic acid cause flaking of the scalp in susceptible individuals. In immunodeficiency states such as acquired immune deficiency syndrome, increased *Malassezia* proliferation is observed resulting in severe seborrheic dermatitis.[35-37] Thomas, et al. reported that non-capsulated viable form of *M.globosa* caused an increased production of IL-6, IL-8 and IL-1α, and a decrease in intracellular IL-10, while the capsulated forms of *Malassezia* yeasts induced limited or no production of inflammatory cytokines, and increased intracellular IL-10, thus supporting the hypothesis that the lipid layer of *Malassezia* species modulates cytokine production by keratinocytes.[38] It has also been studied that there is a difference in the ability to induce cytokine production by the human keratinocytes, among the various species of *Malassezia* resulting in difference in the inflammatory response. Some *Malassezia* yeasts stimulate IL-8 production by human keratinocytes, resulting in a neutrophilic infiltrate in seborrheic dermatitis and malassezia folliculitis.[39]

Box 7.8: Malassezia species

- *M. globosa, M. restricta, M. furfur, M. sympodialis, M. slooffiae, M. obtusa, M. nana, M. dermatis, M. japonica, M.yamatonsis, M. pachydermatis and M. equi*

Treatment of pityriasis capitis comprises frequent use of shampoos and lotions containing azoles namely, ketaconazole, fluconazole, climbazole, ciclopiroxolamine, 1% terbinafine lotion, zinc pyrithione (anti-fungal and anti mitotic), keratolytics, such as 2% salicylic acid, 2% sulfur, tar, selenium sulfide (anti-seborrheic) and combinations of azoles (ketoconazole, sertaconazole) with zinc pyrithione. Short contact period of 5–7 minutes is to be advised while using these topical antifungal lotions or shampoos. Topical corticosteroids such as fluocinonide gel or solution is to be used only for a short term. Systemic antifungals such as ketoconazole, fluconazole and itraconazole are to be given to patients who are refractory to topical formulations. Oral ketoconazole 200 mg daily in an empty stomach for 4 weeks or itraconazole 200 mg/day for 7 days have been found to be effective in the treatment of seborrheic dermatitis.[24,40-42]

Malassezia folliculitis is characterized by the presence of itchy perifollicular papules and pustules over the upper trunk and back, most often in adolescents and young adults. Exact etiopathogenesis is not known. Usually *Malassezia* are present in the stratum corneum. In the case of pityrosporum folliculitis, these organisms are found in the ostium, central and deep segments of the hair follicle. Plugging of the follicle followed by *Malassezia* proliferation with the end result of cell mediated response and activation of alternate complement pathway leads to folliculitis.[43,44] Bacterial folliculitis and acne vulgaris may have a close resemblance to malassezia folliculitis. However, itching is present in the latter condition.

Histopathology reveals hyperkeratosis with dilatation of the pilosebaceous follicles. Spherical to oval budding yeast forms are present within the infundibulum, at the dilated orifice of the lumen of the follicle and occasionally in the perifollicular dermis and these are better visualized with special stains such as PAS (purple). Inflammatory infiltrate is seen both within and around the infundibulum of the follicle.[18] Systemic antifungals namely ketoconazole and itraconazole along with topical ketoconazole lotion are effective in the management of this condition. Ketoconazole 200 mg once a day for 4 weeks or itraconazole 200 mg daily for a period of 2 weeks result in a good clinical response.[24,45]

Conclusion

Among the trichomycoses, infections that are caused by dermatophytes can be completely cured with systemic antifungal agents given for the appropriate duration. There is no complete cure for pityrosporum capitis/ seborrheic dermatitis because of the multiple factors involved in the etiopathogenesis. Long-term treatment is warranted, as these conditions are of chronic nature. Piedra which is less common compared to tinea capitis and seborrheic dermatitis, is amenable to treatment, though may recur at times.

References

1. Verma S, Heffernan MP. Superficial fungal infection: Dermatophytosis, onychcmycosis, piedra. In: Wolff K, Goldsmith LA, Katz SI, Gilchrest BA, Paller AS, Leffell DJ, (eds). Fitzpatrick's Dermatology in General Medicine, 7th edn. New York: McGraw Hill. Health Profession & Division. 2008; pp. 1807-21.
2. Hay, RJ, Ashbee HR., Mycology. In: Burns T, Breathnach S, Cox N, Griffiths C, (eds). Textbook of Dermatology, 8th edn. West Sussex: Wiley Blackwell. 2010;pp. 36.1-36.93.
3. Elewski, BE. Tinea capitis: a current perspective. J Am Acad Dermatol. 2000;42(1) Part1:1-20.
4. Elewski B. Tinea capitis. Dermatol clin. 1996;14(1):23-31.
5. Kanwar AJ, De D. Superficial fungal infections: Tinea capitis. In: Valia RG, Valia AR (eds). Textbook of Dermatology, 3rd edn. Mumbai: Bhalani publishing house. 2008;pp.252-97.
6. Larralde M, Gomar B, Boggio P, Abad ME, Pagotto B. Neonatal Kerion Celsi: Report of three cases. Pediatr dermatol [online] 2010 Jul-Aug [cited 2010 Jul 20];27(4):p.361-63. Available from: http://onlinelibrary.wiley.com.
7. Romano C, Gianni C, Papini M. Tinea capitis in infants less than 1 year of age. Pediatric dermatology [online] 2002 Feb [cited 2002 Feb12];18(6):p.465-68. Available from: http://onlinelibrary.wiley.com.
8. Kamalam A. Observations on the gamut/galaxy of the fungal infections in Tamil Nadu State. Kavaka. 1984;12:15-36.
9. Rippon JW (ed). Cutaneous infections, dermatophytosis and dermatomycosis. Medical Mycology, 3rd edn. Philadelphia: W.B. Saunders. 1988;pp. 169-275.
10. Sentamilselvi G. Dermatophytosis. In: Sentamilselvi G, Janaki VR, Janaki C. The Handbook of Dermatomycology and Colour Atlas. 1st edn. Chennai: Dr G Sentamilselvi. 2006;pp. 9-15.
11. Kamalam A, Thambiah AS. Tinea capitis in South Indian families. Mykosen. 1979;22(7):251-54.
12. Kamalam A, Thambiah AS. Tinea capitis, endemic disease in Madras. Mycopathologica. 1980;71:45-51.
13. Kamalam A, Nanjappa Chetty G, Balasubramanian N, Chandrasekaran N, Thambiah AS. Tinea capitis in a moslem school. Indian Journal of Medical Research, 1979:70:41-43.
14. Chandrasekaran N, Kamalam A, Thambiah AS. Tinea capitis in an anglo-indian school. Tropical and Geographical Medicine. 1981;33:253-55.
15. Ergin S, Ergin C, Erdogan BS, Kaleli I, Evliyaoglu D. An experience from an outbreak of tinea capitis gladiatorum due to *Trichophyton tonsurans*. Clin Exp Dermatol. 2006;31(2):212-4.
16. Paller AS, Mancini AJ (eds). Skin disorders due to fungi. Hurwitz Clinical Pediatric Dermatology, 4th edn. Edinburgh: Elsevier Saunders. 2011;pp. 390-415.
17. Joshi R. Adamson's fringe Horatio George Adamson and Kligman's experiments and observations on tinea capitis. Int Journal of Trichology. 2011;3(1):14-19.
18. Hinshaw M, Longley JB. Fungal diseases. In: Elder DE, Elenitsas R, Johnson Jr BL, Murphy GF, Xu X. (eds). Lever's histopathology of the skin, 10th edn. New Delhi: Wolters Kluwer health. 2010;pp. 591-620.
19. Jahangir M, Hussain I, Khurshid, Haroon TS. A clinico-etiological correlation in tinea capitis. Int Journal of Dermatol. 1999;38(4):275-78.
20. Schwartz RA. Majocchi granuloma. 2011 [cited 2011 May 27]. Available from: http://e-medicine. medscape.com/article/1092601.
21. David Weedon (Ed). Mycoses and algal infections. Weedon's Skin Pathology, 3rd edn. China: Churchill Livingstone. 2010;pp. 581-606.
22. Padhye AA, Summerbell RC. The dermatophytes. In: Merz WG, Hay RJ (eds). Medical mycology. Topley Wilson's microbiology and microbial infections, 10th edn. London: Hodder Arnold. 2005;pp. 220-43.
23. Akbaba M, Ilkit M, Sutoluk Z, Ates A, Zorba H. Comparison of hair brush, tooth brush and cotton swab methods for diagnosing asymptomatic dermatophyte scalp carriage. JEADV. 2008;22(3):356-362.
24. Weeks J, Moser SA, Elewski BE. Superficial cutaneous fungal infections. In: Dismukes WE, Pappas PG, Sobel JD (eds). Clinical Mycology. Newyork: Oxford University Press. 2003;pp. 367-89.
25. Gupta AK. Systemic antifungal agents. In: Wolverton SE. (ed). Comprehensive Dermatologic Drug Therapy. 2nd edn. Philadelphia: Saunders. 2010;p.75-99.
26. Kakourou T, Uksal U. Guidelines for the management of tinea capitis in children. Pediatr Dermatol. 2010;27(3):226-8.
27. Gupta AK, Albreski D, Del Rosso JQ, Konnikov N. The use of the new oral antifungal agents, itraconazole, terbinafine and fluconazole to treat onychomycosis and other dermatomycoses. Curr Probl Dermatol. 2001;13(4):220-46.
28. Gupta AK, Adam P. Terbinafine pulse therapy is effective in tinea Capitis. Pediatr dermatol [online] 1998 [cited 2009 Mar 16];15(1):56–58. Available from: http://onlinelibrary.wiley.com.
29. Gupta AK, Adamiak A, Cooper EA. Efficacy and safety of terbinafine in children. JEADV. 2003;17(6):627-40.
30. Chander J. Piedra: Textbook of Medical Mycology. 3rd edn. New delhi: Mehta publishers. 2010;pp.114-19.
31. Ghorpade A, Ramanan C. White piedra. JEADV. 1994;3(2): 169-73.

32. Roshan A, Janaki C, Parveen B. White piedra in a mother and a daughter. Int Journal of Trichology. 2009;1(2):140-1.
33. Sentamilselvi G, janaki C, Murugusundaram S. Trichomycoses. Int Journal of Trichology. 2009;1(2):100-7.
34. Tajima M, Sugita T, Nishikawa A, Tsuboi R. Molecular Analysis of Malassezia Microflora in Seborrheic Dermatitis Patients: Comparison with Other Diseases and Healthy Subjects. J Invest Dermatol. 2008;128:345-51.
35. Ro BI, Dawson TL. The Role of Sebaceous Gland Activity and Scalp Microfloral Metabolism in the Etiology of Seborrheic Dermatitis and Dandruff. J Invest Dermato Symposium Proceedings. 2005;10:194-7.
36. Dawson Jr TL. Malassezia globosa and restricta: Breakthrough Understanding of the Etiology and Treatment of Dandruff and Seborrheic Dermatitis through Whole-Genome Analysis. J Invest Dermatol Symposium Proceedings. 2007;12:15-9.
37. DeAngelis YM, Gemmer CM, Kaczvinsky JR, Kenneally DC, Schwartz JR and Dawson Jr TL. Three Etiologic Facets of Dandruff and Seborrheic Dermatitis: Malassezia Fungi, Sebaceous Lipids, and Individual Sensitivity. J Invest Dermatol Symposium Proceedings. 2005;10:295-7.
38. Thomas DS, Ingham E, Bojar RA, Holland KT. *In vitro* modulation of human keratinocyte pro- and anti-inflammatory cytokine production by the capsule of *Malassezia* species. FEMS Immunol Medical Microbiol. 2008;54(2):203-14.
39. Watanabe S, Kano R, Sato H, Nakamura Y, Hasegawa A. The Effects of Malassezia Yeasts on Cytokine Production by Human Keratinocytes. J Invest Dermatol. 2001;116:769-73.
40. Jones JB. Seborrhoeic dermatitis. Eczema, lichenification, prurigo and erthroderma. In: Burns TS, Cox N, Griffiths C (eds). Textbook of Dermatology, 8th edn. Wiley Blackwell, West Sussex. 2010;23.1-51.
41. Gupta AK, Bluhm R, Cooper EA, Summerbell RC, Batra R. Seborrhoeic dermatitis. Dermatol clin. 2003;21:401-12.
42. Gupta AK, Bluhm R. Seborrhoeic dermatitis. JEADV. 2004;18:13-26.
43. Inamadar AC, Palit A. The genus Malassezia and human disease. Indian J Dermatol Venereol Leprol. 2003;69:265-70.
44. Bower SM, Hogan DJ, Mason SH. Malassezia (Pityrosporum) folliculitis. [cited 2012 Jan 23]. Available from: http://e-medicine. medscape.com/article/1091037.
45. Janik MP, Heffernan MP. Yeast infections: candidiasis and pityriasis (tinea) versicolor. In: Wolff K, Goldsmith LA, Katz SI, Gilchrest BA, Paller AS, Leffell DJ (eds). Fitzpatrick's Dermatology in General Medicine, 7th edn. New york: McGraw Hill Health Profession and Division. 2008;pp. 1822-30. fbf

8

Pediculosis Capitis

Savitha AS

"There is no more difficult art to acquire than the art of observation."

—*William Osler*

Introduction

Pediculosis capitis also known as head lice or cooties is an infestation of the scalp by head louse *Pediculus humanus* var *capitis* **(Box 8.1)**. The oldest known nits are about 10,000 years old. [1] Lice are ectoparasites, i.e. they live on the surface of the hosts and belong to the order Anoplura. They feed on human blood after piercing the skin and its saliva is the cause for pruritus. A louse can survive outside the human host for approximately 10 days.

Structure

The head louse is a wingless parasite, white to gray in color. The body is elongated, flattened, 1–2 mm in length. The abdomen is segmented and attached to 3 pairs of clawed legs. The female louse is larger in comparison to the male. The mouth is small consisting of 6 hooklets which aid in feeding. The head louse feeds for approximately 5 times per day, each feed lasting for 35–45 minutes **(Figure 8.1)**.

Life Cycle

The life cycle of the head louse lasts for 30-35 days. A mature female louse lays about 300 eggs at the rate of 5–9 per day, which are white and 1 mm in size. The eggs are laid at the base of the hair shaft, 1–2 mm away from the scalp which provides a suitable temperature for incubation, and hatch by 8–10 days.[2] The nit is enclosed by a tough and porous cap known as the operculum. This porous sheath permits gas exchange while the nymph develops in this casing. The nymph nodes 3 times over 10–15 days before reaching the adult form, while the adult louse survives for 30–50 days. On an average 20 lice are present during an infestation located characteristically, in the post-auricular area and posterior hairline **(Figure 8.2)**.

Box 8.1: *Pediculus humanus* capitis	
Kingdom: Animalia	
Phylum: Arthropoda	Class: Insecta
Order: Pthiraptera	Suborder: Anoplura
Family: Pediculidae	Genus: *Pediculus*
Species: *Pediculus humanus*	Sub species: *Pediculus humanus* capitis

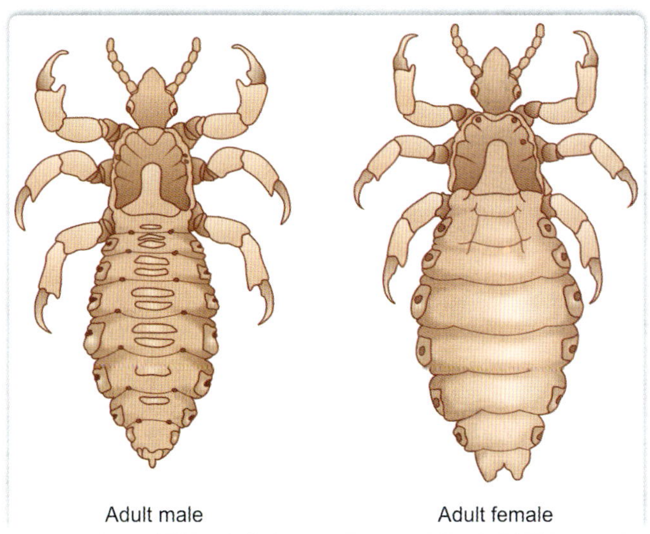

Fig. 8.1: Diagram of adult male and female louse

Epidemiology

Girls are at a higher risk of head louse infestation than boys because of social behavior (e.g. social acceptance of close physical contact; sharing of hats, combs). Children aged

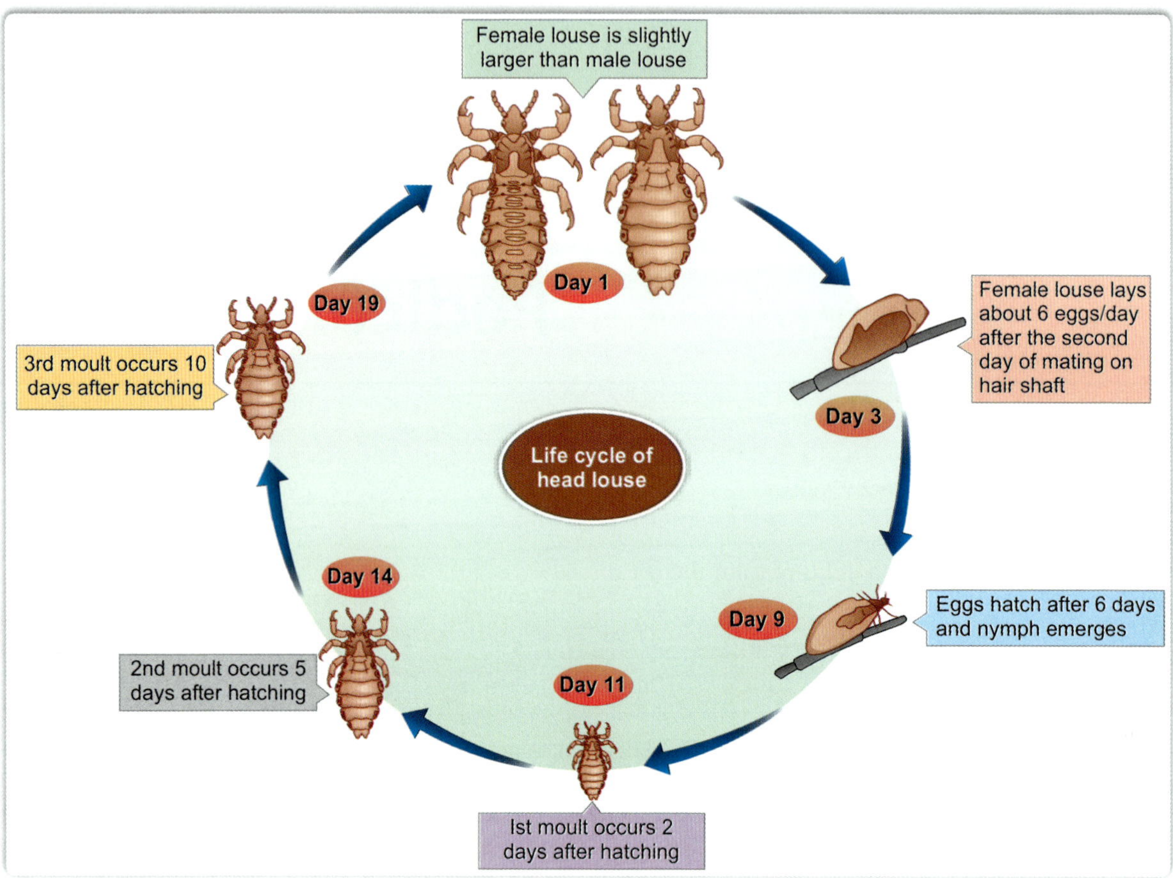

Fig. 8.2: Life cycle of head louse

3–11 years are likely to get infested with head lice because of close contact in classrooms and day care facilities. Head lice are much less common after puberty.

Risk Factors for Transmission

Pediculosis is transmitted by close personal contact and fomites (combs, hats, towels, bed covers, pillows). Overcrowding increases the risk of transmission. Hair combing may expel the louse more than 1 meter from the host.[2] They are unable to move on smooth surfaces like glass or plastic **(Box 8.2)**.

Clinical Features

Parents or teachers in school or care takers usually notice nits on the scalp. Pruritus is the initial presentation which is worse at night, when the lice are feeding. Pruritus begins 2–6 weeks after the first infestation but much sooner during repeated infestations. Though the entire scalp may be involved, infestation is usually confined to suboccipital and retroauricular area. The suboccipital depression is called the louse pit **(Box 8.3)**. Impetigo and enlargement of post-auricular and cervical lymph nodes are the other features. A generalized exanthem rarely accompanies louse infestation (pityriasis rosea-like pediculid) **(Box 8.4)**. On examination, nits attached to the hair shaft cannot be dislodged easily.

Box 8.2: Risk factors for louse infestation

- Young age
- Overcrowding
- Close personal contact
- Fomites—combs, caps, pillows, towels
- Hair combing

Box 8.3: Louse pit

- Suboccipital depression
- Infestation is usually confined to suboccipital and retroauricular area

Box 8.4: Clinical features of louse infestation

- Pruritus
- Impetigo
- Enlargement of post-auricular and cervical nodes
- Generalized exanthem
- Pityriasis rosea–like pediculid
- Plica polonica
- Firmly attached nits to hair shaft

Demonstration of live louse is difficult as they move rapidly through dry hair. Wetting hair and usage of a fine toothed comb is useful to dislodge eggs and live lice. Since human scalp hair grows at a rate of approximately 10 mm/month (0.37 mm/day), the distance of nits from the scalp can be used to estimate the duration of infestation. Nits found several millimeters from the scalp are nonviable empty egg cases **(Figure 8.3)**. They indicate chronic infestation. The composition of the nit sheath is similar to that of human hair, so agents designed to unravel the nit sheath may also damage hair.[3]

Wood's lamp examination shows white fluorescence with nits. "Entodermoscopy" is a new term employed for dermoscopy of skin infections and infestations, recently introduced by Zalaudek, et al.[4] In vivo dermoscopic findings with noncontact handheld dermoscope of pediculosis capitis shows ovoid brown nits with nymphs, while empty cases are translucent with plane and fissured free ending.[5]

Differential Diagnosis

For nits

1. Dried hair spray- can easily be dislodged
2. Hair casts—Hair casts are ring like remnants of the inner root sheath of the hair follicle. They are amorphous and freely moveable along the hair fiber **(Box 8.5)**
3. White piedra—KOH mount shows fungal elements
4. Seborrheic dermatitis—yellow greasy scales
5. Acne necrotica
6. Impetigo
7. Hair shaft disorders like monilethrix, trichorrhexis nodosa

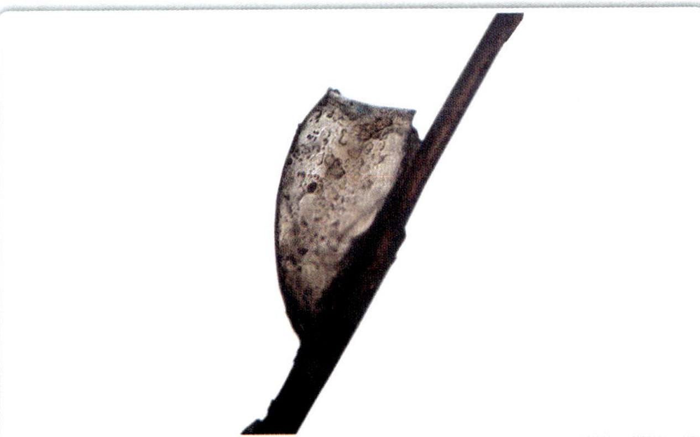

Fig. 8.3: Empty nit case attached to hair shaft

Box 8.5: Hair casts vs nits

- *Hair cast:* Amorphous ring like remnants of the inner root sheath of the hair follicle freely moveable along the hair fiber
- *Nits:* A proteinaceous sheath that encloses the egg laid 1–2 mm above scalp level, enclosing hair shaft and egg except operculum
- Composition of nit sheath is similar to hair shaft
- Distance of nit from scalp is an index of duration of infestation

Treatment (Table 8.1)

General Measures

Patient education regarding the infestation and stressing on retreatment after 7–10 days. Close contacts should be examined and treated. Fomite control has to be instructed. Sharing of combs and towels should be avoided. Young nits have no nervous system , so are immune to neurotoxic pesticides. Careful combing and removal of all nits from the hair as well as cleaning of other articles (i.e. hair accessories, towels, bedding, and clothing) are essential steps to prevent reinfestation. It may be beneficial to launder potential fomites (e.g. towels, pillowcases, sheets, hats, toys) in hot water, followed by machine drying using the hottest cycle. Temperatures exceeding 131°F (55°C) for more than 5 minutes kill eggs, nymphs, and mature lice. Items that are not machine washable, may be placed in a dryer at high heat for 30 minutes. Dry cleaning may be an effective alternative.

Since adult lice cannot survive for long when separated from the host and eggs that hatch in 6–10 days will die without a blood meal, carefully sealing potential fomites in plastic bags for 2 weeks can be effective. This technique works well for objects, such as stuffed toys, that do not tolerate laundering or dry cleaning. Vacuuming selected areas of the home, such as couches used by infested patients, is recommended by some as an adjunctive control measure. Secondary infection should be managed first.

Topical Therapy (Table 8. 2)

1. **Permethrin:** Shampoos, permethrin 1% rinse, permethrin 5% lotion/cream rinse/liquid. Apply to washed and dried hair, leave on for 10 minutes, rinse and

Table 8.1: Management of pediculosis capitis

General measures	Patient education Treatment of close contacts Fomite control Removal of nits mechanically
Topical therapy	Permethrin 1% and 5% Malathion 0.5% Gamma benzene hexachloride Ivermectin Spinosad 0.9% Benzyl alcohol Dimethicone lotion—4%
Oral drugs	Ivermectin Levamisole Albendazole Trimethoprim-sulfamethoxazole

comb out nits and eggs. Application to dry hair reduces the dilution of the medication. Single application is usually curative. Shampooing should be avoided for 24 hours afterward. Side effects include mild and transient burning and stinging (10%). Permethrin acts as a neurotoxin by depolarizing nerve cell membranes of parasites. Delayed repolarization results in paralysis of nerves in the exoskeletal respiratory muscles of parasite leading to death. Permethrin is the drug of choice recommended by most authorities especially for infants older than 2 months and small children. The residual effect on hair persists for several hair wash cycles. Permethrin is effective against adult lice and nymphs but not effective against nits (eggs). A fine-toothed comb is an important adjunct to remove nits.

2. **Malathion:** Malathion has proved to be more ovicidal than permethrin. It is an irreversible cholinesterase inhibitor that is hydrolyzed and therefore detoxified rapidly by mammals but not by insects; it is both ovicidal and pediculicidal. It binds to hair and provides some residual protection after therapy. Malathion is available as 0.5% and 1% aqueous-based lotions, 0.5% cream. Apply to dry hair, leave on for 8–12 hours . Side effects include local irritation, contact hypersensitivity reaction, conjunctivitis if accidental contact with eyes. Cautions—malathion is inflammable: avoid hair dryer and smoking.
3. **Lindane/Gamma benzene hexachloride:** Apply shampoo on dry hair; leave on for 4 minutes, lather, rinse, remove nits with fine comb. One time application is usually sufficient. Contraindications includes premature neonates (< 28 days) (increased absorption), uncontrolled seizure disorder, hypersensitivity and skin conditions that may increase systemic absorption.
4. **Ivermectin:** A single 10-minute application without nit combing, causes parasite death by selective binding to the glutamate-gated chloride channels located in invertebrate nerve and muscle cells. Rare side effects like eye irritation and skin burning sensation may be seen. Plasma levels following topical administration are much lower than those observed following per oral (PO) administration.
5. **Spinosad:** Spinosad is recommended for the treatment of head louse infestation in patients aged 4 years and older. The product is applied to dry hair as a cream rinse, left for 10 minutes, followed by shampooing. Spinosad has ovicidal activity which overcomes the need for manual removal of nits.[6] Spinosad causes neuronal excitation in insects, followed by hyperexcitation, paralysis, and death. This agent is available as a 0.9% suspension.
6. **Benzyl alcohol:** This agent works by clogging the respiratory spiracles of the louse. It is recommended in patients 6 months of age and older.[7,8] The lotion is applied for 10 minutes 1 week apart, to kill the lice which have molted following the first application, since it is ineffective against nits. Benzyl alcohol lotion is a safe alternative compared to lindane and malathion due to its physical action.
7. **4% dimethicone lotion:** A silicone-based lotion believed to disrupt the louse's ability to manage water.[9]

Other occlusive therapy techniques such as vinegar, mayonnaise, petroleum jelly, olive oil, butter, isopropyl alcohol, and water submersion as long as 6 hours have been advocated, but most have not been scientifically evaluated. However, a dry-on, suffocation-based pediculicide lotion was found to be effective in open trials.[10] Essential oils demonstrate variable efficacy and may be contact allergens.

Most studies have shown that mechanical removal alone (i.e. wet-combing every 2–3 days for a minimum of 2 weeks - Bug busting method) **(Box 8.6)** is not as effective as mechanical removal combined with a pediculicide.[11]

Emergence of resistance to over the counter medications has been reported. Knockdown resistance (KDR) is a common mechanism of resistance that manifests as lack of immobilization of the lice. Responsible gene mutations (T929I and L932F) have been identified and can be used to screen for KDR.[12]

Oral Agents

1. **Ivermectin**—ivermectin binds selectively with glutamate gated chloride ion channels in invertebrate nerve and muscle cells, causing cell death. It is not effective against nits. Dosage is 200 mcg/kg PO once; may require 1–2 additional doses repeated after 7 days.
2. **Levamisole**—3.5 mg/kg once daily for 10 days.
3. **Albendazole**—400 mg per day for 3 days. But topical permethrin is better than albendazole.
4. **Trimethoprim-sulfamethoxazole** was initially reported to be effective; however, controlled studies have shown only minimal eradication. Cotrimoxazole kills the adult lice by destroying the bacteria in the gut of the louse on which they are dependent for synthesis of vitamin B.[13]

Box 8.6: Bug busting method

Principle: Lice cannot move to another host within 7 days after hatching, and cannot reproduce within 10 days, and all eggs hatch within 7 to 10 days.

Therefore, if all young lice are combed out a few days after hatching, the infestation can be eradicated

Table 8.2: Topical agents used in pediculosis capitis

Name	Mechanism of action	Method of application	Preparations
Permethrin	It is a neurotoxin, acts by depolarizing nerve cell membranes of parasites. Delayed repolarization results in paralysis of nerves in the exoskeletal respiratory muscles of parasite leading to death	Apply to washed and dried hair, leave on for 10 min, rinse and comb out nits and eggs	1% rinse, 5%- Lotion/cream rinse/ liquid.
Malathion	Irreversible cholinesterase inhibitor that is hydrolyzed and therefore detoxified rapidly by mammals but not by insects	Apply to dry hair, leave on for 8–12 hours	0.5% and 1% aqueous-based lotions, 0.5% cream.
Gamma benzene hexachloride	Stimulates the nervous system of parasite causing seizures and death	Apply shampoo on dry hair; leave on for 4 minutes, lather, rinse, remove nits with fine comb. One time application is usually sufficient	1% lotion, shampoo
Ivermectin	Causes parasite death by selective binding to the glutamate-gated chloride channels located in invertebrate nerve and muscle cells	A single 10-minute application without nit combing	0.5%
Spinosad	Causes neuronal excitation in insects, followed by hyperexcitation, paralysis, and death	Applied to dry hair as a cream rinse, left for 10 minutes, followed by shampooing	0.9% suspension
Benzyl alcohol	Works by clogging the respiratory spiracles of the louse	Applied for 10 minutes 1 week apart, to kill the lice which have molted following the first application, since it is ineffective against nits	5% lotion
Dimethicone lotion	Silicone-based lotion believed to disrupt the louse's ability to manage water	Applied for 12–17 hours	4% lotion

Complications

1. Secondary bacterial infection
2. Social embarrassment
3. Plica polonica—severe infestation with matting of the hair due to pus and exudates
4. Id reaction—pediculid[14]

Prognosis

Treatments are highly effective in killing nymphs and mature lice but less effective against eggs. Appropriate therapy produces a cure in more than 90% of cases after single application.

Causes of therapeutic failure are given in **Box 8.7**.

Box 8.7: Causes for therapeutic failure

- Misdiagnosis
- Inappropriate treatment
- Noncompliance
- Insufficient application of pediculicide
- Lack of ovicidal activity of pediculicide and failure to re-treat in 7–10 days
- Lack of removal of live nits
- Lack of environmental eradication
- Reinfestation
- Resistance to pediculicide

For treatment failures, ivermectin may be used in nonpregnant or non-breastfeeding woman and in children weighing more than 15 kg.

References

1. Araujo A, Ferreira LF, Guidon N, et al. Ten thousand years of head lice infection. Parasitol Today. Jul 2000;16(7):269.
2. Fournier PE, Ndihokubwayo JB, Guidran J, et al. Human pathogens in body and head lice. Emerg Infect Dis. 2002;8:1515-8.
3. Burkhart CN, Burkhart CG. Head lice: scientific assessment of the nit sheath with clinical ramifications and therapeutic options. J Am Acad Dermatol. Jul 2005;53(1):129-33.
4. Zalaudek I, Giacomel J, Cabo H, Di Stefani A, Ferrara G, Hofmann-Wellenhof R, et al. Entodermoscopy: a new tool for diagnosing skin infections and infestations. Dermatology. 2008;216:14-23.
5. Di Stefani A, Hofmann-Wellenhof R, Zalaudek I. Dermoscopy for diagnosis and treatment monitoring of pediculosis capitis. J Am Acad Dermatol. 2006;54:909-11.
6. Stough D, Shellabarger S, Quiring J, Gabrielsen AA Jr. Efficacy and safety of spinosad and permethrin creme rinses for pediculosis capitis (head lice). Pediatrics. Sep 2009;124(3):e389-95.
7. Pearlman DL. A simple treatment for head lice: dry-on, suffocation-based pediculicide. Pediatrics. Sep 2004;114(3):e275-9.

8. Pearlman DL. Nuvo lotion and the future of head-lice treatment. Pediatrics. May 2005;115(5):1452-3.
9. Burgess IF, Brown CM, Lee PN. Treatment of head louse infestation with 4% dimeticone lotion: randomised controlled equivalence trial. BMJ. Jun 18 2005;330(7505):1423.
10. Pearlman DL. A simple treatment for head lice: dry-on, suffocation-based pediculicide. Pediatrics. Sep 2004;114(3):e275-9
11. Roberts RJ, Casey D, Morgan DA, Petrovic M. Comparison of wet combing with malathion for treatment of head lice in the UK: a pragmatic randomised controlled trial. Lancet. Aug 12 2000;356(9229):540-4.
12. William D James, Timothy G Berger, Dirk M Elston (eds). Andrews diseases of the skin, clinical dermatology, 10th edn. Elsiever, saunders. p 447.
13. Burns DA. Action of cotrimoxazole on head lice (letter). Br J Dermatol. 1987;117:399.
14. Brenner S, Ophir J, Krakowski A. Pediculid - an unusual id reaction to pediculosis capitis. Dermatologica. 1984;168: 189-91.

9

Scalp Disorders: Itchy and Scaly Scalp

Manjunath Shenoy M

"Happiness is having a scratch for every itch."

—*Ogden Nash*

Introduction

Itching is a skin sensation that causes a desire to scratch. It is a body's response to the presence of some harmful stimulation which may require immediate attention. It is a symptom that is subjective in nature and poorly localized, and its neuro-anatomy includes receptors, peripheral and central nerves, spinal pathways, and several brain regions **(Box 9.1)**.[1] Scalp is an easily accessible site and there are a number of conditions that provoke pruritus. It is often distressing or uncontrollable, and is a cause of social embarrassment. Hairiness of the scalp makes an itchy scalp diagnostically and therapeutically challenging especially when other body parts are uninvolved. This chapter briefly deals with many such conditions which will able physicians to understand the pathophysiology, diagnostic significance and management.

Shedding of keratinocytes from the scalp may be an indication of a simple dry scalp or a pathological condition. In most pathological conditions, it is associated with signs of inflammation and hence pruritus is a constant symptom. Certain conditions like seborrheic dermatitis are very common affecting half of the population, whereas others like pityriasis amiantacea are associated with massive accumulation or shedding of scales leading to significant discomfort.

Box 9.1: Itch

It is a symptom that is subjective in nature and poorly localized, and its neuro-anatomy includes receptors, peripheral and central nerves, spinal pathways, and several brain regions

Pathophysiology of Itch (Pruritus)

Scalp, like face, is a sebum rich zone. Sebum is composed of a complex mixture of squalene, wax esters, cholesterol esters, triglycerides, and free cholesterol. Triglycerides produce free fatty acids (FFA) by catalytic reactions induced by bacterial hydrolases. Proinflammatory FFAs are capable of irritating the skin. Lipid chemical composition can be significantly altered in different skin diseases like atopic dermatitis, seborrheic dermatitis and psoriasis, thus explaining variable pruritis in these conditions. Stratum corneum has a higher water barrier function compared to the face or extremities, thus induces protective barrier function against exogenous factors like infections and irritants.[2]

Pruritus can be triggered by a wide range of known and unknown stimuli. Receptors for pruritus are both slow and fast adapting, and they include Merkel discs and free nerve endings.[1] It is generally believed that the slow-conducting unmyelinated C fibers are the transmitters of pruritus in humans. Recent advances in neurobiology of pruritus have shown that these fibers do not appear to play an important role in the modulation of chronic pruritus. Non-histaminergic unknown pathways may also contribute to the conduction of pruriginous impulses, and serotonin and endogenous opioids play an important role in systemic pruritus.[3] Pruritus can also be triggered by cytokines, proteases, serotonin, prostaglandins, neuropeptides, endogenous opioids and substance P **(Figure 9.1)**. Similar to the chronic pain, central sensitization of pruritus contributes to the abnormal modulation of chronic pruritus. Scratching stimulates A-delta myelinated sensory fibers and temporarily blocks the pruriginous sensation.[3] Neuronal toll like receptors expressed in neuronal and non-neuronal

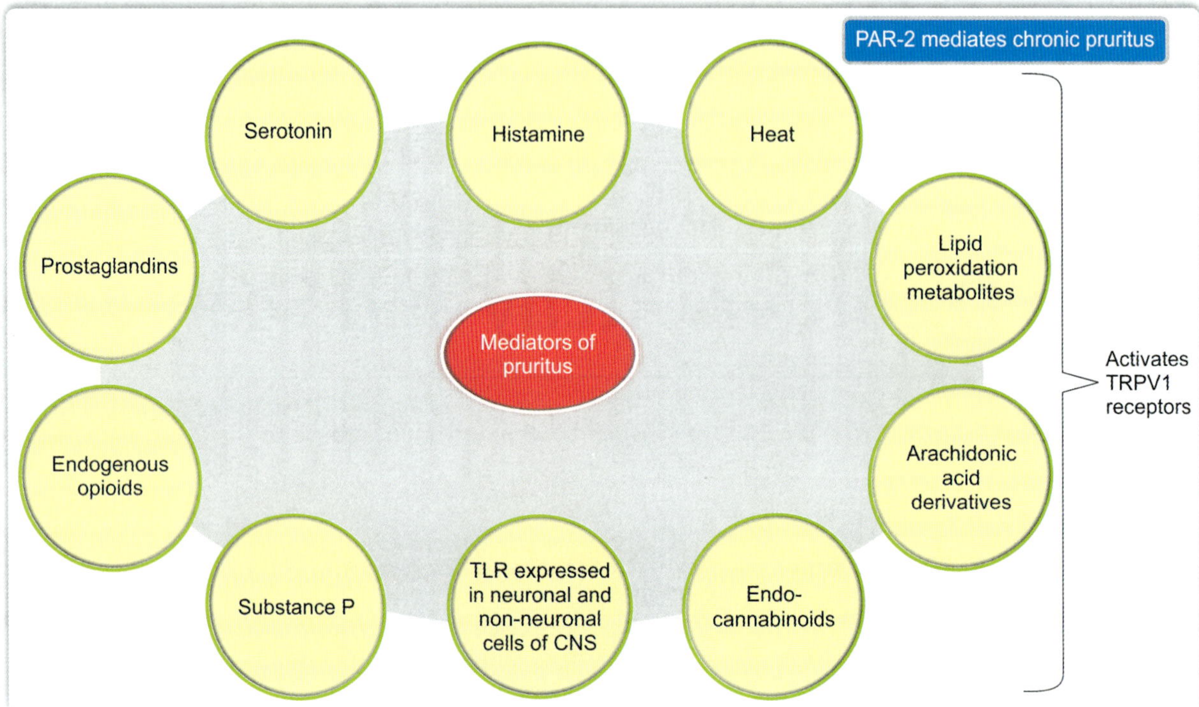

Fig. 9.1: Mediators of pruritus
Abbreviations: TLR, Toll like receptors; TRPV1, Transient receptor potential vanilloid 1

cells of CNS are also now considered as new players in the processing of pain and itch by increasing the excitability of primary sensory neurons.[4] Understanding these newer pathways will open a new avenue for the management of clinical pain and itch.

Histamine released from the mast cells is the most important itch mediator and can induce pruritus via H1 and H4 receptors on nerve fibers, whereas H3 receptors appear to be involved in the suppression of pruritus. Mast cells can also induce pruritus directly through the release of mediators like cytokines chymase and tryptase **(Box 9.2)**. Opioids and their receptors in the skin is a neuronal communication between pain and itch-transmitting neurons that underlies the role of opioids in pruritus. PAR-2 (protease activated receptor 2), a G-protein coupled receptor, plays a major role in mediating chronic pruritus. TRPV1 receptor is activated by heat, acidosis, arachidonic acid derivatives, lipid peroxidation metabolites, and endo-cannabinoids which causes burning pain, itching and heat sensation. Cannabinoid receptors mediate the psychopharmacological action of marijuana itch.[2]

Box 9.2: Mast cells mediators and pruritus

- Mast cell releases histamine, chymase and tryptase (mediators)
- Histamine induces pruritus via H1 and H4 receptors on nerve fibers, whereas H3 receptors causes suppression of pruritus

The scalp has a complex neuroanatomy with abundance of sensory neural end organs in the pilosebaceous unit and dermal vasculature. Understanding the neurobiology of scalp and hair follicles, and mediators of pruritus can provide a putative mechanism for scalp itch.[2] The sensory innervation of the scalp is conducted through branches from the trigeminal nerve, cervical plexus and dorsal rami of the cervical nerves **(Figure 9.2)**. Free nerve endings innervating the hair follicles are the A-delta (thinly myelinated) or C fibers (unmyelinated), that arise from the superficial nerve plexus; and they terminate in the connective tissue

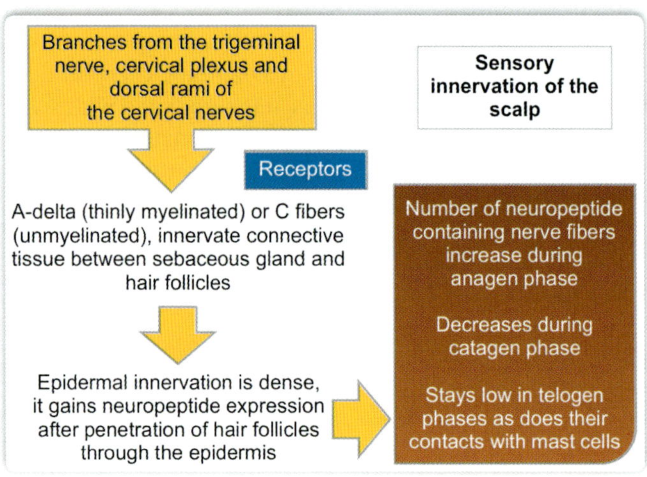

Fig. 9.2: Sensory innervations of scalp

between the sebaceous gland and hair follicles. Epidermal innervation is very dense, but it decreases and gains neuropeptide expression after penetration of hair follicles through the epidermis. Number of neuropeptide containing nerve fibers increase during the anagen phase, decreases during the catagen phase, and stays low in the telogen phase as does their contacts with mast cells. Although the scalp is considered extremely itchy in many inflammatory diseases, the experimental studies in humans were not able to demonstrate lower itch thresholds on the scalp. Scalp is not the most innervated organ too.

Clinical Characteristics

Scalp pruritus has many causes; some patients may have more than one cause while in others no definite underlying disease can be identified. There is no definite classification for causes of itchy scalp. In a proposed classification of causes of pruritus, disorders were divided into three groups; pruritus on diseased (inflamed) skin (group I), pruritus on non-diseased (non-inflamed) skin (group II), and pruritus presenting with severe chronic secondary scratch lesions (group III) **(Box 9.3)**.[5] Underlying diseases are further classified into different categories: dermatological diseases, systemic diseases, drug-induced pruritus, neurological and psychiatric diseases. Similar classification may also yield useful insight into causes of itchy scalp. First and second groups of disorders are well documented on the scalp. Inflamed scalp disorders are almost always associated with scaly lesions.

There are certain disorders that are associated with severe scaling with or without pruritus. Degree of pruritus is highly variable. Often they are resistant to any form of therapy. The list of such disorders is given in **Tables 9.1 and 9.2**.

Some of the more common causes are discussed here.

Box 9.3: Proposed classification of causes of pruritus

- Group I: Pruritus on diseased (inflamed) skin
- Group II: Pruritus on non-diseased (non-inflamed) skin
- Group III: Pruritus presenting with severe chronic secondary scratch lesions

Table 9.1: Causes of itchy (pruritic) scalp

Pruritus on inflamed scalp	Infections and infestations	Folliculitis, tinea, pediculosis, scabies, varicella, herpes zoster, herpes simplex, HIV/AIDS disease
	Inflammatory disorders	Atopic dermatitis, psoriasis, seborrheic dermatitis, pityriasis amiantacea, discoid lupus, Darier disease
	Autoimmune disorders	Dermatitis herpetiformis, pemphigus
	Others	Urticaria, drug rashes, post zoster neuralgia, lichen simplex nuche
Pruritus on non-inflamed scalp	Systemic disorders	Pruritus due to renal, hepatic, hematologic and metabolic disorders, Hodgkin's and non-Hodgkin's lymphoma, drug induced
	Psychiatric and psycho-somatic disorders	Depression, anxiety disorders, obsessive-compulsive disorders, schizophrenia, tactile hallucinosis, delusional parasitosis, somatoform and dissociative disorders

Table 9.2: List of common scaly disorders of scalp with salient features

Psoriasis	Psoriasis is a common scalp disease that appears as silvery white scale on inflamed scalp skin in round or oval plaques. Scalp is a common site but lesions may be found in the post-auricular and external auditory canal area and usually in other body parts. Amount of scaling may vary and scratching results in easy bleeding (Auspitz sign). Psoriasis does not generally cause hair loss
Pityriasis amiantacea	A heavy scaling condition with scales resembling asbestos, giving rise to the name amiantacea. Cause may not be detectable or may be found in association with psoriasis and seborrheic dermatitis. Scalp scales stick to the hair or the hair is stuck to the scalp
Seborrheic dermatitis (pityriasis capitis)	Pityriasis capitis (dandruff) is a common problem associated with excessive shedding of dead skin cells from the stratum corneum. It is thought to be associated with an abundance of pityrosporum ovale yeasts on the scalp and its interaction with scalp skin. It is a common social or self-esteem related problem due to associated scaling and scalp pruritus
Tinea capitis	Ectothrix dermatophytes *M. audouinii* or *M. canis* cause seborrheic form of tinea capitis with prominent scaly scalp with minimal inflammation. Hairs in the affected area discolor, become lusterless and break off. The "black dot" form of tinea capitis is caused by the endothrix fungi *T. tonsurans* and *T. violaceum* is also least inflammatory and cause scaly form of tinea capitis. Hairs are broken at the level of the scalp leaving behind a patch of alopecia with grouped black dots
Discoid lupus erythematosus (DLE)	DLE lesions on the scalp can form large, confluent, disfiguring atrophic plaques of cicatricial alopecia with adherent scales. Scale, if lifted from the advancing margins of the lesions show keratotic spikes resembling carpet tacks (the "carpet tack" sign)
Darier disease	Scalp and other seborrheic areas are typically affected in Darier disease with greasy keratotic papules that form scaly, crusted, and confluent plaques that can be extensive
Atopic dermatitis	Scaly scalp is a common manifestation of childhood atopic dermatitis and is associated with severe pruritus of the scalp. Infra and retroauricular dermatitis with fissuring may be associated

Seborrheic Dermatitis

Seborrheic dermatitis is a result of complex interaction between *Malassezia* yeast, sebum and host immune system. The commonest presentation of seborrheic dermatitis is scalp pruritus and scaling; at least 50% of the population suffer from seborrheic dermatitis sometime in their lifetime. There are two forms of seborrheic dermatitis: infantile and adult.

In the infantile form, frontal and parietal scalp regions are usually affected with greasy thick crust (cradle cap) often showing fissuring. It usually occurs between the first 2 and 6 weeks of life, but may persist until puberty.

Adult form is characterized by erythema and greasy scaling that favor scalp, ears, face, chest, and inter-scapular area. Pruritus may be severe particularly on the scalp and in the auditory canal. It may be a cutaneous marker of human immunodeficiency virus infection when it is severe, atypical and resistant to treatment.

Psoriasis

Scalp psoriasis can be an isolated entity or a part of generalized psoriasis. Involvement can be in the form of localized erythematous round or oval plaques or more diffuse and extending into the scalp margins **(Figure 9.3)**. Pruritus is variable and scratching may lead to bleeding (Auspitz sign).

A common clinical entity known as sebopsoriasis presents with erythematous plaques with greasy scales located in the seborrheic areas like scalp, glabella, nasolabial folds and intertriginous areas. In the absence of typical psoriasis elsewhere, distinction from seborrheic dermatitis is difficult. Sebopsoriasis may represent a modification of seborrheic dermatitis by the genetic background of psoriasis **(Box 9.4)**.[6]

Scalp psoriasis is sometimes indistinguishable from seborrheic dermatitis. **Table 9.3** will summarize a few features that may be invaluable. Dermatoscopy may also be helpful **(Table 9.4)**.

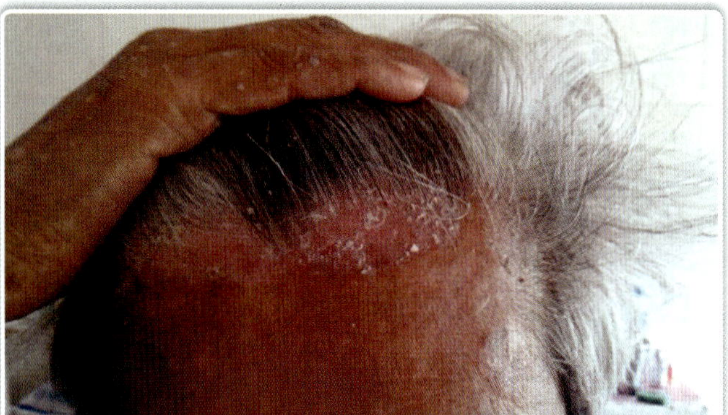

Figure 9.3: Corona psoriatica: scaling in scalp psoriasis extending onto glabrous skin (*Courtesy:* Department of Dermatology, STD and Leprosy, BMCRI, Bengaluru)

Atopic Dermatitis

Atopic dermatitis (AD) is a chronically relapsing cutaneous disease that commonly presents during infancy and early childhood. Abnormalities in skin barrier function, immunologic dysregulation, genetic predisposition and allergen sensitization are among the various pathogenetic mechanisms of AD. Classically it presents with facial and extensor dermatitis in infants and early childhood and involvement of flexural folds of the extremities in older children and adults.

Approximately half of childhood atopic dermatitis manifests with scaling and pruritus of the scalp [7]; this aspect is not highlighted in the literature. Apart from scalp dermatitis, infra-auricular and retro-auricular dermatitis with fissuring was also commonly observed in the infantile phase of AD and can be an important diagnostic clue.[8]

Contact Dermatitis

Scalp may be relatively resistant to allergic sensitization, possibly due to skin thickness, dilutional effect of perspiration, presence of follicular hair units and variations in vascularity.[6] Scalp is often exposed to allergens like hair dyes, surfactants and fragrances, but still the incidence of contact dermatitis seems to be less frequent. Often they elicit dermatitis in the adjacent areas like hairline, eyelids,

Box 9.4: Sebopsoriasis

- May represent a modification of seborrheic dermatitis by the genetic background of psoriasis
- Erythematous plaques with greasy scales located in the seborrheic areas
- Distinction from psoriasis difficult in absence of classic psoriatic lesion

Table 9.3: Differences between scalp psoriasis and seborrheic dermatitis

Scalp psoriasis	*Seborrheic dermatitis*
Erythematous scaly plaques with silvery white scales	Oily skin with yellowish greasy scales; faint erythema
Thick scales and attempt to remove leads to bleeding	Finer scales, when severe may feel crusty
Patches may extend beyond hair margin	Rarely extend beyond hair margin
Variable itching	Severe itching
Psoriasis is usually seen elsewhere on the body	Often limited to scalp but sometimes seen in other seborrheic areas

Table 9.4: Procedural/laboratory diagnosis in itchy scaly scalp

Diagnostic test	*Indications*	*Findings*
Wood's lamp examination	Suspected tinea capitis	Emits green fluorescence in ectothrix-type tinea capitis (*Microsporum* speics.); can also help for specimen collection that has a higher likelihood of yielding a positive culture
Dermatoscopy	To distinguish between psoriasis and seborrheic dermatitis	Scalp psoriasis; red dots, globules, twisted red loops, and glomerular vessels; seborrheic dermatitis depicts arborizing vessels and atypical red vessels with the absence of red dots and globules[11]
Potassium hydroxide (KOH) mount of scales or hairs	Suspected tinea capitis	Confirms tinea capitis if fungal elements are detectable and also shows the pattern of infection, i.e. Ectothrix or Endothrix
Fungal culture	Suspected tinea capitis	Detects the causative agent
Patch test	Suspected contact dermatitis	Detects or confirms the clinically suspected contact dermatitis
Skin biopsy/histopathology	In scarring alopecia (DLE, lichen planus), psoriasis, Darier disease	Histopathology is diagnostic
Immunofluorescence	Dermatitis herpetiformis	Granular IgA deposits in the basement membrane zone

and post-auricular areas. Other causes should be ruled out before diagnosing patient with contact dermatitis of scalp.

Most common cause of contact dermatitis of scalp is the para-phenylenediamine (PPD) from hair dyes. It is often severe allergic contact dermatitis (ACD) and present acutely after allergen exposure in a previously sensitized individual.

Pityriasis Amiantacea (Box 9.5)

Also known as Tinea amiantacea or asbestos scalp is the disease of the scalp in which heavy thick, tenacious scales extend onto the hairs and bind together. Pityriasis amiantacea seems to be a reaction of the scalp to various inflammatory dermatoses with or without an evident cause. It may occur at any age but more common in children. Attempt to remove off the scales can lead to scarring alopecia. It may be most frequently observed as a sequelae of psoriasis, and seborrheic dermatitis[10] but also of pyogenic infections or atopic dermatitis. It is not usually followed by atrophy, scarring or alopecia.

Lichen Planus

Lichen planus of the scalp may present as lichen planopilaris (follicular lichen planus). Pruritic, multiple patches of scaring alopecia with follicular hyperkeratosis and erythema at the margin of the patches is the typical presentation. Evidence of lichen planus may be present at the classical areas like ankles and wrist. Patches of follicular papules with development of areas of alopecia on the scalp, eyebrows, axillary and pubic areas may be seen, described as Graham-Little syndrome **(Box 9.6 and Figure 9.4)**.

Box 9.5: Asbestos scalp (tinea amiantacea/pityriasis amiantacea)

- Reaction of the scalp to various inflammatory dermatoses with or without an evident cause
- Sequelae of psoriasis, seborrheic dermatitis, atopic dermatitis, pyogenic infections
- Thick, tenacious scales extend onto the hairs and bind together
- No atrophy, scarring, or alopecia

Box 9.6: Graham Little Piccardi syndrome

Triad
- Cicatricial alopecia of the scalp with or without follicular plugging
- Loss of axillary and pubic hair without obvious scarring
- Widespread keratosis pilaris

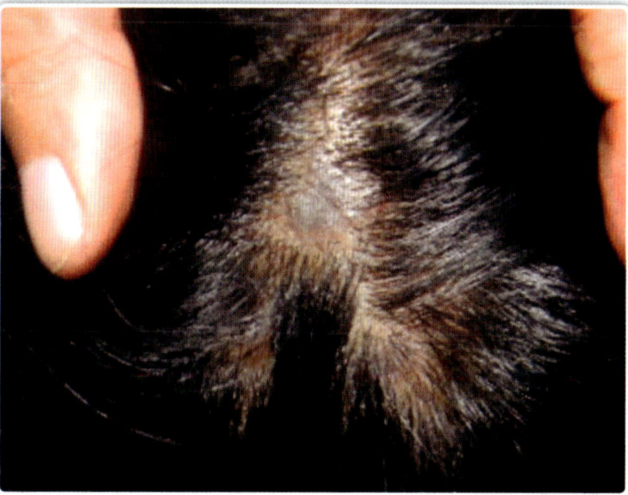

Figure 9.4: Lichen planus of scalp (*Courtesy:* Department of Dermatology, STD and Leprosy, BMCRI, Bengaluru)

Frontal Fibrosing Alopecia

Frontal fibrosing alopecia refers to a fronto-temporal hairline recession and loss of eyebrows in association with perifollicular erythema seen typically in post-menopausal women. Scalp biopsy histologically resembles lichen planopilaris.

Pediculosis Capitis

Pediculosis capitis is a common itchy scalp disease of school children especially girls, typically presents with nits most often found in the occipital and retroauricular regions. Pruritus is due to a hypersensitivity reaction to louse or its products. Tiny hemorrhagic crusts, excoriations, secondary impetigo and lymphadenopathy are also commonly seen.

Lichen Simplex

It is a chronic, severely pruritic disorder characterized by presence of single or few lichenified plaques in which the skin is thickened and accentuated skin markings are seen. Scalp and the nape of neck are among the most common sites of involvement. It is intensely pruritic which may be continuous or paroxysmal. It is more common in adult females, psychological and emotional factors are implicated in the pathogenesis.

Sensitive Scalp

Sensitive scalp is an extension of sensitive skin to this anatomical location. It is characterized by subjective complaints of discomfort without predictable classical visible signs of inflammation. Triggering factors may be shampoos, pollution, heat and emotional factors.[9] It may be a common entity and is reported with high frequency in French population.

Bullous Disorders

Pemphigus and dermatitis herpetiformis are common disorders among the autoimmune bullous disorders that cause scalp lesions and pruritus. In pemphigus, scalp may be one of the earliest cutaneous sites of involvement **(Figure 9.5).** Almost all cases are associated with lesions in other parts of body. Erosions on scalp may sometimes have a tendency to develop excessive granulation tissue and form vegetating lesions. Dermatitis herpetiformis is characterized by the presence of intensely pruritic papulovesicular eruptions. Characteristic lesions are papules,

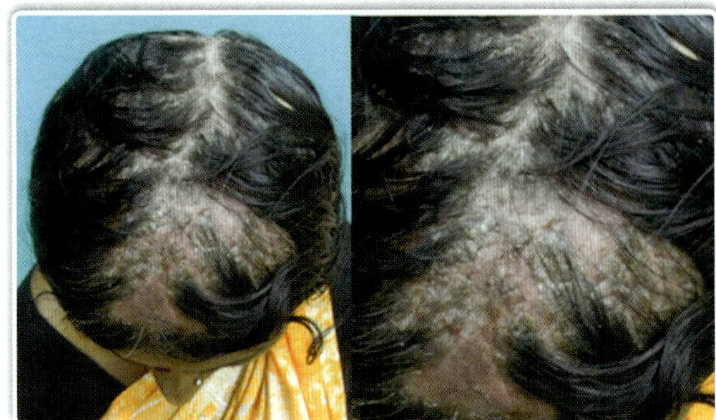

Figure 9.5: Thick crusts in pemphigus vulgaris
(*Courtesy:* Department of Dermatology, STD and Leprosy, BMCRI, Bengaluru)

Table 9.5: Principles of treatment of itchy and scaly scalp

Objective	*Diseases*	*Therapy*
Removal of scales and crusts	Seborrheic dermatitis, psoriasis, pityriasis amiantacea, Darier disease, atopic dermatitis, tinea capitis	Shampoos containing selenium sulfide, anti-fungals (Ketoconazole, sertaconazole, fluconazole, climbazole, ciclopirox olamine), zinc pyrithione, salicylic acid or coal tar
Reduction of erythema	Seborrheic dermatitis, psoriasis, pityriasis amiantacea, atopic dermatitis, contact dermatitis	Creams or lotions containing antifungals, steroids, coal tar, vitamin D analogues or calcineurin inhibitors
Reduction of itching	Seborrheic dermatitis, psoriasis, p.amiantacea, atopic dermatitis, contact dermatitis, folliculitis, pediculosis, lichen simplex, sensitive scalp, dermatitis herpetiformis	Reduction of scales and erythema results in reduced itching. Systemic therapy with antihistamines or specific disease targeted treatment shall be considered
Inhibiting yeast colonization	Seborrheic dermatitis	Topical antifungal therapy and in refractory cases oral antifungals ketoconazole and itraconazole
Treatment of infections/ infestations	Folliculitis, tinea capitis, herpes, pediculosis, scabies	Specific antibiotic, antifungal, antiviral or antiparasitic therapy
Prevention of scarring	DLE, lichen planus	Specific systemic and topical therapies
Systemic therapy	Psoriasis, dermatitis herpetiformis and other auto-immune bullous disorders, pruritus due to systemic and psychosomatic disorders	Proper evaluation and appropriate pharmacological therapy shall be considered in these conditions

urticaria-like plaques and most commonly small vesicles. Scalp and posterior nuchal lines are common sites of appearance of lesions and other sites include elbows, knees, buttocks, shoulders, and sacral areas.

Diagnosis

Diagnosis of itchy scaly scalp is often evident on clinical examination alone and generally laboratory investigations are not required. Diagnostic challenges are limited primarily when signs are minimal or not evident **(Algorithms 9.1 and 9.2).** However, pruritus may be a distressing symptom even in cases where signs may be very minimal. Such cases may also be therapeutically challenging. A list of investigations is summarized in **Table 9.4** with their significance.

Treatment

Pruritic and scaly scalp is a significant discomfort to afflicted individuals and it needs an early attention. It can be a cause of social embarrassment and may impact quality of life. In general, disorders of scalp are more difficult to treat due to the anatomical reasons. Hairy scalp makes it difficult to apply topical creams and ointments, and uniform spreading may be difficult. Lotions are hence preferred mode of topical drug

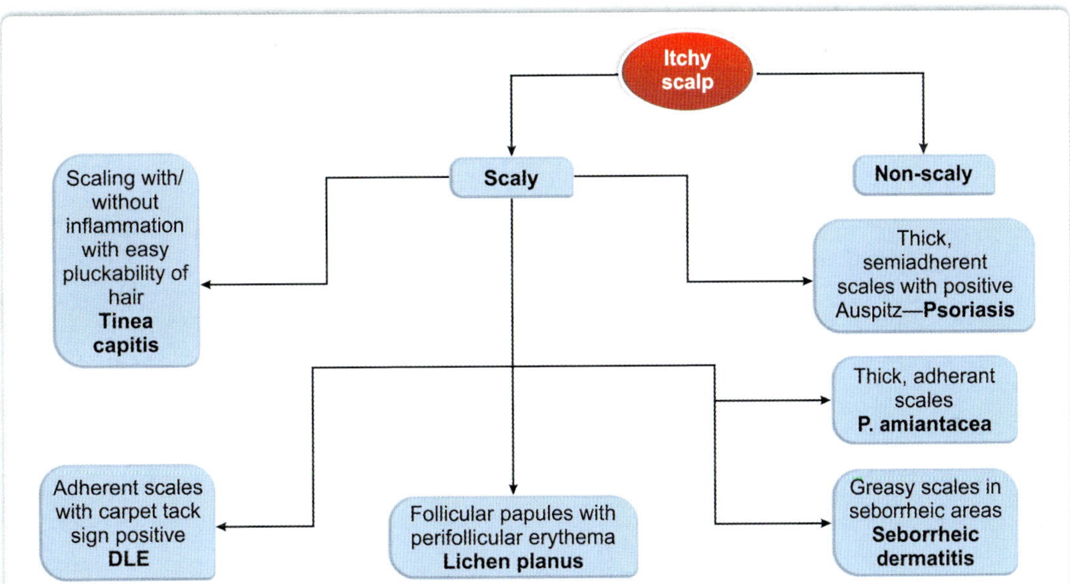

Algorithm 9.1: Algorithm showing approach to scaly itchy scalp: Clinical clues

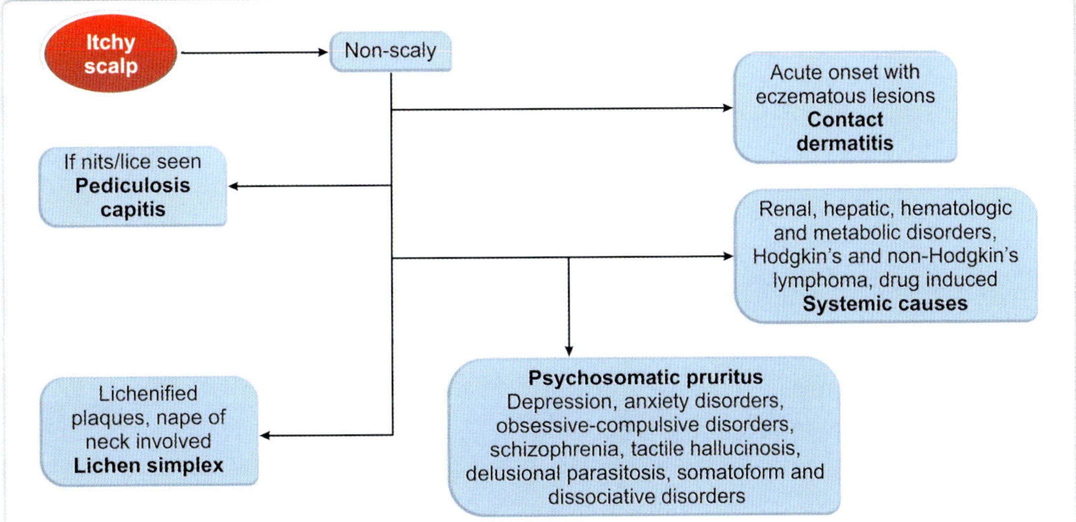

Algorithm 9.2: Algorithm showing approach to non-scaly itchy scalp: Clinical clues

Box 9.7: Preferred topical drug delivery vehicle—scalp

- Lotions: Uniform spread
- Shampoos: To remove scales and crusts

delivery **(Box 9.7)**. Shampoos are generally used to remove scales and crust in all patients. Further management depends on the diagnosis and severity of the disease. Chronic nature of most of the diseases should be discussed with the patients and that therapy is often long standing and is directed towards controlling the disease rather than curing it.

There is no universally effective anti-itch treatment for scalp pruritus since pathophysiology of itch in most disorders is unclear. For any other cutaneous disorders, anti-pruritic therapy is often directed against a variety of targets, including the barrier repair, immune system, nervous system and others.[12] Topical therapy is the mainstay of management and systemic therapy is indicated for resistant or widespread diseases. Commonly used antiitch medications are antiinfective agents, anti-inflammatory agents (steroids, tacrolimus, coal tar), and keratolytics. Future prospects of proper understanding of the pathological mechanisms of itch, targeting specific mediators or neuronal pathways are promising approach to more effective management of pruritus.[13]

Principles of treatment of itchy and scaly scalp are summarized in the **Table 9.5**.

Seborrheic Dermatitis

Mild diseases are treated with antifungal shampoos which work as cleansers for the scaling and may reduce scalp colonization of *Malassezia* yeasts. Severe disease is often treated with topical steroids or salicylic acid preparations. Oral antifungals and isotretinoin can help in severe and resistant diseases.

Ketoconazole, an imidazole antifungal agent with activity against *Malassezia* species and possibly with a mild direct anti-inflammatory effect[14], is the most frequently employed shampoo preparation for seborrheic dermatitis. Ketoconazole 2% shampoo is more effective and better tolerated than selenium sulfide 2.5% shampoo.[15] It is used twice weekly over a usual duration of 4 weeks; intermittent use such as once weekly, has been shown to be effective in preventing relapse. Salicyclic acid and coal tar shampoos may be used for adjunctive benefit but their efficacy has not been well studied. Topical corticosteroids are considered as first line or second line treatment depending on the severity, however there is relative lack of evidence for their usage too **(Box 9.8)**. Milder potency steroids like desonide are preferred over more potent and found to be globally effective in managing scalp seborrheic dermatitis.[16] Pimecrolimus cream was also found effective in decreasing severity of erythema, pruritus and scaling.[17]

Box 9.8: Steroids in seborrheic dermatitis

- Relative lack of evidence for their usage
- Depending on the severity to be used sparingly
- Topical corticosteroids are considered
- Milder potency steroids like desonide are preferred over more potent

Psoriasis

Scalp psoriasis is a difficult to treat condition. Topically coal tar in shampoo or solution has been used primarily in psoriasis. It probably exerts its effect by inhibiting DNA synthesis and mitosis in epidermal cells. It may also have antipruritic and vasoconstrictive effects if used for long duration. Reported adverse effects include bad odor, contact dermatitis, erythema, burning sensation, folliculitis and pigmentation **(Figure 9.6)**. Salicylic acid is used alone as a keratolytic or with coal tar to improve penetration. It is used in concentrations of 3 to 5%. Dithranol should be used cautiously since it can discolor the hairs. Topical steroid alone or with salicylic acid is very effective to reduce inflammation and thickness of lesions. It may cause atrophy and folliculitis as adverse events. Calcipotriol with betamethasone dipropionate gel was also found very effective, and it can be used as a twice weekly maintenance

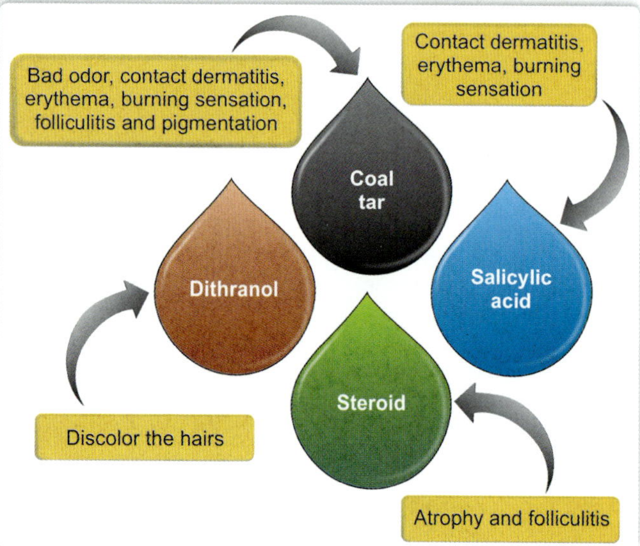

Fig. 9.6: Schematic representation of common side effects of topical agents in scalp psoriasis

for scalp psoriasis.[18] Phototherapy is also effective alone or in combination with topical treatments. Hairline psoriasis may be treated with excimer laser; rapid improvement of hairline psoriasis using a regimen of 308 nm excimer laser with clobetasol spray has been reported.[19] Comb devices can be used to deliver phototherapy to hairy scalp as a portable device to be used at home.[20] Systemic treatment with methotrexate, retinoids or ciclosporin may be considered if indicated.

Pityriasis Amiantacea

It is often a reaction pattern of the scalp in association with conditions like psoriasis or seborrheic dermatitis. It is more common in children and is chronic, however may improve with age. Keratolytics like salicylic acid and topical steroids are used to induce remissions. Tinea capitis should be ruled out in every case. There are no guidelines or recommendations for treatment of pityriasis amiantacea. Sometimes the condition can be very severe and frustrating with necessitation for systemic treatment; infliximab has been used with success.[21]

Atopic Dermatitis

Apart from avoidance of trigger factors in patients with atopic eczema, hydration of skin with the help of suitable emollients is the baseline therapy. Dietary management, psychological support and indoor environmental control are complementary.[22] Scalp lesions are more frequent in children and it is generally managed with mild steroid lotions or calcineurin inhibitors.

Tinea Capitis

Tinea capitis is caused by variety of dermatophytic agents and response to therapy may vary in every case. All infections in hair bearing areas should be treated with oral antifungals because certain dermatophytes are capable of penetrating the hairs. The standard treatment of tinea capitis is griseofulvin, but itraconazole, fluconazole and terbinafine also appear to be safe, effective, and may reduce treatment duration.

Parasitic Diseases

Synthetic pyrethroid compound permethrin used in a 1% cream rinse, which is left on scalp for 10 minutes and then washed of, is the treatment of choice for pediculosis. 5% cream can be used for resistant cases and also for scabies. Ivermectin is an effective oral drug for both pediculosis and scabies.

Bullous Disorders

Pemphigus is generally a severe disease and requires treatment with systemic steroids in high doses, often with an adjuvant like azathioprine, cyclophosphamide or mycophenolate mofetil. There is a tendency for secondary infections which also needs to be addressed. Dermatitis herpetiformis usually responds adequately to dapsone. Therapy for both the condition is long standing.

Darier Disease

Typical keratotic papules on scalp are often complicated by inflammation with severe crusting along with secondary infections. Cleansing with shampoos and application of topical antifungal or antibacterial may help. Topical steroids and tacrolimus may benefit and may temporarily relieve symptoms. Definite treatment includes oral retinoids like acetretin but relapses always known to occur.

References

1. Langner MD, Maibach HI. Pruritus measurement and treatment.Clin Exp Dermatol. 2009;34(3):285-8.
2. Bin Saif GA, Ericson ME, Yosipovitch G. The itchy scalp-scratching for an explanation. Exp Dermatol. 2011; 20(12):959-68.
3. Cunha PR, DelfiniFilho O. Pruritus: still a challenge. An Bras Dermatol. 2012;87(5):735-41.
4. Liu T, Gao YJ, Ji RR.Emerging role of Toll-like receptors in the control of pain and itch.Neurosci Bull. 2012;28(2):131-44.
5. Ständer S, Weisshaar E, Mettang T, Szepietowski JC, Carstens E, Ikoma A, et al. A clinical classification of itch: a position paper of the International Forum for the Study of Itch. Acta Derm Venereol. 2007;87(4):291-4.
6. Lowell Goldsmith, Stephen Katz, Barbara Gilchrest, Amy Paller, David Leffell, Klaus Wolff. Fitzpatrick's Dermatology in General Medicine. McGrw hill Medical. 2012.
7. Williams JV, Eichenfield LF, Burke BL, Barnes-Eley M, Friedlander SF. Prevalence of scalp scaling in prepubertal children. Pediatrics. 2005;115(1).
8. Shi M, Zhang H, Chen X, Guo Y, Tao J, Qi H, et al. Clinical features of atopic dermatitis in a hospital-based setting in China. J Eur Acad Dermatol Venereol. 2011;25(10): 1206-12.
9. Godse K, Zawar V. Sensitive scalp. Int J Trichology. 2012; 4(2):102-4.
10. Abdel-Hamid IA, Agha SA, Moustafa YM, El-Labban AM. Pityriasisamiantacea: a clinical and etiopathologic study of 85 patients. Int J Dermatol. 2003;42(4):260-4.

11. Kim GW, Jung HJ, Ko HC, Kim MB, Lee WJ, Lee SJ, et al. Dermoscopy can be useful in differentiating scalp psoriasis from seborrhoeic dermatitis. Br J Dermatol. 2011;164(3): 652-6.
12. Elmariah SB, Lerner EA. Topical therapies for pruritus.Semin Cutan Med Surg. 2011;30(2):118-26.
13. Tey HL, Yosipovitch GG. Targeted treatment of pruritus - a look into the future Br J Dermatol. 2011;165(1):5-17.
14. Del Rosso JQ. Adult seborrheic dermatitis: a status report on practical topical management. J Clin Aesthet Dermatol. 2011;4(5):32-8.
15. Danby FW, Maddin WS, Margesson LJ, et al. A randomized, double-blind, placebo-controlled trial of ketoconazole 2% shampoo versus selenium sulfide 2.5% shampoo in the treatment of moderate to severe dandruff. J Am Acad Dermatol. 1993;29:1008-12.
16. KircikLH.Treatment of scalp and facialseborrheic dermatitis with desonide hydrogel 0.05%. J Clin Aesthet Dermatol. 2009;2(2):32-6.
17. Ang-Tiu CU, Meghrajani CF, Maano CC. Pimecrolimus 1% cream for the treatment of seborrheic dermatitis: a systematic review of randomized controlled trials.Expert Rev Clin Pharmacol. 2012;5(1):91-7.
18. Saraceno R, Camplone G, D'Agostino M, De Simone C, Di Cesare A, Filosa G, et al. Efficacy and maintenance strategies of two-compound formulation calcipotriol and betamethasone dipropionate gel (Xamiol® gel) in the treatment of scalp psoriasis: results from a study in 885 patients.J Dermatolog Treat. 2013. [Epub ahead of print]
19. Wong JW, Kamangar F, Nguyen TV, Koo JY. Excimer laser therapy for hairline psoriasis: a useful addition to the scalp psoriasis treatment algorithm. Skin Therapy Lett. 2012;17(5):6-9.
20. Caccialanza M, Piccinno R, Cappio F, Rozza M, Mainardi L. Phototherapy of psoriasis of the scalp. Results in 21 patients treated with a special portable ultraviolet rays lamp]. G Ital Dermatol Venereol. 1989;124(11-12).
21. Pham RK, Chan CS, Hsu S. Treatment of pityriasis amiantacea with infliximab. Dermatol Online J. 2009;15(12):13.
22. Lee SI, Kim J, Han Y, Ahn K. A proposal: Atopic Dermatitis Organizer (ADO) guideline for children. Asia Pac Allergy. 2011;1(2):53-63.

10

Alopecia Areata

Eshini Perera, Rodney Sinclair

"Diseases can be diagnosed from the specific character of the symptoms of each."

—*Galen*

Epidemiology

Alopecia areata (AA) is a common non-scarring alopecia that occurs in 0.1–0.2% of the general population and accounts for 0.7–3% of all cases seen in dermatology practice.[1,2] The disease is an inflammatory condition that manifests in the hair follicles and can occur in the nails in up to 66% patients.[3] AA occurs in all races and both genders equally, although it is thought that there may be a male preponderance in the adult population.[4] Prevalence rates peak between the ages of twenty to forty years of life, however up to 60% of patients with AA will present with their first patch before the age of twenty years **(Box 10.1)**.[5,6]

Etiology

The AA is most likely an organ-specific autoimmune disease. Gene association studies confirm a genetic predisposition. Environmental triggers are postulated, but none have been confirmed.

Genetics

Family studies in AA found that 28% of patients have at least one affected family member[7] and the AA concordance rate in monozygotic twins ranges between 42 and 55%.[8] 139 single nucleotide polymorphisms have been identified in 8 regions of the genome.[9] These polymorphisms (IL2/IL21, IL2RA, CTLA4, IK2F4, HLA, NK-activating ligands, ILBP6, ULBP6, STX17, PRDX5) were found to be associated with T cells or the hair follicles. In addition, there was a region of strong association on the cyctomegalovirus UL16-binding protein gene cluster (ULBP).[9] This gene cluster encodes the activating ligands of natural killer cell receptor NKG2D. ULBP3 expression was found to be upregulated in lesions of AA. The authors of this study implicated the ULBP ligand upregulation in triggering autoimmunity **(Box 10.2)**.

Box 10.1: Epidemiology

- Incidence: 0.1–2%
- Equal incidence in both sexes
- Onset: 20–40 years

Autoimmunity (Figure 10.1)

Autoimmunity is believed to play a central role in the development of AA. Patients with AA have been found to have an increased frequency of hair follicle-specific autoantibodies.[10] The inferior portion of the normal hair follicle is an "immune privileged" site which is protected from surveillance by T cells.[11] Major histocompatibility complex (MHC) class I and II molecules that bind and present pathogens to the immune system, are not expressed in normal hair follicle epithelium. In AA, however, this immune privileged site is compromised. There is an increased MHC I and II complexes and increased expression of adhesion molecules ICAM-2 and ELAM-1 surrounding the perivascular and peribulbar hair follicular epithelium.[12]

Further evidence for the role autoimmunity in AA is supported by a number of findings.

Box 10.2: UL 16 binding protein (ULBP)

- Cytomegalovirus UL16-binding protein gene cluster
- This gene cluster encodes activating ligands of natural killer cell receptor NKG2D
- ULBP3 expression was found to be upregulated in lesions of AA
- ULBP ligand upregulation triggers autoimmunity

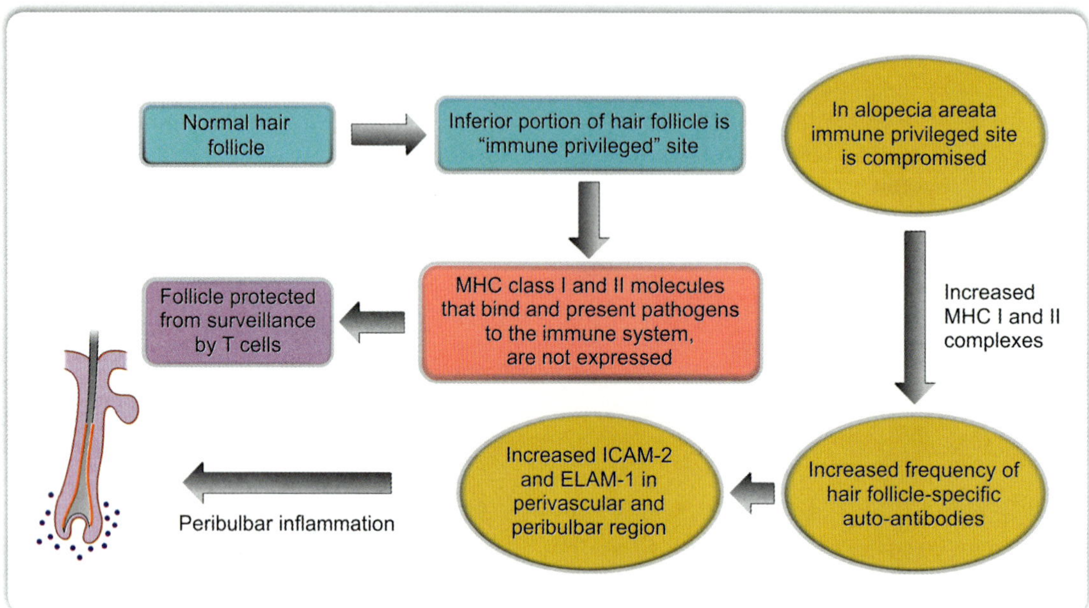

Fig. 10.1: Schematic representation of role of autoimmunity in alopecia areata

1. Murine skin graft experiment illustrate that AA is induced by T cells that recognize hair follicle antigens. The skin of patients affected with AA was grafted to severe combined immunodeficient (SCID) mice and this resulted in hair growth. T lymphocytes, which were isolated from the affected patient and cultured with hair follicle homogenate, were injected into the SCID mice and this resulted in hair loss. T lymphocytes which were not cultured in the hair follicle homogenate did not produce hair loss.[13]
2. Associations with personal and family history of thyroid disease (18.3% of patients with AA), vitiligo (2.8%) and dermatitis (5.6%).[14]
3. Subcutaneous injection of lymph node cells from mice affected with AA into normal mice resulted in the development of AA.[15]
4. Depletion of CD8+ cells in rats affected with AA induced hair regrowth within 29 days.[16]
5. Infiltration of antigen presenting cells around the affected hair follicle.[17]
6. The ability of immunosuppressive agents in promoting hair growth.[18]

Clinical Presentation

Clinically, AA presents as an area of well circumscribed patches of sudden hair loss. Patches up to 2 cm in diameter may appear overnight and then extend circumferentially at a rate of around 1 cm per week. The initial loss is by hair breakage, close to or just below the surface of the skin. Hair remnants are visible as black dots on dermoscopy. While any hair-bearing area may be affected, 90%[5, 7] of lesions occur on the scalp. The skin over the affected areas may have no overt epidermal changes except for some mild erythema and atrophy.

Exclamation mark hairs, dystrophic hairs with fractured tips, are commonly seen around the margins of the hair loss **(Box 10.3)**. AA can also present as diffuse hair loss.

AA can be divided into a number of classifications based on the extent of hair loss or variations of presentations **(Table 10.1)**.

Nail Changes

Nail changes can occur in 10–66% of patients with AA.[3] Presentation may be limited to 1 or more nails. Nail changes occur more commonly in children (12%) compared to adults (3.3%) and in more severe forms of AA.[19] The presence of nail disease confers a poorer prognosis; however the severity of nail disease does not correlate temporally with the severity of hair loss.

Nail presentations include superficial pitting, trachyonychia (sand paper nails), leukonychia and Beau's lines. In severe disease red lunulae can be seen **(Box 10.4)**.

Box 10.3: Exclamation hair

- 2–4 mm long broken hair
- Shafts of which reduce progressively in thickness and pigmentation towards the bulb end
- Seen at the margins of a new or expanding patch

Table 10.1: Morphological classification of alopecia areata

Type	*Description*
Patchy AA	This is the most common presentation of AA. Hair loss is localized and patchy **(Figure 10.2A)**
AA totalis	Total hair loss on the scalp.
AA universalis	Complete hair loss of all hair-bearing areas **(Figure 10.3)**
Acute diffuse and total alopecia (ADTA)	ADTA may present as a short clinical course ranging from acute hair loss to total baldness. The prognosis is favorable and there is rapid resolution of the condition—at times without treatment
Diffuse AA	Diffuse hair loss which can mimic telogen effluvium
Ophiasis	Hair loss is localized to the sides of the scalp and the nape **(Figure 10.4A)**
Sisaipho	Hair loss spares the sides of the scalp and the nape. This presentation is rare **(Figure 10.4B)**
Reticular patches	Several patches of AA may coalesce to form a reticular pattern **(Figure 10.2B)**

Box 10.4: Nail changes in alopecia areata

- 'Scotch plaid' effect or 'ripples'
  - Superficial, uniform, minute pits
  - Arranged regularly along and across the nail
- Red or mottled lunulae
- Nail thinning and ridging
- Beau's lines
- Leukonychia
- Trachyonychia.

Differential Diagnosis

There are multiple disease entities which resemble AA **(Table 10.2)**. Tinea capitis and trichotillomania (TTM) both produce hair breakage and patchy hair loss. In tinea capitis the scalp skin may be scaly. In trichotillomania the border of the alopecia is angular rather than circular. On the upper eyelashes these 2 conditions may be impossible to distinguish. The clinician will need to rely on the natural evolution of the alopecia to make a diagnosis. TTM does not occur on the lower eyelashes.

Physical Examination

The diagnosis of AA is made on clinical grounds and a good physical examination is imperative to distinguish between the differentials. **Table 10.3** lists suggested physical examination techniques for the assessment of suspected AA.

Assessing the Severity of Disease

A quantitative assessment of hair loss on the scalp can be made by calculating the severity of alopecia tool score (SALT score).[21] The scalp is divided in the 4 surface area proportions:

- Vertex (40%)
- Right scalp (18%)
- Left scalp (18%)
- Posterior scalp (24%).

The score is then calculated by summating the percentage of hair loss in each area by the surface area percentages.

The SALT scores are calculated at baseline and then during treatment to assess the proportion of regrowth achieved.

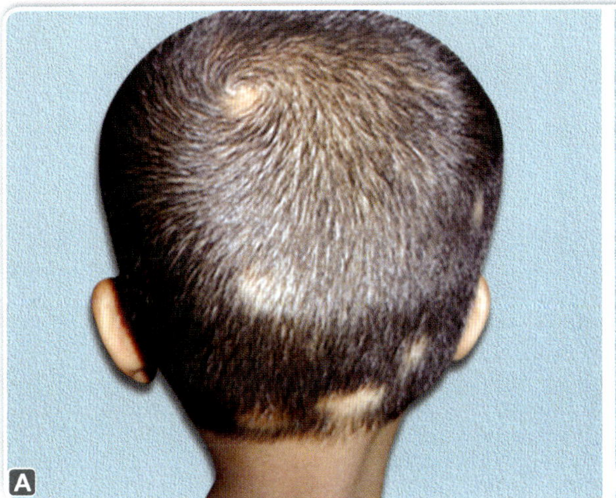

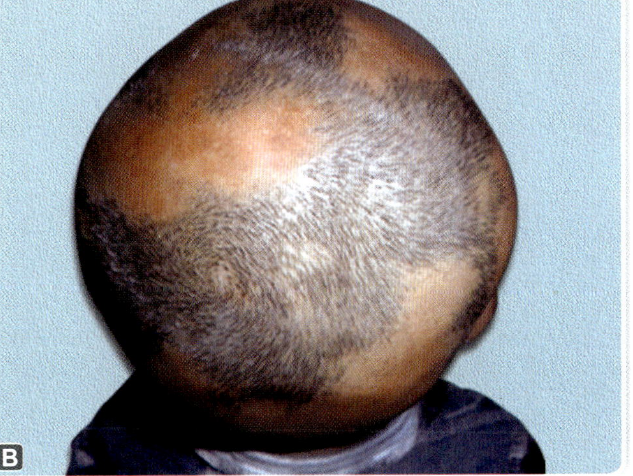

Figs 10.2A and B: (A) Patchy pattern; (B) Reticulate pattern (*Courtesy:* Department of Dermatology, STD and Leprosy, BMCRI, Bengaluru)

Investigations

Diagnosis of AA is usually made on clinical examination and routine tests are not indicated. If there is uncertainity regarding the diagnosis a scalp biopsy may be performed. Fungal culture, lupus serology and syphilis serology can also be done to exclude other differentials.

Histopathology

The histopathological features vary depending on the stage of the disease. Histopathological presentation of AA can be divided into 4 parameters: Acute, subacute, chronic and recovery stage **(Table 10.4)**.

Management

Psychological Support

The morbidity of alopecia areata is psychological rather than physical. Adolescent boys are especially vulnerable due the inability to conceal even small patches. In contrast, women with long hair may be able to conceal up to 50% hair loss through styling alone. Alopecia has profound effects on quality of life and social functioning. Often patients are physically healthy, but may suffer from considerable psychological sequelae. AA may affect patient's self-image including functioning, emotions, self-confidence and stigmatization. AA has been found to be associated with anxiety and depression[23] which can in turn impact the patients physical health. In Australia, a number of cases of youth suicide have been attributed directly to alopecia areata (Personal communication Chelsea Campbell, AAAF).

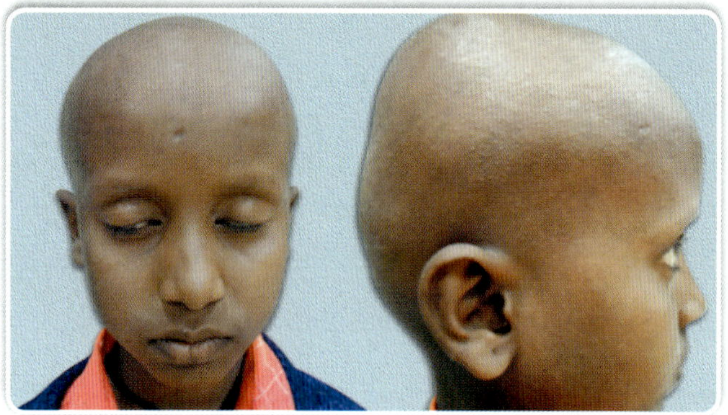

Fig. 10.3: Alopecia universalis (*Courtesy:* Department of Dermatology, STD and Leprosy, BMCRI, Bengaluru)

It is important to take into account the different coping strategies each patient may have in order to assist the depth of psychological support needed to adjust to the illness.

Successful treatment of AA should include focusing on the psychological impact. Clinicians should ensure that patients have adequate social support. A number of support services exist in the community and aim to educate and increase awareness of AA.

While spontaneous remission will occur in up to 50% of patients in 1 year[24], most people seek active treatment. Also the natural evolution of alopecia areata, with multilocular disease evolving over a period of months rather than occurring simultaneously, suggests that the presence of active disease could increase the risk of subsequent patches. While this contention is unproven, the authors favor active treatment. Course of regrowth of hair is given in **Box 10.5**.

Pharmacological Management

High dose oral corticosteroids are highly effective in regrowing hair and preventing relapse, however the associated side-effects makes many patients unwilling to take them and many physician reluctant to prescribe them.

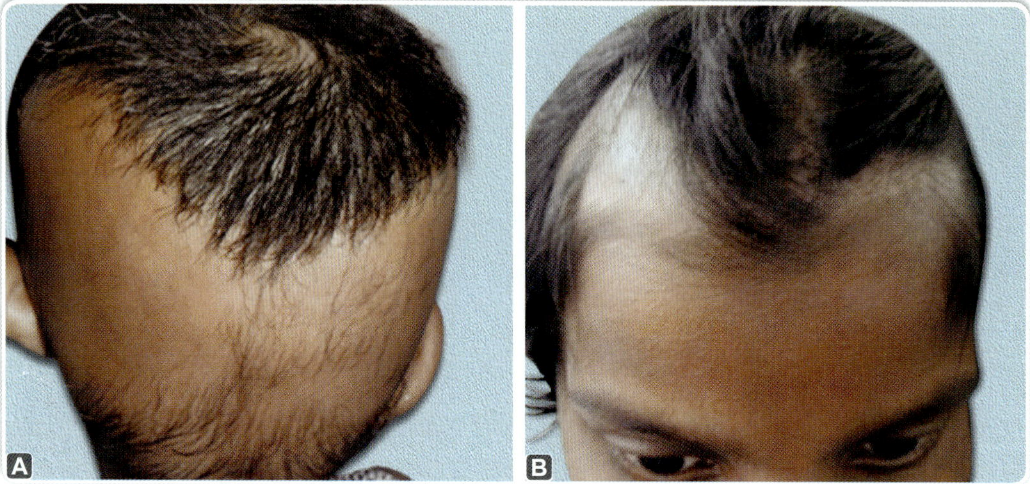

Figs 10.4A and B: (A) Ophiasis; (B) Sisaipho (*Courtesy:* Department of Dermatology, STD and Leprosy, BMCRI, Bengaluru)

Table 10.2: Differential diagnosis of alopecia areata

Differential	Presentation and distinguishing features
Tinea capitis	The diagnosis of tinea capitis should be considered particularly in children Scaling and signs of inflammation are present on physical examination
Trichotillomania	Trichotillomania may co-exist with AA Lesions are usually irregular shaped lesions. Other features which can be noted include: ❑ Broken hairs that may vary in length ❑ The lesion surface may not appear smooth due to the variation of length in broken hairs ❑ Affected patches may have a 'wire brush' feeling
Discoid lupus erythematous (DLE)	DLE presents as patchy hair loss associated with pruritus and burning. There may be follicular plugging (hyperkeratosis) within the lesion. In later stages of the disease the lesion may become atrophic
Lichen planopilaris	Lichen planopilaris should be considered in women between the ages of 30 to 60 years. It typically starts on the central scalp and may be associated with pruritus, burning and pain. There may be perifollicular hyperkeratosis and erythema present
Central cicatricial alopecia	Cicatricial alopecia is characterized by patchy hair loss with loss of follicular orifices. Erythema, scaling, pustules and plugging may occur
Congenital triangular alopecia	Often appears after 2 years of age and rarely occurs in adulthood. Scalp biopsy is needed to distinguish between AA and triangular alopecia. Histology reveals a normal number of hair follicles which are vellus or indeterminate
Telogen effluvium	Telogen effluvium (TE) is the main differential diagnosis for diffuse AA. TE is often associated with a precipitant including recent illness, surgery, weight loss or medications. TE can be difficult to differentiate from AA. Usually the history may point towards the diagnosis. Hair loss usually occurs 2 months after the precipitant
Systemic lupus erythematosus	Hair loss is not uncommon in SLE; however hair loss involving greater than 50% of the scalp area is rarely reported
Loose anagen hair syndrome	Mainly occurs in young girls between the age of 2–6 years but may occur in young boys and in adulthood. Hair often appears lustreless. The occiput is usually affected due to repeated friction of the patient's head against a pillow during sleep
Secondary syphilis	Presents commonly as a moth eaten pattern but may also present as diffuse hair loss. May be present with mucosal or cutaneous lesions

Table 10.3: Physical examination for the investigation of alopecia areata

Examination	How to perform examination	Findings
Pull test	Gentle traction is exerted on a small area of hair. If > 10 hairs come out with each pull this is positive. This test should be conducted at the periphery of the lesion to assess the clinical activity[20]	This test is useful for assessing diffuse hair loss. Positive pull tests may be seen in telogen effluvium, loose anagen syndrome and lichen planopilaris
Pluck test	Hair is pulled out by the root and examined under the microscope to determine the phase of growth	This test is particularly useful in distinguishing between telogen effluvium and anagen effluvium In telogen effluvium there is a greater proportion of hairs in telogen phase and conversely in anagen effluvium there is a decrease in the number of telogen phase hairs. In AA, dystrophic anagen hairs may be seen
Daily hair count	Hair from the first morning combing or washing are collected in a bag over 14 days and counted	A count of > 100 is abnormal. However, it is important to note that after shampooing as many as 250 hairs can be lost
Trichoscopy	Hair is visualized under a dermatoscope	In AA hyperkeratotic plugs are characteristically seen (presenting as yellow dots) and exclamation mark hairs may be seen. In SLE scaling of the scalp, telangiectasia and uneven hair shaft diameter can be observed **(Figures 10.5 and 10.6)**.
Nail examination	-	In AA pitting or trachyonychia are commonly seen Nails should be examined to exclude signs of fungal infection. In some cases of telogen effluvium, Beau's lines half way down the nail can be observed which corresponds with a precipitating insult that occurred 2 months prior

Table 10.4: Histological stages of alopecia areata

Stage	*Histological appearance:*
Acute stage	Terminal hairs are surrounded by bulbar lymphocytes, which can take the classical appearance of a swarm of bees[3] **(Figure 10.7)**
Subacute stage	There is an increase in catagen and telogen hairs and a decrease in anagen hairs
Chronic stage	There are decreased terminal and increased miniaturized hairs. Inflammation may be variable. Immunofluorescence studies have shown deposits of C3, IgG and IgM on the basement membrane of the inferior part of the hair follicle[22]
Recovery stage	The number of terminal anagen hairs increase and there is a lack of inflammation

Box 10.5: Regrowth in alopecia areata

- Fine and unpigmented hair initially
- Gradually gains in caliber and color
- Heterochromia of hair
- Hair growth starts in center, extends peripherally
- May remain unpigmented for a long time- leading to poliosis
- Regrowth and extension may occur simultaneously in different regions of the scalp

To date there are no curative therapies available for the treatment of AA. Pharmacological treatments are aimed at arresting the progression of disease, and regrowing bald scalp. Multiple topical, local and systemic treatment options exist, many of which are immunosuppressants or immunomodulators.

Intralesional Corticosteroids (Figure 10.8)

Intralesional corticosteroids are the treatment of choice for patchy hair loss in AA.

In one study, regrowth of hair occurred in 33 out of 34 sites injected with intralesional triamcinolone hexacetonide and in 16 out of 25 sites treated with triamcinolone acetonide.[25]

Triamcinolone acetonide (5–10 mg/mL) and hydrocortisone acetate (25 mg/mL) are the most commonly used intralesional corticosteroids. 0.1 mL of solution is injected into multiple sites 1 cm apart into deep dermis using a 30 gauge needle. This process is repeated every 4–6 weeks. A 5 mg/mL dosage is recommended as the initial concentration for the scalp and 2.5 mg/mL for areas on the face. No more than 20 mL should be injected for each visit. The triamcinolone may be diluted with lignocaine to minimize

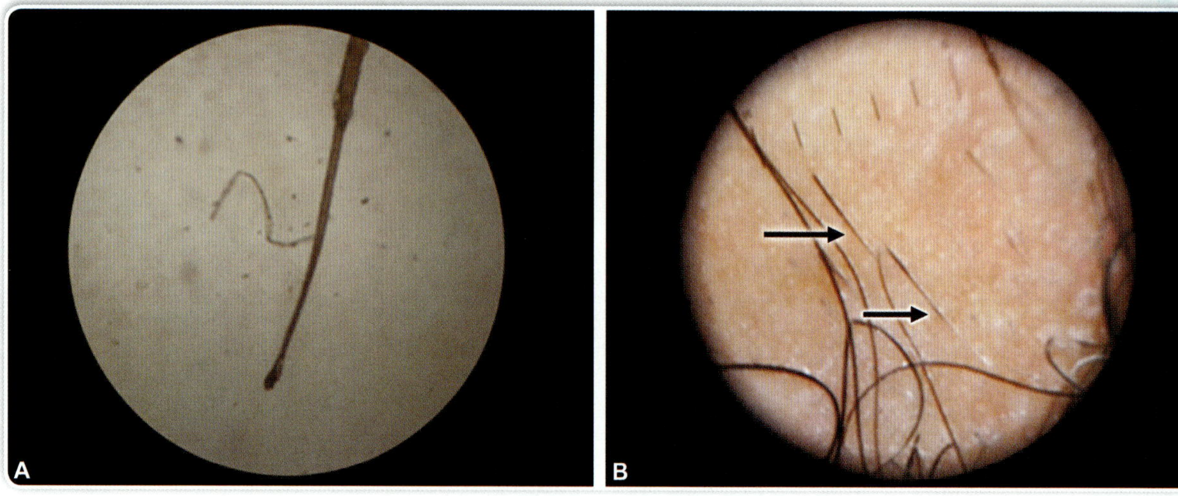

Figs 10.5A and B: Light microscopic and dermoscopic appearance of exclamation hair (*Courtesy:* Department of Dermatology, STD and Leprosy, BMCRI, Bengaluru)

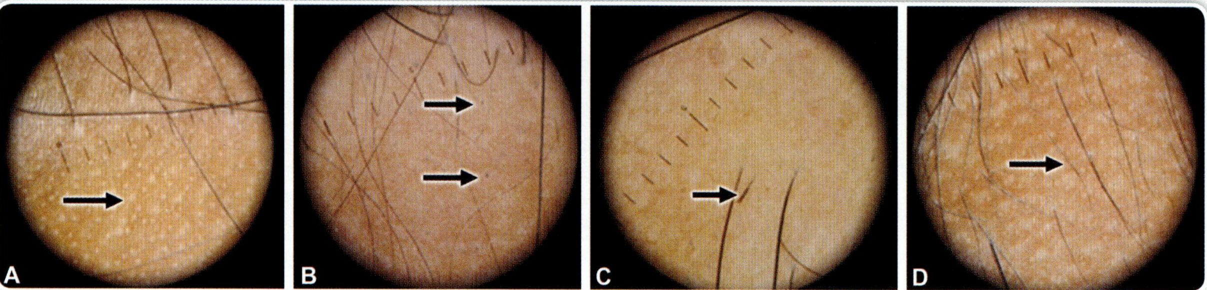

Figs 10.6A to D: Dermoscopic characteristics of alopecia areata. (A) Yellow dots; (B) Black dots; (C) Broken hair; (D) Short vellus hairs (*Courtesy:* Department of Dermatology, STD and Leprosy, BMCRI, Bengaluru)

post-injection discomfort. If there is no improvement over the course of 6 months, or significant atrophy develops, the intralesional corticosteroids should be ceased.

The most common side effect is atrophy of the skin which can be prevented by using smaller volumes or concentrations at each injection site. Other side effects include hypopigmentation, telangiectasia and atrophy. In addition, injections near the eyebrow carry a theoretical risk of cataracts and raised intracranial pressure. Dermal atrophy usually recovers over 3 to 6 months, provided there is no further injection into the site.

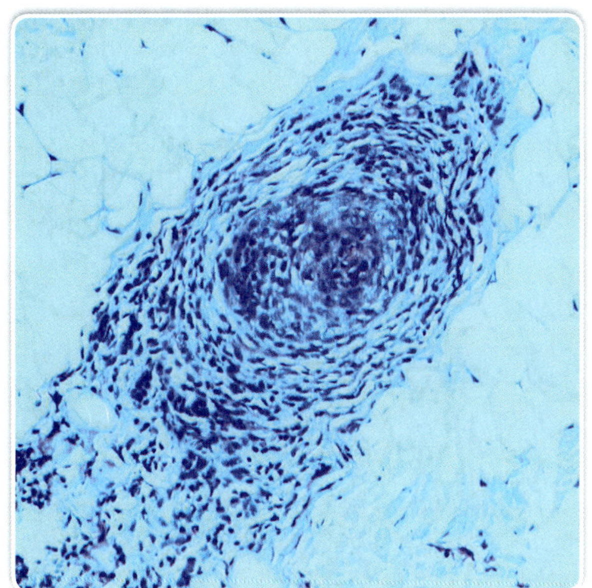

Fig. 10.7: "Swarm of Bees" appearance on H and E staining (*Courtesy:* Department of Dermatology, STD and Leprosy, BMCRI, Bengaluru)

Systemic Corticosteroids

Systemic corticosteroids are highly effective in the treatment of AA. Short term use up to 3 months is generally well tolerated. The chronic nature of the alopecia areata may encourage the chronic use of corticosteroids. Chronic corticosteroid use is toxic. The use of systemic corticosteroids is not justified due to side effects and the high relapse rate, except in severe cases. In one study of 18 patients 38.9% had satisfactory regrowth from systemic corticosteroids however all of the patients relapsed once the corticosteroids were tapered.[26]

For treatment naïve patients a high starting dose is used and tapered by 30% every 2 to 3 weeks. Prednisolone may be given at a starting dosage of 0.5 mg/kg/day.

Higher doses might be associated with aseptic necrosis of the femoral head. For patients who have previously responded to oral corticosteroids, lower starting doses are commonly used.

Use of corticosteroids, particularly at high doses over a long period of time, carries a risk of suppressing the hypothalamic-pituitary-adrenal axis which in turn may cause variations of blood pressure and may increase blood sugar levels. In addition, patients are at risk of developing conditions like psychosis, cataract, glaucoma, peptic ulcer disease or osteoporosis. Pulse corticosteroid therapy has be trialled in an attempt to minimize the risk of steroid related side-effects and there have been reports of successful therapy with 250 mg IV methylprednisolone for 3 days in patchy AA.[27, 28]

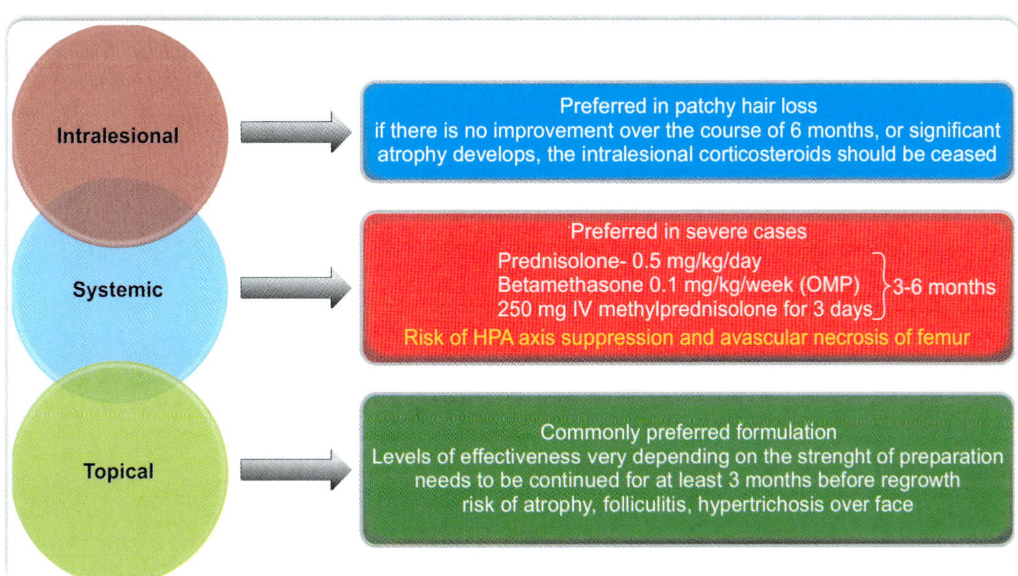

Fig. 10.8: Modalities of steroid use in alopecia areata
Abbreviation: OMP, Oral mini-pulse

Topical Corticosteroids

Topical corticosteroids are commonly used to treat AA. The levels of effectiveness vary depending on the strength of the preparation. Treatment with topical corticosteroids needs to be continued for at least 3 months before regrowth is seen. Common adverse reactions to topical steroids include atrophy of skin, telangiectasia and folliculitis. More success is seen in children than in adults. Children responders commonly develop hypertrichosis of the forehead and face.

Psoralen and Ultraviolet A

Psoralen and ultraviolet A light (PUVA) deplete inflammatory cell infiltrate and can produce satisfactory regrowth in patients with AA totalis and AA universalis with relatively low relapse rates (21% of participants studied over five years).[29]

Another study conducted by Mohamed et al showed topical 8-methoxypsoralen and UVA at doses of 8–42 J/cm^2 produced an excellent response in 85% of patients, with 50% of patients with AA universalis having 50% regrowth.[30] The most common complaints are erythema and burning of skin.

Minoxidil

Minoxidil is an effective topical preparation that stimulates proliferation at the base of the bulb and differentiation above the dermal papilla.[3] A concentration of 2–5% minoxidil is used twice daily as a topical application to the affected area with good results in patients with mild to moderate AA. Oral minoxidil has also been used in a dose of 5 mg daily.[31]

Topical Immunotherapy

Topical immunotherapy is useful for severe and refractory cases of AA.[32] It is hypothesized that the allergic reaction created by the topical immunotherapy generates suppressor T cells that inhibits an autoimmune reaction against the hair follicle.[33] MHC class I and III molecules have been found to disappear around the hair follicle constituent after treatment with topical immunotherapy.[33] More importantly, after treatment begins, the CD4 to CD8 lymphocyte ratio is modified from 4:1 to 1:1, additionally there is a decrease in the CD6 lymphocytes and Langerhan cells **(Box 10.6)**.[35]

Box 10.6: Principle of topical immunotherapy

- The allergic reaction created by the topical immunotherapy generates suppressor T cells that inhibits an autoimmune reaction against the hair follicle
- The CD4 to CD8 lymphocyte ratio is modified from 4:1 to 1:1
- Decrease in the CD6 lymphocytes and langerhan cells

DPCP and squaric acid dibutyl ester (SADBE) are commonly used topical immunotherapy in the treatment of AA. Both treatments produced considerable regrowth with one study demonstrating a 77% and 64% regrowth rate with DPCP and SADBE respectively.[33] Inosiplex has been used in cases of alopecia totalis and has produced satisfactory results.

Initially patients are sensitized by applying 2% DPCP in acetone or paraffin to a small area on the scalp under waterproof occlusion for 24 to 48 hours. After a fortnight 0.001% solution is applied on the scalp and this concentration is increased weekly until a mild allergic contact dermatitis is seen that produces erythema, pruritus and mild scaling that lasts for 24–48 hours. Weeping and vesiculation indicates that the concentration is too high and should be reduced. Postauricular lymphadenopathy may be painful but indicates a better prognosis for regrowth **(Figure 10.9)**.

Anthralin

The exact mechanism of action of anthralin is largely unknown however it is thought to have immunosuppressive and anti-inflammatory properties via the generation of free radicals.[35]

The 0.5–1% of anthralin cream is applied to the affected areas for a period of 20–30 minutes daily over the first 2 weeks of therapy. Exposure can be built up gradually until erythema and pruritis develop. Common side effects include scaly skin, folliculitis and regional lymphadenopathy which can be easily reversed by withholding the application for several days.

Sulfasalazine

Sulfasalazine via the inhibition of inflammatory cells chemotaxis and cytokine antibody production[36] produce satisfactory results. Hair regrowth rates were found to be 27.3% of complete hair regrowth and 40.9% of partial hair regrowth in AA patients.[37] Recommended dosages are 0.5 gram twice daily for the first month, then 1 gram twice daily for the second month, 1.5 gram for another three months. Its side effect profile includes gastrointestinal distress, headaches, fevers, rash and hematological abnormalities.

Cyclosporine

Cyclosporine can be used alone or in combination with systemic corticosteroids. Its mechanism of action is via inhibition of T cell activation and via depletion of perifollicular lymphocytic infiltrates.[38] Treatment responses have been inconsistent with results ranging from 25 to 88%.[39] Additionally, AA has been found to paradoxically occur in transplant patients using high doses of cyclosporine.[40] Cyclosporin also prolongs the anagen

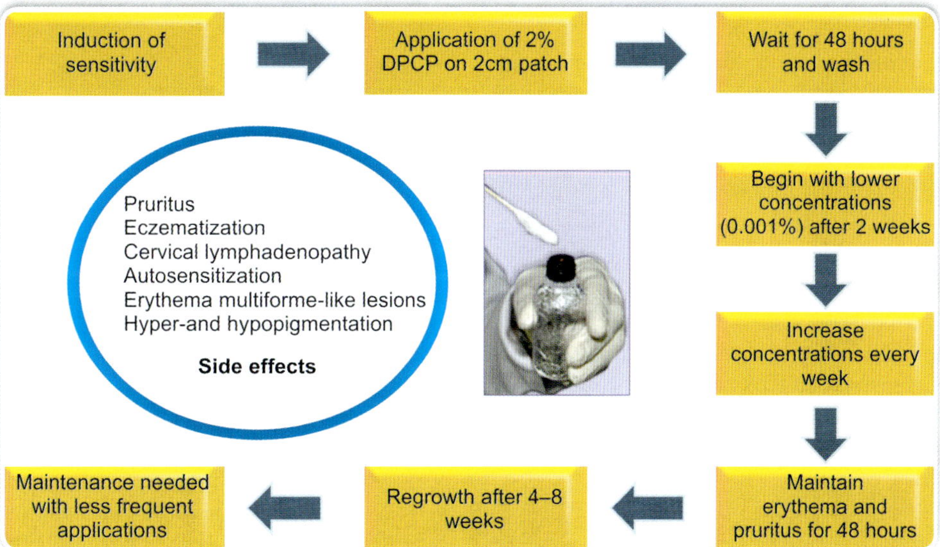

Fig. 10.9: Schematic representation of protocol of contact sensitization

phase of the hair growth cycle causing hypertrichosis as a cutaneous side effect. Other side effects include gingival hyperplasia, nephrotoxicity, hepatotoxicity, headaches and hyperlpidemia.

Calcineurin Inhibitors

Calcineurin inhibitors work by inhibiting the transcription of cytokines and tumor necrosis factor. There have been conflicting results surrounding the efficacy of topical calcineurin inhibitors. One study found that tacrolimus was effective in inducing hair growth in mice[41] while another revealed that no patients responded to tacrolimus over the course of 24 weeks.[42]

Biologic Drugs

There are a number of studies examining biologic therapies, however, to date overall results are disappointing. A study using 50 mg of etanercept twice a week for 24 weeks showed no significant hair regrowth.[43] In addition, a case was reported to have occurred in a patient treated with etanercept.[44] A randomised clinical trial examining 45 patients with chronic severe alopecia showed no significant response to alefacept compared to the placebo.[45] Abetacept, a fusion protein that is comprised of the Fc region of the immunoglobulin IgG1 and fused to the extracellular domain of CTLA-4, has shown promise in murine models of alopecia areata and is currently under investigation in the treatment of human alopecia areata (clinical trials.gov).

Mesotherapy

Mesotherapy is used to improve cutaneous delivery of various pharmaceutical or homeopathic mediations. The compound is administered via multiple subcutaneous injections. There are no randomised control studies that examine the effectiveness of mesotherapy however studies have shown some hair growth in patients using injections of nicotinic acid, vitamin C and pentoxifylline over a 28-week period.[46] Conversely, case studies exist reporting 2 cases of AA, which commenced after mesotherapy using homeopathic compounds.[47]

Laser

Excimer lasers have been investigated as an alternative to photochemotherapy in patients with AA. In a study of 18 patients, using 308-nm excimer laser twice weekly for 12 weeks, regrowth was seen in 17 out of 42 lesions.[48] Similarly 60% of children showed regrowth in patches of AA with the same treatment.[49] While the only adverse event that has been reported thus far has been local erythema, this treatment has never caught on.

Treating Eyelash Alopecia

Topical corticosteroids are rarely used around the eye for fear of cataract and glaucoma. Prostaglandin $F_2\alpha$ analogues such as latanoprost and bimatoprost have recently been employed to improve the appearance of lashes by lengthening and increasing the volume of eyelash hairs. These treatments are typically used for open-angle glaucoma however, eyelash hypertrichosis was noted as a pleasing side effect. Response rates have been variable with one study showing 45% complete or moderate regrowth of eyelashes over 2 years using latanoprost[50] whilst another study showed no significant response to latanoprost or bimatoprost over 16 weeks.[51]

Wigs and Prosthesis

The prognosis of extensive and long standing AA is poor and wigs or prosthesis can be an effective method of coping with the condition. Monofilament acrylic wigs can be constructed to give the appearance of hair growing from the scalp. Synthetic wigs need replacing every 3–4 months. Human hair wigs, in contrast, can last up to 1–2 years if maintained properly.

Hair Transplants and Tattooing

Hair transplants have not been shown to be successful with the only successful procedures being performed on the eyebrows. Other viable options to mask hair loss in the eyebrow region is dermatography or tattooing of the area. False eyelashes can be used in patients with alopecia totalis or alopecia universalis.

Course of Disease

The prognosis for most patients with AA is good given the tendency for spontaneous remission. Patients with long standing extensive AA have a poorer prognosis. In 14–25% of cases AA will progress to alopecia totalis or alopecia universalis.[24] Progression to this stage rarely results in full recovery.

The greatest predictor of long-term outcome in AA is the severity of disease at presentation. Other poor prognostic factors include a positive family history, a long clinical duration of alopecia, presence of nail disease, presence of other autoimmune diseases and a young age of onset. Disease prognosis is also poor in ophiasis and cases where AA develops during childhood **(Table 10.5)**.

Conclusion

In conclusion AA is a common non-scarring alopecia which can affect patients of all ages and races. Although the cause of AA is poorly understood there is a large body of evidence to suggest that genetics and autoimmunity underpin the pathogenesis. The role of immune mediated molecules surrounding the hair follicle has been examined in various mice and rat models and its significance continues to be investigated as a target of existing and novel treatments.

Table 10.5: Poor prognostic factors in alopecia areata

Poor prognostic factors in alopecia areata
❑ Early age of onset
❑ Positive family history
❑ Severe patterns: Ophiasis/reticular/sisaphio/alopecia totalis/ alopecia universalis
❑ Extensive scalp involvement
❑ Recurrent episodes
❑ Loss of eyebrow and eyelashes
❑ Nail involvement: Pitting, dystrophy, onycholysis, anonychia
❑ Associated systemic and genetic disorders
❑ Patchy regrowth of terminal hairs within a patch

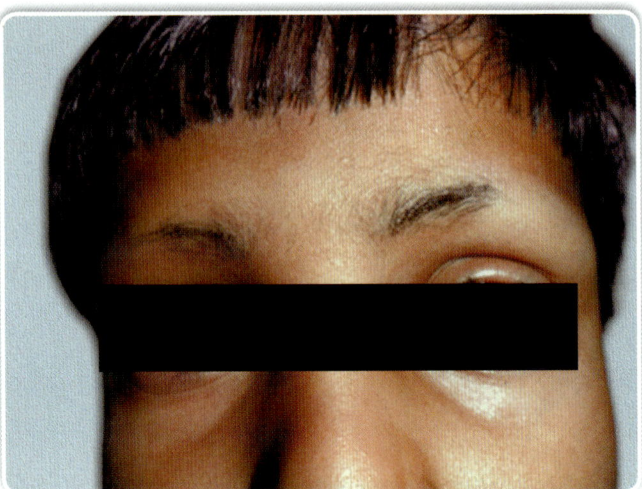

Fig. 10.10: Loss of lateral aspect of eyebrows (*Courtesy:* Department of Dermatology, STD and Leprosy, BMCRI, Bengaluru)

References

1. Safavi K. Prevalence of alopecia areata in the First National Health and Nutrition Examination Survey. Archives of dermatology. 1992;128(5):702. Epub 1992/05/01.
2. Safavi KH, Muller SA, Suman VJ, Moshell AN, Melton LJ, 3rd. Incidence of alopecia areata in Olmsted County, Minnesota, 1975 through 1989. Mayo Clinic proceedings Mayo Clinic. 1995;70(7):628-33.
3. Amin SS, Sachdeva S. Alopecia Areata: An update. Journal of Pakistan Association of Dermatologists. 2013;23(2):209-20.
4. Kyriakis KP, Paltatzidou K, Kosma E, Sofouri E, Tadros A, Rachioti E. Alopecia areata prevalence by gender and age. Journal of the European Academy of Dermatology and Venereology : JEADV. 2009;23(5):572-3. Epub 2008/09/06.
5. Price VH. Alopecia areata: Clinical aspects. The Journal of investigative dermatology. 1991;96(5):68S.
6. Camacho F. Alopecia areata: Clinical features. Dermatopathology. In: Camacho F, Montagna W, editors. Trichology: diseaseas of the pilosebaceous follicle Madrid: Aula Medica Group. 1997;pp.417-40.
7. Alkhalifah A, Alsantali A, Wang E, McElwee KJ, Shapiro J. Alopecia areata update: Part I. Clinical picture, histopathology, and pathogenesis. Journal of the American Academy of Dermatology. 2010;62(2):177-88. quiz 89-90. Epub 2010/02/02.
8. Rodriguez TA, Fernandes KE, Dresser KL, Duvic M, National Alopecia Areata R. Concordance rate of alopecia areata in identical twins supports both genetic and environmental factors. Journal of the American Academy of Dermatology. 2010;62(3):525-7.
9. Petukhova L, Duvic M, Hordinsky M, Norris D, Price V, Shimomura Y, et al. Genome-wide association study in alopecia areata implicates both innate and adaptive immunity. Nature. 2010;466(7302):113-7. Epub 2010/07/03.
10. McElwee KJ, Pickett P, Oliver RF. The DEBR rat, alopecia areata and autoantibodies to the hair follicle. The British Journal of Dermatology. 1996;134(1):55-63. Epub 1996/01/01.

11. Gilhar A, Paus R, Kalish RS. Lymphocytes, neuropeptides, and genes involved in alopecia areata. The Journal of Clinical Investigation. 2007;117(8):2019-27. Epub 2007/08/03.
12. Gilhar A. Collapse of immune privilege in alopecia areata: coincidental or substantial? The Journal of Investigative Dermatology. 2010;130(11):2535-7. Epub 2010/10/15.
13. Gilhar A, Shalaginov R, Assy B, Serafimovich S, Kalish RS. Alopecia areata is a T-lymphocyte mediated autoimmune disease: Lesional human T-lymphocytes transfer alopecia areata to human skin grafts on SCID mice. The Journal of Investigative Dermatology Symposium Proceedings/the Society for Investigative Dermatology, Inc [and] European Society for Dermatological Research. 1999;4(3):207-10. Epub 2000/02/16.
14. Thomas EA, Kadyan RS. Alopecia areata and autoimmunity: a clinical study. Indian Journal of Dermatology. 2008;53(2):70-4. Epub 2008/01/01.
15. McElwee KJ, Freyschmidt-Paul P, Hoffmann R, Kissling S, Hummel S, Vitacolonna M, et al. Transfer of CD8(+) cells induces localized hair loss whereas CD4(+)/CD25(-) cells promote systemic alopecia areata and CD4(+)/CD25(+) cells blockade disease onset in the C3H/HeJ mouse model. The Journal of Investigative Dermatology. 2005;124(5):947-57. Epub 2005/04/28.
16. McElwee KJ, Spiers EM, Oliver RF. In vivo depletion of CD8+ T cells restores hair growth in the DEBR model for alopecia areata. The British Journal of Dermatology. 1996;135(2):211-7. Epub 1996/08/01.
17. Lu W, Shapiro J, Yu M, Barekatain A, Lo B, Finner A, et al. Alopecia areata: Pathogenesis and potential for therapy. Expert Reviews in Molecular Medicine. 2006;8(14):1-19. Epub 2006/06/22.
18. McElwee KJ, Tobin DJ, Bystryn JC, King LE, Jr. Sundberg JP. Alopecia areata: An autoimmune disease? Experimental Dermatology. 1999;8(5):371-9. Epub 1999/10/28.
19. Tosti A, Fanti PA, Morelli R, Bardazzi F. Trachyonychia associated with alopecia areata: A clinical and pathologic study. Journal of the American Academy of Dermatology. 1991;25(2 Pt 1):266-70.
20. Chong AH, Wade M, Sinclair RD. The hair pull test and the hair pluck for analysis of hair abnormalities. Modern Medicine. 1999;42(10):105-8.
21. Olsen EA, Hordinsky MK, Price VH, Roberts JL, Shapiro J, Canfield D, et al. Alopecia areata investigational assessment guidelines—Part II. National Alopecia Areata Foundation. Journal of the American Academy of Dermatology. 2004;51(3):440-7.
22. Igarashi R, Morohashi M, Takeuchi S, Sato Y. Immunofluorescence studies on complement components in the hair follicles of normal scalp and of scalp affected by alopecia areata. Acta Dermato-Venereologica. 1981;61(2):131-5.
23. Hunt N, McHale S. The psychological impact of alopecia. BMJ. 2005;331(7522):951-3. Epub 2005/10/22.
24. Messenger AG, McKillop J, Farrant P, McDonagh AJ, Sladden M. British Association of Dermatologists' guidelines for the management of alopecia areata 2012. Br J Dermatol. 2012;166(5):916-26.
25. Porter D, Burton JL. A comparison of intra-lesional triamcinolone hexacetonide and triamcinolone acetonide in alopecia areata. The British Journal of Dermatology. 1971;85(3):272-3.
26. Alabdulkareem AS, Abahussein AA, Okoro A. Severe alopecia areata treated with systemic corticosteroids. International Journal of Dermatology. 1998;37(8):622-4. Epub 1998/09/10.
27. Friedli A, Labarthe MP, Engelhardt E, Feldmann R, Salomon D, Saurat JH. Pulse methylprednisolone therapy for severe alopecia areata: An open prospective study of 45 patients. Journal of the American Academy of Dermatology. 1998; 39(4 Pt 1):597-602.
28. Perriard-Wolfensberger J, Pasche-Koo F, Mainetti C, Labarthe MP, Salomon D, Saurat JH. Pulse of methylprednisolone in alopecia areata. Dermatology. 1993;187(4):282-5.
29. Whitmont KJ, Cooper AJ. PUVA treatment of alopecia areata totalis and universalis: A retrospective study. The Australasian Journal of Dermatology. 2003;44(2):106-9. Epub 2003/05/20.
30. Mohamed Z, Bhouri A, Jallouli A, Fazaa B, Kamoun MR, Mokhtar I. Alopecia areata treatment with a phototoxic dose of UVA and topical 8-methoxypsoralen. Journal of the European Academy of Dermatology and Venereology : JEADV. 2005;19(5):552-5. Epub 2005/09/17.
31. Fiedler-Weiss VC, Rumsfield J, Buys CM, West DP, Wendrow A. Evaluation of oral minoxidil in the treatment of alopecia areata. Archives of Dermatology. 1987;123(11):1488-90. Epub 1987/11/01.
32. Singh G, Lavanya M. Topical immunotherapy in alopecia areata. International Journal of Trichology. 2010;2(1):36-9. Epub 2010/12/29.
33. Rokhsar CK, Shupack JL, Vafai JJ, Washenik K. Efficacy of topical sensitizers in the treatment of alopecia areata. Journal of the American Academy of Dermatology. 1998;39(5 Pt 1):751-61. Epub 1998/11/12.
34. Majid I, Keen A. Management of alopecia areata: An update. British Journal of Medical Practitioners. 2012;5(3):a 530.
35. Lambelet P, Loliger J, Shroot B. Role of free radicals in the mode of action of anthralin. Skin pharmacology : The official Journal of the Skin Pharmacology Society. 1988;1(2):115-21. Epub 1988/01/01.
36. Rashidi T, Mahd AA. Treatment of persistent alopecia areata with sulfasalazine. International Journal of Dermatology. 2008;47(8):850-2. Epub 2008/08/23.
37. Aghaei S. An uncontrolled, open label study of sulfasalazine in severe alopecia areata. Indian Journal of Dermatology, Venereology and Leprology. 2008;74(6):611-3. Epub 2009/01/28.
38. Gupta AK, Ellis CN, Cooper KD, Nickoloff BJ, Ho VC, Chan LS, et al. Oral cyclosporine for the treatment of alopecia areata. A clinical and immunohistochemical analysis. Journal of the American Academy of Dermatology. 1990;22(2 Pt 1):242-50. Epub 1990/02/01.
39. Wang E, Lee JS, Tang M. Current treatment strategies in pediatric alopecia areata. Indian Journal of Dermatology. 2012;57(6):459-65. Epub 2012/12/19.
40. Phillips MA, Graves JE, Nunley JR. Alopecia areata presenting in 2 kidney-pancreas transplant recipients taking cyclosporine.

Journal of the American Academy of Dermatology. 2005;53(5 Suppl 1):S252-5. Epub 2005/10/18.

41. Yamamoto S, Jiang H, Kato R. Stimulation of hair growth by topical application of FK506, a potent immunosuppressive agent. The Journal of Investigative Dermatology. 1994;102(2):160-4. Epub 1994/02/01.
42. Price VH, Willey A, Chen BK. Topical tacrolimus in alopecia areata. Journal of the American Academy of Dermatology. 2005;52(1):138-9. Epub 2005/01/01.
43. Strober BE, Siu K, Alexis AF, Kim G, Washenik K, Sinha A, et al. Etanercept does not effectively treat moderate to severe alopecia areata: An open-label study. Journal of the American Academy of Dermatology. 2005;52(6):1082-4. Epub 2005/06/02.
44. Pan Y, Rao NA. Alopecia areata during etanercept therapy. Ocular Immunology and Inflammation. 2009;17(2):127-9. Epub 2009/05/05.
45. Strober BE, Menon K, McMichael A, Hordinsky M, Krueger G, Panko J, et al. Alefacept for severe alopecia areata: A randomized, double-blind, placebo-controlled study. Archives of Dermatology. 2009;145(11):1262-6. Epub 2009/11/18.
46. Seetharam KA. Alopecia areata: An update. Indian Journal of Dermatology, Venereology and Leprology. 2013;79(5):563-75. Epub 2013/08/27.
47. Duque-Estrada B, Vincenzi C, Misciali C, Tosti A. Alopecia secondary to mesotherapy. Journal of the American Academy of Dermatology. 2009;61(4):707-9. Epub 2009/07/07.
48. Al-Mutairi N. 308-nm excimer laser for the treatment of alopecia areata. Dermatologic surgery: Official Publication for American Society for Dermatologic Surgery [et al]. 2007;33(12):1483-7. Epub 2007/12/14.
49. Al-Mutairi N. 308-nm excimer laser for the treatment of alopecia areata in children. Pediatric Dermatology. 2009;26(5):547-50. Epub 2009/10/21.
50. Coronel-Perez IM, Rodriguez-Rey EM, Camacho-Martinez FM. Latanoprost in the treatment of eyelash alopecia in alopecia areata universalis. Journal of the European Academy of Dermatology and Venereology : JEADV. 2010;24(4):481-5. Epub 2009/12/24.
51. Roseborough I, Lee H, Chwalek J, Stamper RL, Price VH. Lack of efficacy of topical latanoprost and bimatoprost ophthalmic solutions in promoting eyelash growth in patients with alopecia areata. Journal of the American Academy of Dermatology. 2009;60(4):705-6. Epub 2009/03/19.

ANNEXURE

Ikeda's classification of alopecia areata

- Common (71%)
- Atopic (10%)
- Prehypertensive (4%)
- Autoimmune (5%)

Autoimmune associations

- Endocrine: Hashimoto's thyroiditis, Addison's disease, diabetes mellitus
- Dermatological conditions: Vitiligo, lichen planus, morphea, lichen sclerosus et atrophicus
- Autoimmune disorders: Systemic lupus erythematosus, Sjögren's syndrome, autoimmune hemolytic anemia
- Inflammatory bowel disorders: Ulcerative colitis
- Pernicious anemia
- Myasthenia gravis
- Chronic mucocutaneous candidiasis with endocrinopathy

Coudability sign

- Normal looking hair kinks when forced inwards or bent
- Kink situated 5–10 mm above the surface
- Helps to to differentiate diffuse alopecia areata from other diffuse alopecias

11

Androgenetic Alopecia

Eshini Perera, Rodney Sinclair

"Hair is terribly personal, a tangle of mysterious prejudice. It brings one's self image in focus."

—*Shana Alexander*

Epidemiology

Androgenetic alopecia (AGA) is the most common cause of hair loss. While most noticeable in men, women are also commonly affected. AGA affects roughly 30% of White males by the age of 30 years and 50% by the age of 50 years.[1-3] AGA occurs in all races, however, it is less common in Asians and African-American males. White males are four times more likely that Black males to develop Hamilton stage VIII AGA.[4] The pattern of hair loss is sex dependant. Male pattern hair loss describes the temporal, and vertex balding seen in men due to AGA. Female pattern hair loss (FPHL) describes the mid frontal scalp hair thinning seen in women with AGA. Fifty seven percent of women over the age of 80 are affected with this pattern of hair loss **(Box 11.1)**.[5]

Clinical Presentations

Hair loss typically follows a defined pattern. In males, bitemporal recession of the frontal hairline usually precedes diffuse thinning over the vertex of the scalp which eventually produces vertex baldness. Thinning over the mid frontal scalp eventually joins the receding frontal hairline and vertex bald spot. This highly reproducable pattern of hair loss is illustrated by the Norwood-Hamilton scale **(Figure 11.1)**. The rate of hair loss over the frontal and vertex region may vary producing visual variations. While the scale does not accurately reflect the continuum of hair patterns seen, it is useful in classifying the extent of hair loss.

In FPHL, the anterior hair line is often maintained, or there may be mild bitemporal recession. The severe bitemporal recession seen in men with AGA is not common in women. The usual pattern of hair loss in women is a diffuse reduction in hair density over the crown. A 'Christmas tree' pattern can be observed with widening of the central part line.[6] This hair thinning may extend over the parietal scalp to the ears.[7] This pattern of hair loss seen in females can be observed in the Sinclair scale **(Figure 11.2)**.

Box 11.1: Epidemiology

- Commonest cause of hair loss
- Affects 30% of White males by 30 years and 50% by 50 years
- Males more affected than females
- The pattern of hair loss is sex dependant
- Male pattern hair loss: Temporal, and vertex balding while Female pattern hair loss (FPHL): mid frontal scalp thinning

Etiology

Androgentic alopecia is familial with a complex polygenic mode of inheritance.[8] Polymorphism of the androgen receptor gene, the 5 α reductase gene and 2 other, as yet unidentified genes on chromosomes 3 and 21 have all been associated with premature balding.[9] Twin studies indicate a strong genetic predisposition with minimal environmental modification. Epigenetic modifications that increase the risk of AGA have been postulated.[10]

There is a familial tendency towards androgenetic alopecia and it is thought to have a polygenic mode of inheritance.[8] This tendency is well recognized in males and there is a large body of literature to support this. A study of 54 father and son pairs found that 81.5% of balding sons had fathers with significant balding.[11] Polymorphisms of the androgen receptor gene located on the X-chromosome have been implicated in patients with AGA.[9] A restriction fragment length polymorphism in the androgen receptor gene *Stu1* was found in 98.1% of young bald men and 92.3% of older bald men.[9] The same polymorphisms was also found

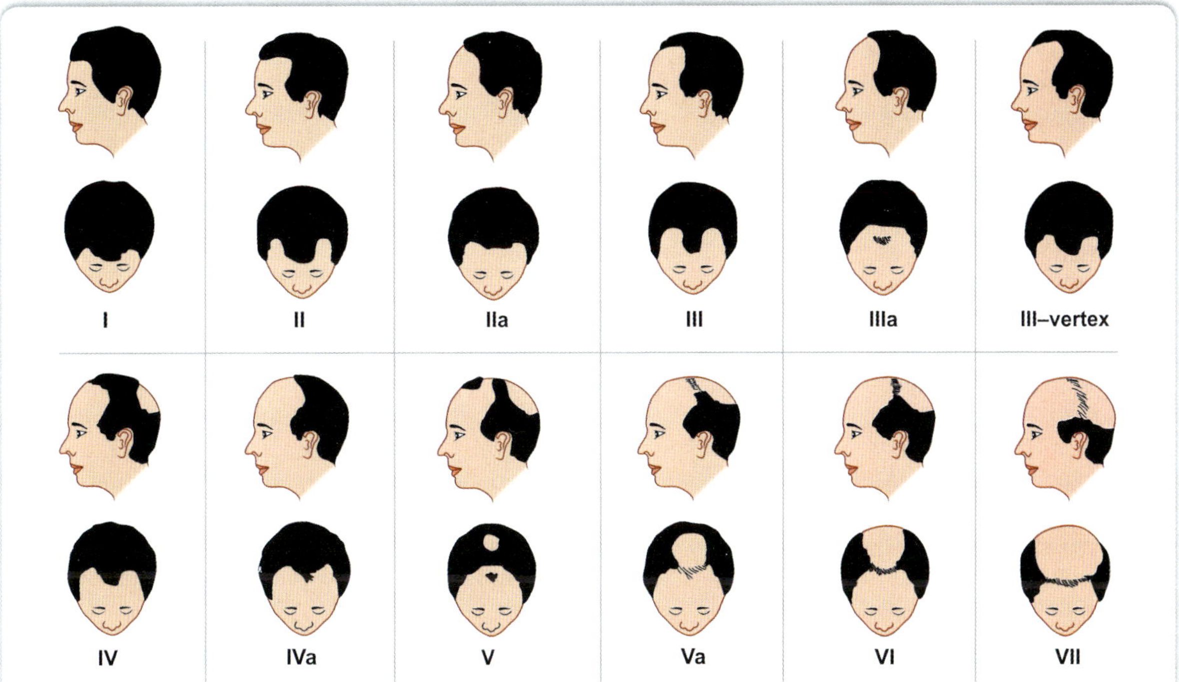

Fig. 11.1: Norwood-Hamilton scale. The following categories are defined as follows: Type I: No hair loss, Type II: Minor recession of the frontal hairline, Type III: Further frontal hair loss, Type III vertex: Significant frontal recession and hair loss from the vertex, Type IV – VI: Further frontal and vertex loss, Type VII: Only the occipital scalp region maintained

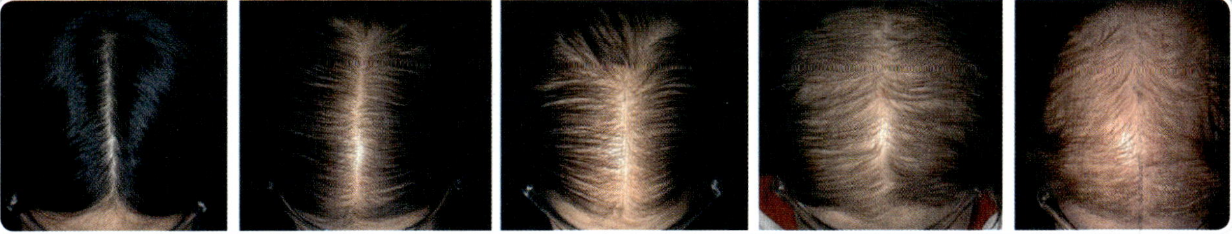

Fig. 11.2: The Sinclair scale

in 77% of non bald men suggesting that while the gene was needed for the development of AGA, the presence of the gene itself was not sufficient for the development of the disease. A number of other genes have been nominated as potentially causing AGA including : SRDA 1, SRDA 5, the insulin gene, the aromatase gene and the gene for Erα estrogen receptor and type II insulin-like growth factor genes, although no associations have been found to date.[8] Furthermore, DNA methylation, adding a methyl group to the cytosine base with in a CpG dinucleotide, of the androgen receptor was found to be increased in occipital hair follicles.[10]

Findings in a study examining patients with Kennedy disease (KD), an X-linked neurodegenerative disease, revealed a reduced risk of AGA in this patient group. KD is associated with partial androgen insensitivity due to functional alteration of the androgen receptor caused by polyglutamine expansion. These findings further support the role of polymorphisms of the androgen receptor gene.[12]

In females, this genetic model is assumed to be the same.[13] It has been suggested that females need a stronger genetic predisposition than men for hair loss to occur. A study of fifty-six women with AGA showed an increased frequency of balding in first degree male relatives over the age of 30 (54%) compared with male relatives of the women in the control group (23%).[14]

Pathogenesis

Androgens can reach the skin through circulation or be manufactured locally. Circulating and locally produced androgens bind to androgen receptors in the hair follicle bulb. These androgens mediate an alteration in the size of the dermal papilla during early anagen that reduces the size of the anagen follicle and of the emerging hair and also reduces the duration of the anagen phase of the hair cycle. In addition the onset of anagen is delayed.

Paradoxical Systemic Effects of Androgens

The effects of circulating androgens on hair follicles are site-specific: Hair on the vertex of the scalp is induced into non-pigmented vellus hairs while pubic, axillary, beard and chest hairs are induced into large terminal hairs. Circulating androgens have no impact on eyebrow or occipital scalp hair.

A study of 10 eunuchs, 10 males castrated at puberty and 34 castrated at adolescence revealed that baldness did not develop in any of the participants.[15] Each participant was then administered intramuscular oral testosterone at a level equivalent to those seen in normal men, and participants who were genetically predisposed subsequently developed baldness.[15] Discontinuation of the testosterone did not reverse the balding.

5α-reductase is an enzyme that converts testosterone to dihydrotestosterone (DHT).[16] DHT is a potent agonist for androgen receptor activation, binding to the receptor with 5 times the avidity of testosterone.[16] Pseudohermaphrodite who have 5α-reductase deficiency have normal levels of testosterone, however they have reduced levels of DHT.[17] Phenotypically they have sparse facial and body hair and lack tendency to develop AGA **(Box 11.2)**.[18] High dose testosterone administered to these individuals did not induce baldness, however it was noted that there was virilization and beard growth.[19] These findings support the notion that the key androgen is DHT.

Local Effects of Androgens

Dermal papilla cells located on the bulb secrete autocrine growth factors in response to testosterone.[20] Testosterone increases the dermal papilla size and thereby increases the hair follicle and hair cortex. The dermal papilla cells on the occiput do not respond in this fashion when exposed to testosterone. Studies involving hair transplantation reveal that scalp hairs from the vertex which are transplanted on the forearm continue to miniaturize at the same rate as the original neighboring hairs on the vertex of the scalp. When occipital scalp hairs are transplanted onto the vertex they continue to maintain their resistance to AGA. These findings support the notion that AGA is dependent on intrinsic factors within each follicle.

Balding and hair-bearing areas of the scalp have different numbers of androgen receptors and 5α-reductase activity, which is associated with the geographical pattern of hair loss. However, the follicle is able to regulate its response to androgens by upregulating 5α-reductase and androgen receptor expression suggesting that these associations are a secondary occurrence.

Box 11.2: 5α-reductase enzyme

- Converts testosterone to dihydrotestosterone
- DHT is a potent agonist for androgen receptor activation, binding to the receptor with 5 times the avidity of testosterone
- Pseudohermaphrodite with 5α-reductase deficiency have reduced levels of DHT

Increased Telogen Hair Count

In AGA the duration of anagen is decreased while the duration of telogen remains the same or increases resulting in a decreased anagen to telogen ratio.[20] The result is that the period of anagen is too short for the hairs to reach the skin surface. Furthermore, the period between the latent component of the telogen phase and anagen regrowth becomes longer reducing the overall number of hairs on the scalp.

Follicular Miniaturization

The dermal papilla is thought to be the target for androgen mediated changes in the hair cycle and for miniaturization of the follicle **(Figure 11.3)**. Papilla size determines the size of the hair bulb and the hair produced. This notion is supported by the relationship between the size of the dermal papilla and the size of the hair matrix. The size of the papilla is largely determined by changes in the cell number, however changes in extracellular matrix and blood supply also affect the size. A study of 42 women revealed that there was an increase in vellus follicle numbers with increasing

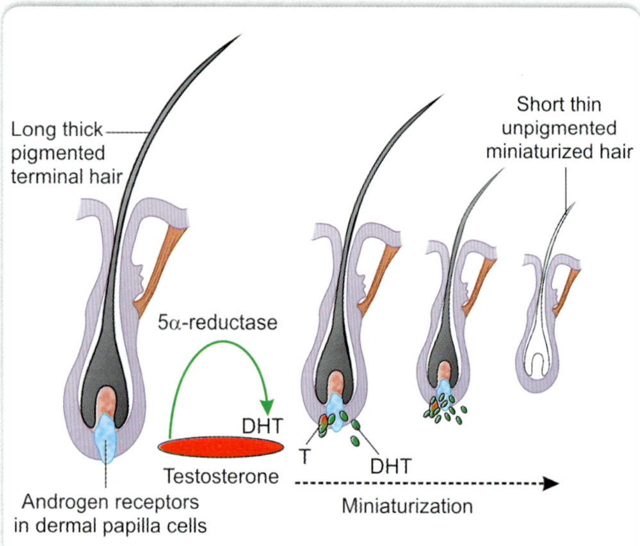

Fig. 11.3: Miniaturization of the hair follicle

severity of hair loss in women confirming that terminal follicles miniaturize.[21]

In AGA there is a decrease in cell numbers that accompanies the miniaturization of hair follicles. The cause of the decrease in dermal papilla cell numbers is unknown but thought to be due to apoptotic cell death, cell displacement or migration of dermal papilla cells into the dermal sheath.

The miniaturization process does not occur continuously during the anagen phase of the hair cycle. Miniaturization takes place in early anagen resulting in a progressive reduction of the follicle size between each cycle. The caliber of the hairs produced from the smaller follicles is reduced and the pigment production decreases. Mean caliber size is reduced from 0.08 mm to <0.06 mm.[22]

Changes in the Follicular Units

Initially, miniaturization affects some but not all of the hairs within an individual follicular unit, so that on affected zones of the scalp each unit has a reduced number of hairs rather than a total absence of hairs. The sparing of one or two hairs within each follicular unit results in diffuse thinning and increased hair shedding that precedes the development of baldness. Eventually, when all the hairs within a follicular unit are lost, a bald scalp becomes apparent.

In contrast, in alopecia areata, which also demonstrates follicular miniaturization, all the hairs within each unit are lost simultaneously leading to instantaneous baldness within affected areas **(Figure 11.4)**.

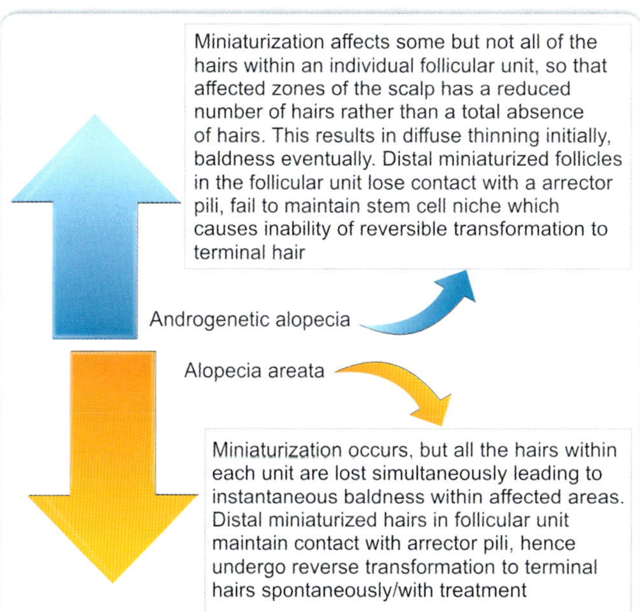

Fig. 11.4: Schematic representation of miniaturization in AGA and alopecia areata

The relationship between hairs within each follicular unit to the arrector pili muscle is also important. The arrector pili muscle inserts into the bulge region where it maintains the epithelial stem cell niche. In most mammals, the hierarchy of hairs within the follicular unit is clearly apparent, with a single primary terminal follicle at the edge of the unit immediately adjacent to the arrector pili muscle, and smaller secondary vellus hairs distally that are often manufactured and destroyed seasonally.

In humans, this hierarchy is not apparent in a normal scalp but becomes so in androgenetic alopecia.[23] The hairs closest to the arrector pili muscle are the most resistant to miniaturization, while those most distal to the muscle miniaturize first. Ultimately, the most distal follicles physically separate from the arrector pili muscle and become unable to maintain their stem cell niche **(Figure 11.5)**. These miniaturized hairs are no longer capable of reverse transformation back into terminal hairs.

In contrast, in alopecia areata, all miniaturized hairs maintain contact with the arrector pili muscle and the condition is potentially fully reversible in people who respond to treatment.[23,24]

Evaluation of hair loss

There is no gold-standard for the diagnosis of early hair loss, however early detection is important given that current treatments for AGA are more effective at arresting the progression of hair loss than stimulating regrowth.[25] Diagnosis of AGA in males is straightforward, however in females the diagnosis may not be so clear-cut. In women, diagnosis of early AGA is aided by use of an epiluminescent microscope **(Figure 11.6)**. Other differentials should be considered including chronic telogen effluvium. A careful history should be obtained from the patient. A history of progressive patterned hair loss is typical in AGA. Information, including family history of AGA and drug history should be collected and a history of menstrual irregularities or hirsutism should be noted in females as this requires further investigation to exclude an underlying cause.

Laboratory investigations are not usually indicated for patients with AGA and diagnosis is made on clinical grounds. However in females who have features of hyperandrogenism, appropriate investigations include FSH, LH, prolactin, serum androgen and estrogen levels, fasting lipids and triglyceride levels.

The scalp should be carefully examined to determine the pattern of hair loss. Concurrent skin diseases should also be identified as conditions like seborrheic dermatitis and photodamage can exacerbate AGA. Furthermore, areas of baldness may also be pigmented due to sun exposure.

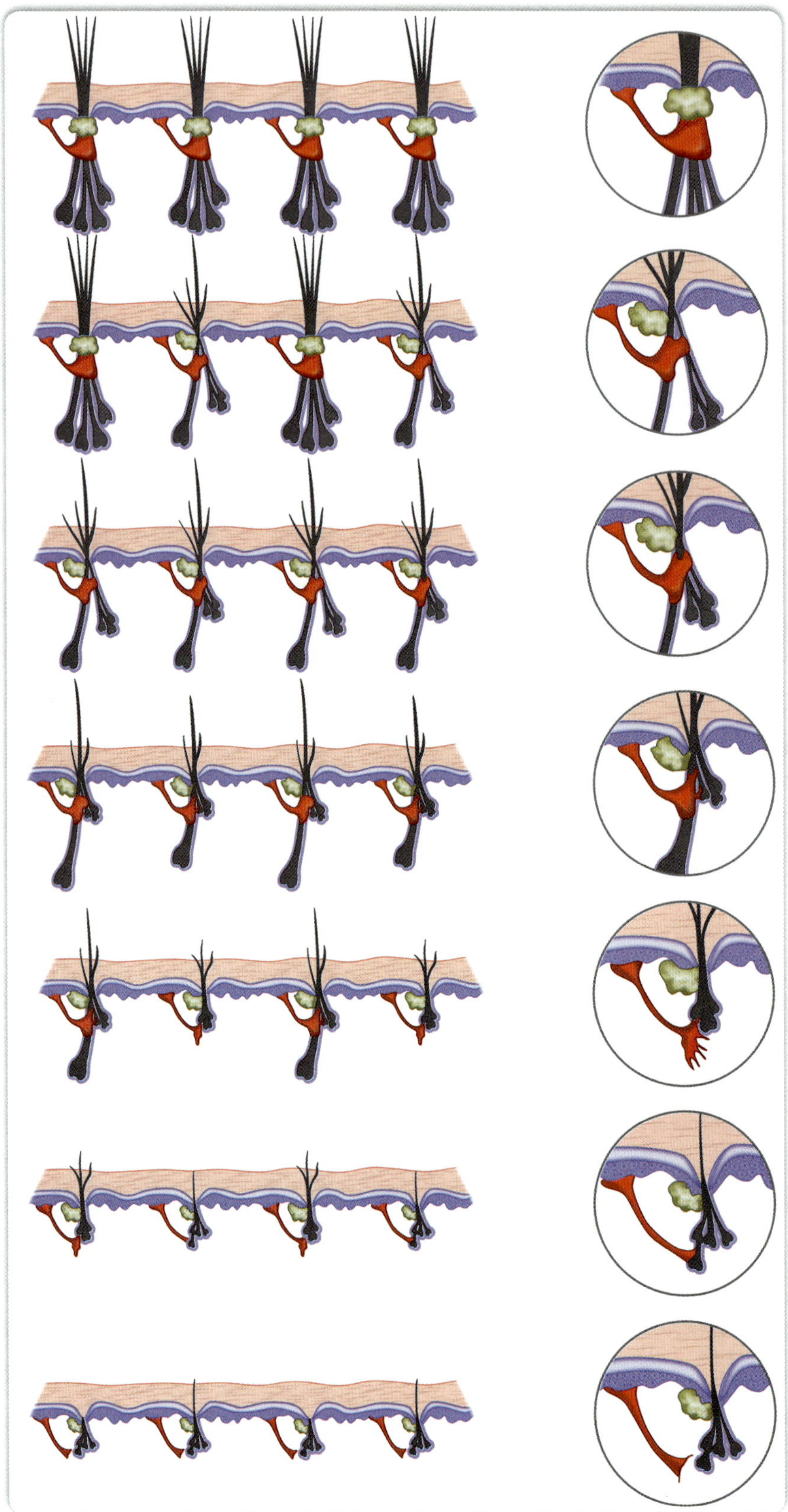

Fig. 11.5: Miniaturization of hairs within a follicular hair unit. Hairs distal to the arrector pili muscle miniaturize first

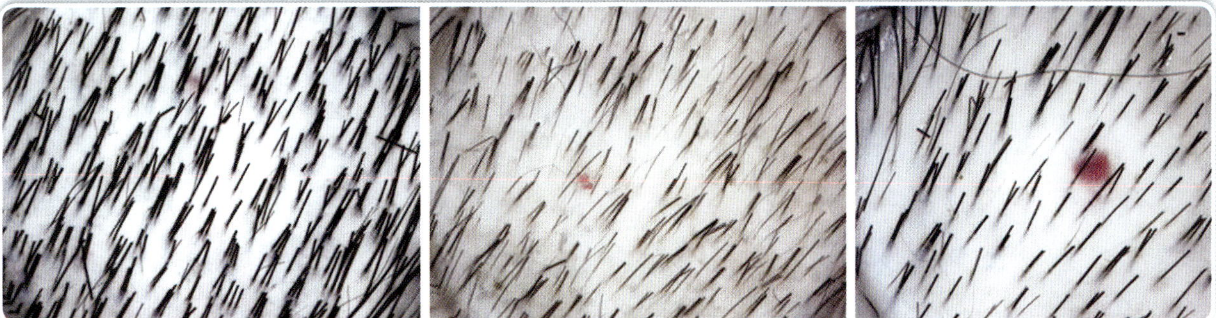

Fig. 11.6: View of scalp in androgenetic alopecia using epiluminescent microscope. The three consecutive images demonstrate the miniaturization and loss of hairs within each follicular unit resulting in progressive hair loss

Table 11.1: Examination findings in the evaluation of androgenetic alopecia

Examination	Description of examination	Findings
Standardized wash test	In this test the patient does not shampoo the hair for 5 days. The hair is then shampooed and washed in a basin and the hair lost from the scalp during the wash is collected. Hairs are then counted and divided into hairs that are less than 3 cm in length and greater than 5 cm in length.	In female pattern hair loss over half the hair is vellus compared to chronic telogen effluvium where only a small proportion of hair is vellus[26]
Pull test	Gentle traction is exerted on a small area of hair. If > 10 percent hairs come out with each pull, this is positive	The pull test is usually negative in AGA. If the pull test is positive then the possibility of other causes of hair loss should be considered. In the case of a diffusely positive pull test, telogen effluvium should be considered
Daily hair count	The number of hairs that are lost can be counted Hair from the first morning combing or washing are collected in a bag over 14 days	If more than 100 hairs are lost per day then the hair bulb should be examined microscopically to differentiate for other causes including telogen effluvium, anagen effluvium and alopecia areata
Trichoscopy	Hair is visualized under a dermatoscope	In AGA a number of features are observable: 1. Hair diameter diversity greater than 20% reflecting hair miniaturization 2. Perifollicular pigmentation roughly 1 mm in diameter 3. Yellow dots can be seen in the transitional zones of AGA 4. Small areas of baldness with exogen hair follicles (empty follicles that represent the delay of anagen after a telogen hair is shed)[27,28]
Contrasting felt examination	A card (black felt on one side and white on the other) is held at the scalp after parting the hair	Miniature hairs in AGA show up on the edge of the felt A short frontal fringe can be seen in telogen effluvium[29]

Listed above **(Table 11.1)** are suggested examinations for the evaluation of hair loss in patients with AGA.

Serial Photography

Serial photographs can be taken of areas affected by hair loss to monitor progress of hair growth and hair follicle density. Patients should be advised to maintain the same hairstyle and color so that progress can be accurately tracked. The canfield technique involves the use of a positioning device to fix the patients chin and forehead **(Figure 11.7)**. A camera, which is mounted is used to take pictures ensuring that the view is the same at each visit.[27]

Scalp Biopsies

Scalp biopsies are not indicated in the diagnosis of AGA. Biopsies, however are useful in distinguishing between chronic telogen effluvium and female pattern hair loss. In females who notice increased hair shedding, a scalp biopsy may reveal early AGA even when clinical symptoms are not apparent. In females, a triple biopsy, i.e. biopsies

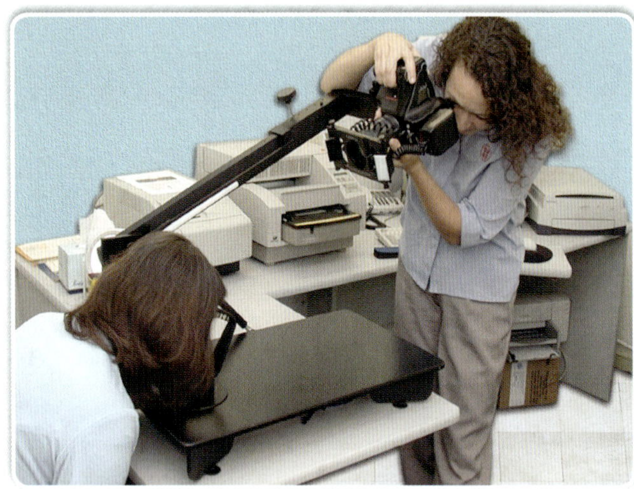

Fig. 11.7: The Canfield technique

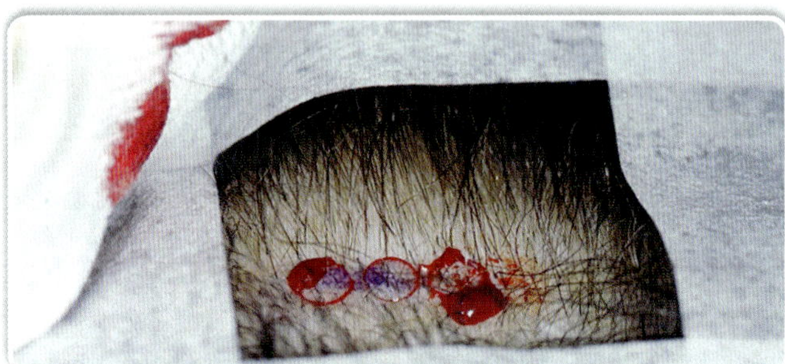

Fig. 11.8: Triple biopsies in a patient with FPHL

at three immediately adjacent sites, is recommended due to the potential to miss the diagnosis on a single biopsy (21% with a single biopsy compared to 2% in a triple biopsy **(Figure 11.8)**.[2]

Histopathology

Biopsies sectioned transversely at the opening of the sebaceous duct show differing hair shaft diameters reflecting the progressive miniaturization of hair follicles. The terminal to vellus ratio in AGA is usually less than 4:1.[27] Biopsies sectioned vertically reveal vellus hair follicles within the papillary dermis while terminal hairs rest in the subcutaneous and reticular dermis.[30] A fibrous tract or a follicular streamer leading to the miniaturized hair indicates the position of the original terminal follicle. Up to 40% of patients may show perifollicular fibrosis on microscopic examination.[2]

Management

Psychological

Addressing the psychological impact of balding on patients is a central process in treating hair loss. The disease is distressing for both men and women, however there is a greater social acceptance of hair loss in men compared to women.[31,32] The loss of hair in women produces greater psychological distress than in men.[31] A study revealed that 52% of women were 'extremely upset' by their hair loss compared to 28% of men.[33,34] Female patients cope by developing compensatory behaviors for example improving other physical features to offset hair loss[35], concealing hair loss and engaging in compulsive activities of reassurance to minimize negative body image.[31] Ultimately, any management plan should take into account the psychological impact and the patient's coping mechanism.

Camouflage Products and Hair Pieces

Products designed to camouflage hair loss are the simplest and cheapest way of treating androgenetic hair loss. Hair building fibers, topical shading and scalp spray thickeners are among the most commonly used camouflaging products **(Table 11.2)**.[36]

These products are resistant to sweating, exercising and swimming. Camouflaging products are recommended for

Table 11.2: Camouflage products

Product	*Explanation*	*Advantages/disadvantages*
Hair building fibers	Keratin fibers are gently shaken from a jar onto exposed areas of the scalp to create the illusion of density	❑ Easily removed with shampoo
Scalp spray thickeners	Scalp spray thickeners work similarly to hair building fibers. Fibers bond to thinning areas of hair adding color and thickness	❑ Messy to use ❑ Staining of clothing and hands ❑ Sticky/greasy ❑ Easily removed with shampoo
Alopecia masking lotion	This is a tinted lotion that can be applied to thinning areas to colour the scalp and create density throughout the area	❑ Does not stain clothing ❑ One tube of lotion will last several months ❑ Easily removed with shampoo
Topical shading	This is a tinted powder that is applied with a sponge- tipped applicator to thinning areas of scalp to create thickness	❑ Used for oily to normal skin and can prevent a shiny scalp

patients with mild to moderate hair loss and can be used in conjunction with topical minoxidil.

For extensive hair loss hairpieces can be used. These are attached to the scalp by tape or hair clips and can be worn throughout the day. In females with advanced hair loss wigs can be used. These can be interwoven or worn over the top of existing hair.

Medical Treatment

Minoxidil

Minoxidil is a piperidinopyrimidine derivative and a potent arteriolar vasodilator.[37] It has been shown to be effective in converting vellus hair to terminal hair in 30% of patients when applied in a 2% solution with a 10% propylene glycol water base.[38,39] 1 mL of the solution is applied to the scalp twice daily. A temporary telogen effluvium may occur in the first 2–8 weeks. Treatment with 5% solution yields superior hair growth compared to the 2% solution in both males and females.[40,41] Foam formulations without propylene glycol cause less cutaneous side effects. There is a higher risk of facial hypertrichosis with the use of 5% formulations in females.[42]

The best response can be seen in men and women who are treated early in the balding process, with a maximum diameter of baldness less than 10 cm and in whom the pre-treatment hair density is in excess of 20 hairs/cm^2.[43] Maximal response is seen in the first 6 months of therapy, benefits thereafter are marginal. To maintain these benefits patients are advised that minoxidil application should be continued for the rest of their life **(Box 11.3)**. Regression of results occurs after 3 months of cessation to the state of baldness that would have occurred if treatment were not applied.[44] Supplementation of minoxidil with spironolactone, in females, produces an additive effect.[45]

Oral Finasteride

Finasteride is a synthetic azo-steroid that is a potent antagonist of 5α-reductase type II.[46] It binds irreversibly to this enzyme to inhibit the conversion of testosterone to DHT. This reduction of DHT production then limits the miniaturization of hair follicles. A dose of 1 mg orally is the optimal dose for treatment of male pattern baldness.[46] At this dosage finasteride has been shown to reduce scalp DHT by 64% and serum DHT by 68%.[47] The side effect profile of finasteride includes decreased libido, erectile dysfunction and depression,[46,48] making some patients hesitant to continue use **(Figure 11.9)**.

An examination of a series of scalp biopsies in patients with AGA revealed that after 12 months of treatment with finasteride, terminal hair count increased and vellus hair counts decreased. The study demonstrated the ability of finasteride to reverse the miniaturization process and encourage growth of terminal hairs.[49]

Conversely topical finasteride use in a 0.05% solution showed no effect on hair regrowth despite reducing the serum DHT by 40%.

Box 11.3: Factors affecting responsiveness with minoxidil

- Early treatment in the balding process, with a maximum diameter of baldness less than 10 cm
- Hair density in excess of 20 hairs/cm^2
- Maximal response is seen in the first 6 months of therapy

Dutasteride

Dutasteride inhibits both type 1 and 2 5α-reductase isoenzymes.[50] It is 100 times more potent in inhibiting the type 1 isoenzyme than finasteride. Dutasteride, 0.5 mg daily, is licensed for the treatment of benign prostatic hyperplasia but, it is not licensed for use in MPHL.[51] Several reports suggest that treatment with dutasteride results in superior hair growth to finasteride and lowers prostate cancer incidence in trials.[50,51] However, it has a longer half-life than finasteride, so its effects on sexual function are potentially more severe and longer lasting. Nonetheless, some physicians prescribe dutasteride off license for MPHL in 0.5 mg twice-weekly dosing schedules. Dutasteride is also a potent teratogen and its use is contraindicated in women of child-bearing age.

Managing Female Pattern Hair Loss

Topical minoxidil induced mild to moderate hair regrowth in 60% of women[52] and can be used alone or in combination with oral anti-androgen therapy.[20] Oral anti-androgen therapies that are thought to be beneficial in preventing progression of AGA in females include cyproterone acetate, spironolactone and flutamide.[6]

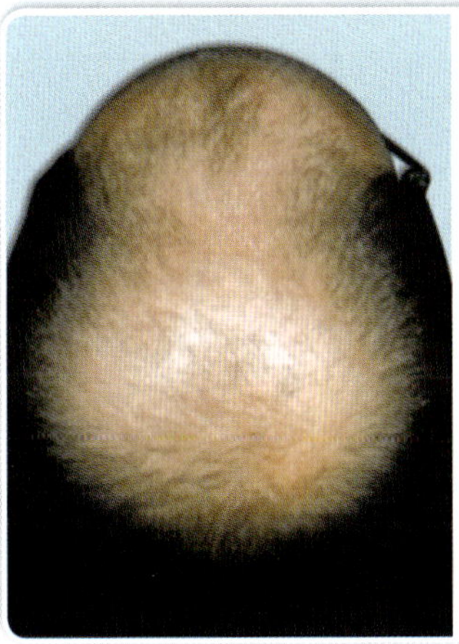
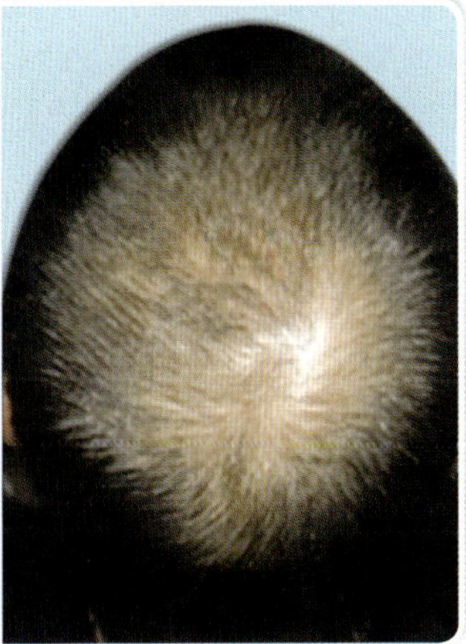

Fig. 11.9: Hair regrowth in a patient using 1 mg of oral finasteride. The first picture illustrates the baseline level of hair loss. The second picture was taken after 5 years

Androgen-dependant treatments are contraindicated in pregnant females due to the risk of causing abnormalities in the genitalia of male fetuses.[31]

Spironolactone

Spironolactone is the most commonly used antiandrogen used to treat female pattern hair loss in the USA.[31] Spironolactone is a synthetic steroid which competitively blocks cytoplasmic receptors for DHT and weakly inhibits androgen biosynthesis.[20] Recommended dosages are between 100–300 mg per day, however most women require a minimum of 200 mg **(Figure 11.10)**.[53] Side effects are dose related and include breast enlargement, menstrual irregularities, electrolyte disturbances and postural hypotension. Regular blood pressure and electrolyte monitoring is recommended during treatment.[54]

Cyproterone Acetate

Cyproterone is an androgen receptor blocker and works by inhibiting gonadotropin-releasing hormone (GnRH).[20] A 12-month randomized trial comparing topical minoxidil 2% and cyproterone acetate demonstrated that cyproterone acetate was more effective in females with signs of hyperandrogenism, while minoxidil was more effective in females without signs of hyperandrogenism.[55] A study comparing spironolactone and cyproterone in females with biopsy confirmed FPHL, showed a comparable level of efficacy between these medications.[56]

The most effective dose is 100 mg/day on day 5–15 of the menstrual cycle.[31] This is supplemented with 50 µg of ethinyl estradiol for days 5–25, however in post-menopausal women cyproterone can be used continuously with or without supplementation of estrogens.[20,31]

Finasteride

Initial studies using finasteride for postmenopausal women with FPHL gave conflicting reports of its efficacy, suggesting that it may be useful predominantly in patients with raised serum testosterone levels. However, a recent study from Korea reported an improvement in hair density and thickness in a group of both pre- and postmenopausal normoandrogenic women treated with finasteride, 5 mg daily.[57] Furthermore, case report of a female who was treated with the same dose also demonstrated successful regrowth after 12 months.[58] In clinical practice, many hair specialists use finasteride off label at a dose of 1–2.5 mg daily **(Figure 11.11)**. Finasteride is teratogenic, and off-label use requires careful patient consent and measures to avoid pregnancy. Reported side effects in women are few but include headache and menstrual irregularity.

Flutamide

Flutamide is an antiandrogen that acts via androgen receptor antagonism.[31] There are studies that suggest, it is superior to cyproterone acetate and spironolactone.[59,60] This is supported by reports in the literature documenting a satisfactory therapeutic response to using flutamide in patients with FPHL that did not respond to spironolactone.[61] Side effects include hepatotoxicity, which limit its use in AGA. However, a more recent prospective cohort study demonstrated that doses lower than 62.5 mg/day have been associated with hepatic tolerability.[62]

Therapies with Uncertain, Unproven or no Efficacy

Ketoconazole Shampoo

A small study showed comparable hair growth in men with AGA using minoxidil 2% to those using ketoconazole shampoo.[63] The mechanism of action is unclear; it may be due to the anti-inflammatory properties of ketoconazole or to its effect on reducing *Malassezia* species (fungal) colonization. It may also disrupt local DHT pathways. The study has never been replicated, and the use of ketoconazole

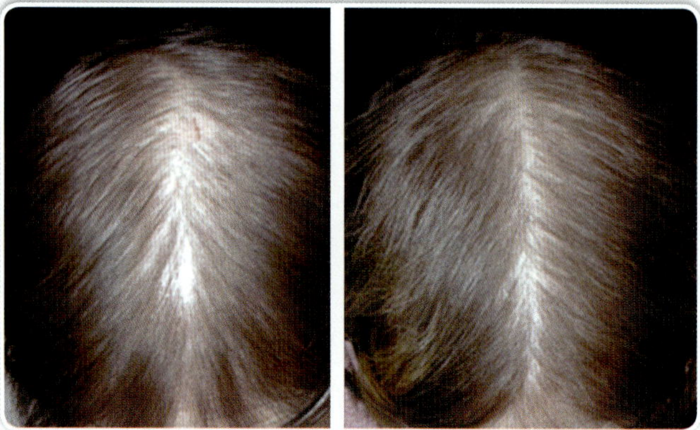

Fig. 11.10: Hair regrowth in a patient using 200 mg oral spironolactone daily. The first picture illustrates the baseline level of hair loss. The second picture was taken after 12 months

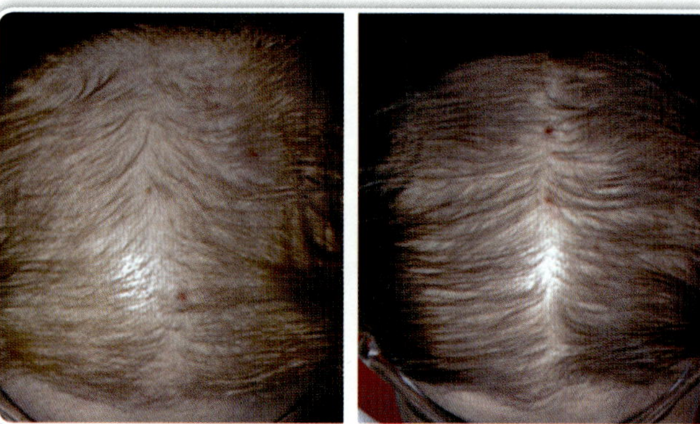

Fig. 11.11: Hair regrowth in a patient using 5 mg oral finasteride daily. The first picture illustrates the baseline level of hair loss. The second picture was taken after 12 months

shampoo is generally only recommended for patients with concomitant seborrheic dermatitis.

Low-level Light Therapy Devices

These resemble hair brushes, claim to stimulate hair growth using low-energy laser light beams. The HairMax LaserComb has a product license from the FDA but there are no published clinical trials regarding its efficacy.

Supplements and Herbal/Natural Remedies

There is a huge array of herbal and vitamin supplements which claim to help hair thinning and loss. Unfortunately, there are few clinical trials to support their use. While some specialists believe that it is beneficial to keep ferritin levels above 70 ng/mL in patients with telogen effluvium, there is no evidence that biotin, tyrosine or procerin are of any benefit in androgenetic alopecia. Saw palmetto is derived from the herb Serenoa repens and is a weak 5α-reductase inhibitor, which has been shown in one poorly conducted clinical trial to increase hair growth in a small number of men with androgenetic alopecia. Many of these products are freely available on the internet.

Scalp Roller

Several manufacturers produce a small microneedle Derma Roller for the scalp, which is marketed to increase the penetration of a topical product (e.g. minoxidil) into the scalp. These rollers may also have a role in stimulating collagen production and putatively encouraging follicle growth. They have not been licensed for use by the FDA and at present there are no clinical trials supporting their use.

Surgery

Surgical treatment options for the treatment of AGA include hair transplant and scalp reduction procedures. Hair transplantation is ideal for patients who have high-density donor hair **(Figure 11.12)**. Male candidates should have just frontal and mid-frontal hair loss while female candidates should have hair loss just over the frontal scalp. Grafts are transplanted into the scalp under local anesthetic over a number of sessions spaced 6 months apart. Results are equally favorable in both males and females.[64] Complications include facial edema, headaches, temporary numbing of scalp and scarring.[64]

Scalp reduction, that is, excising the bald scalp, is a less popular option due to visibility of scars, unpredictability of further hair loss and the need for more than one scalp reduction to address the hair loss.[64] This procedure can be combined with hair transplants to improve the cosmetic appearance.

Conclusion

In conclusion AGA is common cause of hair loss which can affect both males and females. Pathogenesis involves genetic factors, miniaturization of hair follicles, stepwise miniaturization of the hair follicles and local and systemic effects of androgens. Treatment for AGA is focused on the latter in conjunction with topical treatments. Camouflage techniques are a viable and cheap option for disguising hair loss and may ameliorate the psychological distress of balding

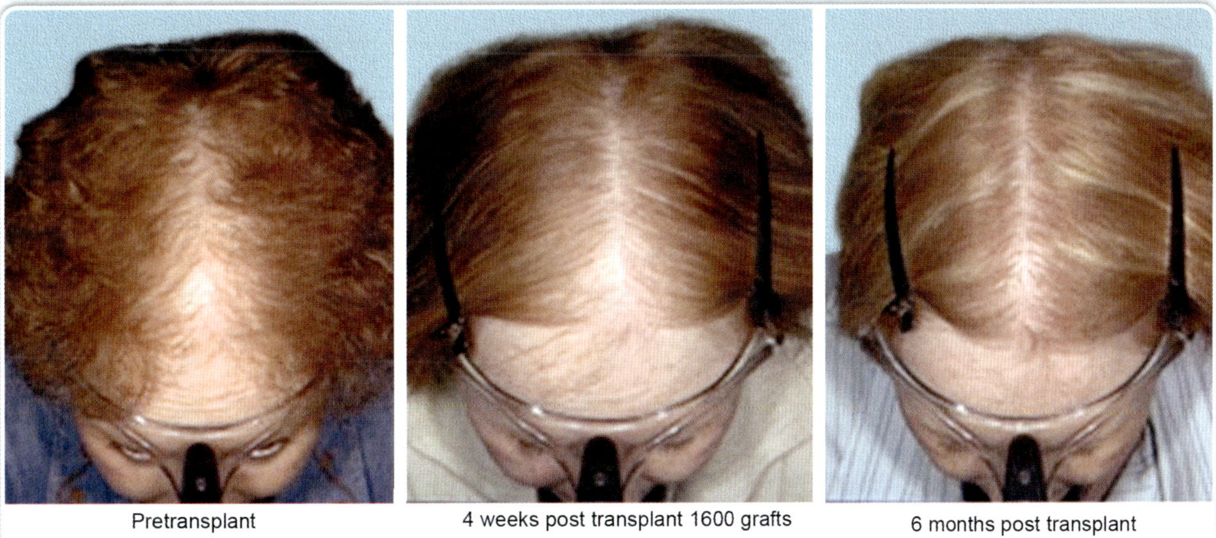

Fig. 11.12: Hair transplant 4 weeks post-transplant with 1600 grafts and 6 months post-transplant

References

1. Ellis JA, Sinclair R, Harrap SB. Androgenetic alopecia: Pathogenesis and potential for therapy. Expert Reviews in Molecular Medicine. 2002;4(22):1-11. Epub 2003/10/31.
2. Sinclair R, Jolley D, Mallari R, Magee J. The reliability of horizontally sectioned scalp biopsies in the diagnosis of chronic diffuse telogen hair loss in women. Journal of the American Academy of Dermatology. 2004;51(2):189-99. Epub 2004/07/29.
3. Severi G, Sinclair R, Hopper JL, English DR, McCredie MR, Boyle P, et al. Androgenetic alopecia in men aged 40-69 years: Prevalence and risk factors. The British Journal of Dermatology. 2003;149(6):1207-13. Epub 2003/12/17.
4. Setty LR. Hair patterns of scalp of white and Negro males. American Journal of Physical Anthropology. 1970;33(1):49-55. Epub 1970/07/01.
5. Gan DC, Sinclair RD. Prevalence of male and female pattern hair loss in Maryborough. The Journal of Investigative Dermatology Symposium Proceedings/the Society for Investigative Dermatology, Inc [and] European Society for Dermatological Research. 2005;10(3):184-9. Epub 2005/12/31.
6. Olsen E. Disorders of hair growth. In: Olsen E, editor. Androgenetic Alopecia. New York: McGraw-Hill. 1994; p.257-84.
7. Ludwig E. Classification of the types of androgenetic alopecia (common baldness) occurring in the female sex. The British Journal of Dermatology. 1977;97(3):247-54. Epub 1977/09/01.
8. Sinclair R. Male pattern androgenetic alopecia. BMJ. 1998;317(7162):865-9. Epub 1998/09/25.
9. Ellis JA, Stebbing M, Harrap SB. Polymorphism of the androgen receptor gene is associated with male pattern baldness. The Journal of Investigative Dermatology. 2001;116(3):452-5. Epub 2001/03/07.
10. Cobb JE, Wong NC, Yip LW, Martinick J, Bosnich R, Sinclair RD, et al. Evidence of increased DNA methylation of the androgen receptor gene in occipital hair follicles from men with androgenetic alopecia. The British Journal of Dermatology. 2011;165(1):210-3. Epub 2011/03/25.
11. Ellis JA, Stebbing M, Harrap SB. Genetic analysis of male pattern baldness and the 5 alpha-reductase genes. The Journal of Investigative Dermatology. 1998;110(6):849-53. Epub 1998/06/10.
12. Sinclair R, Greenland KJ, Egmond S, Hoedemaker C, Chapman A, Zajac JD. Men with Kennedy disease have a reduced risk of androgenetic alopecia. The British Journal of Dermatology. 2007;157(2):290-4. Epub 2007/06/29.
13. Yip L, Rufaut N, Sinclair R. Role of genetics and sex steroid hormones in male androgenetic alopecia and female pattern hair loss: An update of what we now know. The Australasian Journal of Dermatology. 2011;52(2):81-8. Epub 2011/05/25.
14. Smith MA, Wells RS. Male-type alopecia, alopecia areata, and normal hair in women; family histories. Archives of Dermatology. 1964;89:95-8. Epub 1964/01/01.
15. Hamilton JB. Male hormone stimulation is prerequisite and an incitant in common baldness. American Journal of Anatomy. 1942;71(3):451-80.
16. Davison SL, Bell R. Androgen physiology. Seminars in Reproductive Medicine. 2006;24(2):71-7. Epub 2006/04/25.
17. Peterson RE, Imperato-McGinley J, Gautier T, Sturla E. Male pseudohermaphroditism due to steroid 5-alpha-reductase deficiency. The American Journal of Medicine. 1977;62(2):170-91. Epub 1977/02/01.
18. Imperato-McGinley J, Guerrero L, Gautier T, Peterson RE. Steroid 5 alpha-reductase deficiency in man: An inherited form of male pseudohermaphroditism. Science. 1974;186(4170):1213-5. Epub 1974/12/27.
19. Price P, Wass JA, Griffin JE, Leshin M, Savage MO, Large DM, et al. High dose androgen therapy in male pseudohermaphroditism due to 5 alpha-reductase deficiency and disorders of the androgen receptor. The Journal of Clinical Investigation. 1984;74(4):1496-508. Epub 1984/10/01.
20. Sinclair RD, Dawber RP. Androgenetic alopecia in men and women. Clinics in Dermatology. 2001;19(2):167-78. Epub 2001/06/09.
21. Messenger AG, Sinclair R. Follicular miniaturization in female pattern hair loss: Clinicopathological correlations. The British Journal of Dermatology. 2006;155(5):926-30. Epub 2006/10/13.
22. Rushton DH, Ramsay ID, Norris MJ, Gilkes JJ. Natural progression of male pattern baldness in young men. Clinical and Experimental Dermatology. 1991;16(3):188-92. Epub 1991/05/01.
23. Yazdabadi A, Magee J, Harrison S, Sinclair R. The Ludwig pattern of androgenetic alopecia is due to a hierarchy of androgen sensitivity within follicular units that leads to selective miniaturization and a reduction in the number of terminal hairs per follicular unit. The British Journal of Dermatology. 2008;159(6):1300-2. Epub 2008/09/18.
24. Yazdabadi A, Whiting D, Rufaut N, Sinclair R. Miniaturized hairs maintain contact with the arrector pili muscle in alopecia areata but not in androgenetic alopecia: A model for reversible miniaturization and potential for hair regrowth. International Journal of Trichology. 2012;4(3):154-7. Epub 2012/11/28.
25. Norwood OT. Incidence of female androgenetic alopecia (female pattern alopecia). Dermatologic surgery: Official Publication for American Society for Dermatologic Surgery [et al]. 2001;27(1):53-4. Epub 2001/03/07.
26. Rebora A, Guarrera M, Baldari M, Vecchio F. Distinguishing androgenetic alopecia from chronic telogen effluvium when associated in the same patient: A simple noninvasive method. Archives of Dermatology. 2005;141(10):1243-5. Epub 2005/10/19.
27. Dhurat R, Saraogi P. Hair evaluation methods: Merits and demerits. International Journal of Trichology. 2009;1(2):108-19. Epub 2009/07/01.
28. Ross EK, Vincenzi C, Tosti A. Videodermoscopy in the evaluation of hair and scalp disorders. Journal of the American Academy of Dermatology. 2006;55(5):799-806. Epub 2006/10/21.
29. Pierard GE, Pierard-Franchimont C, Marks R, Elsner P. EEMCO guidance for the assessment of hair shedding and alopecia. Skin Pharmacology and Physiology. 2004;17(2):98-110. Epub 2004/02/21.

30. Whiting DA. Diagnostic and predictive value of horizontal sections of scalp biopsy specimens in male pattern androgenetic alopecia. Journal of the American Academy of Dermatology. 1993;28(5 Pt 1):755-63. Epub 1993/05/01.
31. Dinh QQ, Sinclair R. Female pattern hair loss: Current treatment concepts. Clinical Interventions in Aging. 2007;2(2):189-99. Epub 2007/11/30.
32. Biondo S, Sinclair R. Quality of life in Australian women with female pattern hair loss. Open Dermatology Journal [Internet]. 2010 8/9/2013.
33. Cash TF. The psychological effects of androgenetic alopecia in men. Journal of the American Academy of Dermatology. 1992;26(6):926-31. Epub 1992/06/01.
34. Cash TF, Price VH, Savin RC. Psychological effects of androgenetic alopecia on women: Comparisons with balding men and with female control subjects. Journal of the American Academy of Dermatology. 1993;29(4):568-75. Epub 1993/10/01.
35. Cash TF. The psychology of hair loss and its implications for patient care. Clinics in Dermatology. 2001;19(2):161-6. Epub 2001/06/09.
36. Sinclair R, Patel M, Dawson TL, Jr Yazdabadi A, Yip L, Perez A, et al. Hair loss in women: Medical and Cosmetic approaches to increase scalp hair fullness. The British Journal of Dermatology. 2011;165 Suppl 3:12-8. Epub 2011/12/30.
37. Trueb RM. Possibilities and limitations for reversal of age-related hair loss in: Trueb RM, Tobin DJ, editors. Aging Hair. Berlin: Springer-Verlag. 2010;p.193-206.
38. Olsen EA, Weiner MS, Amara IA, DeLong ER. Five-year follow-up of men with androgenetic alopecia treated with topical minoxidil. Journal of the American Academy of Dermatology. 1990;22(4):643-6. Epub 1990/04/01.
39. Rietschel RL, Duncan SH. Safety and efficacy of topical minoxidil in the management of androgenetic alopecia. Journal of the American Academy of Dermatology. 1987;16(3 Pt 2):677-85. Epub 1987/03/01.
40. Lucky AW, Piacquadio DJ, Ditre CM, Dunlap F, Kantor I, Pandya AG, et al. A randomized, placebo-controlled trial of 5% and 2% topical minoxidil solutions in the treatment of female pattern hair loss. Journal of the American Academy of Dermatology. 2004;50(4):541-53. Epub 2004/03/23.
41. Olsen EA, Dunlap FE, Funicella T, Koperski JA, Swinehart JM, Tschen EH, et al. A randomized clinical trial of 5% topical minoxidil versus 2% topical minoxidil and placebo in the treatment of androgenetic alopecia in men. Journal of the American Academy of Dermatology. 2002;47(3):377-85. Epub 2002/08/28.
42. Dawber RP, Rundegren J. Hypertrichosis in females applying minoxidil topical solution and in normal controls. Journal of the European Academy of Dermatology and Venereology: JEADV. 2003;17(3):271-5. Epub 2003/04/19.
43. De Villez RL. Topical minoxidil therapy in hereditary androgenetic alopecia. Archives of Dermatology. 1985;121(2):197-202. Epub 1985/02/01.
44. Olsen EA, DeLong ER, Weiner MS. Long-term follow-up of men with male pattern baldness treated with topical minoxidil. Journal of the American Academy of Dermatology. 1987;16(3 Pt 2):688-95. Epub 1987/03/01.
45. Hoedemaker C, van Egmond S, Sinclair R. Treatment of female pattern hair loss with a combination of spironolactone and minoxidil. The Australasian Journal of Dermatology. 2007;48(1):43-5. Epub 2007/01/16.
46. Roberts JL, Fiedler V, Imperato-McGinley J, Whiting D, Olsen E, Shupack J, et al. Clinical dose ranging studies with finasteride, a type 2, 5alpha-reductase inhibitor, in men with male pattern hair loss. Journal of the American Academy of Dermatology. 1999;41(4):555-63. Epub 1999/09/25.
47. Drake L, Hordinsky M, Fiedler V, Swinehart J, Unger WP, Cotterill PC, et al. The effects of finasteride on scalp skin and serum androgen levels in men with androgenetic alopecia. Journal of the American Academy of Dermatology. 1999;41(4):550-4. Epub 1999/09/25.
48. Irwig MS. Depressive symptoms and suicidal thoughts among former users of finasteride with persistent sexual side effects. The Journal of Clinical Psychiatry. 2012;73(9):1220-3. Epub 2012/09/04.
49. Whiting DA, Waldstreicher J, Sanchez M, Kaufman KD. Measuring reversal of hair miniaturization in androgenetic alopecia by follicular counts in horizontal sections of serial scalp biopsies: Results of finasteride 1 mg treatment of men and postmenopausal women. The Journal of Investigative Dermatology Symposium Proceedings/the Society for Investigative Dermatology, Inc [and] European Society for Dermatological Research. 1999;4(3):282-4. Epub 2000/02/16.
50. Olsen EA, Hordinsky M, Whiting D, Stough D, Hobbs S, Ellis ML, et al. The importance of dual 5alpha-reductase inhibition in the treatment of male pattern hair loss: Results of a randomized placebo-controlled study of dutasteride versus finasteride. Journal of the American Academy of Dermatology. 2006;55(6):1014-23. Epub 2006/11/18.
51. Boyapati A, Sinclair R. Combination therapy with finasteride and low-dose dutasteride in the treatment of androgenetic alopecia. The Australasian Journal of Dermatology. 2013;54(1):49-51. Epub 2012/06/13.
52. DeVillez RL, Jacobs JP, Szpunar CA, Warner ML. Androgenetic alopecia in the female. Treatment with 2% topical minoxidil solution. Archives of Dermatology. 1994;130(3):303-7. Epub 1994/03/01.
53. Adamopoulos DA, Karamertzanis M, Nicopoulou S, Gregoriou A. Beneficial effect of spironolactone on androgenic alopecia. Clinical Endocrinology. 1997;47(6):759-60. Epub 1998/03/14.
54. Rathnayake D, Sinclair R. Innovative use of spironolactone as an antiandrogen in the treatment of female pattern hair loss. Dermatologic Clinics. 2010;28(3):611-8. Epub 2010/06/01.
55. Vexiau P, Chaspoux C, Boudou P, Fiet J, Jouanique C, Hardy N, et al. Effects of minoxidil 2% vs. cyproterone acetate treatment on female androgenetic alopecia: A controlled, 12-month randomized trial. The British Journal of Dermatology. 2002;146(6):992-9. Epub 2002/06/20.
56. Sinclair R, Wewerinke M, Jolley D. Treatment of female pattern hair loss with oral antiandrogens. The British Journal of Dermatology. 2005;152(3):466-73. Epub 2005/03/25.

57. Yeon JH, Jung JY, Choi JW, Kim BJ, Youn SW, Park KC, et al. 5 mg/day finasteride treatment for normoandrogenic Asian women with female pattern hair loss. Journal of the European Academy of Dermatology and Venereology (JEADV). 2011;25(2):211-4. Epub 2010/06/24.
58. Thai KE, Sinclair RD. Finasteride for female androgenetic alopecia. The British Journal of Dermatology. 2002;147(4):812-3. Epub 2002/10/09.
59. Grigoriou O, Papadias C, Konidaris S, Antoniou G, Karakitsos P, Giannikos L. Comparison of flutamide and cyproterone acetate in the treatment of hirsutism: A randomized controlled trial. Gynecological endocrinology: The Official Journal of the International Society of Gynecological Endocrinology. 1996;10(2):119-23. Epub 1996/04/01.
60. Cusan L, Dupont A, Gomez JL. Comparison of flutamide and spironolactone in the treatment of hirstism: A randomized controlled trial. Fertil Steril. 1995;63:680.
61. Yazdabadi A, Sinclair R. Treatment of female pattern hair loss with the androgen receptor antagonist flutamide. The Australasian Journal of Dermatology. 2011;52(2):132-4. Epub 2011/05/25.
62. Paradisi R, Porcu E, Fabbri R, Seracchioli R, Battaglia C, Venturoli S. Prospective cohort study on the effects and tolerability of flutamide in patients with female pattern hair loss. The Annals of Pharmacotherapy. 2011;45(4):469-75. Epub 2011/04/14.
63. Piérard-Franchimont C, De Doncker P, Cauwenbergh G, Piérard GE. Ketoconazole shampoo: Effect of long-term use in androgenic alopecia. Dermatology. 1998;196(4):474-7.
64. Unger WP, Unger RH. Hair transplanting: An important but often forgotten treatment for female pattern hair loss. Journal of the American Academy of Dermatology. 2003;49(5):853-60. Epub 2003/10/25.

12

Hair Loss in Women

Ralph M Trüeb

"A hair in the head is worth two in the brush."

—*Oliver Herford*

Few dermatologic complaints carry as much emotional overtones as hair loss, and in some cases they seem disproportionate to the extent of hair loss, especially in the adult female patient presenting with hair loss. Adding to the patient's worry may be prior negative experiences with physicians, who tend to trivialize complaints of hair loss. This attitude on the part of physicians may result from lack of familiarity with the management of hair loss, thereby making them feel uncomfortable dealing with such patients. However, comprehension of the main types of hair loss and their causes is prerequisite to meeting patients' expectations and providing appropriate patient management. The best way to alleviate the anxiety is to effectively treat the underlying problem. Therefore, it is paramount to address the symptom systematically. In addition to its psychological impact, hair loss may be a manifestation of a more general medical problem. The diagnosis can be established with a detailed patient history focussing on chronology of events, examination of the scalp and pattern of hair loss, a pull test with examination of bulbs of shed hairs, trichoscopy, and few pertinent screening blood tests. In selected cases a scalp biopsy may be required. The most frequent cause of hair loss in women is female androgenetic alopecia, important differential diagnoses include acute and chronic telogen effluvium, and diffuse alopecia areata. Occasionally, patients seeking advice are not necessarily losing hair. In the absence of convincing evidence of hair loss, they are suffering of imaginary hair loss or psychogenic pseudoeffluvium, and thought should be given to an underlying psychological disorder. Once the diagnosis is established, treatment appropriate for that diagnosis is likely to control the hair loss. Finally, appropriate psychological support and education about the basics of the hair cycle, and why considerable patience is required for effective cosmetic recovery, are essential to help limit patient anxiety.

Pathologic Dynamics of Hair Loss

In 1932, Sabouraud originally coined the term "defluvium capillorum" to characterize a sudden type of diffuse hair loss following shortly after a severe emotional shock, while others later applied it to all forms of alopecia. In the late 1950's, Sulzberger differentiated a chronic type of diffuse alopecia in women from acute and reversible hair loss that is attributable to a readily identifiable cause. However, a majority of these patients later turned out to be women with female androgenetic alopecia or diffuse hair loss of unexplored etiology, such as thyroid dysfunction, or malnutrition. In 1960, Guy and Edmundson described a form of "diffuse cyclic hair loss in women" in which no specific trigger was evident. Whatever the cause, the follicle tends to behave in a similar way. To grasp the meaning of this generalization, requires understanding of the hair cycle and its derangements.

The hair follicle is subject to constant turnover in the course of perpetual cycles through phases of proliferation (anagen), involution (catagen), and resting (telogen), with regeneration in the successive hair cycle: It is a major characteristic of *anagen* that not only the hair shaft is growing but that most epithelial hair follicle compartments undergo proliferation, with the hair matrix keratinocytes showing the highest proliferative activity. During *catagen*, hair follicles enter a process of involution that is characterized by a burst of programmed cell death (apoptosis) in the majority of follicular keratinocytes. The resulting shortening of the regressing epithelial strand is associated with an upwards movement of the follicle. In *telogen*, the hair shaft matures into a club hair, which is held tightly in the bulbous base of the follicular epithelium, before it is eventually shed. It is still unresolved whether shedding of the telogen hair (teloptosis) is an active, regulated process or represents a passive event that occurs at the onset of subsequent anagen, as the new hair grows in.

Cyclic hair growth activity occurs in a random mosaic pattern with each follicle possessing its own individual control mechanism over the evolution and triggering of the successive phases, though systemic factors, such as the hormonal system, cytokines and growth factors, as well as external factors linked to the environment, such as toxins, and deficiencies of nutrient, vitamins and energy, have influence.

Finally, there are considerable variations in length of these phases depending on the body site location, with the duration of anagen determining the type of hair produced, particularly its length. On the scalp, hairs remain in anagen for a 2- to 6-year period of time, whereas that of telogen is approximately 100 days, resulting in a ratio of anagen to telogen hairs of 9:1. On average, the amount of new scalp hair formation matches the amount that is shed, thereby maintaining a consistent covering. With a range of 75,000 to 150,000 hairs on the head, the reported average daily telogen hair shedding varies from 35 to 180 hairs. In general, the anagen phase is longer in women than in men.

Many factors can lead to pathologically increased hair loss. Disease states that cause hair loss are categorized according to whether the hair loss is diffuse or localized, and to whether the follicle remains intact or is destroyed and replaced by scar. Except for the scarring alopecias, hair loss represents a disorder of hair follicle cycling.

Dystrophic anagen effluvium is hair loss that results from the shedding of large numbers of hairs from the anagen phase of growth. The common pathogenesis which unites the different etiologies of dystrophic anagen effluvium is a direct insult to the rapidly dividing bulb matrix cells. They stop the reproduction of matrix cells, but evidently mitotic inhibition alone is not sufficient to force the follicle into catagen, but merely causes it to suspend operations. The abrupt cessation of mitotic activity leads to the weakening of the partially keratinized, proximal portion of the hair shaft, its narrowing and subsequent breakage within the hair canal and shedding. The morphological consequence is the dystrophic anagen hair with a tapered proximal end and lack of root sheath.

Telogen effluvium is hair loss that results from the increased shedding of hairs from the telogen phase of growth. In 1961 Kligman revealed the pathodynamics of one common pattern of response of hair follicles to a variety of insults and named it telogen effluvium. On the basis of changes in different phases of the follicular cycle, Headington later proposed classification of telogen effluvium into five functional types based on changes in different phases of the hair cycle:

In *immediate anagen release*, follicles that would normally complete a longer cycle by remaining in anagen prematurely enter telogen. It is a very common form of telogen effluvium, typically occurring after periods of physiologic stress including episodes of high fever. In fever, the pyrogens, basically circulating cytokines, drive the hair follicle keratinocytes into apoptosis initiating catagen with following telogen. Because the shedding is dependent on transition from anagen through catagen and telogen with subsequent release of telogen hairs, hair loss occurs 3 to 4 months after the inciting event.

In *delayed anagen release*, hair follicles remain in prolonged anagen rather than cycling into telogen. When finally released from anagen, the clinical sign of increased shedding of telogen hair will be found. This type of telogen effluvium underlies postpartum hair loss.

In *immediate telogen release*, hair follicles normally programmed for release of the club hair after an interval of usually 100 days after the end of anagen, are prematurely stimulated to cycle into anagen. There is premature teloptosis. This type of telogen effluvium underlies the shedding of hair upon initiation of therapy with topical minoxidil (shedding phase).

In *delayed telogen release*, hair follicles remain in prolonged telogen rather than being shed and recycling into anagen. When finally teloptosis sets in, again the clinical sign of increased shedding of club hairs is observed. This process underlies moulting in mammals and possibly mild telogen effluvia following travel from low-daylight to high-daylight conditions.

Finally, a *short anagen phase* (without synchronization) results in a slight but persistent telogen effluvium in association with decreased hair length. This may occur as an isolated disorder in otherwise healthy children (short anagen syndrome), far more frequent is acquired progressive shortening of anagen due to androgenetic alopecia.

Etiologies and Clinical Presentations

A simple office technique for evaluation of hair loss is to pull gently on the patient's hair (hair pull test). Normally, one can come away with up to five hairs, but with pathologic hair loss this number is increased (positive hair pull). In diffuse hair loss the hair pull test is positive in both the vertex area and margins of the scalp. Diffuse hair loss is further classified by the types of hairs that are shed, in particular whether they are anagen hairs (anagen effluvium) or telogen hairs (telogen effluvium).

Dystrophic Anagen Effluvium

Causes for dystrophic anagen effluvium are antineoplastic drugs (chemotherapy-induced alopecia), radiation (radiation-induced alopecia), environmental or occupational exposure to toxins (toxic alopecia), and alopecia areata.

Chemotherapy-induced alopecia is understood to be the consequence of a direct toxic insult to the rapidly dividing bulb matrix cells of the hair follicle during anagen. The consequence is hair shedding, that usually begins at 1–3 weeks and is complete at 1–2 months after initiation of chemotherapy. Since normally up to 90% of scalp hair is in anagen, hair loss is usually copious and the resulting alopecia is quite obvious.

The incidence and severity of the hair loss are variable and related to the particular chemotherapeutic protocol. Multiple classes of anticancer drugs induce alopecia with frequencies of chemotherapy-induced alopecia differing for the four major drug classes: over 80% for antimicrotubule agents, e.g. paclitaxel, 60–100% for topoisomerase inhibitors, e.g. doxorubicin, over 60% for alkylators, e.g. cyclophosphamide, and 10–50% for antimetabolites, e.g. 5-fluorouracil plus leucovorin. Combination therapy consisting of two or more agents usually produces higher incidences of a more severe chemotherapy-induced alopecia compared to single agent therapy.

Chemotherapy-induced alopecia is usually reversible with hair regrowth typically occurring after a delay of 3–6 months. In a number of patients, the regrown hair shows changes in color and/or structure and texture. In some cases, the hair growth may remain reduced. Ultimately, permanent alopecia following chemotherapy with busulphan after bone marrow transplantation has been reported: risk factors include chronic graft-versus-host reaction, prior exposure to X-ray, and older age of patients. More recently, permanent scalp alopecia related to breast cancer chemotherapy by sequential fluorouracil/epirubicin/cyclophosphamide (FEC) and docetaxel has been reported. Often the alopecia is sustained through subsequent long-term treatment with aromatose inhibitors in women with pre-existing female androgenetic alopecia (**Figure 12.1**).

Radiation-induced alopecia may either be reversible or permanent. Radiation-induced temporary epilation may be observed following neuroradiologically guided embolization procedures. Permanent alopecia occurs with > 30 Gy of deep X-rays, or > 50 Gy of soft X-rays.

Toxic alopecia from occupational exposure to hazardous chemicals has decreased over the years due to more stringent government regulations. More recently, interest has focussed on mild aggressions from toxic metals of the environment. Many heavy metals are capable of disrupting the formation of the hair shaft through covalent binding with the sulfhydryl groups in keratin: thallium, mercury, arsenic, copper, cadmium and bismuth. A study conducted 1979 in Belgium reported diffuse alopecia related to ingestion of toxic metals in 36 of 78 patients with diffuse alopecia. Toxic metals in abnormal amount in blood and urine were observed only when >10% of hair bulbs were dystrophic. Copper was involved in 17 alopecias, arsenic in 12, mercury in five, and cadmium in two. Copper intoxication was found to be related to ingestion of tap water containing a high concentration of copper salts, presumably from low pH, presence of chelating agents, or connection of electrical ground wires to copper water pipes, which caused sufficient flow of electrical current to ionize the metal.

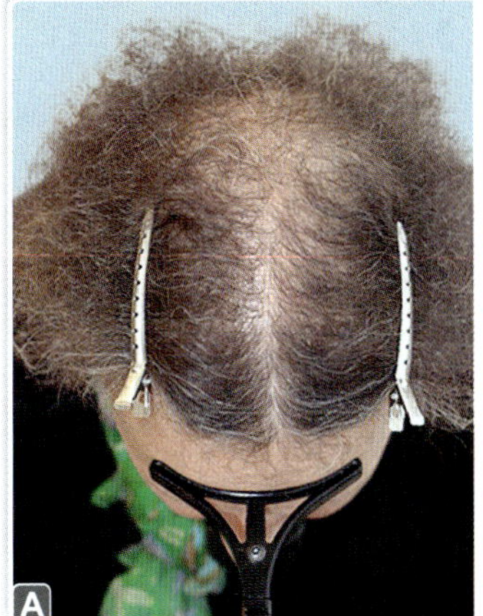

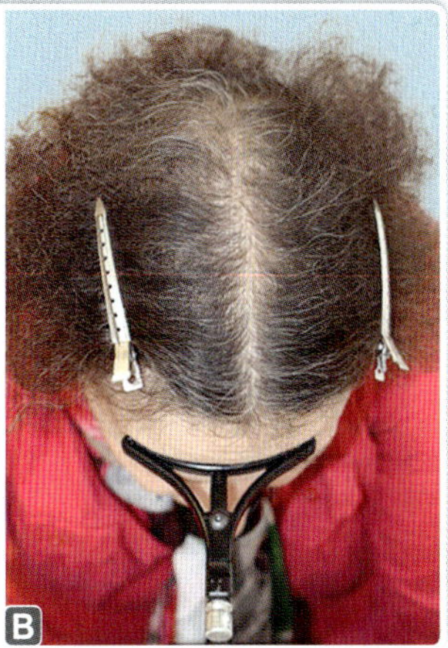

Figs 12.1A and B: Postchemotherapy alopecia combined with female androgenetic alopecia under aromatase inhibition. Successful treatment of alopecia with 5% topical minoxidil

Adverse effects related to dental amalgam, including hair loss, have also been the subject of recent attention. In one study, mercury levels in blood and urine correlated with the number of amalgam surfaces, indicating the release of mercury from dental amalgam restorations. Since the mercury levels were far below those where negative health effects would be expected and were similar in patients with complaints self-related to dental amalgam restorations and healthy control individuals, mercury was not found to be a likely cause of the impaired health reported by the patients. In another study, assays of mercury in urine samples of patients with "amalgam illness" indicated that the exposure was far below the levels at which symptoms could be indicated by psychometric tests. Psychologic investigation indicated that the symptoms were psychosomatic. All patients had experienced important psychic trauma in close correlation with the first appearance of symptoms.

Alopecia areata probably represents the most frequent cause of anagen dystrophic effluvium, either localized

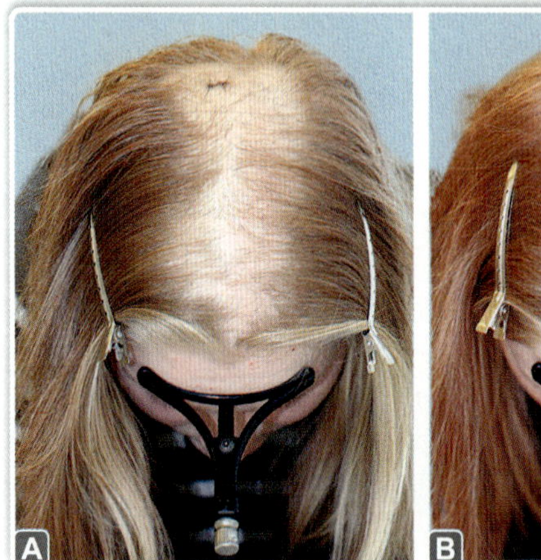

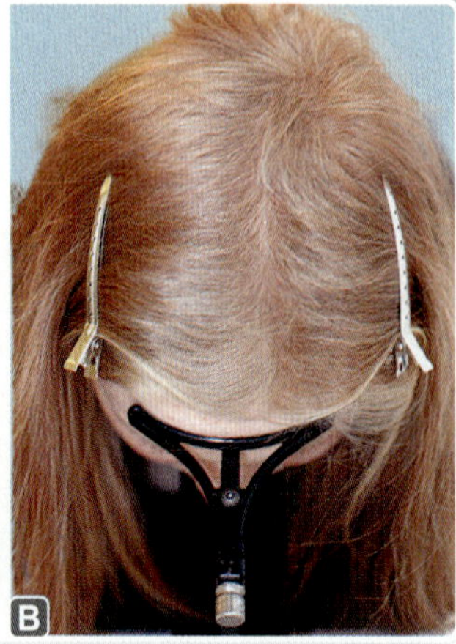

Figs 12.2A and B: Diffuse alopecia areata of female androgenetic type (pattern alopecia areata). Successful treatment with intravenous methylprednisolone pulse therapy within first 6 months of hair loss and topical 5% minoxidil

or diffuse, occurring in the otherwise healthy child or adult. Alopecia areata is regarded to be an organ-specific autoimmune disease, with the hair follicle being the target of autoimmunity. The cytokines generated by a peribulbar lymphocytic infiltrate cause apoptosis of the hair follicle keratinocytes. In its diffuse and patterned variant it may pose differential diagnostic problems to diffuse alopecia and female androgenetic alopecia, respectively (**Figure 12.2**).

Telogen Effluvium

Most patients with hair loss seen in clinical practice present with telogen effluvium. As telogen hairs have a depigmented bulb, examination of shed or pulled hairs with the naked eye will usually clarify this.

Acute telogen effluvium presents as a diffuse, non-patterned hair loss from the scalp that occurs around 3 months after a triggering event, and is usually self-limiting within 6 months by definition. Severe febrile illness, childbirth, accidental trauma or surgical operations with a large hemorrhage, a crash diet, or severe emotional distress are among the most common causes. Hair loss is usually <50% of scalp hair. The diffuse hair loss from the scalp may produce thinning of hair all over the scalp, but frequently manifests with bitemporal hair thinning. Reassuring patients that they are not going bald, and that the telogen effluvium is temporary is usually sufficient.

The literature on the subject of *psychogenic hair loss* has been more confounding than helpful. The presence of emotional stress is not indisputable proof of its having incited the patient's hair loss. The relationship may also be the inverse. Nevertheless, recent studies suggest that women who experience high stress are more likely to experience hair loss. Moreover, in a murine model, experimental stress has been shown to inhibit hair growth, indicating the existence of a brain-hair follicle axis.

Chronic telogen effluvium has been defined as diffuse telogen hair loss that persisits > 6 months. In Kligman's original description, telogen effluvium is an acute and diffuse hair loss brought about by a variety of triggers. Clinical experience, however, suggests that chronic telogen effluvium also exists. Diffuse shedding of telogen hairs that persists >6 months either represents a primary disorder and is then a diagnosis of exclusion, or it is secondary to a variety of systemic disorders: iron deficiency, other dietary deficiencies (protein-calorie malnutrition, zinc deficiency), thyroid disease, other metabolic diseases (chronic renal or liver failure, advanced malignancy, pancreatic disease and upper gastrointestinal disorder with malabsorption), systemic lupus erythematosus, other connective tissue disorders (dermatomyositis), HIV infection, and drug-induced telogen hair loss.

Apart from iron deficiency as cause of diffuse hair loss, all others are less common, though the literature concerning iron deficiency remains controversial. Rushton has reported iron deficiency in a majority of women presenting with diffuse hair loss, but this probably has been overestimated, since more recent data suggest that in most women with chronic telogen effluvium, no direct relationship between serum ferritin levels within the lower normal range and hair loss exists.

While chronic telogen effluvium may be triggered by an acute telogen effluvium, in *primary chronic telogen effluvium* no specific trigger is evident. It predominantly affects women, while men with short hair tend not to notice increased hair shedding. The presentation of this type of diffuse hair loss tends to be distinctive, and was first described in detail by Guy and Edmundson as "diffuse cyclic hair loss in women", and revived by Whiting in 1996, who additionally characterized the histopathologic features.

The typical patient with primary chronic telogen effluvium is a vigorous otherwise healthy woman between 30 and 60 with a full, thick head of hair. On examination there is some bitemporal recession and a positive hair pull test equally over the vertex and occiput. There is no widening of the central part, as is common in androgenetic alopecia. Nevertheless, patients are adamant that they previously had more hair and are distressed by the prospect of going bald. Many frequently bring large balls of hair for inspection, but despite this do not show any obvious balding. The condition tends to run a fluctuating course, in the long run the disorder appears to be self-limiting. It has been proposed that this disorder may be due to synchronization phenomena of the hair cycle, shortening of the anagen phase, or premature teloptosis.

It is important to reassure patients with primary chronic telogen effluvium that this condition represents exaggerated shedding rather than actual hair loss. As often happens in skin diseases in women, guilt feelings about cosmetics come out. Shampoos and hair colorants are blamed. While absence of effects of shampoos on hair loss rates has been demonstrated, telogen effluvium after allergic contact dermatitis of the scalp has been reported.

Androgenetic Alopecia

Androgenetic alopecia, also referred to as male-pattern hair loss or common baldness in men, and as female-pattern hair loss in women, affects at least 50% of men by the age of 50 years, and up to 70% of all males in later life. Estimates of its prevalence in women have varied widely, though recent studies claim that six percent of women aged under 50 years are affected, increasing to a proportion of 30–40% of women aged 70 years and over.

The hair loss is heritable, androgen-dependent, and occurs in a defined pattern. It is assumed that the genetically predisposed hair follicles are the target for androgen-stimulated hair follicle miniaturization, leading to gradual replacement of large, pigmented hairs (terminal hairs) by barely visible, depigmented hairs (vellus hairs) in affected areas. The result is a progressive decline in visible scalp hair density.

Androgenetic alopecia is characterized by progressive shortening of the duration of anagen with successive hair cycles, leading to decreased numbers of hair in anagen at any given time, and progressive follicular miniaturization with conversion of terminal to vellus-like follicles. The result is increased shedding of short-lived telogen hairs (telogen effluvium), while the affected hair follicles produce shorter, finer hairs that cover the scalp poorly.

While male pattern hair loss is characterized by its typical bitemporal recession of hair and balding vertex, female pattern hair loss is set apart by its rather diffuse thinning of the crown and a usually intact frontal hairline (**Figure 12.3**).

Recent literature suggests that patterned hair loss may have different mechanisms in men and in women. Because the androgen dependence of hair loss in all women with this type of alopecia has not been sufficiently demonstrated, and it has been observed in the absence of circulating androgens, the term female pattern hair loss has been proposed to replace androgenetic alopecia when applied in women. Nevertheless, female pattern hair loss shares with androgenetic alopecia the histolopathologic feature of hair follicle miniaturization: A terminal to vellus ratio of < 4:1 on a horizontally sectioned 4 mm scalp biopsy is diagnostic of androgenetic alopecia, while a ratio > 7:1 suggests chronic telogen effluvium (**Box 12.1**).

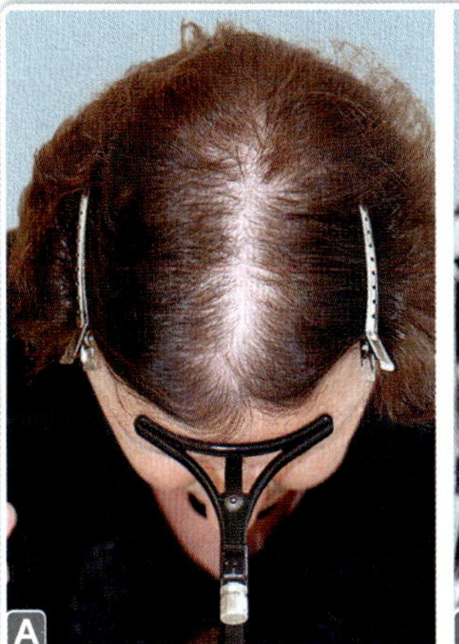

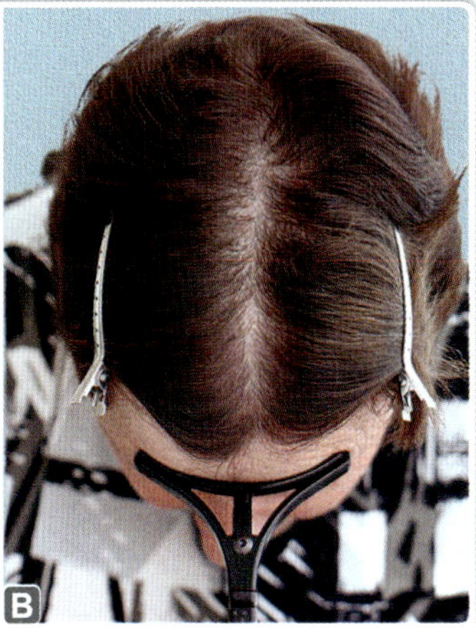

Figs 12.3A and B: Female androgenetic alopecia. Successful treatment with 5% topical minoxidil

Box 12.1: Histopathology of AGA and FPHL

A terminal to vellus ratio of <4:1 is diagnostic of androgenetic alopecia, while a ratio >7:1 suggests chronic telogen effluvium.

From a clinical point of view, male pattern hair loss with its characteristic bitemporal recession of hair and balding vertex has been set apart from female pattern hair loss with a rather diffuse thinning of the crown and intact frontal hairline, as originally characterized by Ludwig. While affected men predominantly present with the male pattern, the female pattern is more characteristic for women. Nevertheless, considerable overlap exists, the reason for which alternative classification schemes to the Hamilton-Norwood scale for male pattern alopecia and the Ludwig scale for female pattern alopecia have been proposed. Moreover, Venning and Dawber have found that 13% of premenopausal women and 37% of postmenopausal women present with the male pattern of androgenetic alopecia (**Figure 12.4**).

Again, there are further clinical subtypes of female androgenetic alopecia depending on the scalp area involved. Besides the classical Ludwig type with diffuse thinning of the centroparietal scalp and intact frontal hair line (female pattern hair loss), there is the Olsen type with frontal thinning in the form of a Christmas tree with its base at the frontal hairline (Christmas tree pattern), a more diffuse thinning of the hair, first described by Sulzberger and further characterized by Rushton as diffuse androgen-dependent alopecia in women (Sulzberger or Rushton type), and a type localized to the vertex, or "widow's cap" alopecia, with tendency to affect the older age group.

Androgenetic alopecia that is clinically manifest between the ages of 10 and 20 is called premature alopecia or alopecia praecox. In children before puberty it presents in both females and males exclusively with the female pattern (**Box 12.2**).

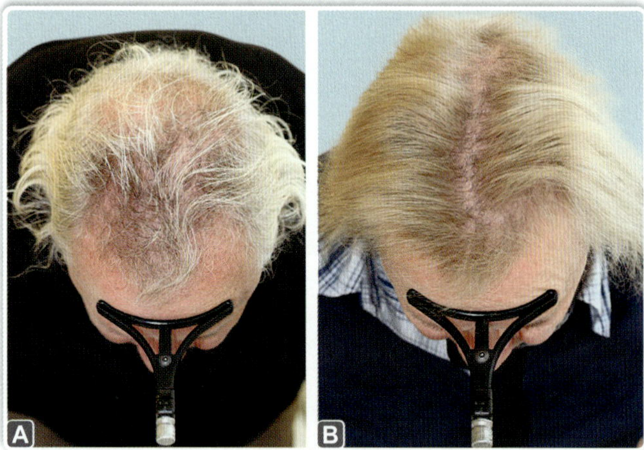

Figs 12.4A and B: Male pattern androgenetic alopecia in a postmenopausal woman. Successful treatment with a combination therapy of 5 mg oral finasteride with 5% topical minoxidil

Box 12.2: Alopecia praecox

Androgenetic alopecia that is clinically manifest between the ages of 10 and 20

Postpartum Hair Loss

During the second half of pregnancy, the percentage of anagen hairs increases from the normal 85% to 95%, at this time also the percentage of hairs of large shaft diameter is higher than in non-pregnant women of the same age. After partuition the follicles, in which anagen has been prolonged, rapidly enter catagen and then telogen, with an increased shedding of hair evident after 3–4 months (postpartum effluvium). Most women will return to their usual hair growth cycle between 6 and 12 months after birth. Postpartum hair loss usually returns the hair to pre-pregnancy thickness, unless it leads over to female androgenetic alopecia.

In case of persistent postpartum effluvium (> 12 months), excessive hair loss may be caused by common conditions, such as female androgenetic alopecia, iron deficiency, or hypothyroidism. Lesser common conditions include persistent hyperprolactinemia (Chiari-Frommel syndrome) and postpartum hypopituitarism (Sheehan syndrome) caused by pituitary necrosis due to blood loss and hypovolemic shock during childbirth.

Menopause

Menopause is based on the cessation of hormone production by the ovaries, in this case of the hormones which make reproduction possible and may influence sexual behavior. The resultant decreased levels of circulating estrogen impacts the entire cascade of a woman's reproductive functioning, from brain to skin. Estrogens clearly have an important function in many components of human skin including the epidermis, dermis, vasculature, hair follicle, sebaceous, eccrine and apocrine glands, having significant roles in skin aging, pigmentation, hair growth, and sebum production.

The typical age range for the occurrence of menopause is between the age of 45 and 55. The average age of menopause varies according to geographic location. In the Western world, the average age of menopause is 51 years, in some developing countries, such as India and the Philippines, the median age of natural menopause is earlier, at 44 years.

Dermatologic problems postmenopausal women encounter include: atrophy, dryness, pruritus, loss of resilience and pliability, easily traumatized skin, dry hair, and alopecia. Post-menopausal women show an increased tendency towards male pattern hair loss. Those effects are currently understood to be due to low estrogen levels.

Senescent Alopecia

Senile involutional or senescent alopecia has been defined as non-androgen-dependent hair thinning found in those over 60 years of age. Much like androgenetic alopecia, it involves a progressive decrease in the number of anagen follicles and hair diameter. It frequently occurs together with androgenetic alopecia, further complicating its delineation from the latter.

In their study on aging and hair cycles over an exceptionally long duration of 8 to 14 years, Courtois, et al. found a reduction in the duration of hair growth and in the diameter of hair shafts, and a prolongation of the interval separating the loss of a hair in telogen and the emergence of a replacement hair in anagen (latency phase). These phenomena resemble those observed in the course of androgenetic alopecia, although their development is less marked, suggesting androgenetic alopecia a premature aging phenomenon. This aging process was evidenced by a reduction in the number of hairs per unit area and deterioration in the quality of scalp hair. The reduction in density was manifested to different degrees in different individuals. It amounted to less than 10% in 10 years in the individuals with the least alopecia, and was much more pronounced in the balding subjects. The maximal length of hair diminished as the subjects aged, in parallel the hairs became finer. However, among non-balding subjects, there was a tendency for the proportion of thicker hairs to increase. Finally, aging did not appear to follow a perfectly regular course over time. Periods of stability, or even partial remission, alternated with periods of more marked evolution, reflecting perhaps the influence of individual factors such as the subject's general health, lifestyle, and risk factors for accelerated aging.

Recent data comparing androgenetic alopecia and senescent alopecia using microarray analysis have demonstrated significant differences in the gene expression patterns suggesting they represent different entities. In androgenetic alopecia, genes required for anagen onset (Wnt-beta-catenin, TGF-alpha, TGF-beta, Stat-3, Stat-1), epithelial signal to dermal papilla (PPARd, IGF-1), hair shaft differentiation (Notch, Msx2, KRTs, KAPs), and anagen maintenance (Msx2, Activin, IGF-1) were downregulated, and genes for catagen (BDNF, BMP2, BMP7, VDR, IL-1, ER) and telogen induction and maintenance (VDR, RAR) were upregulated. In senescent alopecia, genes involved in epithelial signal to dermal papilla (FGF5), actin cytoskeleton (DST, ACTN2, TNNI3, PARVB) and mitochondrial function (JAK2, PRKD3, AK2, TRAP1, TRIO, ATP12A, MLL4, STK22B) were downregulated, while oxidative stress and inflammatory response genes were upregulated.

Experimental evidence supports the hypothesis that oxidative stress plays a major role in the aging process. As early as 1956, Harman, et al. first proposed this "free radical theory of aging". Today it is one of the most widely accepted theories used to explain mechanisms underlying the aging process. Free radicals are highly reactive molecules with unpaired electrons that can directly damage various cellular structural membranes, lipids, proteins, and DNA. The damaging effects of these reactive oxygen species are induced internally during normal metabolism and externally through exposure to various oxidative stresses from the environment. The body possesses endogenous defense mechanisms, such as anti-oxidative enzymes (superoxide dismutase, catalase, glutathione peroxidase) and non-enzymatic anti-oxidative molecules (vitamin E, vitamin C, glutathione, ubiquinone), protecting it from free radicals by reducing and neutralizing them. With age, the production of free radicals increases, while the endogenous defence mechanisms decrease. This imbalance leads to the progressive damage of cellular structures, presumably resulting in the aging phenotype.

Ultimately, studies have also focused on the role of oxidative stress for the evolution of androgenetic alopecia. Naito, et al. analyzed the effect of the lipid peroxides on hair follicles, and observed that the topical application of linolein hydroperoxides, one of the lipid peroxides, lead to the early onset of the catagen phase in murine hair cycles. Furthermore, they found that lipid peroxides induced apoptosis of hair follicle cells. They also induced apoptosis in human epidermal keratinocytes by up-regulating apoptosis-related genes. These results indicate that lipid peroxides, which can cause free radicals, induce the apoptosis of hair follicle cells, and this is followed by early onset of the catagen phase.

Bahta, et al. cultured dermal hair papilla cells (DPC) from balding and non-balding scalp and demonstrated that balding DPCs grow slower in vitro than non-balding DPCs. Loss of proliferative capacity of balding DPCs was associated with changes in cell morphology, expression of senescence-associated beta-galactosidase, decreased expression of proliferating cell nuclear antigen and Bmi-1, upregulation of p16 (INK4a)/pRb and nuclear expression of markers of oxidative stress and DNA damage including heat shock protein-27, super oxide dismutase catalase, ataxia-telangiectasia-mutated kinase (ATM), and ATM- and Rad3-related protein. The finding of premature senescence of balding DPC in vitro in association with expression of p16 (INK4a)/pRB suggests that balding DPCs are particularly sensitive to environmental stress.

Seasonality of Hair Growth and Shedding

A number of otherwise healthy women with or without clinical alopecia complain of recurrent hair loss, despite at times successful therapy. To test the hypothesis that periodicity in shedding of hair reflects seasonal changes in human hair growth, we performed a retrospective study of 823 otherwise healthy women with telogen effluvium during a period of 6 years, and demonstrated the existence of overall annual periodicity in the growth and shedding of hair, manifested by a maximal proportion of telogen hairs in July. Taking a telogen phase duration of approximately 100 days into account, one would expect shedding of these hairs by autumn. A second peak seems to exist, although less pronounced, in April. The telogen rate was lowest towards the beginning of February.

The cyclical activities of the hair follicle is the mechanism by which mammals change their coat of hair to meet the exigencies of growth, seasonal changes in the ambient environment and, perhaps, normal wear and tear. It seems likely that environmental factors, such as the photoperiod, mediate through the optic pathway and the neuroendocrine system coat phenotype and function to photoperiod-dependent environmental changes. The fact that human hair follicles, just as those of other mammals, undergo cyclical activity and are influenced by hormones, implies that human hair is not unaffected by these phenomena. From an evolutionary point of view, the maintenance of the low winter level of hair shedding and the postponement of hair fall until the end of summer might, perhaps, be postulated as having a selective advantage with respect to isolation of the head against the cold in winter, and protection of the scalp against the midday sun in summer, respectively.

Most importantly, the existence of seasonal fluctuations in hair growth and shedding complicates the assessment of pharmacological effects. Awareness of these fluctuations is prerequisite to providing the correct cause and prognosis to the patient, ensuring patient compliance with therapy, but also has potentially serious implications for investigations with new hair growth promoting agents. Depending on the stage of periodicity in growth and shedding of hair for a particular subject, the heterogenicity of included subjects may be enough to distort the clinical efficacy results and the perceived benefit of an investigational agent. In the active stage of seasonal telogen effluvium, the involved hair follicles would probably fail to respond to the therapeutic agent, which may cause a false-negative result. In the recovery stage, the increased amounts of spontaneously regrowing hair might be interpreted falsely as a positive result.

Inflammatory Phenomena and Scarring

The limited success rate of treatment of androgenetic alopecia with minoxidil and finasteride means that further pathogenic pathways may be taken into account. On histologic examination of scalp biopsies, the miniaturization of terminal hairs is frequently associated with perifollicular lymphocytic infiltration, and eventually fibrosis. Therefore it is conceivable that the role of this microscopic follicular inflammation causing fibrosis below the shortened balding follicle has been underestimated, though it seems likely that this would prevent the follicle to reform a terminal hair follicle.

The implication of microscopic follicular inflammation in the pathogenesis of androgenetic alopecia has emerged from several independent studies. An early study referred to an inflammatory infiltrate of activated T cells and macrophages in the upper third of the hair follicles, associated with an enlargement of the follicular dermal sheath composed of collagen bundles (perifollicular fibrosis), in regions of actively progressing alopecia. Horizontal section studies of scalp biopsies indicated that the perifollicular fibrosis is generally mild, consisting of loose, concentric layers of collagen that must be distinguished from cicatricial alopecia. Bernard, et al. proposed the term follicular microinflammation, because the process involves a slow, subtle, and indolent course, in contrast to the inflammatory and destructive process in the classical inflammatory scarring alopecias.

The significance of follicular microinflammation and fibrosis in androgenetic alopecia remains controversial. However, morphometric studies in male patients with androgenetic alopecia treated with topical minoxidil showed that 55% of those with microinflammation had regrowth in response to treatment, in comparison to 77% in those patients without inflammation and fibrosis.

Postmenopausal Frontal Fibrosing Alopecia

Postmenopausal frontal fibrosing alopecia represents a peculiar condition predominantly, but not exclusively affecting women in postmenopause. Originally reported by Kossard, postmenopausal frontal fibrosing alopecia presents with a symmetric, marginal alopecia along the frontal and frontal-temporal hairline, often with concomitant thinning or complete loss of the eyebrows. Affected women typically present with the complaint of asymptomatic, progressive recession of their frontal hairline. The affected scalp skin is pale and smooth with loss of follicular orifices, often perifollicular erythema and follicular keratinization is observed marking the underlying inflammatory process. Histopathologic examination of affected scalp shows a reduced number of hair follicles, which have been replaced by fibrous tracts, and a perifollicular, lymphocytic, lichenoid infiltrate that is typical of lichen planopilaris. Since Kossard's original description in 1994 the number of cases of postmenopausal frontal fibrosing alopecia has exploded exponentially worldwide, while its etiology remains obscure. Hormone replacement therapy does not appear to alter the course and progression of this condition.

Fibrosing Alopecia in a Pattern Distribution

Alopecia in a pattern distribution is a common event associated with androgenetic hair loss and aging. Although it is regarded as a pathologic process by some physicians and many affected patients, by others it is considered a genetically determined physiologic event in the lives of most men and women. The same controversy applies to the histological finding of inflammatory cells in the vicinity of the upper hair follicle in androgenetic alopecia in as much as it remains uncertain whether this phenomenon is still a physiologic event or already reflects a pathologic process. Clinically, androgenetic alopecia is usually a noninflammatory and nonscarring process that eventually leads to permanent hair loss of the affected scalp.

In our original description of fibrosing alopecia in a pattern distribution, patients displayed progressive scarring alopecia in a pattern distribution (**Figure 12.5**). Close clinical examination reveals obliteration of follicular orifices, perifollicular erythema, and follicular keratosis limited to the area of androgenetic hair loss. Histological findings of androgenetic alopecia, i.e. increased numbers of miniaturized hair follicles with underlying fibrous streamers, are evident in the majority of patients and associated with a perifollicular lymphocytic infiltrate. A pattern of follicular interface dermatitis targeting

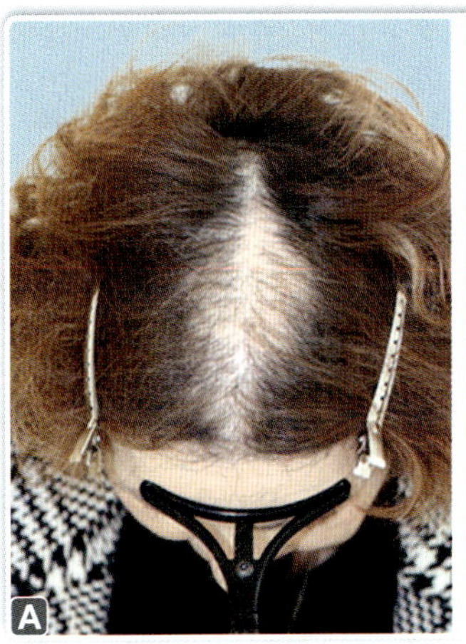

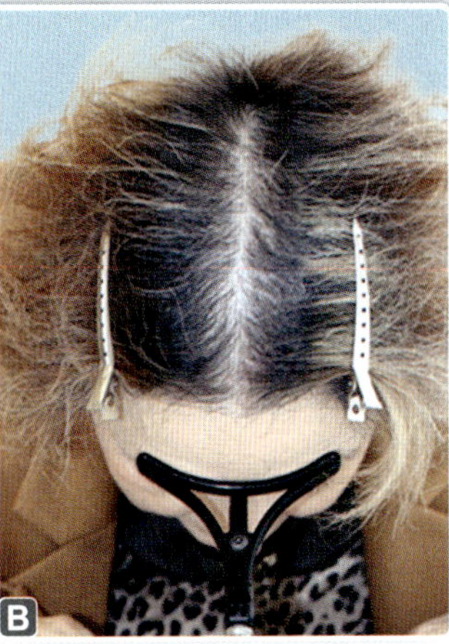

Figs 12.5A and B: Fibrosing alopecia in a pattern distribution. Successful treatment with compound of 5% topical minoxidil and 0.2% trimacinolone acetonide and autologous hair transplantation

the upper follicle is found in early lesions, whereas perifollicular lamellar fibrosis and the presence of selectively fibrosed follicular tracts characterize late lesions.

The pattern distribution and histological findings share features with Kossard's postmenopausal frontal fibrosing alopecia. The clinical presentation in these women might mimic male pattern alopecia because it produces frontal recession of the hairline, but it is associated with clinical evidence of scarring. Kossard, et al. later interpreted this type of alopecia as a frontal variant of lichen planopilaris on the basis of histopathologic and immunohistochemical studies.

Considerable overlap exists among postmenopausal frontal fibrosing alopecia, lichen planopilaris, and fibrosing alopecia in a pattern distribution. Postmenopausal frontal fibrosing alopecia has been described in association with lichen planus elsewhere (oral cavity), and we observed postmenopausal frontal fibrosing alopecia-type changes in patients with fibrosing alopecia in a pattern distribution.

Acute Diffuse and Total Alopecia of the Female Scalp

In 2002 Sato-Kuwamora, et al. suggested naming a peculiar type of inflammatory noncicatricial alopecia that is characterized by marked female predominance and a uniquely short clinical course "acute diffuse and total alopecia of the female scalp". It is basically identical with a subtype of alopecia areata presenting with diffuse hair loss as originally proposed in the German literature by Braun-Falco and Zaun 40 years earlier in 1962.

Diffuse alopecia areata or alopecia areata "incognita" (yet another synonymous designation proposed by Rebora in 1987) represents an uncommon variety of alopecia areata characterized by diffuse hair shedding in the absence of typical patches. The condition usually affects women over 40 years of age, who complain of diffuse alopecia and are often misdiagnosed as having telogen effluvium. Presence of yellow dots and short regrowing miniaturized hairs seen in the terminal hair-bearing scalp are an important clue to the diagnosis. The diagnosis is usually confirmed by histopathology.

Yet another variant of diffuse alopecia areata is canities subita or the *Marie Antoinette syndrome* that designates the condition in which scalp hair suddenly turns white. The eponym alludes to the wretched French Queen Marie Antoinette (1755–1793), whose hair allegedly turned white the night before her last walk to the guillotine during the French Revolution. The term canities subita has also been used for this disorder.

Although the actual incidence is rare, this stigmatizing phenomenon has captured storytellers' imagination like few other afflictions as a sign of grave sorrow. More modern accounts refer to the turning white of hair in survivors of bomb attacks during World War II. We reported a 54-year-old woman who initially presented with a single circular hairless patch of alopecia areata. Although she was successfully treated with topical steroids (betamethasone with dimethyl sulfoxide), her entire scalp hair suddenly turned white within a few weeks. She was completely healthy, allegedly did not notice any loss of hair during the change of color, and underwent no frightful experience.

Today, the syndrome is interpreted as an acute episode of diffuse alopecia areata in which the very sudden "overnight" graying is caused by the preferential loss of pigmented hair in this supposedly immune-mediated disorder. This observation has led some experts to hypothesize that the autoimmune target in alopecia areata may be related to the melanin pigment system.

Chronic diffuse alopecia areata is particularly rare. Patients present with profound hair loss, but often are not actively shedding. The alopecia may have a slightly reticular pattern. Where no patch of alopecia coexists as a clue to the diagnosis, a biopsy is usually required to establish the diagnosis. Optimal specimens include two 4 mm punch biopsy specimens from the vertex submitted for horizontal and vertical embedding. The histologic features depend on the stage of the disease, and biopsy specimens of clinically active alopecia areata show peribulbar lymphocytic infiltrates around anagen follicles. Especially in biopsy specimens from long-standing areas of alopecia areata with an increased number of telogen follicles and follicular miniaturization, the histology is sometimes equivocal, since a light perifollicular lymphocytic infiltrate can be a non-specific histologic finding.

A response with hair regrowth to systemic corticosteroid treatment, either as intravenous pulse therapy with methylprednisolone or as oral minipulse therapy with betamethasone usually establishes the diagnosis of alopecia areata.

Psychogenic Pseudoeffluvium

Ultimately, patients seeking advice for hair loss are not necessarily balding. When they have normally dense scalp hair, and absence of any convincing evidence of hair loss, they are regarded as suffering of "imaginary hair loss" or psychogenic pseudoeffluvium. In these cases thought should be given to underlying psychological disorders. It is important to question women who complain of excessive hair loss while no evidence of alopecia is evident on examination about depression and marital difficulties.

Mild instances of *alopecia phobia* are common in connection with depressive disorder.

Some extremely hair-conscious patients are capable of fierce fits of hair brushing or *telogen mania*, which is perhaps a modified form of obsessive-compulsive disorder.

Finally, the physician should be aware of the potential seriousness of *body dysmorphic disorder* and *delusion of alopecia*, both nearly psychotic states. In addition to the relentless complaint of hair loss, patients suffering from body dysmorphic disorder adopt obsessional, repetitive ritualistic behavior, and may come to spend the majority of the day in front of a mirror, repeatedly checking their hair. Another aspect of this behavior is a constant need for reassurance about the hair, not only from the immediate family but also from the medical profession and from dermatologists in particular. These patients may become the most demanding types of patient to try to manage.

The more recently described *Dorian Gray syndrome* denotes a cultural and societal phenomenon characterized by an excessive preoccupation with the individual's own appearance accompanied by difficulties coping with the aging process. The syndrome is characterized by a triad of symptoms combining diagnostic signs of dysmorphophobia, narcisistic character traits, and arrests in psychic maturation. Sufferers of Dorian Gray syndrome are heavy users of cosmetic medical procedures and products in an attempt to preserve their youth, including hair growth promoting agents and hair transplantations.

Box 12.3: Dorian Gray syndrome

- A cultural and societal phenomenon characterized by an excessive preoccupation with the individual's own appearance accompanied by difficulties coping with the aging process.
- A triad of symptoms combining diagnostic signs of dysmorphophobia, narcisistic character traits, and arrests in psychic maturation

Tonsure Trichotillomania

Yet another psychopathological condition to be taken into account in the differential diagnosis of patterned hair loss is tonsure trichotillomania. Trichotillomania involves the repetitive, uncontrollable pulling of one's hair, resulting in noticeable hair loss. It represents a disorder of impulse control. The disorder usually begins between early childhood and adolescence. It occurs six to seven times more frequently in children than in adults, before the age of 6 males predominate, thereafter females. Most commonly, scalp hair is pulled, resulting in ill-defined areas of incomplete hair loss. In the affected areas, there are different lengths of hair, short, longer, and normal. When the hair is pulled in the centroparietal area of the scalp, sparing the lateral margins and the nape of the neck, a tonsural pattern may result.

While in young children, trichotillomania results from a mild form of frustration in a climate of psychosocial stress, and soon becomes a habitual practice, from puberty onward, trichotillomania is related to more severe pathologic psychodynamics, and prognosis is more guarded, particularly tonsure trichotillomania in the female adolescent.

Associated features may include—excoriations of the scalp, nail biting (onychophagy), and eating hairs (trichophagy) with the risk of gastrointestinal obstruction by a mass of hair (trichobezoar), a complication that has been termed the Rapunzel syndrome.

Adjustment Disorders

Even though most patients with hair disorders experience significant psychological impact, it is usually not of an intensity to qualify as a mental illness, nevertheless, some patients have difficulties adjusting to hair loss. As a result, the individual may have difficulty with his or her mood and behavior. From a psychopathological point of view, adjustment disorders may result from the stressful event of hair loss, depending on its acuity, extent, and prognosis.

An adjustment disorder is a debilitating reaction to a stressful event or situation. These symptoms or behaviors are clinically significant as evidenced by either of the following: distress that is in excess of what would be expected, or significant impairment in social, occupational or educational functioning. Adjustment disorders subtypes include: adjustment disorder with depressed mood, with anxiety, with mixed anxiety and depressed mood, with disturbance of conduct, or with mixed disturbance of emotions and conduct.

Associated features may be somatic and/or sexual dysfunction, feelings of guilt and/or obsession.

The best way to alleviate the emotional distress caused by hair disease is to eliminate the hair disease that is causing the problem. If one appreciates the psychosocial impact of hair disease, there is no doubt that appropriate treatment frequently has a huge bearing on the patients' quality of life.

Quantitating Hair Loss

Reliably assessing the actual shedding of hair is a crucial diagnostic point in trichological practice. To fulfill office requirements, the test should be easy, non-invasive and not time-consuming. Many methods have been proposed, but all need standardization.

The *hair pull test* has been found to be a poorly sensitive method, while telogen percentage in the *trichogram* did not correlate with severity of hair loss.

While the *daily hair count* is a cumbersome procedure, it has been proposed that the *wash test* is probably the best method to adopt.

More so, measurement of the effects of treatment need to be quantified reliably. The method should be more sensitive than the wash test, and capable of analyzing relevant parameters of hair growth, which are: hair density, hair diameter, hair growth rate, and anagen/telogen ratio. For this purpose, a technique for office-based use has been developed that combines epiluminiscence microscopy with automatic digital image analysis (TrichoScan).

Global photographic assessment has successfully been established as a standard method for objectively monitoring hair growth in the course of the finasteride trials in men since 1992. Since its introduction the technique has proven to be essential for follow-up of hair loss patients undergoing long-term treatment in daily clinical practice as well. Global photographs represent head shots taken at short distance from the patient, and are therefore different from the close-up photographs used with the TrichoScan technique. For this purpose, the patient's head is positioned in a stereotactic device in which the patient's chin and forehead are fixed, and on which a given camera and flash device are mounted, ensuring that the view, magnification, and lighting are the same at consecutive visits, thus enabling precise follow-up of the same scalp area of interest. The result of global photographs are easily falsified, if photographs are taken with different degrees of flash lighting for each photograph. More light reflectance on the skin and hair can give the impression of less hair, while correspondingly less lighting can give the impression of more hair (**Figures 12.6A and B**). As a result, photographs taken without maintaining consistency in the way the photographs are taken can look very different and bias the results.

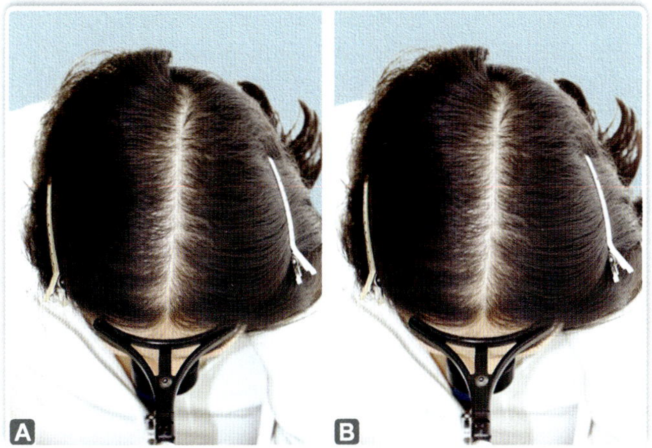

Figs 12.6A and B: (A) Image with more lighting; (B) Image with less lighting

Value of Trichoscopy for Differential Diagnosis

While the standard methods used to diagnose hair and scalp disorders (clinical inspection, pull test, trichogram and biopsy) vary in sensitivity, reproducibility, and invasiveness, recent studies suggest that the use of dermoscopy in the clinical evaluation of hair and scalp disorders improves diagnostic capability beyond simple clinical inspection and reveals novel features of disease, which may extend our clinical and pathogenetic understanding. Dermoscopy of hair and scalp or trichoscopy is gaining popularity as a valuable tool in differential diagnosis of hair and scalp disorders. For trichoscopy in daily clinical practice, a simple dermatoscope (Heine Delta 20® or DermoGenius®) can be used, with alcohol as the interface solution (Kodan® spray, Schulke & Mayr, Vienna, Austria). This method allows viewing of the hair and scalp at high magnifications, and is especially helpful in differentiating diffuse telogen effluvium from female androgenetic alopecia, and from diffuse alopecia areata.

Dermoscopic features of androgenetic alopecia are: hair diameter diversity, peripilar signs, and empty follicles.

Hair diameter diversity or *anisotrichosis* relates to the presence of hairs with different caliber. This finding reflects progressive hair follicle miniaturization due to this condition.

Peripilar signs (peripilar cupular atrophy) are characterized by the presence of a brown halo, roughly 1 mm in diameter, at the follicular ostium around the emerging hair shaft. This finding has been found to be linked to superficial perifollicular lymphocytic infiltrates.

Empty follicles are characterized by empty follicular ostia. They represent the physiological interval of the hair cycle in which the hair follicle remains empty after the telogen hair has been extruded and before a new anagen hair emerges (lag phase or kenogen). During kenogen, the hair follicle rests physiologically, but duration and frequency are greater in female pattern hair loss, possibly accounting for hair thinning.

Dermoscopic features of alopecia areata are: yellow dots, dystrophic hairs, and short regrowing miniaturized hairs.

Yellow dots are characterized by an array of quite monomorphous, though variably sized, yellow to yellow-pink, round or polycyclic dots that are devoid of hair or contain dystrophic or vellus hair. They correspond to dilated follicular infundibula that contain sebaceous and keratinous material.

Dystrophic hairs represent hairs that have fractured tips due to any process inhibiting cell division in the hair matrix. The hair shaft may be fractured before emergence from the scalp and then appears as *cadaverized hair*, or then appears as short *exclamation mark hair*. Dystrophic hairs are typically seen in acute alopecia areata at the active margin, where all types are usually numerous.

Short regrowing miniaturized hairs are a common feature seen in both acute and chronic alopecia areata.

Treatment

Management and prognosis of hair loss depend on the cause and underlying pathomechanism in its relation to the hair growth cycle. Once the diagnosis is established, treatment appropriate for that diagnosis is likely to control the hair loss, e.g. iron deficiency, other dietary deficiencies, thyroid disease, other metabolic or endocrine diseases, systemic lupus erythematosus, other connective tissue disorders, syphilis, other chronic infectious diseases, and drug-induced telogen effluvium.

Drugs known to cause hair loss, such as anticoagulants (heparin, warfarin), oral retinoids (acitretin, isotretinoin), interferon, agents with antithyroid action (carbimazole, propylthiouracil, amiodarone), hypolipidemic agents (fibrates), colchicine, antimetabolites (methotrexate, azathioprine, cyclophosphamide), and hormones with pro-androgen action (norethisterone, levonorgestrel, tibolon) should be discontinued unless they are essential for the patient.

Especially in young women the diet should also be addressed. If anorexia nervosa/bulimia is suspected, the aid of a psychiatrist should be sought, in other cases the informed patient will be happy to abandon any dietary culprit.

While most acute telogen effluvia, particularly those due to acute-onset physiologic events, e.g. postfebrile, postpartum, as well as seasonal telogen effluvium, and the shedding phase upon initiation of topical minoxidil treatment are self-limiting and will undergo normal reversal, the cause of chronic telogen effluvium may be multifactorial and difficult to establish. Differential diagnosis may be complicated through considerable overlap, especially with female pattern hair loss, for instance in postpartum effluvium that does not necessarily return to the same antepartum texture and length of hair. Synchronization phenomena of hair cycling, also on a seasonal basis, seem to be more pronounced in patients with female pattern hair loss, since with a shorter anagen phase a greater proportion of hair follicles will synchronize.

Recommendations for treatment of primary chronic telogen effluvium are scanty, and include topical or systemic corticosteroids, topical minoxidil, and dietary supplements.

Besides an understanding of the pathologic dynamics of hair loss as they relate to the hair growth cycle and intergrity of the hair follicle, insight into a multitude of cause relationships is prerequisite for delivering appropriate patient care. It must be borne in mind that hair loss often does not result from a single cause effect, but from a combination of internal and external factors that all need to be addressed simultaneously in an individualized manner for success, such as: nutrition (proteins, energy, vitamins, and trace metals), hormones, aging, seasonality of hair growth and shedding, cigarette smoking, UV radiation, inflammatory phenomena and hair care.

Ultimately, the problem of multimorbidity has to be taken into account, especially in the elderly population. The term multimorbidity means several concurrent medical conditions within one person. With technologic advances and improvements in medical care, an increasing number of patients survive medical conditions that used to be fatal. This fact combined with the aging of the population means that a growing proportion of patients have multiple concurrent medical conditions. According to a survey done in Canada in 1998, 30% of the population reported suffering from more than one chronic health problem, and the percentage increased with age. In the United States, the prevalence of multimorbidity among those 65 and older has been estimated at 65%. The quantity and quality of hair are closely related to the nutritional, general and mental health state of the individual, while older patients increasingly suffer from a variety of conditions that affect the hair, i.e. nutritional deficiency, endocrine disorders, psychologic problems, and drug-related adverse effects. Sometimes symptoms of overt pathologic conditions are misinterpreted as signs of normal aging, ignored and left untreated.

In taking care of older patients with hair problems, it is important to be suspicious of the possibility of a more general problem underlying the patient's complaint. The increasing number of chronic conditions per patient and the increasing amount of multimorbidity in the elderly population lead to a more complex approach to successful treatment of hair problems in the elderly.

Value of Oral Supplementation Therapy

The quantity and quality of hair are closely related the nutritional state of an individual. Normal supply, uptake, and transport of proteins, calories, trace elements, and vitamins are of fundamental importance in tissues with a high biosynthetic activity such as the hair follicle. Because hair shaft is composed almost entirely of protein, protein component of diet is critical for production of normal healthy hair. The rate of mitosis is sensitive to the calorific value of diet, provided mainly by carbohydrates stored as glycogen in the outer hair root sheath of the follicle. Finally, a sufficient supply of vitamins and trace metals is essential for the biosynthetic and energetic metabolism of the follicle. In instances of protein and calorie malnutrition, deficiency of essential amino acids, of trace elements, and of vitamins, hair growth and pigmentation may be impaired. The effects of nutrition on hair growth have been recognized from observations in inborn errors of metabolism, in deficiency disorders, and from supplementation studies in animals and humans.

The rationale for the use of a dietary supplement based on L-cystine for treatment of hair loss is based on the biochemistry of cystine metabolism, clinical observations in disorders of cystine metabolism and cystine deficiency, and results of animal and human studies. In the 1960s, the role of L-cystine in the production of wool proteins was investigated, and it was found that enrichment of even what appeared to be a normal diet with sulfur-containing amino acids increased wool production in sheep. In the early 1990s, human studies on the effect of dietary supplements containing L-cystine, usually in combination with B-complex vitamins or medicinal yeast that is rich in B-complex vitamins, have been published, exclusively in German language, showing improvements in the trichogram, in hair swelling as a criterion for hair quality, and in the tensile strength of the hair fiber.

We performed a study combining epiluminiscence microscopy with digital image analysis (TrichoScan) to demonstrate that a L-cystine-, medicinal yeast- and B-complex vitamin-based nutrient influences hair growth in otherwise healthy women between 25 and 65 years of age with telogen effluvium: after 6 months of treatment the active compound group showed a statistical significant improvement and normalization of the anagen hair rate, while the placebo group did not. The hair count, hair density, and cumulative hair shaft diameter did not show any changes from the baseline values. Nevertheless, the change in anagen hair rate was sufficient to reflect in clinical outcome, since the appearance of hair growth in the global photographic assessment was judged better, probably due to the increase of the proportion of actively growing hairs in anagen. The mechanism of action is not known, but these data suggest that the active compound has a therapeutic effect probably due to an induction of anagen.

Recently it was also shown that the noxious effect of cigarette smoke in exposed C57BL/6 mice could be abrogated by the oral administration of N-acetylcysteine, an analogue and precursor of L-cysteine and reduced glutathione, as well as by L-cystine, the oxidized form of L-cysteine, which is a key hair component, in combination with vitamin B6, which plays a role in L-cystine incorporation in hair cells. The effect may be related to the glutathione-related detoxification system.

Treatment of Female Androgenetic Alopecia

The aim of therapy in androgenetic alopecia is to increase hair coverage of the scalp and to retard progression of hair thinning.

First line treatment and treatment with the highest level of evidence for female androgenetic alopecia is topical minoxidil. Minoxidil promotes hair growth through increasing the duration of anagen. It causes hair follicles at rest to grow, and enlarges suboptimal follicles. Topical solutions of 2 and 5 percent minoxidil are available for treatment of androgenetic alopecia. Originally developed for treatment of androgenetic alopecia in men, topical minoxidil proved to be more effective in female androgenetic alopecia. In the original studies performed on women by Jacobs, et al. the investigators observed that 44% of patients in the 2% minoxidil group achieved new hair growth compared with 29% in the placebo group. DeVillez, et al. determined that 13% in the minoxidil-treated group had moderate growth and 50% had minimal growth, compared to 6% and 33%, respectively, in the placebo-treated group. Similarly, 60% of patients in the 2% minoxidil group reported new hair growth (20% moderate, 40% minimal) compared with 40% (7% moderate, 33% minimal) in the placebo group. Clinical studies using hair counts as a primary endpoint reported a mean increase in hair growth of 15–33% in the minoxidil-treated groups compared with 9–14% in the vehicle control groups. Using hair weight as the endpoint Price and Menefee found an increase of 42.5% in hair weights in the minoxidil group compared to 1.9% in the controls. In the most recent trial comparing 5% and 2% minoxidil lotion, Lucky, et al. found increases of 18% and 14% respectively in mean non-vellus hair counts after 48 weeks treatment, compared to a 7% increase in the placebo group. The increase in hair counts following treatment with topical minoxidil was noticeable within 8 weeks and peaked after 16 weeks. The 5% topical minoxidil group demonstrated statistical superiority over the 2% topical minoxidil group in the patient assessment of treatment benefit. Both concentrations of topical minoxidil were well tolerated by the women in this trial without evidence of systemic adverse effects. Ultimately, Blume-Peytavi, et al. compared the efficacy of once-daily 5% minoxidil topical foam with twice daily 2% minoxidil topical solution in women with androgenetic alopecia, and demonstrated non-inferiority of once-daily 5% minoxidil topical foam to twice daily 2% minoxidil topical solution for stimulating hair growth. Moreover, 5% minoxidil topical foam was significantly superior to twice daily 2% minoxidil topical solution in participants' agreement with "the treatment does not interfere with styling my hair". The authors concluded that once-daily 5% topical minoxidil foam is associated both aesthetic and practical advantages.

Traditionally, female androgenetic alopecia has been treated with iron supplementation and antiandrogen treatment. In fact, iron deficiency is overestimated as a single cause of hair loss in women, as well as the role of antiandrogens in the treatment of female androgetic alopecia.

Several studies have evaluated the relationship between iron deficiency and hair loss. The various observational studies that evaluated the association between decreased ferritin levels and hair loss have resulted in opposing conclusions. A critical appraisal of available data points to the fact that iron deficiency is probably overestimated as a single cause of hair loss in women. In our study of 181 women complaining of hair loss, we found no association between serum ferritin levels >10 microg/L and hair loss activity in women.

Since Hammerstein's proposition of the use of antiandrogens to treat women with symptoms of hyperandrogenism, such as hirsutism, seborrhea, and alopecia, antiandrogen therapy was established as a treatment of androgenetic alopecia in women. Typically, a high dosage reverse sequential therapy of 100 mg cyproterone acetate (CPA) on the 5–14th days of the menstrual cycle and 40 mcg ethinyl estradiol (E2) on the 5–25th days was used in severe cases, while low dosages of 2 mg CPA and 50 mcg of E2 preparations were used for light cases. More recently, to compare topical minoxidil 2% and CPA in the treatment of female androgenetic alopecia, Vexiau et al randomly assigned sixty-six women for 12 cycles into two groups, 33 received two local applications (2 mL day-1) of topical minoxidil 2% plus combined oral contraceptive and 33 received CPA 52 mg day-1 plus E2 35 microg for 20 of every 28 days. The investigators found that minoxidil treatment was more effective in the absence of other signs of hyperandrogenism, hyperseborrhea, and menstrual cycle modifications when the Body Mass Index (BMI) was low, and when nothing argued in favor of biochemical hyperandrogenism, while CPA treatment was more effective when other signs were present and when the BMI was elevated, factors that favoured a diagnosis of biochemical hyperandrogenism.

Spironolactone is yet another agent with antiandrogenic action considered in the treatment of female androgenetic alopecia. Spironolactone is a competitive inhibitor of aldosterone receptors, that also blocks androgen receptors and increases metabolic clearance of testosterone. It has been widely used to treat hirsutism, but there are no controlled trials of its use in female androgenetic alopecia. Rushton and colleagues reported that women treated for 12 months with spironolactone showed less hair loss than an untreated group, while in an open uncontrolled case series of 80 women treated for 1 year with 200 mg spironolactone daily or CPA, Sinclair, et al. found that 35 (44%) showed improvement in hair growth as assessed by standardised photography.

Moreover, antiandrogen treatment is not without problems. Dose-related side effects of CPA, including weight gain, fatigue, loss of libido, mastodynia, nausea, headaches and depression, are common. Spironolactone may cause breast soreness and menstrual irregularities.

In contrast, finasteride is well-tolerated and probably represents the safer option in postmenopausal and infertile women. Finasteride, an inhibitor of type 2 5α-reductase, inhibits conversion of tesosterone to DHT, resulting in decrease in serum and scalp DHT levels believed to be pathogenic in androgenetic alopecia. 1mg oral finasteride daily has been shown to be effective in prevention and treatment of hair loss in men, and has also proven to be effective in the aging male, though to a lesser degree and with a higher frequency of sexual adverse effects compared to men between 18–40 years. While oral finasteride has unanimously been shown to be effective in treatment of hair loss in men, its efficacy in women remains controversial.

In a double-blind, placebo-controlled, multicenter trial, Price, et al. demonstrated that oral finasteride, 1 mg/d, taken for 1 year did not slow progression of hair loss or promote hair growth, nor improve follicular counts in horizontal sections of scalp biopsies in postmenopausal women with androgenetic alopecia. One explanation might be that the different pattern of hair loss in the majority of women from that usually seen in men may be due to differences in the relative levels of 5α-reductase, aromatase, and androgen receptors in scalp hair follicles in women compared with those in men. Shum, et al. reported 4 cases of hair loss with characteristics of both male and female pattern hair loss in women with hyperandrogenism, in which finasteride improved the alopecia. Their patients differed from those in the trial reported by Price, et al. in that the patients had increased androgen levels, and finasteride was used in a slighty higher dose (1.25 mg/d), and given for a longer period of time (24 to 30 months as opposed to 1 year). On the other hand, Carmina and Lobo did not find finasteride, 5 mg/d, to be effective in treatment of alopecia in hyperandrogenic women. In the so far largest series of 37 pre-menopausal women treated for 1 year with finasteride in doses of 2.5–5 mg daily, Iorizzo, et al. showed some improvement in 62% as assessed by global photography.

Differences in response of women to oral finasteride have led to the suggestion that not all types of female hair loss have the same pathophysiology, i.e. a distinction should be made between alopecia with early (premenopausal) or late (postmenopausal) onset, and with or without hyperandrogenemia. Unfortunately, up to date no predictive factor for response to finasteride treatment has been identified in women with female androgenetic alopecia.

It must be kept in mind that due to teratogenicity for the male fetus, oral finasteride is contraindicated for use in premenopausal women.

Estrogens are primarily marketed in a number of ways to address problems related to hypoestrogenism. According to the indication, oral, transdermal, and topical preparations are available. In an attempt to circumvent problems related to systemic hormonal treatments of female androgenetic alopecia, topical treatment with 17β- and 17α-estradiol have been introduced. 17α-estradiol (alfatradiol) represents a stereoisomer of 17β- estradiol (estradiol) with 100-fold lower estrogenic and 2-fold higher 5α-reductase inhibitory action. Unfortunately, efficacy studies bear a low level of evidence. Moreover, no literature exists comparing efficacy, and safety of topical versus systemic estrogens. Ultimately, in a study involving 103 women comparing alfatradiol to minoxidil, Blume-Peytavi, et al. found minoxidil to be more effective. In contrast to minoxidil, alfatradiol did not result in an increase of hair density or thickness.

Low-level laser therapy (LLLT) has recently emerged as a novel therapy for the treatment of hair loss. It has received considerable media attention and marketing budgets from companies that advertise the devices, but a reservation has been that no independent, peer-reviewed studies had demonstrated its efficacy in this application.

The HairMax LaserComb is a hand-held Class 3R low level laser therapy device that contains a single laser module that emulates 9 beams at a wavelength of 655 nm. The device uses a technique of parting the user's hair by combs that are attached to the device. This improves delivery of distributed laser light to the scalp. The combs are designed so that each of the teeth on the combs aligns with a laser beam. By aligning the teeth with the laser beams, the hair can be parted and the laser energy delivered to the scalp of the user without obstruction by the individual hairs on the scalp.

Avram and Rogers investigated the efficacy of low-level laser therapy in enhancing hair growth. A total of seven patients were exposed to treatment for 3–6 months. Videomicroscopic images were taken at baseline, 3, and 6 months, and analyzed for changes in vellus hair counts, terminal hair counts, and hair shaft diameter. Both videomicroscopic and global images underwent blinded review for evidence of improvement. The results indicated that on average patients had a decrease in the number of vellus hairs, an increase in the number of terminal hairs, and an increase in hair shaft diameter. However, paired i-testing indicated that none of these was statistically significant. Also, blinded evaluation of global images did not support a recognizable improvement.

From our own experience we share with the authors the opinion that low-lever laser therapy represents a safe and promising treatment option for patients who do not respond or are not tolerant to minoxidil. This technology appears to work better for some people than for others. Predictive factors who will most benefit from low-level laser treatment are yet to be determined.

Ultimately, combination treatments with topical minoxidil, nutritional supplements, low-level laser therapy, and appropriate scalp care may act synergistic to enhance hair growth. The scientific rationale for such an approach is given, but there is a need for clinical studies to establish increase in efficacy of combination regimes and adjuvant treatments.

Value of Hair Care

The condition of our hair is important for both our overall appearance and self-pereption. There are no significant differences in the number of hair follicles between men and women, or between different races. Differences in the appearance of hair are due to the type of hair produced by a follicle and to the type of hair care and cosmetics practiced by the individual.

Healthy hair is usually perceived to be shiny hair with a smooth texture and clean-cut end or tapered tips.

For treatment success with pharmacologic agents, patients need to adhere to treatment and have patience. On the other, patients expect immediate results. This is only possible by adding an appropriate hair care regimen to the pharmacologic treatment.

A survey has demonstrated that 70 percent of women are not satisfied with the condition of their hair at least once a week, and 40 percent are unsatisfied with their hair care products. This has to do with the fact that approximately half of women are incapable of determining their hair type correctly and choosing the appropriate hair care and styling products. Women are very well aware of how their hair should ideally look, but are not knowledgeable about the appropriate hair care and cosmetic products. These findings underscore the significance of counselling on appropriate hair care ad cosmetics besides prescribing effective treatment for hair loss.

Moreover, the physician who is knowledgeable of appropriate hair care, will more easily win patient confidence as a prerequisite for patient compliance.

Shampoos are the most commonly used means of managing hair and scalp conditions. Today shampoos are expected to be more than mere cleansing agents. They are expected to not dry out the hair; to produce lather in hard and soft water and when applied to oily hair; to be non-irritating to skin and mucous membranes; to be chemically and physically stable; to possess conditioning benefits; to be biodegradable; and affordable. A shampoo is expected to improve the hair cosmetically while being tailored to the needs of various hair types as well as age and individual habits. Scalp condition is another important factor in individual health and well-being; the scalp should neither be oily nor should dandruff develop. Shampoos have evolved into high-tech products consisting of 10 to 30 ingredients that are combined in precise formulations to meet consumer demands.

Our natural *hair conditioner* is sebum. Excessive removal of sebum in the course of washing the hair and scalp created the need for synthetic sebum-like substances that attempt to supply hair with the positive attributes of sebum while avoiding the greasy appearance of excessive sebum and dirty hair. Hair conditioners aim at: imparting softness, increasing luster and gloss, reducing fly-away, enhancing disentagling facility, and alleviating defects related to certain types of hair and hair treatments.They are available as: shampoos for dry or damaged hair, conditioning (2-in-1) shampoos, and hair conditioners (liquids, creams, pastes, gels).

Finally, *hair styling aids* are intended to maintain hair in fashionable arrangement while improving the quality of hair fibers. Hair styles are in part dictated by the available technology in hair styling products. Hair styling aids aim at maintaining hair in desired position, adding increased hold to hair, creating illusion of fullness, creating a wet, "spiky" look, straightening, conditioning, moisturizing, and adding shine to kinky hair. They are available as: hair spray, hair styling gel, hair sculputuring gel, hair wax, hair mousse, and ethnic styling aids, such as pomade, brilliantine, oil sheen spray, and curl activator.

Autologous Hair Transplantation

Autologous hair transplantation represents the only treatment that can produce substantial improvement in patients with advanced hair loss and can give satisfactory results, as long as the patient has a realistic expectation regarding the treatment results. Hair line design, evaluation of the donor and recipient areas as well as the discussion of graft numbers are basic parts of the hair transplant consultation. There are two donor hair harvesting techniques that are performed under local anesthesia: in one technique, a strip of scalp skin is taken from the occipital area, which then is divided into mini- or micro-grafts, each containing 1–4 hairs. The grafts are then planted into tiny slits in the desired recipient area. The other technique is follicular unit extraction (FUE): multiple follicles are harvested with small 1 mm punches and planted in the target area, avoiding the occipital linear scar of the strip technique. However, FUE is more labor intensive and therefore usually more expensive. A natural looking result can be achieved with both procedures. One or two sessions usually provide a good coverage of a balding recipient area. Final results are usually seen 6–8 months after the surgery.

Hair transplantation is most appropriate in women with pronounced hair loss of limited extent, e.g. the frontal Olsen or Christmas tree pattern, who retain good hair density in the donor site. Hair transplantation is ideally combined with medical treatment to prevent further hair loss and to improve hair growth, density and texture.

Hair Prosthesis

A hair or cranial prosthesis, is a custom-made wig specifically designed for patients who have lost their hair as a result of medical conditions or treatments, such as alopecia totalis, trichotillomania, chemotherapy, or any other clinical disease or treatment resulting in hair loss. The terminology is used when applying for medical insurance or tax deduction status.

Physicians have been prescribing these prostheses since the 1950s. Cranial prostheses do not only have the purpose to disguise hair loss, but also help to protect the unprotected scalp from the sun, and to regulate body temperature.

Many of the manufacturers today are designing excellent high quality wigs that provide comfortable caps, high quality synthetic fibers, durable human hair, and special materials to achieve a secure fit. Many of these products will be extremely light weight and have a very natural appearance.

While wigs cover the whole head, hair pieces and hair integrations intend to complement the proper hair.

Psychological Counseling

Finally, the issue of psychogenic effluvium or of overvalued ideas in relation to the condition of the hair is not always easy to resolve, however it is important to control stress as a complication of hair loss or fear of hair loss. In general, the best way to alleviate the emotional distress caused by a hair disorder is to effectively treat it. Psychotherapy is aimed at any associated symptomatology of depression, regardless of whether there is a causal relationship between the psychiatric findings, hair loss or fear of hair loss, because it is possible that patients who are depressed perceive even normal hair shedding in an exaggerated manner. Patients with anxiety related to the fear of hair loss may also benefit from anxiolytic therapy. In addition, appropriate psychological support is essential to help limit patient anxiety. Patients need to be educated about the basics of the hair cycle, and why usually considerable patience is required for effective cosmetic recovery.

Suggested Reading

Pathologic Dynamics of Hair Loss

1. Barraud-Klenovsek MM, Trüeb RM. Congenital hypotrichosis due to short anagen. Br J Dermatol. 2000;143:612-7.
2. Kligman AM. Pathologic dynamics of human hair loss, I: telogen effluvium. Arch Dermatol. 1961;83:175-98.
3. Kluger N, Jacot W, Frouin E, et al. Permanent scalp alopecia related to breast cancer chemotherapy by sequential fluorouracil/epirubicin/cyclophosphamide (FEC) and docetaxel: a prospective study of 20 patients. Ann Oncol. 2012;23:2879-84.
4. Paus R. Control of the hair cycle and hair diseases as cycling disorders. Curr Opin Dermatol. 1996;3:248-58.
5. Paus R, Cotsarelis G. The biology of hair follicles. N Engl J Med. 1999;341:491-7.
6. Pierard-Franchimont C, Pierard GE. Teloptosis, a turning point in hair shedding biorhythms. Dermatology. 2001;203:115-7.

Telogen Effluvium

7. Aydingoz I, Ferhanoglu B, Guney O. Does tissue iron status have a role in female alopecia? J Eur Acad Dermatol Venereol. 1999;13:65-7.
8. Bregy A, Trueb RM. No association between serum ferritin levels >10 microg/L and hair loss activity in women. Dermatology. 2008;217:1-6.
9. Chartier MB, Hoss DMM. Grant-Kels JM. Approach to the adult female patient with diffuse nonscarring alopecia. J Am Acad Dermatol. 2002;47:809-18.
10. Comaisch S. The thyroid and hair growth. Sem Dermatol. 1985;4:4-8.
11. Guy WB, Edmundson WF. Diffuse cyclic hair loss in women. Arch Dermatol. 1960;81:205-27.
12. Hard S. Non-anemic iron deficiency as an etiologic factor in diffuse loss of hair of the scalp in women. Acta Derm Venereol. 1963:43:562-9.
13. Headington JT. Telogen effluvium. New concepts and review. Arch Dermatol. 1993;129:356-63.
14. Ikeda T, Yamada M. Both telogen effluvium and traction alopecia mainly occur in patients with a condition of alopecia prematura. Acta Dermatol (Kyoto). 1967;62:47.
15. Kantor J, Kessler LJ, Brooks DG, Cotsarelis G. Decreased serum ferritin is associated with alopecia in women. J Invest Dermatol. 2003;121:985-8.
16. Mirmirani P, Hessol N, Maurer T, et al. Prevalence of hair disorders in the women's interagency HIV study (abstract 265). J Invest Dermatol. 2001;117:434.
17. Orme S, Cullen DR, Messenger AG. Diffuse female hair loss: are androgens necessary? Br J Dermatol. 1999;141:521-3.
18. Rebora A. Telogen effluvium. Dermatology. 1997;195:209-12.
19. Reeves JRT, Maibach HI. Drug and chemical induced hair loss. In: Marzulli FN, Maibach HI (eds.) Advances in Modern Toxicology. Hemisphere Publishing Corp., Washington, London. 1977;4:487-500.
20. Rushton DH. Management of hair loss in women. Dermatol Clin. 1993;11:47-53.
21. Rushton DH, Dover R, Sainsbury AW, et al. Iron deficiency is neglected in women's health. Br Med J. 2002;325:1176.
22. Rushton DH, Ramsay ID, James KC. Biochemical and trichological characterization of diffuse alopeca in women. Br J Dermatol. 1990;123:187-19.
23. Rushton DH, Ramsay ID. The importance of adequate serum ferritin levels during oral cyproterone acetate and ethinyl oestradiol treatment of diffuse androgendependent alopecia in women. Clin Endocrinol. 1992;36:421-7.
24. Sinclair R. Diffuse hair loss. Int J Dermatol. 1999;38(Suppl. 1):8-18.
25. Sinclair R. There is no clear association between low serum ferritin and chronic diffuse telogen hair loss. Br J Dermatol. 2002;147:982-4.
26. Spencer LV, Callen JP. Hair loss in systemic disease. Dermatol Clin. 1987;5;565-70.
27. Stroud JP. Diagnosis and management of the hair loss patient. Cutis. 1987;40:272-6.
28. Tosti A, Misciali C, Piraccini BM, et al. Drug-induced hair loss and hair growth. Incidence, management and avoidance. Drug Saf. 1994;10:310-17.
29. Trost LB, Bergfeld WF, Calogeras E. The diagnosis and treatment of iron deficiency and its potential relationship to hair loss. J Am Acad Dermatol. 2006;54:824-44.
30. Trüeb RM. Idiopathic chronic telogen effluvium in women. Hautarzt. 2000;51:899-905.
31. Trüeb RM. Systematic approach to hair loss in women. J Dtsch Dermatol Ges. 2010;8:284-98.
32. Whiting DA. Chronic telogen effluvium: increased scalp hair shedding in middle-aged women. J Am Acad Dermatol. 1996;35:899-906.
33. Wysenbeek AI, Leibovici L, Amit M, Weinberger A. Alopecia in systemic lupus erythematosus. Relation to disease manifestations. J Rheumatol. 1991;18:1185-6.

34. York J, Nicholson T, Minors P, Duncan DF. Stressful life events and loss of hair among adult women, a case-control study. Psychol Rep. 1998;82:1044-6.

Androgenetic Alopecia

35. Bahta AW, Farjo N, Farjo B, Philpott MP. Premature senescence of balding dermal papilla cells in vitro is associated with p16(INK4a) expression. J Invest Dermatol. 2008;128:1088-94.
36. Carlini P, Di Cosimo S, Ferretti G, et al. Alopecia in a premenopausal breast cancer woman treated with letrozole and triptorelin. Ann Oncol. 2003;14:1689-90.
37. Cormia FE. Alopecia from oral contraceptives. JAMA. 1967;201:635-7.
38. Hoffmann R, Happle R. Current understanding of androgenetic alopecia. Part I: etiopathogenesis. Eur J Dermatol. 2000;10:319-26.
39. Kaufman KD. Androgen metabolism as it affects hair growth in androgenetic alopecia. Dermatol Clinics. 1996;14:697-711.
40. Naito A, Midorikawa T, Yoshino T, Ohdera M. Lipid peroxides induce early onset of catagen phase in murine hair cycles. Int J Mol Med. 2008;22:725-9.
41. Norwood OT. Incidence of female androgenetic alopecia (female pattern alopecia). Dermatol Surg. 2001;27:53-54.
42. Ohnemus U, Uenalan M, Conrad F, et al. Hair cycle control by estrogens: catagen induction via estrogen receptor (ER)-alpha is checked by ER beta signaling. Endocrinology. 2005;146:1214-25.
43. Ohnemus U, Uenalan M, Inzunza J, et al. The hair follicle as an estrogen target and source. Enodcr Rev. 2006;27:677-706.
44. Orme S, Cullen DR, Messenger AG. Diffuse female hair loss: are androgens necessary? Br J Dermatol. 1999;141:521-3.
45. Riedel-Baima B, Riedel A. Female pattern hair loss may be triggered by low oestrogen to androgen ratio. Endocr Regul. 2008;42:13-6.
46. Sawaya ME, Price VH. Different levels of 5alpha-reductase type I and II, aromatase, and androgen receptor in hair follicles of women and men with androgenetic alopecia. J Invest Dermatol. 1997;109:296-300.
47. Tosti A, Iorizzo M, Piraccini BM. Androgenetic alopecia in children: report of 20 cases. Br J Dermatol. 2005;152:556-9.
48. Trüeb RM. Molecular mechanisms of androgenetic alopecia. Exp Gerontol. 2002;37:981-90.
49. Venning VA, Dawber RP. Patterned androgenic alopecia in women. J Am Acad Dermatol. 1988;18:1073-7.

Postpartum Hair Loss

50. Cormia FE. Alopecia from oral contraceptives. JAMA. 1967;201:635-7.
51. Lynfield YL. Effect of pregnancy on the human hair cycle. J Invest Dermatol. 1960;35:323-7.
52. Pecoraro V, Barman JM, Astoe I. The normal trichogram of pregnant women. In: Montagna W, Dobson RL (eds.) Advances in Biology of Skin vol. IX, Hair Growth: p. 203, Pergamon Press, Oxford 1969.

Menopause

53. Phillips TJ, Demarcay Z, Sahu M. Hormonal effects on skin aging. Clin Geriatr Med. 2001;17:661-72.
54. Ringa V. Menopause and treatments. Quality of life research. 2000;9:695-707.
55. Thornton MJ. The biological actions of estrogens on skin. Exp Dermatol. 2002;11:487-502.
56. Venning VA, Dawber RP. Patterned androgenic alopecia in women. J Am Acad Dermatol. 1988;18:1073-7.

Senescent Alopecia

57. Courtois M, Loussouarn G, Hourseau C, Grollier JF. Aging and hair cycles. Br J Dermatol. 1995;132:86-93.
58. Harman D. Aging: a theory based on free radical and radiation chemistry. J Gerontol. 1956;11:298-300.
59. Kligman AM. The comparative histopathology of male-pattern baldness and senescent baldness. Clin Dermatol. 1988;6:108-18.
60. Paradi M, Shahee O, Shaza D, et al. Comparison of senescent and androgenetic alopecia using microarray analysis. 5th International Hair Research Societies Meeting, Vancouver 2007. Abstract O-10-3.
61. Tobin DJ, Paus R. Graying: gerontobiology of the hair follicle pigmentary unit. Exp Gerontol. 2001;36:29-54.
62. Trüeb RM. Dermocosmetic aspects of hair and scalp. J Investig Dermatol Symp Proc. 2005;10:289-92.
63. Trüeb RM. Aging of hair. J Cosmet Dermatol. 2005;4:60-72.
64. Trüeb RM. Pharmacologic interventions in aging hair. Clin Interv Aging. 2006;1:121-9.
65. Trüeb RM. Oxidative stress in ageing of hair. Int J Trichology. 2009;1:6-14.
66. van Neste D. Thickness, medullation and growth rate of female scalp hair are subject to significant variation according to pigmentation of scalp location during aging. Eur J Dermatol. 2004;14:28-32.
67. van Neste D, Tobin DJ. Hair cycle and hair pigmentation: dynamic interactions and changes associated with aging. Micron. 2004;35:193-200.

Seasonality of Hair Growth and Shedding

68. Courtois M, Loussouarn G, Hourseau S, Grollier JF. Periodicity in the growth and shedding of hair. Br J Dermatol. 1996;134: 47-54.
69. Kunz M, Seifert B, Trüeb RM. Seasonality of hair shedding in healthy women complaining of hair loss. Dermatology. 2009;219:105-10.
70. Orentreich N. Scalp replacement in man. In: Montagna W, Bobson RL (eds). Advances in Biology of Skin, Vol IX: Hair Growth. Oxford: Pewrgamon. 1969;99-108.

71. Randall VA, Ebling FJG. Seasonal changes in human hair growth. Br J Dermatol. 1991;124:146-51.

Inflammatory Phenomena and Scarring

72. Jaworsky C, Kligman AM, Murphy GF. Characterisation of inflammatory infiltrates in male pattern alopecia: implication for pathogenesis. Br J Dermatol. 1992;127:239-46.
73. Mahé YF, Michelet JF, Billoni N, et al. Androgenetic alopecia and microinflammation. Int J Dermatol. 2000;39:576-84.
74. Philpott MP, Sander DA, Bowen J, Kealey T. Effects of interleukins, colony stimulating factor and tumour necrosis factor on human hair follicle growth in vitro: a possible role for interleukin-1 and tumour necrosis factor-alpha in alopecia areata. Br J Dermatol. 1996;135:942-8.
75. Whiting DA. Diagnostic and predictive value of horizontal sections of scalp biopsy specimens in male pattern androgenetic alopecia. J Am Acad Dermatol. 1993;28:755-63.

Postmenopausal Frontal Fibrosing Alopecia

76. Kossard S. Postmenopausal frontal fibrosing alopecia: scarring alopecia in a pattern distribution. Arch Dermatol. 1994;130:770-4.
77. Kossard S, Lee MS, Wilkinson B. Postmenopausal frontal fibrosing alopecia: a frontal variant of lichen planopilaris. J Am Acad Dermatol. 1997;36:59-66.
78. Trüeb RM, Toricelli R. Lichen planopilaris unter dem Bild einer postmenopausalen frontalen fibrosierenden Alopezie (Kossard). Hautarzt. 1998;49:388-391.

Fibrosing Alopecia in a Pattern Distribution

79. Zinkernagel MS, Trüeb RM. Fibrosing alopecia in a pattern distribution. Patterned lichen planopilaris or androgenetic alopecia with a lichenoid tissue reaction pattern? Arch Dermatol. 2000;136:205-11.

Acute Diffuse and Total Alopecia of the Female Scalp

80. Braun-Falco, Zaun O. Über die Beteiligung des gesamten Capillitiums bei Alopecia areata. Hautarzt. 1962;13:342-8.
81. Ephraim A. On sudden or rapid whitening of the hair. AMA Arch Derm. 1959;79:228-36.
82. Helm F, Milgrom H. Can scalp hair suddenly turn white? a case of canities subita. Arch Dermatol. 1970;102:102-3.
83. Hoffmann E. Sudden turning gray of the hair caused by fright, canities subita psychogenica. Z Haut Geschlechtskr. 1957;22:74-8.
84. Khaitan BK, Mittal R, Verma KK. Extensive alopecia areata treated with betamethasone oral mini-pulse therapy: an open uncontrolled study. Indian J Dermatol Venereol Leprol. 2004;70:350-3.
85. Lew BL, Shin MK, Sim WY. Acute diffuse and total alopecia: A new subtype of alopecia areata with a favorable prognosis. J Am Acad Dermatol. 2009;60:85-93.
86. Nakajima T, Inui S, Itami S. Pulse corticosteroid therapy for alopecia areata: study of 139 patients. Dermatology. 2007;215:320-4.
87. Navarini AA, Nobbe S, Trüeb RM. Marie Antoinette syndrome. Arch Dermatol. 2009;145:656.
88. Paus R, Slominski A, Czarnetzki BM. Is alopecia areata an autoimmune-response against melanogenesis-related proteins, exposed by abnormal MHC class I expression in the anagen hair bulb? Yale J Biol Med. 1993;66:541-54.
89. Rebora A. Alopecia areata incognita: a hypothesis. Dermatologica. 1987;174:214-8.
90. Sato-Kawamura M, Aiba S, Tagami H. Acute diffuse and total alopecia of the female scalp. A new subtype of diffuse alopecia areata that has a favorable prognosis. Dermatology. 2002;205:367-73.

Psychogenic Pseudoeffluvium

91. Brosig B, Kupfer J, Niemeier V, et al. The "Dorian Gray Syndrome": psychodynamic need for hair growth restorers and, other "fountains of youth". Int J Clin Pharmacol Ther. 2001;39:279-83.
92. Cotterill JA. Body dysmorphic disorder. Dermatol Clin. 1996;14:457-63.

Tonsure Trichotillomania

93. Davis-Daneshfar A, Trüeb RM. Tonsur-Trichotillomanie. Hautarzt. 1995;46:804-7.
94. Delsmann BM, Nikolaidis N, Schomacher PH. Trichobezoar als seltene Ursache eines Dünndarmileus. Dtsch Med Wochenschr. 1993;118:1361-4.
95. Sanderson KV. Tonsure trichotillomania. Br J Dermatol. 1970;82:343-50.
96. Van Moffaert M. Localization of self-inflicted dermatological lesions: what do they tell the dermatologist. Acta Derm Venereol Suppl (Stockh). 1991;156:23-7.

Adjustment Disorders

97. Cash TF, Price VH, Savin RC. Psychological effects of androgenetic alopecia on women: comparisons with balding men and with female control subjects. J Am Acad Dermatol. 1993;29:568-75.
98. Cash TF. The psychosocial consequences of androgenetic alopecia: a review of the research literature. Br J Dermatol. 1999;141:398-405.
99. Maffei C, Fossatti A, Rinaldi F, et al. Personality disorders and psychopathologic symptoms in patients with androgenetic alopecia. Arch Dermatol. 1994;130:868-72.

Quantitating Hair Loss

100. Guarrera M, Semino MT, Rebora A. Quantitating hair loss in women: a critical approach. Dermatology. 1997;1997:12-16.
101. Hoffmann R. TrichoScan: combining epiluminiscence microscopy with digital image analysis for the measurement of hair growth in vivo. Eur J Dermatol. 2001;11:362-8.

102. Ihm CW, Lee JY. Evaluation in daily hair counts. Dermatologica. 1991;182:67.
103. Rampini P, Guarrera M, Rampini E, Rebora A. Assessing hair shedding in children. Dermatology. 1999;199:256-7.
104. Seung Ho Lee, Oh Sang Kwon, Jun Gyu Oh, et al. Phototrichogram: Evaluation of Modified Methods with Bleaching and Trichoscan. Seoul, Korea, poster presentation at the European Hair Research Society. June 2004.
105. Van Neste D, Trüeb RM. Critical study of hair growth analysis with computer-assisted methods. J Eur Acad Dermatol Venereol. 2006;20:578-83.

Value of Trichoscopy for Differential Diagnosis

106. de Lacharrière O, Deloche C, Misciali C, et al. Hair diameter diversity: a clinical sign reflecting the follicle miniaturization. Arch Dermatol. 2001;137:641-6.
107. Deloche C, de Lacharrière O, Misciali C, et al. Histological features of peripilar signs associated with androgenetic alopecia. Arch Dermatol Res. 2004;295:422-8.
108. Galliker NA, Trüeb RM. Value of trichoscopy versus trichogram for diagnosis of female androgenetic alopecia. Int J Trichology. 2012;4:19-22.
109. Guarrera M, Rebora A. Anagen hairs may fail to replace telogen hairs in early androgenic female alopecia. Dermatology. 1996;192:28-31.
110. Guarrera M, Rebora A. Kenogen in female androgenetic alopecia. A longitudinal study. Dermatology. 2005;210:18-20.
111. Hidvégi B. Dermoscopy of hair and scalp disorders. Eur J Dermatol. 2008;18:607.
112. Inui S, Nakajima T, Itami S. Dry dermoscopy in clinical treatment of alopecia areata. J Dermatol. 2007;34:635-9.
113. Inui S, Nakajima T, Nakagawa K, Itami S. Clinical significance of dermoscopy in alopecia areata: analysis of 300 cases. Int J Dermatol. 2008;47:688-93.
114. Inui S, Nakajima T, Itami S. Significance of dermoscopy in acute diffuse and total alopecia of the female scalp: review of twenty cases. Dermatology. 2008;217:333-6.
115. Lacarrubba F,Dall'Oglio F,Nasca MR, Micali G. Videodermoscopy enhances diagnostic capability in some forms of hair loss. Am J Clin Dermatol. 2004;5:205-8.
116. Olszewska M, Rudnicka L, Rakowska A, et al. Trichoscopy. Arch Dermatol. 2008;144:1007.
117. Rebora A, Guarrera M. Kenogen. A new phase of the hair cycle? Dermatology. 2002;205:108-10.
118. Ross EK, Vincenzi C, Tosti A. Videodermoscopy in the evaluation of hair and scalp disorders. J Am Acad Dermatol. 2006;55:799-806.
119. Rudnicka L, Olszewska M, Rakowska A, et al. Trichoscopy: a new method for diagnosing hair loss. J Drugs Dermatol. 2008;7:651-4.
120. Sewell LD, Elston DM, Dorion RP. "Anisotrichosis": a novel term to describe pattern alopecia. J Am Acad Dermatol. 2007;56:856.
121. Toncić RJ, Lipozencić J, Pastar Z. Videodermoscopy in the evaluation of hair and scalp disorders. Acta Dermatovenerol Croat. 2007;15:116-8.
122. Tosti A, Whiting D, Iorizzo M, et al. The role of scalp dermoscopy in the diagnosis of alopecia areata incognita. J Am Acad Dermatol. 2008;59:64-7.
123. Tosti A. Dermoscopy of hair and scalp disorders with clinical and pathological correlations. Informa healthcare, Andover, Hampshire, UK 2007.

Value of Oral Supplementation Therapy

124. Ahrens J. Systemische Behandlung des diffusen Haarausfalls. Therapiewoche Schweiz. 1994;10:551-4.
125. Budde J, Tronnier H, Rahlfs VW, Frei-Kleiner S. Systemische Therapie von diffusem Effluvium und Haarstrukturschäden. Hautarzt. 1993;44:380-4.
126. D'Agostini F, Fiallo P, Pennisi TM, De Flora S. Chemoprevention of smoke-induced alopecia in mice by oral administration of L-cystine and vitamin B6. J Dermatol Sci. 2007;46:189-98.
127. Frenkel MJ, Gillepsie JM, Reis PJ. Factors influencing the biosynthesis of the tyrosine-rich proteins of wool. Aust J Biol Sci. 1974;27:31-8.
128. Gillespie JM, Reis PJ. Dietary regulated biosynthesis of high-sulfur wool proteins. Bioche. J. 1966;98:669-77.
129. Gummer CL. Diet and hair loss. Semin Dermatol. 1985;4:35-9.
130. Lengg N, Heidecker B, Seifert B, Trüeb RM. Dietary supplement increases anagen hair rate in women with telogen effluvium: results of a double-blind placebo-controlled trial. Therapy. 2007;4:59-65.
131. Petri H, Perchalla P, Tronnier H. Die Wirksamkeit einer medikamentösen Therapie bei Haarstrukturschäden und diffusen Effluvien-vergleichende Doppelblindstudie. Schweiz Rundsch Med Prax. 1990;79:1457-62.
132. Reis PJ, Tunks DA, Sharry LF. Plasma amino acid patterns in sheep receiving abomasal infusions of methionine and cystine. Aust J Biol Sci. 1973;26:635-44.
133. Rushton DH. Nutritional factors and hair loss. Clin Exp Dermatol. 2002;27:396-404.

Treatment of Female Androgenetic Alopecia

134. Avram MR, Rogers NE. The use of low-level light for hair growth: part I. J Cosmet Laser Ther. 2009;11:110-7.
135. Blume-Peytavi U, Hillmann K, Dietz E, et al. A randomized, single-blind trial of 5% minoxidil foam once daily versus 2% minoxidil solution twice daily in the treatment of androgenetic alopecia in women. J Am Acad Dermatol. 2011;65:1126-34.
136. Blume-Peytavi U, Kunte C, Krisp A, et al. Comparison of the efficacy and safety of topical minoxidil and topical alfatradiol in the treatment of androgenetic alopecia in women. J Dtsch Dermatol Ges. 2007;5:391-5.
137. Carmina E, Lobo RA. Treatment of hyperandrogenic alopecia in women. Fertility and Sterility. 2003;79:91-5.
138. DeVillez RL, Jacobs JP, Szpunar CA, Warner ML. Androgenetic alopecia in the female. Treatment with 2% topical minoxidil solution. Arch Dermatol. 1994;130:303-7.
139. Iorizzo M, Vincenzi C, Voudouris S, et al. Finasteride treatment of female pattern hair loss. Arch Dermatol. 2006;142:298-302.
140. Jacobs JP, Szpunar CA, Warner ML. Use of topical minoxidil therapy for androgenetic alopecia in women. Int J Dermatol. 1993;32:758-62.

141. Leavitt M, Charles G, Heyman E, Michaels D. HairMax LaserComb laser phototherapy device in the treatment of male androgenetic alopecia: A randomized, double-blind, sham device-controlled, multicentre trial. Clin Drug Investig. 2009;29:283-92.
142. Lucky AW, Piacquadio DJ, Ditre CM, et al. A randomized, placebo-controlled trial of 5% and 2% topical minoxidil solutions in the treatment of female pattern hair loss. J Am Acad Dermatol. 2004;50:541-53.
143. Moltz L, Schwartz U, Hammerstein J. Clinical use of antiandrogens in the female. Gynakologe. 1980;13:1-17.
144. Olsen EA. Topical minoxidil in the treatment of androgenetic alopecia in women. Cutis. 1991;48:243-8.
145. Price VH. Treatment of hair loss. N Engl J Med. 1999;341: 964-73.
146. Price VH, Menefee E. Quantitative estimation of hair growth. I. androgenetic alopecia in women: effect of minoxidil. J Invest Dermatol. 1990;95:683-7.
147. Price VH, Roberts JL, Hordinsky M, et al. Lack of efficacy of finasteride in postmenopausal women with androgenetic alopecia. J Am Acad Dermatol. 2000;43:768-7.
148. Rushton DH, Futterweit W, Kingsley D, et al. Quantitative assessment of spironolactone treatment in women with diffuse androgen-dependent alopecia. J Soc Cosmet Chem. 1991;42:317-25.
149. Sawaya ME, Shapiro J. Androgenetic alopecia. New approved and unapproved treatments. Dermatol Clinics. 2000;18:47-61.
150. Shum KW, Cullen DR, Messenger AG. Hair loss in women with hyperandrogenism: four cases responding to finasteride. J Am Acad Dermatol. 2002;47:733-9.
151. Sinclair R, Wewerinke M, Jolley D. Treatment of female pattern hair loss with oral antiandrogens. Br J Dermatol. 2005;152:466-73.
152. Trüeb RM; Swiss Trichology Study Group. Finasteride treatment of patterned hair loss in normoandrogenic postmenopausal women. Dermatology. 2004;209:202-7.
153. Vexiau P, Chaspoux C, Boudou P, et al. Effects of minoxidil 2% vs. cyproterone acetate treatment on female androgenetic alopecia: a controlled, 12-month randomized trial. Br J Dermatol. 2002;146:992-9.
154. Whiting DA, Jacobson C. Treatment of female androgenetic alopecia with minoxidil 2%. Int J Dermatol. 1992;31:800-4.
155. Whiting DA, Waldstreicher J, Sanchez M, Kaufman KD. Measuring reversal of hair miniaturization in androgenetic alopecia by follicular counts in horizontal sections of serial scalp biopsies: results of finasteride 1 mg treatment of men and postmenopausal women. J Invest Dermatol Symp Proc. 1999;4:282-4.

Value of Hair Care

156. Bouillon C. Shampoos. Clin Dermatol. 1996;14:113-21.
157. Rushton H, Gummer CL, Flasch H. 2-in-1 shampoo technology: state of the art shampoo and conditioner in one. Skin Parmacology. 1994;7:78-83.
158. Shapiro J, Maddin S. Medicated shampoos. Clin Dermatol. 1996;14:123-8.
159. Sinclair R. Healthy hair: what is it? J Invest Dermatol Symp Proc. 2007;12:2-5.
160. Trüeb RM. Dermocosmetic aspects of hair and scalp. J Investig Dermatol Sympos Proc. 2005;10:289-92.
161. Trüeb RM. Shampoos: ingredients, efficacy and adverse effects. J Dtsch Dermatol Ges. 2007;5:356-65.
162. Urbano CC. 50 years of hair care development. Cosmet Toiletries. 1995;110:85-104.

Autologous Hair Transplantation

163. Unger WP, Unger RH. Hair transplanting: an important but often forgotten treatment for female pattern hair loss. J Am Acad Dermatol. 2003;49:853-60.

Psychological Counseling

164. Neumann M, Scheffer C, Tauschel D, Lutz G, Wirtz M, Edelhäuser F. Physician empathy: Definition, outcome-relevance and its measurement in patient care and medical education. GMS Z Med Ausbild. 2012;29:Doc11.
165. Teutsch C. Patient-doctor communication. Med Clin North Am. 2003;87:1115-45.
166. Trüeb RM, Swiss Trichology Study Group. Interaction between the medical profession, hairdressers and the media in the management of hair loss. Hautarzt. 2000;51:729-32.

13

Telogen Effluvium

Neelima Sharma, S Sacchidanand

"Acute disease is an act of god, of chronic disease the patient himself is the author."

—*Thomas Sydenham*

Definition

Telogen effluvium (TE), the term first coined in 1961 by Kligman, is a form of non-scarring alopecia characterized by diffuse scalp hair thinning in response to a trigger that causes abnormal hair cycling with a premature conversion of anagen follicles to telogen follicles.[1-3]

As TE is a reactive process, it should be considered a medical sign, and the cause diligently looked for.[2,4]

Burden

As many cases of TE are subclinical, the true incidence in the community is not known. However, it is the most common cause of diffuse hair loss for which an individual often seeks treatment.[5] TE can occur at any age. Most of the adults experience an episode of TE at some point in their life time. TE is likely the most common cause of hair loss in children.[6] Even infants in the first months of life often experience an episode of TE.[4]

The TE can occur in either sex, however as postpartum state is a common trigger, women experience it more often as compared to men. Also, women find hair shedding more troublesome than men, thus more women seek treatment **(Box 13.1)**.[4]

Box 13.1: Epidemiology

- One of the leading causes of diffuse hair loss
- Physiological: Postpartum, early infancy
- Women more affected than men

Impact on the Individual

Though TE is a benign self-limiting condition, it has a substantial psychological impact on those affected. Hair loss provokes anxiety and distress (more profound than its objective severity would appear to justify) leading to a reduction of quality of life and secondary morbidity. It has been observed that in some individuals, the psychological burden of hair loss may be similar to that caused by severe chronic or life-threatening diseases.[7]

Triggers

A wide variety of triggers are known to incite TE **(Table 13.1)**. In approximately one-third of cases, it is not possible to identify the precipitating event.[5]

Physiological Condition

Postpartum Effluvium (Box 13.2)

Postpartum TE, also known as telogen gravidarum, is a universal phenomenon that occurs 2 to 4 months after child birth but it is often subclinical.[8,9] The prevalence of postpartum TE is higher in multiparas, in women giving birth after 38 weeks of gestational age, with cesarean section delivery, and in women who gain more weight during pregnancy.[3] Most cases of postpartum TE resolve, with regrowth being visible by 6 months; however, persistent shedding may be experienced by some women resulting in diffuse alopecia. This is because after pregnancy some hairs may not revert to an asynchronous growth pattern seen in normal adult hair follicles.[9] In such patients, female pattern hair loss has to be ruled out, as postpartum TE can unmask androgenetic alopecia.[2]

Table 13.1: Causes of telogen effluvium

❑ Physiological conditions	❑ Postpartum effluvium ❑ TE with prolonged breastfeeding ❑ Newborn alopecia
❑ Dietary triggers	❑ Protein-calorie restriction: Weight loss diets such as crash diets, chronic starvation ❑ Fatty acid deficiency: Malabsorption, deficient intake ❑ Trace element deficiencies: Iron, zinc, copper ❑ Vitamin deficiencies: Biotin, vitamin D, C, B_{12}, folate
❑ Stress	❑ Febrile illness ❑ Chronic illness such as malignancy, systemic lupus erythematosus, hepatic failure, renal failure, HIV, etc. ❑ Major surgery ❑ Major trauma ❑ Psychological stress
❑ Endocrine dysfunction	❑ Hypo or hyperthyroidism
❑ Inflammatory scalp disease	❑ Seborrheic dermatitis ❑ Contact dermatitis ❑ Psoriasis
❑ Drugs and supplements	❑ Androgens ❑ Anticoagulants especially heparin ❑ Anticonvulsants such as valproic acid and carbamazepine ❑ Antidepressants such as selective serotonin reuptake inhibitors ❑ Anthelmintic such as albendazole ❑ Antipsychotics such as lithium ❑ Angiotensin-converting enzyme inhibitors such as captopril and enalapril ❑ Azoles such as fluconazole and ketaconazole in large doses ❑ Beta-blockers such as propranolol ❑ Cytostatic agents in low doses ❑ Dopamine agonists such as bromocriptine ❑ Estrogen antagonists such as tamoxifen ❑ Hormone replacement therapy ❑ Minoxidil ❑ Oral contraceptive pills – Changing or discontinuation of oral contraceptives – Intake of oral contraceptives with androgenic progesterones, testosterone, or depot progesterone ❑ Retinoids ❑ Statins ❑ Vaccines such as bivalent human papilloma virus (HPV) vaccine
❑ Intoxication	❑ Thallium ❑ Mercury ❑ Arsenic ❑ Gold

Box 13.2: Telogen gravidarum

- Postpartum telogen effluvium occurs 2 to 4 months after child birth due to failure of hairs to revert to asynchronous growth pattern
- Risk group: Multiparous, women giving birth after 38 weeks gestational age, with cesarean section delivery, and women who gain more weight during pregnancy
- Subclinical; regrowth being visible by 6 months

TE with Prolonged Breastfeeding

In women who prolong breastfeeding, the shedding following childbirth may persist and become chronic. The factors implicated in persistence of hair shedding include reduction in estrogen levels, elevated prolactin levels, and deficiency of iron, zinc, biotin and fatty acids.[2]

Newborn Alopecia (Figures 13.1 and 13.2)

Newborns may experience a physiological form of telogen effluvium, which may present as diffuse hair loss or neonatal occipital alopecia, 2 to 3 months after birth. During embryogenesis, the development of hair follicles on the fetal scalp begins in the 3rd month of gestation. By 5th month of gestation, the whole scalp is covered with anagen hair. At about 7 to 8 months of gestation, the hair follicles enter telogen phase and the first hairs may be shed in utero. However, often, the newborn retains the hair until birth. After birth these hair abruptly enter telogen phase and are shed. Hair follicles gradually return to anagen phase, producing pigmented terminal hair.[10]

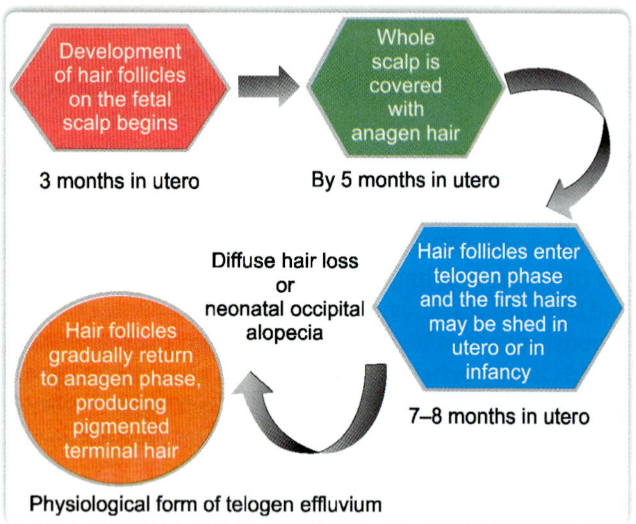

Fig. 13.1: Schematic representation of pathophysiology of newborn alopecia

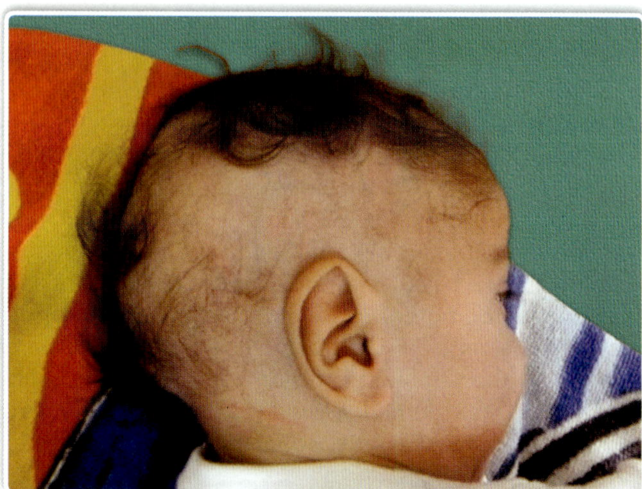

Fig. 13.2: Neonatal occipital alopecia (*Courtesy:* Department of Dermatology, STD and Leprosy, BMCRI, Bengaluru)

Dietary Triggers

Nutritional deficiencies, especially protein, calorie, fatty acids and trace elements, can contribute to increased hair shedding by weakening hair shafts that cause breakage to the hair and slow regrowth. Hair problems that are caused by nutritional deficiencies can be corrected by a proper diet.[5]

Protein-Calorie Restrictions

Chronic starvation (illness-related, marasmus, kwashiorkor), conditions associated with negative nitrogen balance and crash diets cause protein-calorie deficiency. This is known to induce diffuse telogen hair loss. If not corrected, the diameter, size and density of hair follicles diminishes, thereby making the hair thin and fine **(Figure 13.3)**. In long-standing cases, trichodystrophies have been described, with the hair becoming sparse, fragile, short, fine, and light-colored.[2,8]

Fatty Acid Deficiency

Malabsorption syndromes, pancreatic disease, chronic illness, inadequate intake and parenteral nutrition result in fatty acid deficiencies that may precipitate telogen hair shedding.[8] In addition, the hair becomes dry, fragile and light colored.[2]

Iron Deficiency

Iron deficiency is the world's most common nutritional deficiency. It can manifest with or without anemia. Deficient dietary intake is the most common cause in both sexes, with menorrhagia being an additional causative factor in women.[11] Several published studies suggests a relationship between iron deficiency and hair loss. Iron deficiency anemia has been reported in as many as 72% of women presenting with diffuse telogen hair loss, and the patients treated with oral iron had regrowth of their hair associated with normalization of their iron stores. Nearly 90% of women with anemia have diffuse telogen hair loss.[12] The relationship between iron deficiency with no anemia or only mild anemia and chronic diffuse hair loss is, however, more complex and controversial. Serum ferritin concentration is an indicator of the status of iron stores and has a greater predictive value than other tests of iron status, such as transferrin saturation and erythrocyte zinc protoporphyrin.[12] Some studies have shown that serum ferritin concentrations may be a factor in diffuse hair loss in non anemic, iron deficient women. The mean ferritin levels in patients with TE were found to be statistically significantly lower than levels in women without hair loss.[5] Other studies however, report no direct relationship between low serum ferritin and hair loss. These studies refute the usefulness of serum ferritin in the routine investigation of women with chronic diffuse telogen hair loss.[5]

The possible explanations of effect of iron on hair growth, and loss of telogen hair in iron deficiency could be **(Figure 13.4)**.[5,12]

- Being the most rapidly proliferating cells in the body, the hair follicle matrix cells have lower levels of ferritin and higher levels of free iron.
- Iron is required as a cofactor for ribonucleotide reductase, the rate-limiting enzyme for DNA synthesis. Iron depletion could prevent proper function of this enzyme, resulting in inhibition of proliferation.

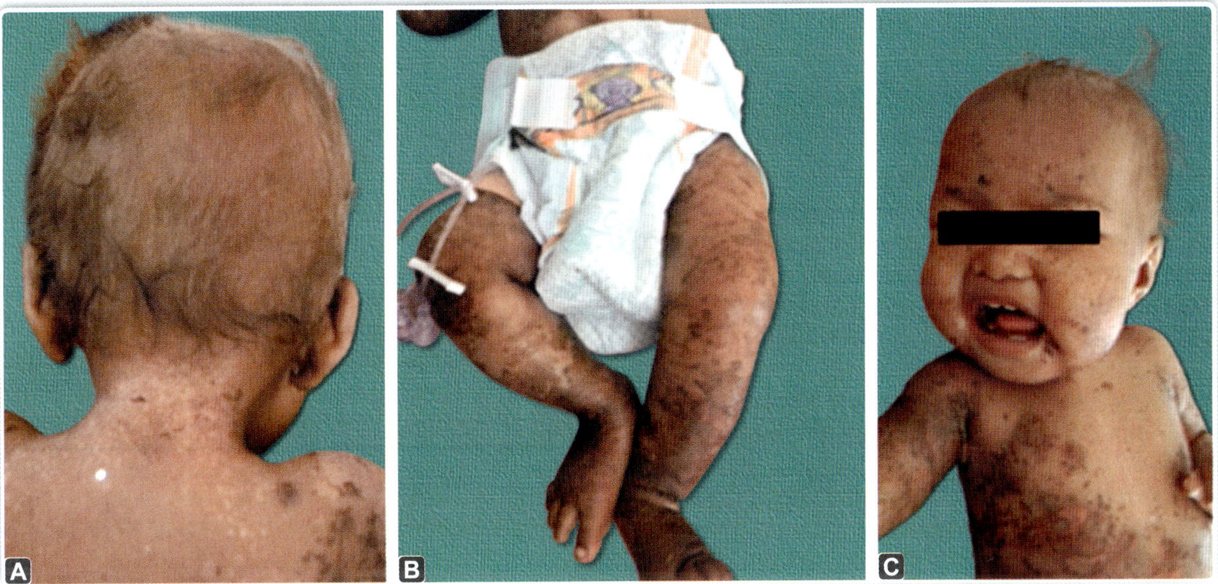

Figs 13.3A to C: Child with protein energy malnutrition: (A) Diffuse hair loss; (B) Flaky paint dermatosis; (C) Irritable child (*Courtesy:* Department of Dermatology, STD and Leprosy, BMCRI, Bengaluru)

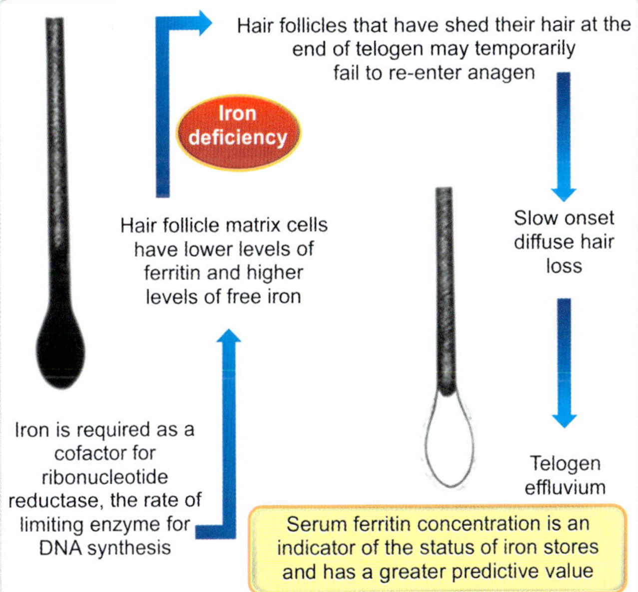

Fig. 13.4: Schematic representation of proposed role of iron in telogen effluvium

- The hair follicles that have shed their hair at the end of telogen may temporarily fail to re-enter anagen leading to a slow onset diffuse hair loss.

Zinc Deficiency

Zinc is a mineral that promotes cell reproduction, tissue growth and repair. It also acts in the maintenance of the sebaceous glands attached to hair follicles. Zinc deficiency, both congenital and acquired, may cause hair loss, and lead to sparse, dry and brittle hair.[5] Low levels of zinc can be associated with reduced absorption of unsaturated fatty acids and impaired metabolism. The acquired zinc deficiency is mainly due to dietary restriction, parenteral nutrition, excessive iron supplementation, and vitamin A deficiency.[2] As with iron, the relationship between zinc deficiency and telogen effluvium is controversial. Some studies found no evidence to support low serum zinc concentrations in the TE patients. The low zinc levels found on routine screening of patients with diffuse telogen hair loss is probably an incidental finding. Hence, diffuse hair shedding with no other symptoms or signs is never due to zinc deficiency.[5]

Copper Deficiency

Copper is a trace mineral that is essential for the formation of hemoglobin and is needed to carry oxygen in red blood cells. Copper deficiency can weaken the hair shaft and cause increased hair shedding.[5]

Biotin Deficiency

Biotin is an essential vitamin that complements hair and nail growth. Biotin deficiency is reported with pregnancy, prolonged breastfeeding, parenteral nutrition, and excessive raw egg white ingestion.[2] Biotin deficiency can result in alopecia, but this is a very rare cause of hair loss.[8]

Vitamin D Deficiency

Vitamin D is an essential vitamin in cell growth. Studies have shown that low vitamin D3, can induce follicular cycling alteration and produce TE.[2,8]

Other vitamins implicated in TE include folate, vitamin B_{12} and vitamin C. These help in effective utilization of iron **(Box 13.3)**.

Stress

Stress such as febrile illness, chronic systemic illness, surgery, trauma, hemorrhage, and emotional stress are known to trigger TE. Hair loss in turn may cause stress, inducing a self-perpetuating vicious cycle.[7]

Animal studies have shown stress to exert profound hair growth inhibitory, catagen-inducing and hair-damaging pro-inflammatory effects.[7] Studies have shown that stress inhibits murine hair follicle keratinocyte proliferation, prematurely induces intrafollicular keratinocyte apoptosis and hair follicle regression (catagen), and triggers mast cell-dependent neurogenic inflammation.[13] These effects are modulated predominantly by substance P and nerve growth factors. The other mediators include corticotropin releasing hormone, catecholamines, prolactin, adrenocorticotropic hormone (ACTH), beta-endorphins, glucocorticoids, etc. Hair follicle has been identified as the prominent peripheral target organ for these mediators. In addition, the hair follicles can itself generate many stress mediators and express cognate receptors, resulting in local modulation of stress response, possible as a part of skin stress system.[7]

Human studies have shown expression of cognate receptors (NK1) on the gene and protein level, hair growth inhibition and premature catagen induction by substance P, downregulation of NK1, and up-regulation of substance P-degrading enzymes in the hair follicle epithelium. Hence, the possible mechanisms by which the stress mediators especially substance P inhibits hair growth in humans include **(Figure 13.5)**.[13]

- Downregulation of pro-proliferative signaling in hair follicle keratinocytes
- Deleterious neurogenic inflammation induced by activation of perifollicular mast cells
- Activation of catagen-inductive growth factor cascades
- Enhanced immune attack on the no longer immune-privileged hair follicle epithelium.

Endocrine Dysfunction

Nearly 18 to 50% of women having either hypothyroidism or hyperthyroidism experience diffuse telogen hair loss that is usually reversible once the euthyroid state is restored. However, it has to be noted that treatment of thyroid dysfunction would initially cause profound telogen shedding.[2]

Inflammatory Scalp Diseases

Inflammatory disorders of the scalp such as dandruff, seborrheic dermatitis, psoriasis and contact dermatitis are known to trigger TE. They may precede or accompany telogen effluvium. Though the exact pathogenesis is not known, microinflammation of the hair follicle and cytokine release during inflammatory process may be responsible for hair shedding.[8,14,15]

Drugs and Supplements

A variety of drugs have been implicated in TE **(Table 13.1)**. It is, however, important to establish the temporal association between the onset of hair loss and commencement/change of dose of medication. Drug-induced TE begins about 12 weeks after starting the drug and continues while on the drug. As there are many triggers for TE as already discussed, a thorough exclusion of these potential confounders is necessary before the hair loss can be blamed on the medication.[8,16]

Box 13.3: Micronutrients implicated in telogen effluvium

- Iron
- Zinc
- Biotin
- Copper
- Folate
- Vitamins D, B_{12} and C

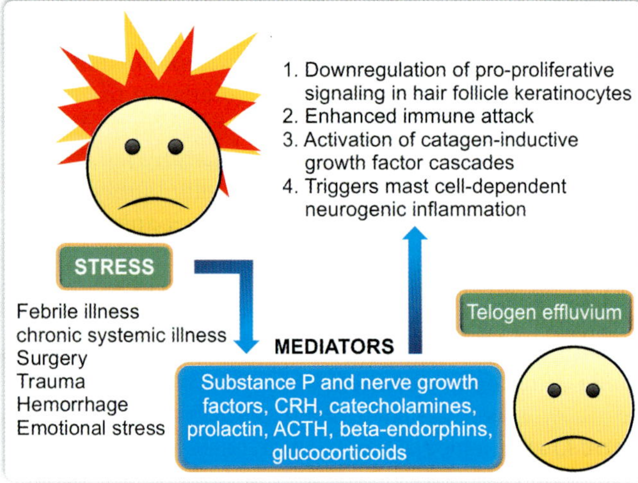

Fig. 13.5: Schematic representation of role of stress in telogen effluvium

Pathogenesis

The asynchronous growth pattern of the scalp hair is well established. Hence, it is normal to shed 25 to 100 hairs daily. Any alteration of the hair growth cycle manifests as increased shedding of scalp hair. In TE, the excessive shedding occurs due to a premature conversion of anagen follicles to telogen follicles, with the primary insult being at the level of dermal papillae. It is observed that nearly 7% to 25% of anagen follicles convert into telogen follicles **(Figure 13.6)**.[2]

In chronic or long-standing cases, the anagen cycle gradually shortens resulting in thinner and shorter hair. As regeneration is determined by the bulge area, the inciting event that involves the bulge area will affect regeneration.[2]

Classification

There are 2 ways of classifying TE: Functionally **(Box 13.4)** and clinically.

Functional Classification

Based on the changes in different phases of hair cycles, TE is classified into 5 functional types:[9]

1. *Immediate anagen release:* In this, the follicles are stimulated to leave the anagen phase and enter the telogen phase prematurely. This is seen following physiological stress and drug intake. This is short lasting, and reversal occurs with return of normal hair cycling.
2. *Delayed anagen release:* This is responsible for TE occurring in the postpartum period, as during pregnancy the follicles remain in prolonged anagen phase rather than cycling into the telogen phase. Following delivery there is a telogen conversion of large number of follicles resulting in increased shedding.
3. *Short anagen syndrome:* This is characterized by shortening of anagen phase and persistent shedding of telogen hair. This is responsible for chronic telogen effluvium, where the cause cannot be identified.
4. *Immediate telogen release:* This occurs due to shortening of telogen phase, with release of club hairs, as the follicles are stimulated to re-enter anagen phase. The effluvium seen after use of minoxidil is due to immediate telogen release.
5. *Delayed telogen release:* This occurs after a prolonged telogen phase followed by transition to anagen phase.

Clinical Classification

Clinically, TE can be classified as acute TE, and chronic telogen hair loss.

The symptom of TE is increased shedding and development of diffuse alopecia over period of several months. Patients with TE usually present with an increased number of hairs in their hairbrush or shower. Though the scalp hair is often involved, patients may also complain of thinning of hair in other body areas such as axilla and

Box 13.4: Functional classification of telogen effluvium

1. Immediate anagen release
2. Delayed anagen release
3. Short anagen syndrome
4. Immediate telogen release
5. Delayed telogen release

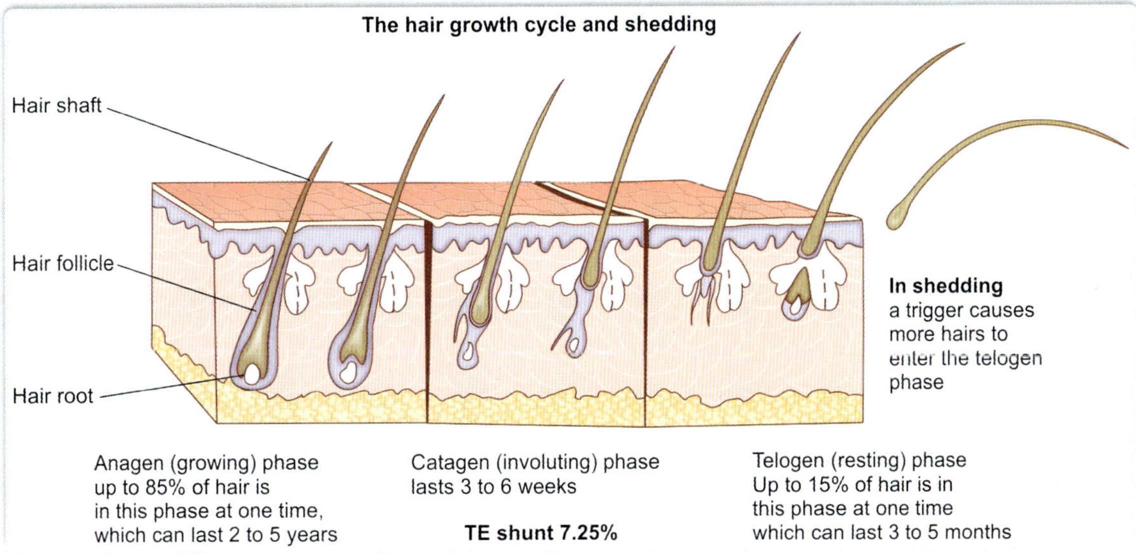

Fig. 13.6: Hair growth and shedding

legs.[2,17] In most of the cases, if the triggers are managed, the hair follicles can recover.[18] It is common for a patient of TE to complain of scalp dysesthesia or a sensation of "pain in the hair", i.e. trichodynia, which often coexists with psychopathologic findings, such as depression and anxiety.[19]

1. ***Acute telogen effluvium***
   Acute TE or classical TE is a self-limiting condition characterized by an abrupt onset of diffuse generalized shedding of telogen hairs. Nearly 100 to 1000 hairs may be lost every day. If the condition persists for only a short time, then thinning is not seen. If large numbers of hair are shed, then the patient may notice generalized reduction in hair density. Complete baldness however does not occur.[18]
   It is important to establish a connect between the triggering event and shedding. Acute TE usually starts 2 weeks after a trigger, peaks between 6–8 weeks and then tapers off, if the trigger is removed or treated. Spontaneous regrowth is not visible for 4–6 months.[2]
2. ***Chronic telogen hair loss***
   Chronic telogen hair loss refers to telogen hair shedding persisting for longer than 6 months. There are 2 variants of chronic telogen hair loss.
   a. *Chronic diffuse telogen hair loss* **(Figures 13.7 and 13.8)**
   This always results from either prolonged sequential or repetitive triggers. The shedding is less pronounced as compared to that observed with acute TE.[8] In long-standing cases, the hair regrowth is diminished leading to chronic diffuse alopecia.[2] To be a true cause of chronic diffuse telogen hair loss, it is vital to establish the relationship between the trigger and the hair loss. It is important to rule out other causes of increased shedding and diffuse alopecia, especially androgenetic alopecia. Among the various causes, thyroid abnormalities including hypo and hyperthyroidism, and nutritional deficiencies particularly iron, zinc, protein and essential fatty acid deficiencies are often responsible for chronic diffuse telogen hair loss.[12, 18]
   b. *Chronic telogen effluvium*
   Chronic TE is a primary, idiopathic and often self-limiting condition first described in 1996 by David Whiting. It is characterized by an abrupt onset of excessive, alarming, diffuse, generalized shedding of hair in women aged 30–60 years; though there are occasional reports of it being diagnosed in men.[18,20] The patient often gives a history of ability to grow their hair very long in childhood, and report a high hair density prior to the onset of hair loss. They complain of shedding chunks of hair during shampooing, combing, on floor and pillow, and

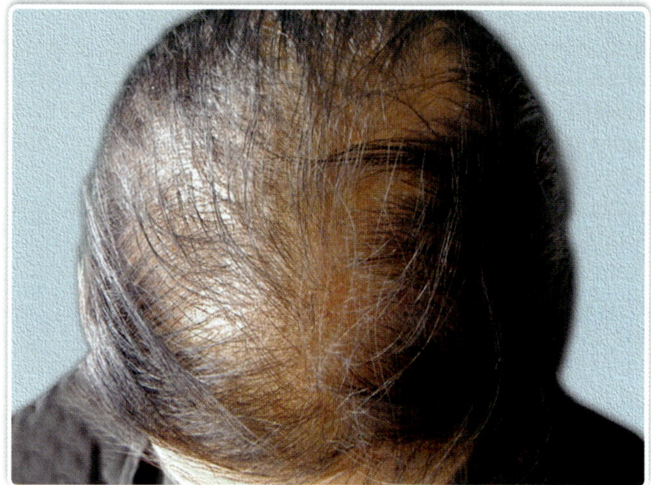

Fig. 13.7: Chronic telogen effluvium
(*Courtesy:* Department of Dermatology, STD and Leprosy, BMCRI, Bengaluru)

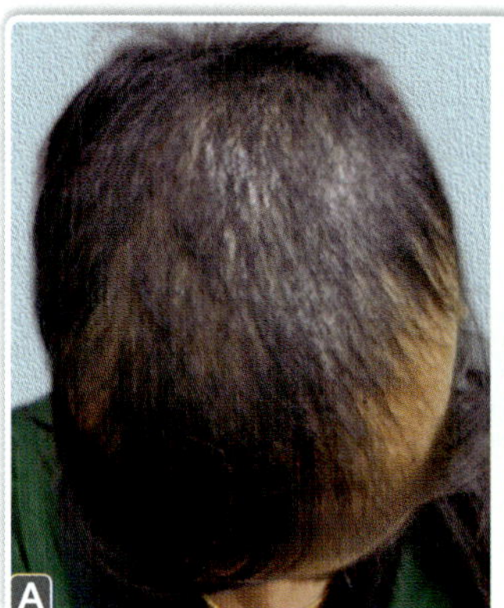

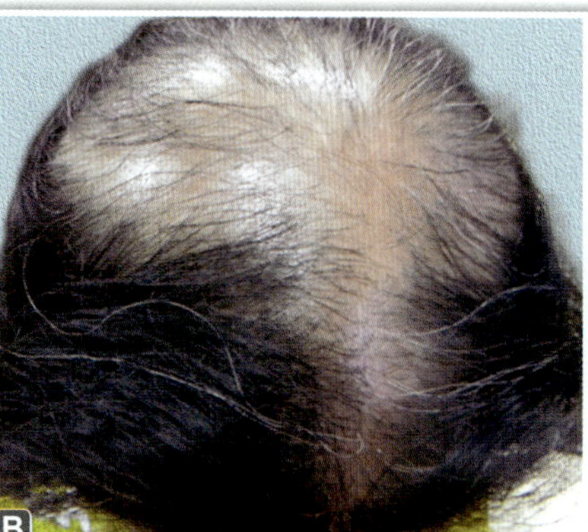

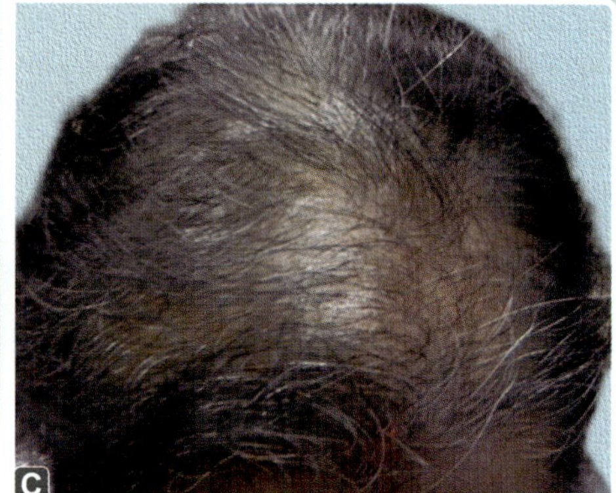

Figs 13.8A to C: (A) Chronic diffuse telogen effluvium; (B and C) Female pattern hair loss **(Refer Table 13.3)**
(*Courtesy:* Department of Dermatology, STD and Leprosy, BMCRI, Bengaluru)

may bring a hand full of hair to corroborate the complaint of excessive shedding. Though there is no obvious diffuse thinning or visible widening of the central parting line or miniaturization, many women do notice a reduction in the volume of their braid thickness. Moderate to severe bitemporal recession may be seen. Chronic TE runs a prolonged fluctuating course that spans over several years. It may resolve spontaneously in 3–10 years. In order to diagnose chronic TE, ruling out causes of chronic diffuse hair loss, including androgenetic alopecia is a must.[1, 18]

Diagnosis

A detailed history that includes time of onset, duration of shedding, estimation of percentage of thinning, identification of triggers and their temporal relation to hair loss is vital in diagnosing TE.[8]

Physical Examination

Scalp Examination

Examination of scalp for features of dandruff and other inflammatory conditions is essential. A Wood's lamp examination would help in identification of scaling and presence of pityrosporum.[2] A dermatoscope (trichoscope) could be used to visualize the scalp skin and hair. Empty follicles and numerous short regrowing hairs of normal thickness (>0.03 mm) are the most common findings in TE. The dermatoscopic diagnosis of chronic telogen effluvium is based on exclusion rather than fulfillment of specific trichoscopic criteria. The critical feature is the presence of less than 20% hair diameter variability **(Figure 13.9)**.[21]

Examination of other body areas for hair loss needs to be done. Nail examination could give a clue to the time of the triggering event or onset of the TE. Beau's lines, especially on the thumb and great toenail, can indicate a thinning of the nail plate in response to a stress such as medical illness, fever, and surgery. Pallor and koilonychia is a sign of anemia. Thickening of the nail, convex nail and onycholysis is indicative of thyroid disease.[2]

Assessment of Hair Shedding

Hair Collection

In this, the patient is asked to collect shed hair daily for two weeks. A morning collection done during hair grooming is usually simplest. These hairs are then counted and examined. The interpretation is described in **Table 13.2.**[2]

Hair Pull Test

The hair pull test helps to determine the ongoing activity and severity of hair loss. In TE, the hair pull test is strongly positive on the entire scalp (including occiput), with more than 10% telogen hair being extracted, especially if the patient has not shampooed the hairs for more than 24 hours. Recent shampooing or vigorous combing gives rise to a false negative hair pull test. Hence, it is advisable to ask the patient not to wash the hair, preferably for 5 days or at least 2 days prior to examination.[2,18]

Trichogram

About 50 hairs are plucked using a rubber-tipped forceps, and examined under the microscope. This test provides

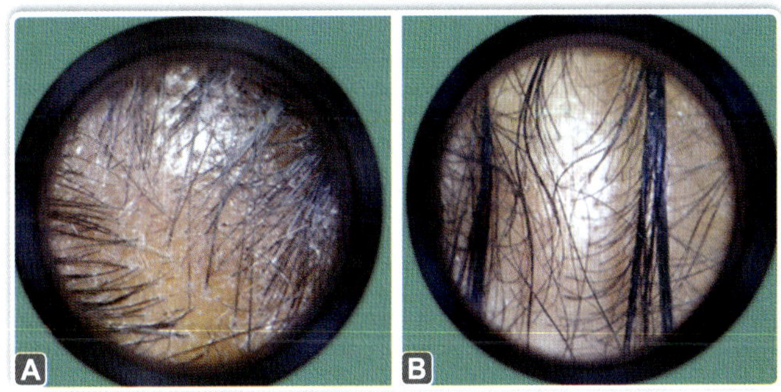

Figs 13.9A and B: Dermoscopic appearance in telogen effluvium (A) Perifollicular fibrosis; (B) Varied diameter of the shaft without increased miniaturized hairs
(*Courtesy:* Department of Dermatology, STD and Leprosy, BMCRI, Bengaluru)

Table 13.2: Interpretation of hair collection

Amount and type of hair	*Interpretation*
Collection of > 100 club hairs/day	Telogen effluvium
Collection of hairs > 100 hairs/day with many hairs being < 3 cm with distal tapering	Telogen hair loss associated with androgenetic alopecia
Collection of < 100 hairs/day	Androgenetic alopecia
Collection of dystrophic telogen hair with an adherent epithelial envelope	Telogen hair loss due to cytotoxic drug or alopecia areata
Normal telogen hair with adherent epithelial envelop	Inflammatory alopecia such as lichen planopilaris or tinea capitis or discoid lupus erythematosus

additional information, such as hair diameters and the anagen-telogen ratio. In TE, there is a significant reduction in anagen: Telogen ratio. Usually, >25% of the plucked hairs are telogen hairs in acute phase.[18]

Phototrichogram

In this, all hairs within 2 cm^2 area are trimmed 1 mm from the scalp skin surface and photographed on day 1, 3 and 7 to assess the rate of hair growth, hair density and rate of shedding.

Wash test

After a 5-day abstention from shampooing, the patients wash and rinse their hair in a basin whose hole is covered by gauze to entrap the lost hairs. Hairs are then collected in a paper envelope and examined. Counting of total number of telogen hairs and vellus hairs (≤ 3 cm) has been reported as a good tool to differentiate between chronic TE and female pattern hair loss.[2,18]

Laboratory Work-up

Tests in TE need to be ordered based on the patient's history and clinical findings. The preliminary investigations include complete blood count, serum ferritin levels, erythrocyte sedimentation rate (ESR), thyroid screen (TSH, T3, T4, and if needed microsomal antibodies), serum vitamin D levels and serum zinc levels.[2] Ferritin levels below 60 ng/mL with normal erythrocyte sedimentation rate (ESR) present high specificity and predictive value (> 90%) for iron deficiency. As ferritin is an acute-phase protein, the levels may be normal, despite the individual having iron deficiency, in inflammation or infection; hence interpretation should always be done taking the ESR into consideration.[4,22]

The extended laboratory work-up would depend on the history, clinical findings and results of the preliminary tests. Vitamin B_{12} levels may have to be assessed, and gastroenterology work-up done in cases of malabsorption. If metabolic syndrome or renal or liver disease is suspected, a comprehensive metabolic panel would have to be done. If the history and physical examination suggest lupus erythematosus or syphilis, serologic testing can be ordered. If features of hyperandrogenism are present or if a hormonal cause for TE is suspected, then an androgen screen (free testosterone levels, dehydroepiandrosterone sulfate (DHEAS), estradiol, prolactin, FSH, LH, 17-OH progesterone) has to be performed.[2,8]

Scalp Biopsy

Scalp biopsy is indicated when there is lack of identifiable triggers, chronic hair loss, miniaturized hair shafts, and failure to exclude alopecia areata. Two 4-mm biopsy specimens are recommended to provide for adequate horizontal and vertical sectioning.[8] In TE, the biopsy shows normal histology except for an increase in the telogen follicles **(Figure13.10)**. The normal telogen count ranges from 6 to 13%. The proportion of normal telogen follicles in excess of 15% is suggestive of TE, while a level of 25% or more is considered definitive. There is no variation in the terminal: vellus ratio (normal 7:1), diameter of hair shaft, and sebaceous gland density. Usually, there is no evidence of inflammation or follicular fibrous tract in TE.[18,22]

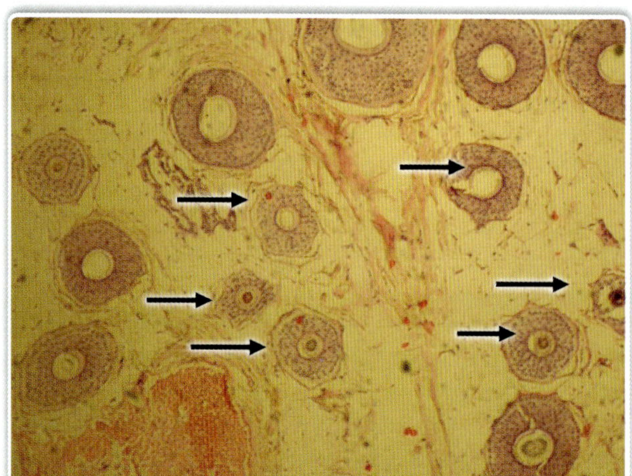

Fig. 13.10A: Histopathology showing increased miniaturized hair follicles in female pattern hair loss

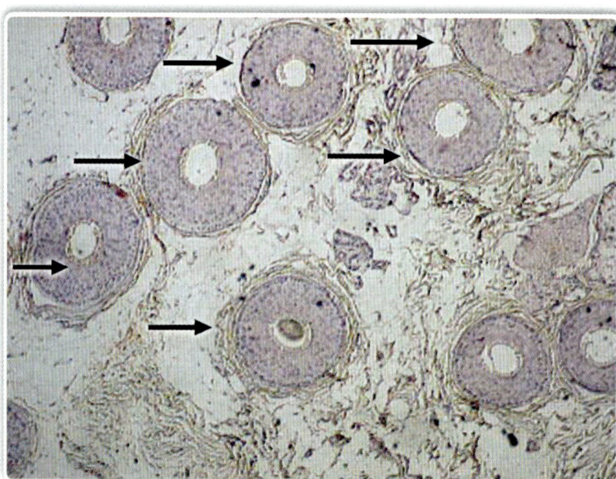

Fig. 13.10B: Histopathology showing numerous telogen hair follicles in telogen effluvium
(*Courtesy:* Department of Dermatology, STD and Leprosy, BMCRI, Bengaluru)

Differential Diagnosis

One of the most important differential diagnoses of TE is early androgenetic alopecia, as this can present with episodic telogen shedding before the distinctive pattern of hair loss is seen. In women, chronic TE needs to be differentiated from female pattern hair loss. In rare instances, diffuse alopecia areata may mimic TE.[8,18]

Table 13.3 lists the differentiating features of TE, chronic TE, female pattern hair loss and diffuse alopecia areata.[18,23]

Treatment

The most important aspects in the management of TE are patient education and removal/treatment/inhibition of triggers. Other topical and systemic agents have been tried with varying efficacy.

Patient Education

Patient education forms a key part of management of TE. The education should include understanding of normal hair cycle, the relationship between triggers and timing of hair loss, and natural history of TE. A diary could be maintained to identify the triggers and patient should be instructed to record any stresses, medication intake or dose changes, and other triggers. It is important to explain to the patient that despite removal/treatment of triggers, increased shedding may continue for up to 6 months. Regrowth would be noticed 3 to 6 months after elimination of the triggers, but it may take 1 to 1.5 years for a cosmetically significant regrowth to appear.[8]

Management of Triggers

Nutritional deficiencies, thyroid disease, systemic illness, and infections, which are common triggers, should be treated. If a drug is suspected, then it should be stopped or changed.

Nutritional Supplement

As nutritional deficiency is one of the most common trigger of TE, balanced diet has to be advocated.[8] In patients with protein-calorie deficiency, protein supplementation has shown to improve the quality of hair. Among amino acid support, evidence is in favor of L-cystine, administration of which has shown to increase hair fiber diameter.[2] The role of essential amino acids in anemia is well known. L-lysine appears to play a role in iron and zinc uptake **(Box 13.5)**. Adding L-lysine (1.5–2 g/day) to existing iron supplementation has shown to result in a significant

Table 13.3: Differentiating features of TE, chronic TE, female pattern hair loss and diffuse alopecia areata

Features	*TE*	*Chronic TE*	*Female pattern hair loss*	*Diffuse alopecia areata*
Age on onset	Any age	30 to 60 years of age	Puberty or older	Any age
Onset	Abrupt	Abrupt	Gradual progressive	Abrupt, waxes and wanes
Hair shedding	Prominent	Alarming	Minimal or absent	Prominent
Possible cause or Association	Underlying trigger	Idiopathic	Multifactorial, hormones, polycystic ovarian disease	Autoimmune, thyroid disease
Appearance	Diffuse hair loss	Diffuse hair loss, reduced braid thickness, absence of widening of central parting line, moderate to severe bitemporal recession	Sparse hair in central scalp, widening of central parting line, patterned thinning	Thinning, abrupt bare patches, exclamation mark hairs, nail pitting
Hair pull test	Strongly positive throughout the scalp	Positive throughout the scalp in active phase	Usually negative	Positive
Microscope analysis	Telogen hair	Telogen hair	-	Dystrophic hair
Dermatoscopy	No variation in shaft diameter	No variation in shaft diameter, no miniaturization	Marked variation in shaft diameter, miniaturization present	Exclamatory mark hairs - tapered hairs with dark thick broken tips
Scalp biopsy	Increased telogen hair, normal terminal: Vellus ratio 7:1, no miniaturization	Increased telogen hair, normal terminal: Vellus ratio, no miniaturization	Low terminal: Vellus ratio < 4:1, miniaturization present	Peribulbar lymphocytic infiltrate (swarm of bees)

Box 13.5: L-lysine

- Has a role in iron and zinc uptake
- Increases hair fiber diameter
- Dosage 1.5–2 g/day to existing iron supplementation shown to result in a significant increase in the mean serum ferritin concentration

Box 13.6: Zinc supplementation and paradoxical hair loss

- High serum levels during supplementation can result in deficiency of copper, iron and calcium, leading to hairfall
- Recommended dose:
  - Children and infants is 0.5–1 mg of elemental zinc/kg/day
  - Adults 25–50 mg/day of elemental zinc

increase in the mean serum ferritin concentration.[24] In malabsorptions, correction of underlying cause and fatty acid supplements have shown to reverse TE.[8]

In iron deficiency, addition of iron rich diet and iron supplements has to be done. When on supplements, hemoglobin and ferritin have to be monitored regularly every 6 to 8 weeks. The target should be to achieve a hemoglobin level of >13g/dL and serum ferritin concentration ≥ 70 ng/mL with a normal ESR.[2,8,24] Vitamin C supplements could be given along with iron supplements to increase the absorption of iron. Alternatively, the patient may be instructed to take iron supplements with vitamin C rich foods such as citrus fruits, amla, guava, etc.

Biotin and zinc supplementation has shown to support hair regrowth in TE. The dose of biotin in TE is 3–5 mg per day. When used with zinc supplementation there is a complimentary hair growth effect.[2,8] Oral zinc supplements assist in iron absorption, and have anti-inflammatory and antiandrogenic activity. In zinc deficiency, the recommended dose in children and infants is 0.5–1 mg of elemental zinc/kg/day and in adults 25–50 mg/day of elemental zinc. It is important to regularly monitor zinc levels while supplementing as high serum levels can result in deficiency of copper, iron and calcium, leading to hair fall **(Box 13.6)**. It is not necessary to correct subclinical zinc deficiency, as zinc supplementation in this condition would not stop the increase shedding.[2,5]

In case of a diagnosed vitamin D deficiency, the recommendation is 50,000 IU once a week for 6 weeks for infants and children, and 50,000 IU once weekly for 8 weeks for adults.[25]

Treatment of Underlying Scalp Inflammation

Antifungal shampoos containing ketoconazole or zinc pyrithione have shown to partially reverse TE and enhance hair growth. If the seborrhea does not adequately respond to topical medications, then oral fluconazole or oral terbinafine could be used. If there is associated erythema and scalp inflammation, then anti-inflammatory agents such as topical steroids or topical calcineurin inhibitors (pimecrolimus, tacrolimus) need to be considered.[2]

Specific Treatments

TE being a self-limiting condition ideally may not need specific drug therapy for hair regrowth, however the psychological trauma from hair shedding should not be underestimated. It is, hence, advisable to adopt a treatment strategy to inhibit exogen, so that the hair shafts would be retained in the follicles until new hair growth occurs to an acceptable length.

Minoxidil

Topical minoxidil has been used in TE anticipating that it would prolong anagen phase, thus preventing the premature onset of catagen, which forms the basis of TE. Topical minoxidil should be avoided during lactation.[7,18]

Botanicals and Topical Supplements

Many botanical hair care and hair growth-promoter products containing vitamins, antioxidants, amino acids, proteins, and fatty acids claim to induce vasodilatation, angiogenesis and reduce inflammation. Herbal extracts of *Butea monosperma, Butea frondosa* and *Butea parviflora* inhibit hair follicular degeneration, extend the anagen phase of the hair growth cycle, prevent the massive apoptosis in the proximal hair bulb and help in the multiplication of hair fiber cells with the stimulation of anagen phase, reducing the catagen and telogen phases.[26] Treatment with these herbs has shown to improve the tensile strength of hair, mean number of hairs lost after one-minute combing, and hair follicle count in a selected shaved scalp area in TE.[27]

Some studies have shown that the combined use of a shampoo and hair lotion, formulated with vitamins and zinc, shortens the course of acute telogen effluvium.[5]

Growth Factors

The hair follicle undergoes a life-long cyclic transformation regulated by many growth factors. These include vascular endothelial growth factor (VEGF), epidermal growth factor (EGF), insulin like growth factor-1 (IGF-1), platelet derived growth factor–4 (PDGF -4) and fibroblast growth factor (FGF).[28] These growth factors could prevent dermal

BOX 13.7: Mechanism of action of growth factors

- Prevent dermal papilla apoptosis
- Prolong anagen phase
- Delay catagen and telogen

papilla apoptosis, prolong anagen phase, delay catagen and telogen, eventually reducing diffuse hair loss (most studies have been done in androgenetic alopecia) **(Box 13.7)**.[28]

For the management of TE, it is better to choose growth factors such as VEGF and PDGF-4 that promote vasodilatation and angiogenesis to maintain hair bulb vascularization, as the telogen phase is associated with disappearance of vascular network in hair dermal papilla.[29,30]

These growth factors can be obtained from autologous platelet rich plasma administration or commercially available preparations such as brevetted vegetal extract RTH16.[29,30]

Camouflage and Scalp Prosthesis

Variety of methods, such as hair styling, scalp prostheses such as hair extensions and fringes, and scalp coloring products such as tints, powders, lotions, and sprays could be used for diffuse alopecia.[2]

Surgery

Hair transplant is not an option for TE, as spontaneous regrowth often occur. However, it could be considered in patients with significant diffuse thinning.[4]

References

1. Messenger AG, de Berker DAR, Sinclair RD. Disorders of hair. In: Burns T, Breathnach S, Cox N, Griffiths C, editors. Rook's Textbook of Dermatology. 8th edn. Wiley-Blackwell. 2010;pp. 66.27-66.31.
2. Bergfeld WF. Telogen effluvium. In: McMichael ABJ, Hordinsky MK, editors. Hair and scalp diseases. Medical, surgical, and cosmetic treatments. Informa healthcare. 2008;pp. 119-135.
3. Seo HD, Chung BS, Choi KC, Shin BS. A clinical study of prevalence of telogen effluvium after childbirth. Korean J Dermatol. 2009;47(2):127-131.
4. Hughes ECW. Telogen Effluvium [Online]. 2012 Mar 27 [cited 2013 March 21]. Available from: URL: emedicine.medscape.com/article.
5. Hamad AMW, Said AF, Abd El Hamid AA. Role of some trace elements in the pathogenesis of telogen effluvium in Egyptian females. J Egypt Women Dermatol Soc. 2010;7:44-48.
6. Sardana K, Mahajan S, Sarkar R, Mendiratta V, Bhushan P, Koranne RV, et al. The spectrum of skin disease among Indian children. Ped Dermatol. 2009;26(1):6-13.
7. Hadshiew IM, Foitzik K, Arck PC, Paus R. Burden of hair loss: Stress and the underestimated psychosocial impact of telogen effluvium and androgenetic alopecia. J Invest Dermatol. 2004;123:455-457.
8. Harrison S, Bergfeld W. Diffuse hair loss: Its triggers and management. Cleveland Clin J Med. 2009;76:361-367.
9. Headington JT. Telogen effluvium. New concepts and review. Arch Dermatol. 1993;129(3):356-363.
10. Kim MS, Na CH, Choi H, Shin BS. Prevalence and factors associated with neonatal occipital alopecia: A retrospective study. Ann Dermatol. 2011;23(3):288-292.
11. Trost LB, Bergfeld WF, Calogeras E. The diagnosis and treatment of iron deficiency and its potential relationship to hair loss. J Am Acad Dermatol. 2006;54(5):824-44.
12. Sarkar P, Raghunatha H, Harish MR, Shashikumar BM. A case control study to determine the correlation between serum ferritin levels and chronic telogen effluvium in a tertiary hospital, Mandya. Biochemistry. 2013;4(2):1-7.
13. Peters EMJ, Liotiri S, Bodo´ E, Hagen E, Bı´ro´ T, Arck PC, et al. Probing the effects of stress mediators on the human hair follicle. Substance P holds central position. Am J Pathol. 2007;171:1872-1886.
14. Tosti A, Piraccini BM, van Neste DJ. Telogen effluvium after allergic contact dermatitis of the scalp. Arch Dermatol. 2001;137(2):187-90.
15. Piérard-Franchimont C, Petit L, Loussouarn G, Saint-Léger D, Piérard GE. The hair eclipse phenomenon: Sharpening the focus on the hair cycle chronobiology. Int J Cosmet Sci. 2003;25(6):295-9.
16. Patel M, Harrison S, Sinclair R. Drugs and hair loss. Dermatol Clin. 2013;31(1):67-73.
17. Mounsey AL, Reed SW. Diagnosing and treating hair loss. Am Fam Physician. 2009;80(4):356-362, 373-374.
18. Shrivastava SB. Diffuse hair loss in an adult female: Approach to diagnosis and management. Indian J Dermatol Venereol Leprol. 2009;75:20-8.
19. Baldari M, Montinari M, Guarrera M, Rebora A. Trichodynia is a distinguishing symptom of telogen effluvium. J Eur Acad Dermatol Venereol. 2009;23(6):733-4.
20. Thai KE, Sinclair RD. Chronic telogen effluvium in a man. J Am Acad Dermatol. 2002;47(4):605-7.
21. Miteva M, Tosti A. Hair and scalp dermatoscopy. J Am Acad Dermatol 10.1016/j.jaad.2012.02.013.
22. Werner B, Mulinari-Brenner F. Clinical and histological challenge in the differential diagnosis of diffuse alopecia: Female androgenetic alopecia, telogen effluvium and alopecia areata-Part II. An Bras Dermatol. 2012;87(6):884-890.
23. Shapiro J. Hair loss in women. N Engl J Med. 2007;357:1620-30.
24. Rushton DH. Nutritional factors and hair loss. Clinical and Experimental Dermatology. 2002;27:396-404.
25. Holick MF, Binkley NC, Bischoff-Ferrari HA, Gordon CM, Henley DA, Heaney RP, et al. Evaluation, treatment, and prevention of vitamin D deficiency: An Endocrine Society Clinical Practice Guideline. J Clin Endocrinol Metab. 2011;96:1-20.
26. Agarwal U, Deepa HS, Hegde S. An open clinical study to evaluate safety and efficacy of Hairzone® solution in

the management of diffuse hair loss. Indian J Clin Pract. 2010;21(7):308-311.
27. Rawal R, Kolhapure SA. Evaluation of the efficacy and safety of "Hair Loss Cream (PCPB Hair Cream)" in the management of telogen effluvium. Indian J Clin Pract. 2005;16(5):19-26.
28. Rinaldi F, Sorbellini E, Coscera T. The role of platelet rich plasma to control anagen phase: Evaluation in vitro and in vivo in hair transplant and hair treatment. Int J Trichol. 2011;3:supplement.
29. Reese RJ. Autologous platelet rich plasma. What do we know? Important concepts relevant to hair restoration surgery. Hair Transplant Forum Intl. 2010;20(1):14-17.
30. Lachgar S, Charveron M, Gall Y, Bonafe JL. RTH 16, is a potent modulator of VEGF expression (protein and gene) in human hair cultured dermal papilla cells in vitro [poster].Centre de Recherche Europeen Sur la Peau Pierre Fabre. Toulouse, France.

14

Hair and Endocrine System

Neelima Sharma

"Diagnosis means finding the cause of a disorder, not just giving it a name."

—*Sydney Walker III*

Introduction

Hundred years ago, the term "hormone" was coined by Starling to describe secretin, a substance secreted by the small intestine into the bloodstream to stimulate pancreatic secretion.[1] Over years, the understanding of endocrine system was that of a network of organs and glands, which produced and released hormones. Advances in medicine resulted in a change in concept, with endocrine system now being regarded as organized communities in which the cells emit, receive and coordinate molecular signals from established endocrine organs, other distant sources, their neighbors, and themselves.[2] Taking this new understanding into consideration, the skin is also an endocrine system. Within the skin, the pilosebaceous unit is the main factory for hormone production. Evidence has shown that hair follicles are not just targets but also producers of hormones.[3] The hair follicle is a target tissue for endocrine signals such as androgens, estrogens, glucocorticoids, thyroid hormones, adrenocorticotropic hormone (ACTH), thymic hormone, corticotrophin-releasing hormone (CRH), melanocortins, parathyroid hormone and parathyroid hormone-related protein, insulin, prolactin, melatonin, vitamin D, retinoids, catecholamines and prostaglandins, to name a few. It is also a site for hormone metabolism especially androgens, estrogens and prostaglandins. In addition, it also serves as a non-classical, peripheral production site for a wide range of steroid and neurohormones. Normal human scalp hair follicles in anagen synthesize CRH, ACTH, cortisol, melatonin, and prolactin. They also express erythropoietin and its receptor. Finally, hair follicles display a fully functional peripheral equivalent of the hypothalamus-pituitary-adrenal axis.[4,5]

Table 14.1 lists the biosynthesis of hormones and expression of hormone receptors in human hair follicle.[3]

Table 14.1: Biosynthesis of hormones and expression of hormone receptors in hair follicle of man

Hormones biosynthesized	*Positive expression of hormone receptors*
❑ ACTH ❑ Adrenomedullin ❑ Alpha-MSH ❑ Androgens ❑ Chorionic gonadotropin (hCG) ❑ Cortisol releasing hormone (CRH) ❑ Endothelin ❑ Erythropoietin ❑ Estrogens ❑ Fibroblast growth factor ❑ Glucocorticoid ❑ Hepatic growth factor ❑ Leptin ❑ Luteinizing hormone (LH) ❑ Melatonin ❑ Parathyroid hormone related protein (PTHrP) ❑ Platelet derived growth factor (PDGF) ❑ Progesterone ❑ Prolactin ❑ Prostaglandins ❑ Resistin ❑ Retinoids ❑ Serotonin ❑ Transforming growth factor-beta (TGF-β) ❑ Vascular growth factor	❑ Aldosterone receptor ❑ Androgen receptor ❑ Calcitonin receptor-like receptor ❑ CRH-R2 ❑ Endothelin receptor ❑ Epidermal growth factor receptor ❑ Erythropoietin receptor ❑ Estrogen receptor ❑ Fibroblast growth factor receptor ❑ Glucocorticoid receptor ❑ Growth hormone receptor ❑ hCG receptor ❑ Hepatic growth factor receptor ❑ IGF-I receptor ❑ Leptin receptor ❑ Luteinizing hormone receptor ❑ MC 1R ❑ MCR-1, MCR-5 ❑ Melatonin receptors ❑ PDGF receptor ❑ Progesterone receptor ❑ Prolactin receptor ❑ Retinoid receptors ❑ Somatostatin receptor 1-5 ❑ Thyroxine receptor ❑ Transforming growth factor—beta receptor ❑ Vitamin D3 receptors

Androgens

Androgens are sex steroids, with testosterone being the predominant androgen in man. Androgens directly or indirectly affect almost all body systems during fetal and pubertal development, and in adult life. In men, most of the testosterone is produced in the testis.[1] However, skin is a major site of testosterone formation in women.[6]

James Hamilton, an American anatomist, was the first to establish the importance of androgens in human hair growth. He observed that castration before puberty prevented beard and axillary hair growth, while castration after puberty reduced hair growth in both areas.[7] Androgens are now recognized as the main regulator of changes in human hair growth.[8]

Synthesis

Majority, i.e. 95% of circulating testosterone in men is derived from testicular secretion. Cholesterol needed for testosterone biosynthesis can be obtained from circulating cholesterol, or synthesized within the cell. Testosterone can be synthesized from cholesterol by two pathways, namely, the Δ-5 pathway and the Δ-4 pathway **(Figure 14.1)**. In the human testis, the Δ5 pathway predominates. The delivery of cholesterol to the inner mitochondrial membrane for side chain cleavage, the rate-limiting step in testosterone biosynthesis, is under the control of luteinizing hormone (LH). The secretion of testosterone is regulated by the hypothalamic-pituitary-gonadal axis (HPA). Hypothalamic release of GnRH stimulates the anterior pituitary to release LH, which in turn stimulates the testes to synthesize testosterone. Testosterone secretion has pulsatile, diurnal, and circannual rhythms; the highest concentrations are observed in the hours after waking, and lower concentrations are observed in the afternoon and evening. Testosterone concentrations can vary considerably in a given patient due to the diurnal rhythm and the pulsatile nature of testosterone secretion. The other androgens synthesized include dehydroepiandrosterone (DHEA) and androstenedione, which are weak androgens.[1]

The skin is not capable of de novo synthesis of androgens from cholesterol. However, skin contains all the enzymes necessary to convert the prohormones DHEA and androstenedione into testosterone and the most potent androgen, dihydrotestosterone (DHT).[6]

Androgen Transport

Once released into circulation, most of the testosterone is bound to either sex hormone binding globulin (SHBG) or albumin. Only 0.5% to 3.0% of testosterone is unbound. In men, about 50–68% is bound to albumin and 30% to 45% to SHBG. In women, about 25% is bound to albumin and 70% of circulating testosterone is bound to SHBG. Bioavailable testosterone refers to free or unbound testosterone plus the albumin-bound fraction.[1]

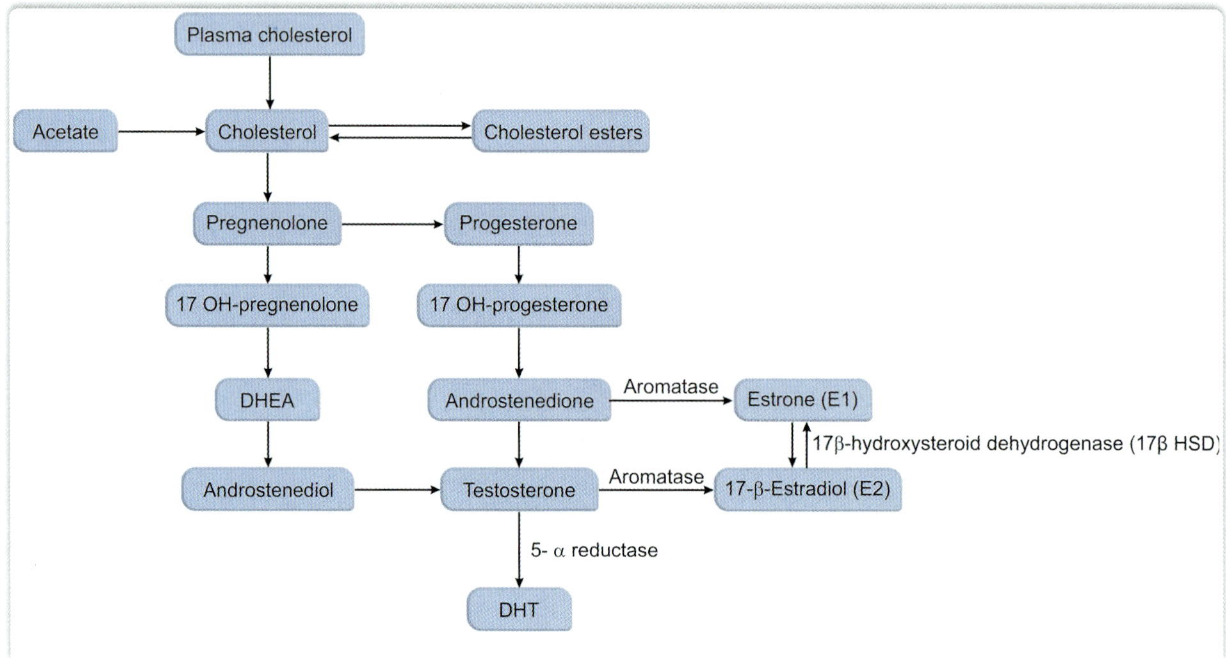

Fig. 14.1: Schematic representation of biosynthesis of sex steroids
Abbreviations: DHEA: Dehydroepiandrosterone; DHT: Dihydrotestosterone

SHBG is a glycoprotein, synthesized in the liver, which possesses high-affinity binding for testosterone and estradiol. It is a major transport protein for sex steroids in plasma. The production of SHBG is regulated by insulin, thyroid hormones, dietary factors, androgens, and estrogens. Androgen administration, obesity, hyperinsulinemic states, and nephrotic syndrome are associated with low SHBG concentrations. Hyperthyroidism, chronic inflammatory states, and aging are associated with high SHBG concentrations **(Box 14.1)**.[1]

Peripheral Conversion

The biological activity of testosterone on target tissues is affected in large part by its conversion to DHT by 5-α reductase, which is a microsomal NADPH-dependent enzyme. Testosterone and DHT stimulate 5-α reductase mRNA and 5-α reductase activity, an effect mediated through the androgen receptor. Two forms of 5-α reductase have been cloned and characterized. Type 1 5-α reductase isoenzyme is expressed in many nongenital tissues and is the major form present in the skin. Its biological role has not been fully ascertained, though it is suggested that it plays a role in progesterone metabolism at the end of pregnancy. Type 2 5-α reductase isoenzyme is expressed in the prostate and other genital tissues. It has also been localized by immunohistochemistry to hair follicles of human scalp; specifically to the innermost portion of the outer root sheath and the proximal inner root sheath. Type 2 5-α reductase isoenzyme has been implicated in the pathophysiology of benign prostatic hypertrophy, hirsutism, and androgenetic alopecia **(Figure 14.2)**.[1,6]

Box 14.1: SHBG: Sex hormone binding globulin

1. Glycoprotein, synthesized in the liver, which possesses high-affinity binding for testosterone and estradiol
2. Major transport protein for sex steroids in plasma
3. Production of SHBG is regulated by insulin, thyroid hormones, dietary factors, androgens, and estrogens
4. Androgen administration, obesity, hyperinsulinemic states, and the nephrotic syndrome are associated with low SHBG concentrations
5. Hyperthyroidism, chronic inflammatory states, and aging are associated with high SHBG concentrations

Androgen Metabolism

In the body, DHT is reduced to 3-androstenediol, which, after conjugation with glucuronic acid, is excreted in urine. Plasma and urine levels of 3-androstanediol glucuronide are the most precise clinical indicators of the extent of testosterone transformation to DHT.[9]

The androgen-sensitive skin appendages that include hair follicles metabolize androgens in a characteristic pattern; Type 2 17β-HSD mRNA expression has been reported in outer root sheath cells of cultured human hair, and type 3 17β-HSD expressions in beard and axillary dermal papilla cells from both sexes. The former favors inactivation of estrogen and the latter formation of testosterone.[6]

Mode of Action

The action of androgens is triggered by binding to the androgen receptor, which is a member of the subfamily of steroid hormone receptors that includes the progesterone, mineralocorticoid, and glucocorticoid receptors. Both testosterone and DHT bind to the same high-affinity androgen receptor. Once testosterone or DHT is bound to the androgen receptor, the substrate-receptor complex

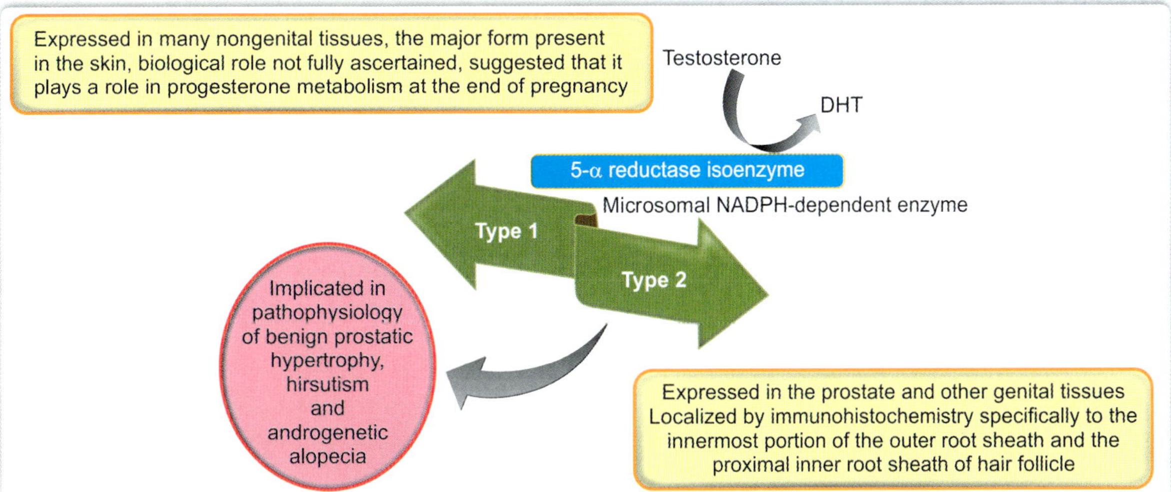

Fig. 14.2: Schematic representation of isoenzymes of 5-α reductase enzyme and its respective functions

binds to the androgen receptor response element and regulates gene expression by acting as a transcription factor. The DHT-receptor complex appears to be the more effective complex at activating gene transcription and may also be capable of activating genes that the testosterone-receptor complex cannot activate.[6]

In the skin, the androgen receptors are primarily localized to dermal papilla, sebaceous epithelium, and eccrine sweat epithelium.[6] The number and activity of androgen receptors in the dermal papilla cells can be affected by various factors. Reduction in the number of androgen receptors by 30–40% is seen with long term use of retinoic acid. Vitamin B_6 reduces the extent of protein synthesis observed after androgen receptor activation by 35–40%. Calreticulin, a polypeptide analogous to an intracellular calcium-binding protein, prevents binding of the androgen-receptor complex.[9]

The mesenchyme-derived dermal papilla plays an important regulatory role in the follicle, altering many parameters and determining the type of hair produced. As per Randall's hypothesis, the androgens enter the follicle via the dermal papilla's capillaries, bind to androgen receptors within the dermal papilla cells and trigger the expression of hormone responsive genes. This then alters the paracrine factors (soluble mitogenic factors or extracellular matrix components) produced by the dermal papilla cells which regulate the growth and activity of the other cell types in the follicle such as follicular keratinocytes, melanocytes, endothelial cells of the blood vessel capillaries and dermal papilla cells themselves **(Box 14.2)**.[8] By doing so, androgens alter the size and diameter of the hair follicle and modify the duration of the hair growth cycle such as stimulation of matrix cell division and differentiation in most areas, and inhibition in parietal region, leading to follicle atrophy **(Box 14.2)**.[9]

Paradoxical Effect on Hair Follicle

Androgens have diverse effects on hair in different body regions. Effects vary from essentially nonexistent (e.g. on eye-lashes), weak (on temporal and suboccipital region hair), moderate (on extremity hair), or strong (on facial, parietal region, pubic, chest, and axillary hair).[9] After puberty androgens promote transformation of tiny, unpigmented vellus follicles to terminal ones, forming larger pigmented hairs, in many areas, such as the axilla.

> **Box 14.2:** Randall's hypothesis
>
> Androgens enter the follicle via the dermal papilla's capillaries, bind to androgen receptors within the dermal papilla cells and trigger the expression of hormone responsive genes which then alters paracrine factors produced by dermal papilla cells

Androgens can also cause the opposite transformation on the scalp leading to the replacement of terminal hairs by vellus hairs and the gradual onset of androgenetic alopecia. This paradox **(Figure 14.3)** appears to be a unique hormonal effect probably resulting from differential gene expression within hair follicles caused during embryogenesis.[10]

Clinical Relevance

Hirsutism in women and androgenetic alopecia in both sexes are the two main clinical conditions of hair growth involving androgens.

Androgenetic Alopecia

Androgenetic alopecia (AGA) is the most common hair loss disorder, affecting both men and women. It is characterized by nonscarring progressive miniaturization of the hair follicle in response to androgens with a usually characteristic patterned distribution in genetically predisposed men and women. In men, AGA typically shows a pattern distribution, with frontotemporal recession and vertex baldness, as described by Hamilton-Norwood **(Figure 14.4)**.[11]

In women, AGA presents either as diffuse thinning of the crown region with preservation of the frontal hairline (as described by Ludwig) or thinning and widening of the central part of the scalp with breach of frontal hairline or thinning associated with bitemporal recession. Majority of women with AGA have physiological hormonal levels, hence the development of AGA is due to higher levels of 5-α reductase, higher androgen receptors, and lower levels of cytochrome P450 (which converts testosterone to estrogen). However, if irregular menstrual cycle, amenorrhea,infertility, miscarriages, signs of hyperandrogenism and seborrhoea are present then hormonal dysregulation, such as polycystic ovary syndrome needs to be ruled out.[11,12]

Hirsutism

Hirsutism, defined as the presence of excessive terminal hair in androgen-dependent areas, is a common disorder affecting up to 8% of women. Hirsutism is a sign of increased androgen action on hair follicles, from increased circulating levels of androgens (endogenous or exogenous) or increased sensitivity of hair follicles to normal levels of circulating androgens. Increased androgen effect that results in hirsutism can be familial, idiopathic, or caused by excess androgen secretion by the ovary (e.g., tumors, polycystic ovary syndrome [PCOS]), excess secretion of androgens (Dehydroepiandrosterone sulfate [DHEAS] by adrenal glands (e.g., congenital adrenal hyperplasia [CAH], Cushing's syndrome, tumor), or exogenous pharmacologic sources of androgens.[13]

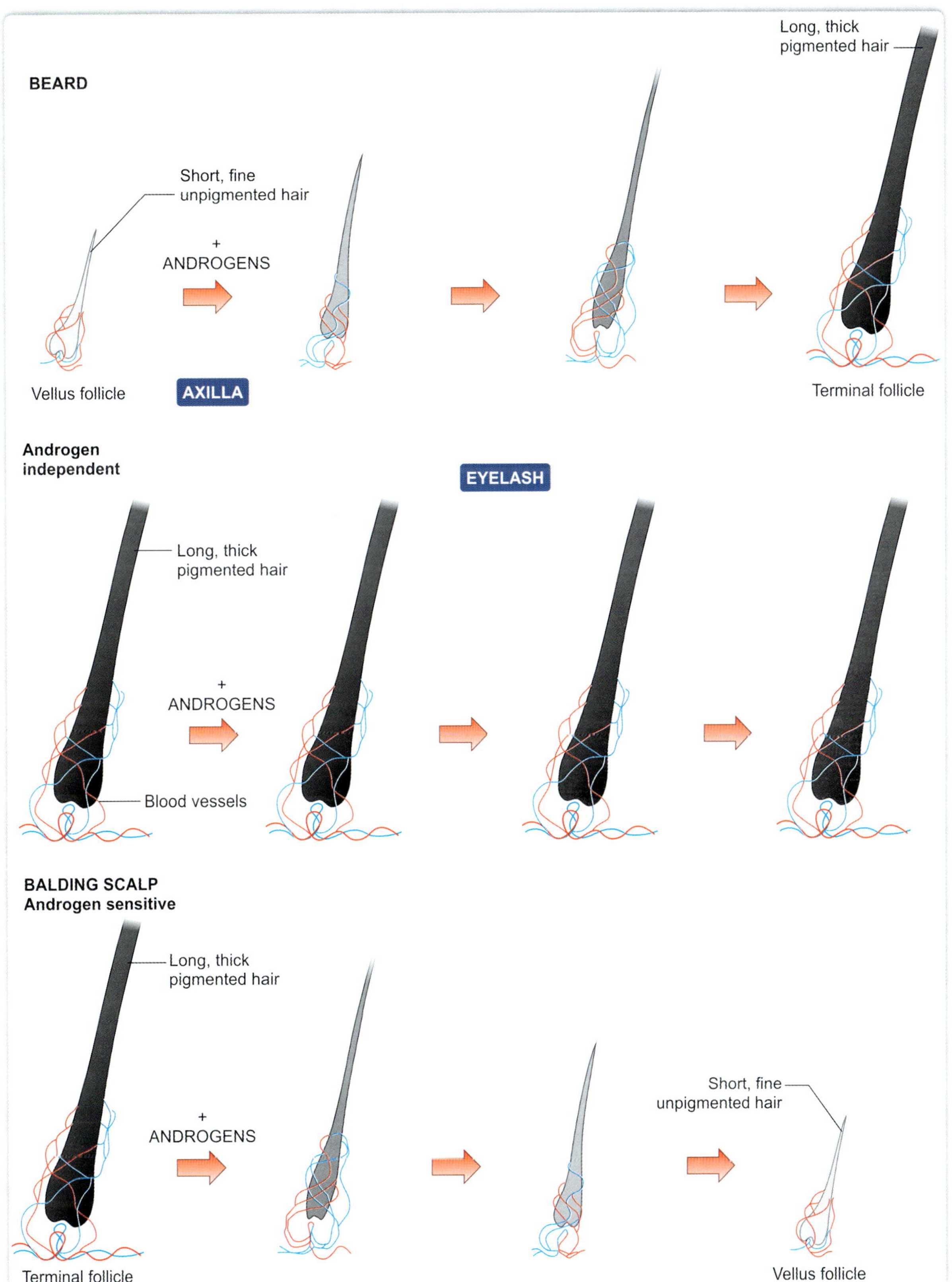

Fig. 14.3: Paradoxical action of androgen on hair

Diagnostic Tests

In men, hormonal work-up may not be needed. In women, the diagnostic testing should examine levels of serum testosterone, 17 hydroxyprogesterone, DHEA, prolactin, estradiol, FSH and LH. The measurements should be taken between 08.00 AM and 09.00 AM, ideally between the second and fifth days of the menstrual cycle. If the patient is on oral contraceptives, then a minimum pause in hormonal contraception has to be 2 months. In both sexes, it is advisable to look for insulin resistance **(Box 14.3)**.[11-13]

Management

Disorders of hair growth involving androgens excess could be managed as follows:[9]

1. By decreasing androgen production: Androgen production can be decreased either surgically (removal of hormone-producing ovarian or adrenal tumor) or with drugs. Ketoconazole is an inhibitor of androgen biosynthesis and also an androgen receptor blocker. Cortisone is the preferred treatment in androgen excess resulting from adrenal cortex hyperplasia. Inhibition of hypophyseal release of gonadotropins by gonadorelin analogs such as leuprolide or goserelin efficiently controls the excess androgen production in polycystic ovarian dystrophy. Simultaneous administration of estrogen (during the first 21 days of the menstrual cycle) and progesterone (from 12th to 21st days of the cycle) is mandatory while the patient is on gonadorelin analogs, in order to reduce the side-effects such as menstrual irregularities, flushes and osteoporosis.
2. By blocking testosterone transformation to DHT: This can be achieved by use of 5-α reductase inhibitors such as finasteride or dutasteride.
3. By blocking androgen receptors: This can be achieved by use of drugs such as spironolactone or flutamide.

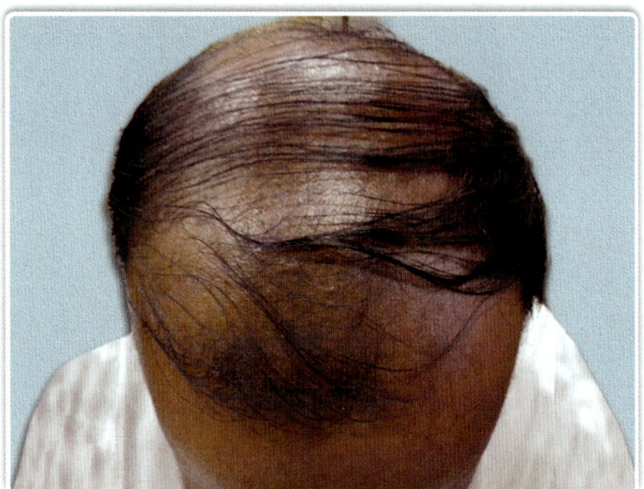

Fig. 14.4: Androgenetic alopecia
(*Courtesy:* Department of Dermatology, STD and Leprosy, BMCRI, Bengaluru)

Box 14.3: Hormonal workup in women

1. Estimate levels of serum testosterone, 17 hydroxyprogesterone, DHEA, prolactin, estradiol, FSH and LH
2. Blood sample drawn between 08.00 AM and 09.00 AM
3. Ideally between the second and fifth days of the menstrual cycle
4. If the patient is on oral contraceptives, then a minimum pause in hormonal contraception has to be 2 months

Hair Disorders in Menopause

Postmenopausal hair loss occurs due to ageing, in conjunction with hormonal changes. There is reduction of the anagen phase and regression of scalp hair to finer, vellus hair caused by androgen, leading to female pattern hair loss. However, not all women have elevated androgen levels, indicating that other androgen-independent mechanisms may be involved. Topical minoxidil is suitable for treating post-menopausal women with or without hyperandrogenism because it works via an androgen-independent mechanism. Systemic antiandrogens, androgen antagonists or enzyme inhibitors, which inhibit the synthesis of potent androgens, such as cyproterone acetate 50 mg/day, finasteride 2.5 mg/day could also be considered. Alternative therapies such as black cohosh that have weak estrogen-like effects can be considered in post-menopausal women.[14]

Another type of hair loss seen in postmenopausal women is the frontal fibrosing alopecia, a form of cicatricial alopecia. Although there is no proof of a hormonal basis, some response has been reported in a few patients following androgen-dependent therapy. Dutasteride has demonstrated efficacy in the treatment of post-menopausal frontal fibrosing alopecia.[14]

Hirsutism can also arise following menopause. The other causes that need to be ruled out when a postmenopausal woman presents with hirsutism include hyperandrogenism caused by adrenal ganglioneuroma, ovarian hyperthecosis, ovarian neoplasms, and androgen therapy including testosterone therapy and androgen-estrogen hormone therapy. Cases of severe virilization in post-menopausal women with nonmalignant etiology have also been reported, but are rare. The treatment of hirsutism in postmenopausal women includes oral contraceptives, anti-androgen therapies, eflornithine and direct methods of hair removal.[14]

Estrogen

Estrogen is the predominant steroid responsible for development of secondary sexual characteristics in girls and women. Most of the estrogen in the premenopausal years is produced in the ovary. The skin constitutes the largest non-reproductive target on which estrogen acts.[15]

Estrogens and estrogen metabolism are as important as androgens in male and female hair biology. The pioneering work by Ebling, in the late 1950s, showed an increase in mitotic rate in the epidermis of both rodents and man by estrogens. This encouraged the concept that "female" hormones (estrogens, prolactin, or progesterone) influence the hair growth cycle.[16]

Synthesis (Figures 14.4 and 14.5)

As with testosterone, cholesterol is the parent steroid from which estrogens are derived. The final step essentially requires androgens as substrates. Several forms of estrogen act within the body, namely, estradiol (E2), estrone, and estriol. Estradiol is the most potent whereas estriol is the least potent.[15]

In males, the total E2 production rate ranges from 35 to 45 g per day, of which 15–20% originates from the testes. About 60% of circulating E2 is thought to arise from peripheral aromatization of testosterone, whereas 20% is formed by reduction of estrone. Estrone can also be directly produced and released by the adrenals. In premenopausal women, the main biosynthesis of estrogen occurs in the ovary, with small amounts being produced by the adrenals. During pregnancy, the placenta is responsible for production of substantial amounts of estrogens. In postmenopausal women, estrogen is mainly obtained by non-ovarian conversion of androstenedione in the adrenals, liver, adipose tissue, skeletal muscle, kidney, and brain. Isolated human hair follicles harbor the enzymes 5α-reductase, aromatase, and 17β-hydroxysteroid dehydrogenase to control estrogen synthesis in the pilosebaceous unit. As with androgens, the secretion of estrogen is also controlled by the HPA.[15,16]

Estrogen Metabolism

Estrogens are metabolized primarily in the liver and then secreted into the urine. Liver dysfunction is associated with a hyperestrogenemic state.[15]

Mode of Action

Estrogen exerts its actions through estrogen receptors (ER), namely, ERα and ERβ, which belong to the nuclear receptor superfamily. ERα is expressed in major female organs such as ovary, uterus, vagina, mammary gland, and hypothalamus. ERβ is more widely distributed within the skin and skin structures than ERα. In human scalp skin, ERβ is the predominant ER. Within the hair follicle, ERβ is expressed in the nuclei of outer root sheath cells, epithelial matrix cells, dermal papilla cells, and the cells of the specialized bulge region of the outer root sheath. In contrast, ERα is expressed only in dermal papilla cells.[15,16]

After binding to the receptors, estrogens may have two different mechanisms of action. They may exert a genotropic effect regulating the transcription expression of genes directly or indirectly, or may have a cytoplasmic effect activating signaling pathways that affect cell survival and/or modulate other growth factor signaling.[15]

Effect on Hair

Estrogens may act alone or together with androgens on hair follicles. In low doses, estrogen stimulates pubic and axillary hair growth. Estrogen prolongs the growth period of scalp hair by increasing cell proliferation rates and postponing the anagen-telogen transition.[6] E2 exerts paradoxical, site-dependent effects on human hair growth. On occipital hair, E2 may inhibit hair shaft elongation in both sexes. However, a differential response based on the gender is seen with frontotemporal hair **(Box 14.4)**. Among women, the frontotemporal anagen hair shaft elongation is inhibited by E2, whereas it is significantly stimulated in men. However, the major, clinically relevant effect of topical E2 on human scalp hair follicles seems to be the inhibition of catagen.[16]

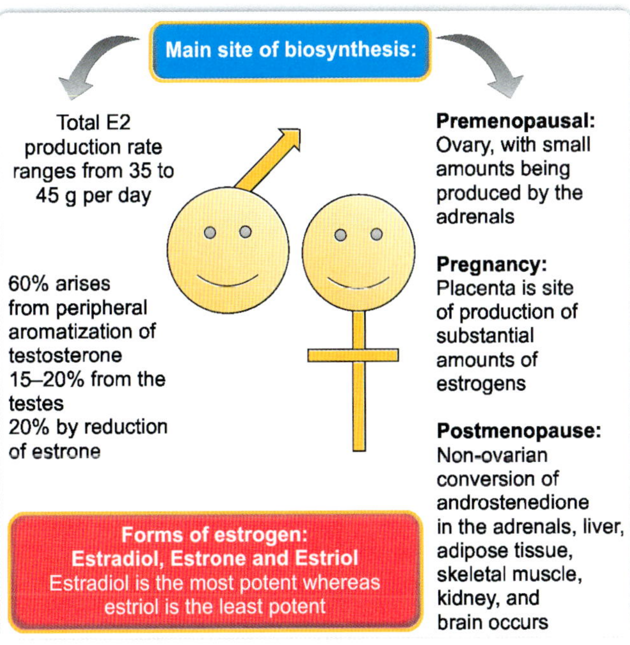

Fig. 14.5: Sites of estrogen synthesis

BOX 14.4: Effects of estrogen on hair follicle

1. Estrogen prolongs the growth period of scalp hair by increasing cell proliferation rates and postponing the anagen-telogen transition
2. E2 exerts paradoxical, site-dependent effects on human hair growth
3. Frontotemporal anagen hair shaft elongation is inhibited by E2 in women, whereas it is significantly stimulated in men

In addition to hair follicle cycling, the intrafollicularly generated estrogens may also play a key role in the enigmatic controls of hair waves, i.e. in the synchronized switches of very large hair follicle populations from one stage of the hair cycle to another.[16]

Clinical Relevance

Estrogens are responsible for development of postpartum effluvium. Large amounts of estrogen secreted by placenta, especially in late pregnancy, cause a high proportion of hair follicles to remain in anagen. The rapid decline in estrogen levels following delivery cause telogen conversion of large number of follicles resulting in increased shedding **(Figure 14.6)**.[6]

For more than half a century estrogens have been used for management of hair disorders such as telogen effluvium, androgenetic alopecia and female pattern hair loss. E2 has been proposed to decrease telogen rate and prolong anagen phase in human scalp skin, justifying the use of topical E2 in the management of hair loss characterized by premature catagen entry, such as androgenetic alopecia and telogen effluvium. Topical solutions containing different formulations of estradiol are available in the market especially for use among women with hair loss. However, caution has to be exercised while using estrogens (both topical and systemic) in men, as unwanted side-effects such as gynecomastia could occur. 17α-estradiol has been found to be relatively safer for use among men. Few reports are available where systemic estrogens administered daily have shown to increase proliferation rate, slow down differentiation and thus postpone telogen effluvium. There was a time when even intralesional stilbene was recommended for the treatment of alopecia areata. However, systemic, double-blind, placebo-controlled, randomized, prospective clinical trials need to be done to establish the role of estrogens in management of hair disorders.[16]

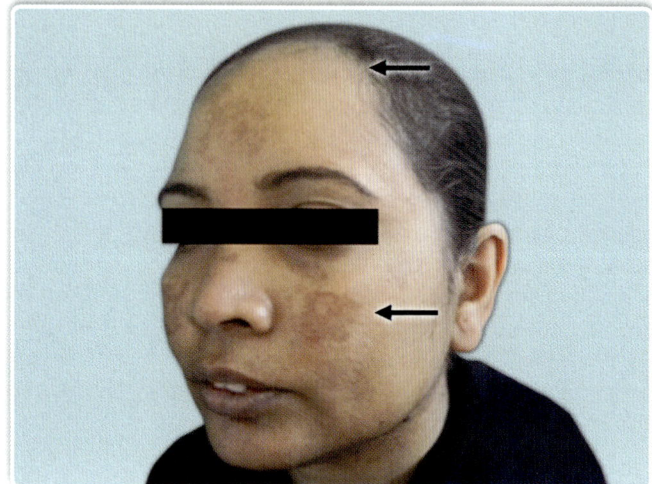

Fig. 14.6: Diffuse hair loss and melasma postpregnancy (*Courtesy:* Department of Dermatology, STD and Leprosy, BMCRI, Bengaluru)

Thyroid Hormones

The thyroid gland is one of the largest of the endocrine organs. Dysfunction and structural abnormalities of the thyroid gland are among the most common diseases of the endocrine glands.[1] It has long been observed that patients with thyroid dysfunction may show prominent hair abnormalities and several in vivo studies have demonstrated hair growth-modulatory effects of thyroid hormone.[17]

Synthesis and Metabolism

Thyroid hormones are produced by the thyroid glands. For the formation of normal quantities of thyroid hormone, an adequate daily dietary intake of iodine (in adults 150 µg/day) is necessary. Within the thyroid, iodide participates in a series of reactions that lead to the synthesis of the active thyroid hormones, namely, thyroxine (T4) and triiodothyronine (T3). Oxidation of thyroidal iodide is mediated by the heme-containing protein thyroid peroxidase (TPO). T4 is secreted from the thyroid gland in about 20-fold more than T3. The metabolic transformations of thyroid hormones in peripheral tissues determine their biologic potency and regulate their biologic effects. Of these, T4 is highest in concentration and the only one that arises solely from direct secretion by the thyroid gland. In normal humans, T3 is also released from the thyroid but approximately 80% is derived from the peripheral tissues. Both hormones are transported in the body bound to plasma proteins, which includes thyroxine-binding globulin (TBG), transthyretin, and albumin. As TBG is the principal T4 and T3-binding protein, any changes in TBG or its binding (due to administration of glucocorticoids, estrogens, androgens, or pregnancy) result in changes in total plasma T4 and T3. The normal ranges for free T4 are 9 to 30 pmol/L (0.7 to 2.5 ng/dL) and for free T3, 3 to 8 pmol/L (0.2 to 0.5 ng/dL). In most situations, a free T4 estimate is all that is required to ascertain the state of thyroid secretion or supply.[1]

The secretion of thyroid hormones is regulated by thyroid stimulating hormone (TSH), secreted by the pituitary gland. TSH serves as the most useful physiologic marker of thyroid hormone action. In normal serum, TSH is present at concentrations between 0.4 and 4.2 mU/L. Circulating TSH displays both pulsatile and circadian variations. TSH secretion is in turn regulated by hypothalamic thyrotropin-releasing hormone (TRH).[1]

Mode of Action

Circulating thyroid hormones enter cells by passive diffusion and bind to the nuclear thyroid hormone receptors (TR) α and β. T3 has a 15-fold higher binding affinity as compared to T4. T4 is also actively transported into the cells (including hair follicles) and then transformed into T3 by the action of intracellular deiodinase. The activated receptor then leads to gene transcription. Thyroid receptors have been localized in human scalp hair follicles in the outer root sheath and dermal papilla.[1,6]

Effect on Hair

A direct modulatory effect of thyroid hormones is observed on the hair follicles, ranging from hair follicle cycling to pigmentation. Hair follicle epithelial cell proliferation, and prolongation of the duration of anagen (due to the down-regulation of TGF-β, the key anagen-inhibitory endogenous growth factor) is brought about by T4 Both T3 and T4 down-regulate apoptosis, modulate keratins, and stimulate intrafollicular melanin synthesis. However, thyroid hormones do not have stimulatory effect on hair shaft growth **(Box 14.5)**.[17]

Clinical Relevance (Figure 14.7)

Thyroid dysfunctions could result in telogen effluvium, or be associated with female pattern hair loss and alopecia areata. Hence, it is advisable to screen all individuals presenting with hair loss for thyroid dysfunction.[17]

Hypothyroidism is associated with telogen effluvium, and dry, brittle, dull hair shafts. Due to premature catagen induction, a diffuse alopecia occurs with a greater proportion of hair follicles in telogen. Hyperthyroidism also leads to effluvium, together with thinned hair shaft diameter and brittle, greasy hair, despite an apparently increased hair matrix proliferation. Hair shafts of patients with hyperthyroidism also show substantially reduced tensile strength. Early graying has been claimed to be related to autoimmune thyroid disease, hypothyroidism, and hyperthyroidism, whereas darkening of gray/white hair may occur in some patients after thyroxin supplementation.[17]

It is important to look for structural abnormalities of thyroid gland in hair disorder, even if the patient is euthyroid. Physical examination of the thyroid is a safe, noninvasive and rapidly performed procedure that is commonly used to assess the thyroid for size, shape, consistency, tenderness and the presence of nodularity. The patient is seated in good light with the neck relaxed. If any abnormality is detected on physical examination, an ultrasonography could be ordered **(Box 14.6)**.[18]

Vitamin D

Vitamin D and its metabolites are not true vitamins; instead they are considered to be hormones and hormone precursors, since in the proper biologic setting, they can be synthesized

Box 14.5: Effect of thyroid hormones on hair follicle

T4:
- Causes hair follicle epithelial cell proliferation, and prolongation of the duration of anagen (due to the down-regulation of TGF-β, the key anagen-inhibitory endogenous growth factor)

T3 and T4
- Down-regulate apoptosis, modulate keratins, and stimulate intrafollicular melanin synthesis
- Thyroid hormones do not have stimulatory effect on hair shaft growth

Box 14.6: Thyroid examination

1. Examine in good light with neck relaxed
2. Locate the thyroid isthmus just caudal to the cricoid cartilage with gentle pressure of thumb
3. The thumb is then moved laterally, without release of gentle pressure, to locate the lobes of the thyroid by pressing it against the trachea as the patient swallows sips of water

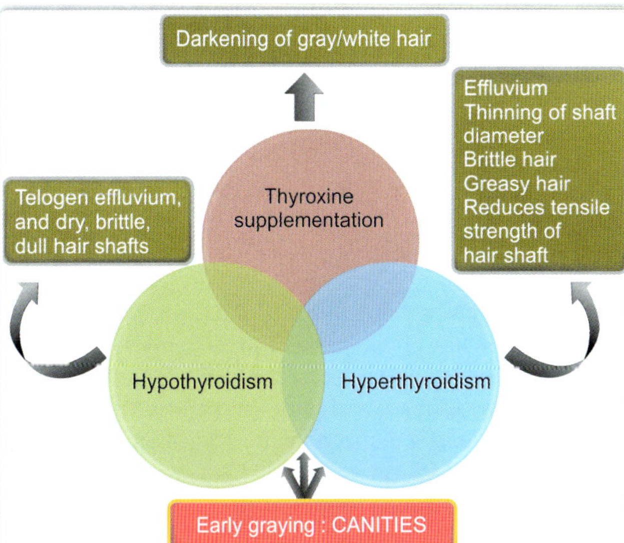

Fig. 14.7: Thyroid states and associated hair disorders

endogenously. 1,25-dihydroxyvitamin D is the major steroid hormone involved in mineral ion homeostasis regulation.[1]

Synthesis and Metabolism of Vitamin D

Vitamin D can be synthesized either from ultraviolet radiation following sun exposure or can be obtained from dietary sources such as egg yolk, fish, and fortified products. As melanin and use of sunblocks reduces the magnitude of solar exposure, an increased reliance on dietary sources of vitamin D has been observed in the last few decades.[1]

Vitamin D, absorbed from the intestine or synthesized in the skin, enters circulation and is bound to vitamin D-binding protein, which is synthesized in the liver. It is then acted upon by the cytochrome P450-like enzymes in the liver and is 25-hydroxylated. This 25-hydroxyvitamin D is the major circulating and storage form of vitamin D. The mature hormone, 1,25-dihydroxyvitamin D is formed in the kidney by another hydroxylation in the presence of 25-hydroxyvitamin D-1α-hydroxylase enzyme. This enzyme is induced by parathyroid hormone and hypophosphatemia and inhibited by calcium and 1,25-dihydroxy vitamin D.[1]

Vitamin D metabolites are inactivated by an additional hydroxylation step and these polar metabolites are secreted into the bile and reabsorbed via the enterohepatic circulation.[1]

Mode of Action

Vitamin D exerts its biologic functions by binding to a nuclear receptor (VDR), which then regulates transcription of DNA into RNA. The affinity of the receptor for 1,25-dihydroxy vitamin D is approximately 3-times higher than that for other vitamin D metabolites. The VDR is expressed in a wide range of cells and tissues including keratinocytes. In hair follicle, VDRs are expressed in the mesodermal papilla cells and the outer root sheath of epidermal keratinocytes. The effects of vitamin D and the VDR on keratinocytes are particularly intriguing. Alopecia is seen with mutant VDRs but is not a feature of vitamin D deficiency; thus, the effects of the VDR on the hair follicle are ligand-independent.[1,19]

Effect on Hair (Box 14.7)

VDR may play a vital role in the postnatal maintenance of the hair follicle. In late anagen and catagen there is an increase in VDR, which is associated with decreased proliferation and increased differentiation of the keratinocytes. These changes are thought to promote the progression of the hair cycle.[19]

Animal studies have shown that VDR, independent of vitamin D3 hormone, plays an important role in the hair follicle cycle, specifically anagen initiation.[19]

Box 14.7: Effects of vitamin D on hair follicle

1. Helps in initiation and maintenance of the postnatal hair follicle
2. Decreases proliferation and increases differentiation of the keratinocytes in late anagen and catagen which promotes progression of the hair cycle

Clinical Relevance

As absence of VDR leads to alopecia, VDR gene polymorphisms may be the causative factor in alopecia areata. Mutations in VDR are responsible for alopecia in patients with type IIA vitamin D dependent rickets and generalized atrichia. These patients have normal hair at birth, but lose their hair between 1 to 3 months of age. On histology, a normal infundibular portion of the hair follicle is seen; however, the lower two-thirds of the hair follicle, below the level of the sebaceous gland is replaced by irregular epithelial structures and dermal cysts. This indicates that normal function of VDR is essential for initiation of the first postnatal hair cycle.[19]

The use of sunblocks has resulted in majority of population being vitamin D deficient.[1] Whether this deficiency plays a role in hair loss needs further investigation. As of now, there are only a few clinical studies available to elaborate the role of vitamin D in hair cycle. Vitamin D has shown to play a protective role in chemotherapy-induced alopecia especially that caused by paclitaxel and cyclophosphamide. Another potential application for vitamin D is in hair loss due to scalp psoriasis, which is associated with an increased telogen to anagen ratio. It has been suggested that an optimal concentration of vitamin D is necessary to delay the aging phenomena, including hair loss. Low concentrations of vitamin D3 have shown to stimulate hair growth. However, high concentration and longer contact has an inhibitory effect on hair follicle growth.[9,19]

Prolactin

Prolactin (PRL), primarily secreted by the pituitary gland, acts as a hormone systemically and as a cytokine locally. PRL is also produced in various other tissues, including the skin. The pituitary PRL expression and secretion is stimulated by oxytocin, thyrotropin-releasing hormone, or estradiol, and inhibited by dopamine or bromocriptine. Normal adult serum PRL levels are about 10–25 g/L in women and 10–20 g/L in men. PRL secretion is pulsatile, with the highest secretory peaks occurring during rapid eye movement sleep. Peak serum PRL levels (up to 30 g/L) occur between 4:00 and 6:00 am. Transient elevation of serum PRL levels are seen after exercise, meals, sexual intercourse, minor surgical procedures, general anesthesia, chest wall injury, acute myocardial infarction, and other forms of acute stress. Marked elevation of PRL occurs during pregnancy, with the levels declining rapidly within 2 weeks of parturition. The basal PRL levels remain elevated during lactation. Marked elevation of PRL levels indicate pituitary tumors, i.e. prolactinoma. Small elevations of serum PRL are more common and often caused by drugs, hypothyroidism, or renal failure.[1,20]

Mode of Action

PRL acts via high-affinity cognate membrane receptors. The PRL receptor (PRLR) is a member of the type I cytokine receptor family that also includes GH and interleukin (IL) 6 receptors. The main functions of PRL are to induce and maintain lactation, decrease reproductive function, and suppress sexual drive. In the ovary, PRL blocks folliculogenesis and inhibits granulosa cell aromatase activity, leading to hypoestrogenism and anovulation. PRL also has a luteolytic effect, generating a shortened, or inadequate, luteal phase of the menstrual cycle. In men, attenuated LH secretion leads to low testosterone levels and decreased spermatogenesis. These hormonal changes decrease libido and reduce fertility. In addition to these classical functions, PRL is implicated in more than 300 distinct biological activities such as regulation of fat metabolism, stimulation of insulin secretion, immunomodulation, stimulation of sebum production, melanin synthesis, etc.[1,20]

Effect on Hair (Box 14.8)

The human scalp hair follicles in anagen VI phase express both PRL and PRLRs on the mRNA and protein. It has been observed that high-dose PRL in men results in significant inhibition of hair shaft elongation and hair bulb keratinocyte proliferation, along with stimulation of premature catagen and increased hair bulb keratinocyte apoptosis. Hence, human scalp hair follicles are both a target and a source of prolactin, which serves as an autocrine and/or paracrine promoter of apoptosis-driven hair follicle regression.[20]

Clinical Relevance

Patients with hyperprolactinemia may complain of telogen effluvium, due to the catagen-inducing effects of PRL on human hair growth. Among women, hyperprolactinemia (also seen as a part of polycystic ovarian syndrome) is associated with female pattern hair loss and hirsutism. These patients may benefit from PRLR antagonists; however, it has to be proven by structured trials.[20]

Box 14.8: Effects of prolactin on hair follicle

High-dose PRL in men results in
1. Significant inhibition of hair shaft elongation
2. Hair bulb keratinocyte proliferation
3. Stimulation of premature catagen
4. Increased hair bulb keratinocyte apoptosis

Growth Hormone and Insulin-like Growth Factor

Growth hormone (GH), the most abundant anterior pituitary hormone, has a pulsatile secretion, with highest peak levels occurring at night, generally correlating with sleep onset. With ageing, a decline in secretion of GH occurs. GH is an important factor for organ growth and cell differentiation. GH exerts direct effects in target tissues via the GH receptors. The GH receptor has been found in hair follicles and the acini of sebaceous glands by immunohistochemistry. GH enhances androgen effects on hair growth and is likely to be involved in sebaceous gland development. It stimulates differentiation of sebocytes and augments the effect of DHT on sebaceous lipid synthesis.[1,6]

Many of the physiologic effects of GH are also mediated indirectly through insulin-like growth factor-I (IGF-I), a potent growth and differentiation factor. IGF-I has also been detected in hair follicles, with the IGF-I receptor being localized to the outer root sheath and matrix cells of the hair bulb. IGF-I at physiological doses is essential for hair follicle growth by preventing them from entering the catagen phase.[6]

Clinical Relevance

Growth hormone (GH) replacement therapy in GH-deficient children augments sexual hair growth and in GH-deficient adult men augments androgen effects on hair growth.[6]

A positive association between high IGF-1 levels and the likelihood of vertex baldness in men has been suggested.[6]

Insulin

Insulin is a hormone produced by the beta cells of the pancreatic islets. The key regulator of insulin secretion is glucose. Insulin acts by binding to its receptor. It stimulates recruitment of intracellular signaling molecules resulting in the widespread metabolic and mitogenic effects.[1]

Insulin resistance indicates the presence of an impaired biologic response to either exogenously administered or endogenously secreted insulin. Insulin resistance is manifested by decreased insulin-stimulated glucose transport and metabolism in adipocytes and skeletal muscle, and by impaired suppression of hepatic glucose output. There is a strong influence of environmental factors such as weight, body fat (especially abdominal), physical activity, and medications on the genetic predisposition to insulin resistance. Insulin resistant individuals are predisposed to impaired glucose tolerance and diabetes.

In addition to diabetes, insulin resistance is implicated in polycystic ovarian syndrome, obesity and metabolic syndrome.[1,12,13]

Effect on Hair

In vitro studies have demonstrated that insulin at supraphysiological doses is essential for hair follicle growth. The hair follicles are shown to prematurely enter into a catagen-like state in the absence of insulin. This action of insulin could be mediated through the IGF-1 receptor as insulin acts as an IGF-1 surrogate.[6]

Clinical Relevance

The hair growth is retarded in diabetes mellitus and accelerated by insulin treatment.[6] Insulin resistance is thought to be linked to androgenetic alopecia, particularly premature androgenetic alopecia, in men. It has also been observed that women with insulin resistance have significantly increased risk for female pattern hair loss **(Box 14.9 and Figure 14.8)**.[21]

Box 14.9: Insulin resistance (IR) and hair growth

1. Hair growth is retarded in diabetes mellitus
2. IR causes premature androgenetic alopecia (men)
3. Increases risk for female pattern hair loss
4. HAIR-AN syndrome:
   Hyperandrogenism, insulin resistance and acanthosis nigricans

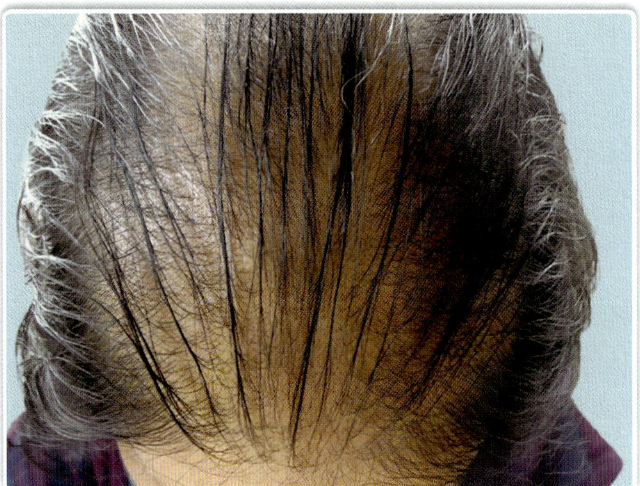

Fig. 14.8: Female pattern hair loss in a postmenopausal patient with diabetes mellitus
(*Courtesy:* Department of Dermatology, STD and Leprosy, BMCRI, Bengaluru)

Parathyroid Hormone

Parathyroid hormone (PTH), secreted by the 4 parathyroid glands situated posterior to thyroid glands, primarily is responsible for maintenance of extracellular fluid calcium concentration.[1]

Parathyroid hormone-related protein (PTHrP) is a protein, produced by various cell types including skin and hair (PTHrP is produced by cells of the inner root sheath of the hair follicle), which exhibits considerable functional and structural homology to PTH. PTHrP, as a paracrine factor, is thought to be produced, act and be destroyed locally within tissues. Both PTH and PTHrP bind to and activate the PTH/PTHrP receptor, causing biological effects on calcium and phosphorus metabolism. PTHrP exerts important developmental influences on fetal bone development and in adult physiology. However, except in disease states such as paraneoplastic syndromes, it does not have any influence in calcium homeostasis in adults.[1,22]

In vivo and animal studies have shown that PTH and PTHrP may influence the proliferation and differentiation of epidermis and hair follicle. Animal studies have shown that PTH increases the total number of visible hair shafts and hair length. PTH has shown to accelerate anagen development in telogen follicles, either by replacing the natural anagen initiation signal or counteracting PTHrP as a "brake" on anagen development. Alternatively, PTH may directly antagonize the natural catagen inhibition signals. These findings could lead to the development of PTH analogs and PTHrP analogs for treating hair loss; however, large clinical studies need to be done **(Box 14.10)**.[22]

Box 14.10: Effect of parathyroid hormone on hair follicle

1. Accelerates anagen development in telogen follicles, either by replacing natural anagen initiation signal or counteracting PTHrP as a "brake" on anagen development
2. Directly antagonizes the natural catagen inhibition signals

Melatonin

Melatonin is a hormone secreted by the pineal gland, a pea-sized organ near the centre of the brain. Melatonin has a strong diurnal pattern, with high output at night and low melatonin output during the day. Melatonin is a primary physiological driver of the daily metabolic, awake/sleep cycle. Melatonin plays a vital role in functions such as sleep, learning, free radical scavenging, maintaining immune system health and mediating hormone functions, to name a few.[1,23]

In addition to the pineal gland, melatonin is also produced by various structures including hair follicles. Catecholamines enhance the melatonin production in hair follicle and pineal gland. Melatonin is thought to play an essential role in hair physiology. Studies have shown that it down-regulates both apoptosis and estrogen receptor-alpha expression. Melatonin's additional potency as a free radical scavenger and DNA repair inducer may make the highly active anagen hair bulb to exploit melatonin synthesis as a self-cytoprotective strategy.[23] Melatonin 0.1% applied topically on the scalp once daily for 6 months has shown to improve hair counts in women with androgenetic alopecia and diffuse alopecia.[24]

Glucocorticoids

Glucocorticoids (e.g. cortisol) are corticosteroid hormones produced by the adrenal cortex. Acting via specific nuclear receptors, i.e. glucocorticoid receptors (GR), they regulate physiologic stress response. The production of glucocorticoids is under the control of the hypothalamic-pituitary-adrenal (HPA) axis. Under stress, the hypothalamus produces corticotrophin releasing hormone (CRH) that stimulates the release of adrenocorticotropic hormone (ACTH) from the pituitary gland. ACTH stimulation initiates steroidogenesis.[1,25]

Hair follicles can synthesize and secrete cortisol. Recent research has shown that epidermal keratinocytes can synthesize de novo cortisol and the enzymes steroid 11β-hydroxylase and 11β-hydroxysteroid dehydrogenase 2. These enzymes catalyze the interconversion of active cortisol and inactive cortisone, thus controlling the biological availability of active hormone.[25] At low doses, cortisol augments the proliferative effects of IGF-1. Hence, glucocorticoids can induce hair growth, as seen in Cushing's disease and steroid therapy.[6]

Corticotropin Releasing Factor

Corticotropin releasing hormone (CRF) is the central trigger of HPA, and the key component of the endocrine and neuroimmune responses to stress. In human scalp hair follicles, CRF up-regulates transcription of pro-opiomelanocortin (POMC) and immunoreactivity of ACTH and α-melanocyte-stimulating hormone (MSH), and increases cortisol secretion. By acting on the CRF receptor situated in hair follicles, it interrupts hair follicle growth cycle in man. Animal studies have shown that the non-selective CRF receptor antagonist, astressin-B activates hair growth and pigmentation. Therefore, the astressin-B could be explored in chronic stress-related hair loss.[26]

Erythropoietin

Erythropoietin (EPO) is a hormone secreted by the kidneys that primarily serves as an essential growth factor for erythrocyte precursor cells. Recent research has shown that human scalp hair follicles are important extrarenal sources and extrahematopoietic targets of EPO-induced signaling. EPO protein is exclusively produced by outer root sheath keratinocytes of human anagen VI hair follicles. Due to its potent antiapoptotic properties, EPO may serve as an endogenous hair follicle cytoprotectant. Taking this into consideration, an assessment needs to be made whether EPO can be exploited clinically as an anti-hair loss agent, conditions of hypoxia and chemotherapy-induced stress such as chemotherapy-induced alopecia.[27]

Conclusion

Many endocrine disorders such as hypopituitarism, hypothyroidism, hyperthyroidism, hypoparathyroidism, diabetes mellitus, growth hormone deficiency, hyperprolactinaemia, polycystic ovary syndrome, SAHA syndrome, congenital adrenal hyperplasia, Cushing syndrome, or virilising tumours are associated with hair loss.**(Table 14.2)** Hence, when encountered with an individual presenting with hair loss, a detailed history and examination for features of hormonal dysfunction is mandatory. Based on the history and clinical findings, appropriate investigations need to be ordered. It is not advisable to get the complete hormone profile done in all patients. If a hormonal dysfunction is suspected or detected, a multidisciplinary approach along with endocrinologist referral would be apt in managing the patient with hair loss

Table 14.2: Endocrine disorders associated with hair loss

Disorder	Non-trichological clinic features	Hair features
Hypopituitarism	Depends on which specific trophic hormones are lost	Telogen effluvium, androgenetic alopecia
Growth hormone deficiency	In children: Short stature, micropenis, increased fat, high-pitched voice, and a propensity to hypoglycemia In adults: Changes in body composition, lipid metabolism, quality of life and cardiovascular dysfunction	In children: Lack of sexual hair growth
Hypothyroidism	Tiredness, weakness, dry skin, cold intolerance, difficulty in concentration and poor memory, constipation, weight gain with poor appetite, dyspnea, hoarse voice, menorrhagia (later oligomenorrhea or amenorrhea), paresthesia, puffy face, hands, and feet (myxedema)	Telogen effluvium, dry brittle dull hair shafts, diffuse alopecia, early graying, alopecia areata (with autoimmune thyroiditis)

Contd...

Contd...

Disorder	Non-trichological clinic features	Hair features
Hyperthyroidism	Hyperactivity, irritability, heat intolerance and sweating, palpitations, fatigue and weakness, weight loss with increased appetite, diarrhea, oligomenorrhea, loss of libido, tremor, goiter, warm, moist skin	Telogen effluvium, thinned hair shaft diameter, brittle greasy hair
Hypoparathyroidism	Muscle spasms, carpopedal spasm, irritability, depression, psychosis, intestinal cramps, chronic malabsorption, chronic changes in fingernails, lenticular cataracts	Alopecia
Diabetes mellitus	Increased thirst, increased frequency of micturition, fatigue	Androgenetic alopecia, female pattern hair loss
Hyperprolactinemia	In women: Amenorrhea, galactorrhea, and infertility In men: Diminished libido, infertility, and visual loss; long-standing cases lead to osteopenia, reduced muscle mass, and decreased beard growth	Telogen effluvium, female pattern hair loss, hirsutism
Polycystic ovary syndrome	Obesity, irregular menstrual cycles, infertility PCOS is diagnosed when at least two of the following three criteria are met:[28] 1. Oligomenorrhea and/or anovulation 2. Clinical or biochemical symptoms of hyperandrogenemia: Clinically the patient may have hirsutism, female pattern baldness, acne and obesity. Increase of at least of one of the hormones, i.e. total or free testosterone, androstenedione, dehydroepiandrostenedione or its sulfate occurs. A moderate increase 17 hydroxyprogesterone and low concentration of SHBG is often observed 3. Sonographic finding of polycystic ovaries: At least 10 and more follicular cysts of 2–8 mm in diameter are laid subcapsularly in combination with increased stroma need to be seen on sonography	Female pattern hair loss, hirsutism
Congenital adrenal hyperplasia	Oligomenorrhea resembling a polycystic ovary syndrome, virilization of external genitalia	Hirsutism
Cushing syndrome	Weight gain, central obesity, rounded face, fat pad on back of neck ("buffalo hump"), thin and brittle skin, easy bruising, broad and purple stretch marks, acne, decreased libido In women, amenorrhea	Hirsutism, androgenetic alopecia
Virilizing tumors	Change in voice, menstrual irregularities	Hirsutism, female pattern hair loss

References

1. Kronenberg HM, Melmed S, Polonsky KS, Larsen PR, editors. Williams Textbook of Endocrinology. 11th edn. Saunders Elsevier. 2008.
2. Zouboulis CC. Human skin: An independent peripheral endocrine organ. Horm Res. 2000;54:230-42.
3. Chen WC, Zouboulis CC. Hormones and the pilosebaceous unit. Dermato-Endocrinol. 2009;1:2:81-6.
4. Paus R, Kromminga A, Hasse S, Laugsch M, Jelkmann W, Wenzel BE, et al. New frontiers in human hair follicle (neuro-) endocrinology. Experimental Dermatol. 2006;15:643-648.
5. Paus R, Arck P, Tiede S. (Neuro-) endocrinology of epithelial hair follicle stem cells. Molecular Cellular Endocrinol. 2007.
6. Deplewski D, Rosenfield RL. Role of hormones in pilosebaceous unit development. Endocrine Reviews. 2000;21:363-392.
7. Randall VA. Androgens and human hair growth. Clin Endocrinol. 1994;40:439-457.
8. Randall VA, Hibberts NA, Thornton MJ, Merrick AE, Hamada K, Kato S, et al. Do androgens influence hair growth by altering the paracrine factors secreted by dermal papilla cells? Eur J Dermatol. 2001;11(4):315-320.
9. Jankovic SM, Jankovic SV. The control of hair growth. Dermatology Online Journal 4(1): 2. Available at: dermatology-s10.cdlib.org/DOJvol4num1/original/jankovi.html. Accessed on 10 April, 2013.
10. Randall VA, Hibberts NA, Thornton MJ, Hamada K, Merrick AE, Kato S, et al. The hair follicle: A paradoxical androgen target organ. Horm Res. 2000;54(5-6):243-50.
11. Blume-Peytavi U, Blumeyer A, Tosti A, Finner A, Marmol V, Trakatelli M, et al. S1 guideline for diagnostic evaluation in androgenetic alopecia in men, women and adolescents. British J Dermatol. 2011;164:5-15.
12. Thiedke CC. Alopecia in women. Am Fam Physician. 2003;67:1007-14,1017-8.
13. Hunter M H, Carek PJ. Evaluation and treatment of women with hirsutism. Am Fam Physician. 2003;67:2565-72.
14. Blume-Peytavi U, Atkin S, Gieler U, Grimalt R. Skin academy: Hair, skin, hormones and menopause—current status/ knowledge on the management of hair disorders in menopausal women. Eur J Dermatol. 2012;22(3):310-8.
15. Hall G, Phillips TJ. Estrogen and skin: The effects of estrogen, menopause, and hormone replacement therapy on the skin. J Am Acad Dermatol. 2005;53:555-68.

16. Ohnemus U, Uenalan M, Inzunza J, Gustafsson J, Paus R. The hair follicle as an estrogen target and source. Endocrine Reviews. 2006;27:677-706.
17. Beek NV, Bodo E, Kromminga A, Gaspar E, Meyer A, Zmijewski MA, et al. Thyroid hormones directly alter human hair follicle functions: Anagen prolongation and stimulation of both hair matrix keratinocyte proliferation and hair pigmentation. J Clin Endocrinol Metab. 2008;93:4381-8.
18. Sicco KL, McGuire S, English JC. A retrospective study of thyroid structural abnormalities in alopecia patients. Dermato-Endocrinology. 2011;3(3):251-4.
19. Amor KT, Rashid RM, Mirmirani P. Does D matter? The role of vitamin D in hair disorders and hair follicle cycling. Dermatol Online J. 2010 16 (2). Available at: dermatology.cdlib.org/1602/reviews/vitamind/rashid.html. Accessed on 5 May, 2013.
20. Foitzik K, Langan EA, Paus R. Prolactin and the skin: A dermatological perspective on an ancient pleiotropic peptide hormone. J Invest Dermatol. 2009;129:1071-87.
21. Matilainen V, Laaksoa M, Hirssoa P, Koskelad P, Rajalaa U, Keinänen-Kiukaanniem S. Hair loss, insulin resistance, and heredity in middle-aged women. a population-based study. Eur Preventive Cardiol. 2003;10(3):227-31.
22. Schilli MB, Ray S, Paus R, Obi-Tabot E, Holick MF. Control of hair growth with parathyroid hormone. J Invest Dermatol. 1997;108:928-932.
23. Fischer TW, Slominski A, Tobin DJ, Paus R. Melatonin and the hair follicle. J Pineal Res. 2008;44(1):1-15.
24. Fischer TW, Burmeister G, Schmidt HW, Elsner P. Melatonin increases anagen hair rate in women with androgenetic alopecia or diffuse alopecia: Results of a pilot randomized controlled trial. Br J Dermatol. 2004;150(2):341-5.
25. Perez P. Glucocorticoid receptors, epidermal homeostasis and hair follicle differentiation. Dermato-Endocrinol. 2011;3(3):166-74.
26. Wang L, Million M, Rivier J, Rivier C, Craft N, Stenzel-Poore MP, et al. CRF receptor antagonist astressin-b reverses and prevents alopecia in crf over-expressing mice. PLoS One. 2011;6(2). Available at: e16377. doi:10.1371/journal.pone.0016377.
27. Bodo E, Kromminga A, Funk W, Laugsch M, Duske U, Jelkmann W, et al. Human hair follicles are an extrarenal source and a nonhematopoietic target of erythropoietin. The FASEB J. 2007;21(12):3346-54.
28. Dušková M, Stárka L. The existence of a male equivalent of the polycystic ovary syndrome - the present state of the issue. Prague Medical Report. 2006;107(1):17-25.

15

Cicatricial Alopecia

Ashok Kumar Jaiswal, TS Nagesh

"Scars speak more loudly than the sword that caused them."
—*Paulo Coelho*

Introduction

As man ascends the ladder of evolution, the physiological function of hair decreases and it becomes localized over some particular sites of the body unlike other mammals or plifiers. The psychologic importance of hair to man is in inverse ratio to its physical function. Scalp hair is a major social and sexual display of human body. For women, the crowning glory of decently exposable feminity and for men, a traditional symbol of masculinity. So, in humans, hair is of minimal functional benefit, but is all important for personal adornment.

The term alopecia comes from the Greek word 'alopekia' (a fox, because partial baldness is common in that animal) meaning lack of hair or baldness in areas where hair ordinarily would be found. Generally, this means a loss of terminal hair on the scalp, since hair loss elsewhere is less frequent and less conspicuous.

The term 'cicatricia' comes from Latin word 'cicatrix', meaning scar. Cicatricial or scarring alopecias are a group of disorders leading to permanent hair loss. The essential features of all cicatricial alopecias are visible loss of follicular ostia, clinically and destruction of the hair follicle, histopathologically. Cicatricial alopecia can be primary or secondary. Primary group involves specific targeting of the hair follicle unit for destruction. In contrast, hair follicle destruction in secondary scarring alopecia occurs as "collateral damage" to a nonspecific disruption of the dermis. The inflammatory infiltrate typically involves the permanent portion of the hair follicle which houses the bulge region that contains the follicular stem cell reservoir.[1]

Epidemiology

Cicatricial alopecia is a relatively uncommon condition accounting for 3–7% of the dermatologic consultations for alopecia.[2] Not many race-based studies are available, however central centrifugal cicatricial alopecia is believed to be predominant in adults of African origin. The majority of patients are over the age of 20 years, and most are women, probably because they are more concerned about the loss of scalp hair.

Classification

The history of cicatricial alopecias has been covered in detail by several authors including Brocq, Laymon, Degos , Gay Prieto and Pinkus.[3-7] Confusion concerning the entities is as evident today as it was historically. Inability to agree on descriptive terminology has resulted in a plethora of synonyms.

The main criteria of classification of scarring alopecias since the turn of the 20th century had been on the basis of etiology. Recently, North American Hair Research Society has proposed a working classification of cicatricial alopecia based on the histological findings.[8] A modified combined classification based on both etiology and histopathology is shown in **Table 15.1**. This classification is currently used as a guide for both diagnosis and treatment.

This chapter will focus mainly on primary cicatricial alopecias.

Table 15.1: Classification of cicatricial alopecia[9]

Primary cicatricial alopecia			
Inflammatory	Lymphocytic	Chronic cutaneous lupus erythematosus Lichen planopilaris (LPP)	
			Classic LPP Graham-Little syndrome Frontal fibrosing alopecia
		Pseudopelade of Brocq Central centrifugal cicatricial alopecia Alopecia mucinosa Keratosis pilaris spinulosa decalvans	
	Neutrophilic	Folliculitis decalvans (including tufted folliculitis) Dissecting cellulitis/folliculitis	
	Mixed	Acne keloidalis Acne necrotica	
	Non-specific or end-stage cicatricial alopecia		
Secondary cicatricial alopecia			
Traumatic	Radiodermatitis Mechanical trauma Postoperative (e.g. flap necrosis) Burns Accidental alopecia Dermatitis artefacta Traction alopecia Hot comb alopecia		
Sclerosing disorders	Morphea Scleroderma Lichen sclerosus Sclerodermoid porphyria cutanea tarda Chronic graft-versus-host disease		
Granulomatous	Sarcoidosis Necrobiosis lipoidica Infectious granulomas		
Infectious	Bacterial	Folliculitis Carbuncle/furuncle	
	Fungal	Kerion Favus Tinea capitis (rarely scarring)	
	Viral	Shingles Varicella HIV	
	Protozoal	Leishmaniasis	
	Treponemal	Syphilis	
	Mycobacterial	Tuberculosis	
Neoplastic	Benign	Cylindroma Other adnexal tumors	
	Malignant	Primary	Basal cell carcinoma Squamous cell carcinoma Cutaneous T-cell lymphoma
		Secondary	Renal, breast, lung, gastrointestinal lymphoma, leukemia

Contd...

Contd...

Developmental defects and hereditary disorders			
	Aplasia cutis Facial hemiatrophy (Romberg's syndrome) Epidermal naevi Hair follicle hamartomas Incontinentia pigmenti Focal dermal hypoplasia of Goltz Porokeratosis of Mibelli Ichthyosis Epidermolysis bullosa Polyostotic fibrous dysplasia Conradi–Hünermann syndrome (chondrodysplasia punctata)		

Primary Cicatricial Alopecia

Lichen Planopilaris (Syn: Lichen planus et acuminatus atrophicans; Follicular lichen planus)

Lichen planopilaris (LPP) is the prototypical lymphocytic cicatricial alopecia. The disorder was labeled lichen planopilaris by Pringle in 1897.[10] Little and Feldman described the condition under the names 'folliculitis decalvans et atrophicans' and 'lichen planus et acuminatus atrophicans' respectively.[11,12] Later in 1953, Silver et al expressed the belief that, both the conditions are one and the same as that recognized and fully described by Pringle in 1897.[13]

Etiology

LPP remains a dark etiologic mystery. The present evidence, which is necessarily circumstantial, suggests that lichen planus, LPP, frontal fibrosing alopecia and Graham- Little syndrome are variants of the same process.

Clinical Features (Box 15.1)

LPP is usually seen between the ages of 30 and 60 years. The disease is diagnosed considerably more often in women than in men. The features of lichen planus may occur before, during, or after the onset of scalp involvement. The occurrence of associated lichen planus varies in reports from 17% to 50% of patients with LPP.[14] It is usually an insidious process. Subjective symptoms often include patchy hair loss with itching, pain and burning sensation. Scalp is involved in about 40%, with the vertex being chiefly involved.[15] Recent scalp lesions may show violaceous papules, perifollicular erythema and scaling **(Figure 15.1)**. These papules are replaced by follicular plugs and scarring.[9] Most frequently, multiple small areas of white scarring are seen which may coalesce and enlarge to involve larger areas. The center of the patch is smooth and devoid of follicular ostia with conspicuous follicular plugging at the periphery. The hair at the margins of the extending patches can be easily pulled, which shows twisted anagen hair. Erythema and edema with adherent scales and dilated hair follicular orifices may be seen in some patients **(Figure 15.2)**. In late cases, the appearance is that of end stage nonspecific

Box 15.1: Course of LPP lesions

- Scalp is involved in about 40%, esp vertex
- Violaceous papules, perifollicular erythema and scaling
- Papules are replaced by follicular plugs and scarring
- Multiple small areas of white scarring are seen which coalesce and enlarge to involve larger areas
- The center of the patch is smooth and devoid of follicular ostia with conspicuous follicular plugging at the periphery. The hair at the margins of the extending patches can be easily pulled, which shows twisted anagen hair

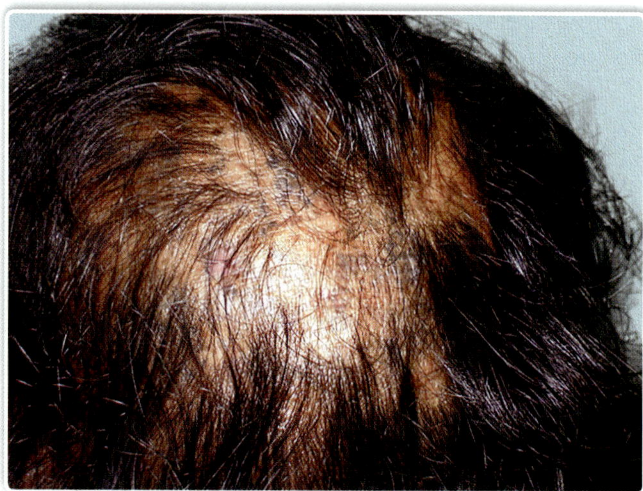

Fig. 15.1: Lichen planopilaris. Scarring alopecia and violaceous papules

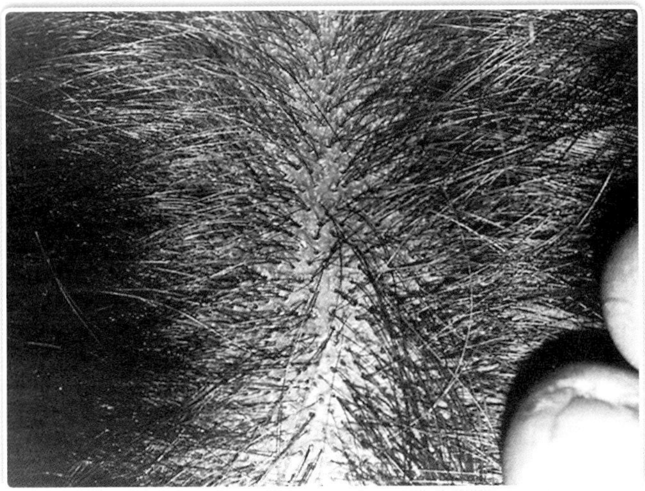

Fig. 15.2: Lichen planopilaris. Dilated follicular openings

cicatricial alopecia **(Figure 15.3)**. The course of LPP in most cases is very slow.

Pathology

The histopathologic picture of LPP is essentially that of lichen planus, but the characteristic changes involve the follicles and perifollicular areas.[16] The initial abnormality is in the epidermis; fibrillar changes in the basal cells lead to the formation of colloid bodies. The hair follicles are dilated and filled with a keratotic plug which is more commonly cup shaped. Hypergranulosis within the affected infundibula is characteristic. A lichenoid lymphocytic infiltrate surrounds the follicle, especially involving the upper portion (infundibulum and isthmus). Liquefaction degeneration and invasion of the infiltrate into the basal cell layer is seen. Over time, there is flattened epidermis, perifollicular fibrosis with complete disappearance of hair and sebaceous glands, mild perivascular infiltrate and remnants of arrector pili muscles **(Figure 15.4)**. End-stage LPP shows loss of elastic fibers in a superficial dermal wedge-shaped scar, which is better demarcated with elastic tissue stain. Direct immunofluorescence shows characteristic pattern of grouped globular deposition of IgM adjacent to the follicular epithelium.[17]

Silver et al are of the opinion that, atrophy is due to loss of the pilosebaceous apparatus, probably due to pressure of the perifollicular infiltrate thus interfering with the blood supply and not due to the loss of elastic tissue.[13]

Treatment[9,18,19]

Treatment can be difficult. Potent topical (clobetasol propionate twice daily) and intralesional corticosteroids (triamcinolone acetonide 10mg/cc) are found to be helpful in early lesions with active inflammatory changes. Improvement has also been noted with topical tacrolimus 0.1%. A short course of oral corticosteroids is usually helpful in some cases, but has to be used with caution in chronic progressive disease. Antimalarials such as hydroxychloroquine 200 mg bid for 6–12 months has been tried as a first line of treatment with variable success. Other immunomodulating agents like ciclosporin (3–5 mg/kg/day for 3–5 months), mycophenolate mofetil (0.5 g to 1 g bid for upto 6 months), and low dose methotrexate may be effective in some patients. Various anecdotal reports have shown improvement following the use of Peroxisome Proliferator-Activated Receptor (PPAR) - gamma agonists like pioglitazone (15 mg daily for 3–6 months) and also with oral retinoids.

Fig. 15.3: Lichen planopilaris. Late stage showing smooth, atrophic alopecic patch with pterygium of left ring finger

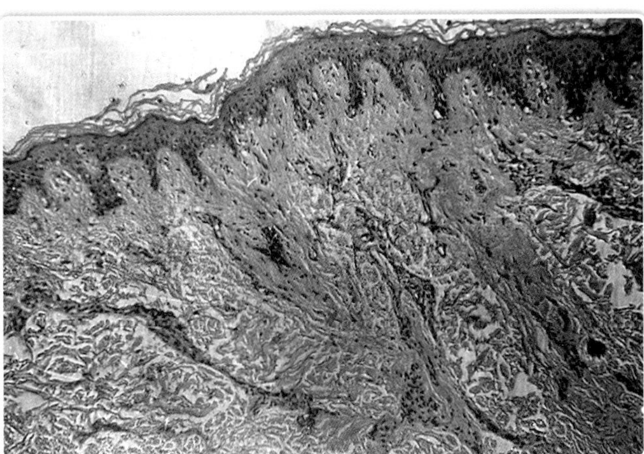

Fig. 15.4: Lichen planopilaris showing atrophy of epidermis, complete obliteration of pilosebaceous structures and scanty inflammatory infiltrate mainly around remnants of hair follicles (low power)

Graham-Little syndrome (Syn: Lassueur Graham- Little syndrome; Piccardi–Lassueur–Little syndrome; Lichen spinulosis et folliculitis decalvans)

This rare syndrome was first described by Graham Little in 1915 in a patient referred to him by Lassueur. Piccardi of Italy had described a similar case a year earlier. It is considered a rare variant of LPP.[14]

The syndrome is seen most often in women between the ages of 30 and 70 years. It is characterized by a triad of cicatricial alopecia of the scalp with prominent follicular plugging, keratosis pilaris like follicular papules and loss of axillary and pubic hair. The loss of axillary and pubic hair may not appear to be cicatricial on clinical examination, but is in fact the result of destruction of the follicles.

The earliest change is usually patchy cicatricial alopecia of the scalp which precedes the widespread keratosis pilaris by months or years. The patches may be associated with pruritus. Keratosis pilaris presents as horny papules of variable extent on the trunk, limbs and occasionally on eyebrows and sides of face.

Treatment

There is no effective treatment. Corticosteroids, ciclosporin and thalidomide have been found to be useful.[17]

Frontal Fibrosing Alopecia

Frontal Fibrosing Alopecia (FFA) was first described by Kossard in 1994.[20] It is considered to be a potential variant of LPP. The condition is characterized by progressive symmetrical frontotemporal recession due to scarring hair loss. The affected skin is pale and shiny in contrast to chronically sun-exposed skin of the upper forehead. Follicular hyperkeratosis with perifollicular erythema can be seen at the hair margin when the disease is active. It is often associated with loss of eyebrows and is regarded as a helpful diagnostic sign. Postmenopausal women are predominantly affected even though it can occur occasionally in premenopausal women and men.[19]

FFA is less symptomatic than LPP with only occasional itching. The band-like frontal recession varies from 1–6 cm and may progress laterally to above and behind the ears and less often to the occipital hairline. Here, the frontal hair line recedes in a straight line rather than bitemporally, in contrast to androgenetic alopecia **(Figure 15.5)**. The natural course of FFA is slow progression over many years, though at times it may spread rapidly. Lichen planus and/or LPP may develop in some patients with FFA.[14]

In view of the distinct clinical presentation of the lymphocytic cicatricial alopecias with similar histopathological features, Price and Mirmirani[14] are of the opinion that FFA is a separate entity and not a variant of LPP.

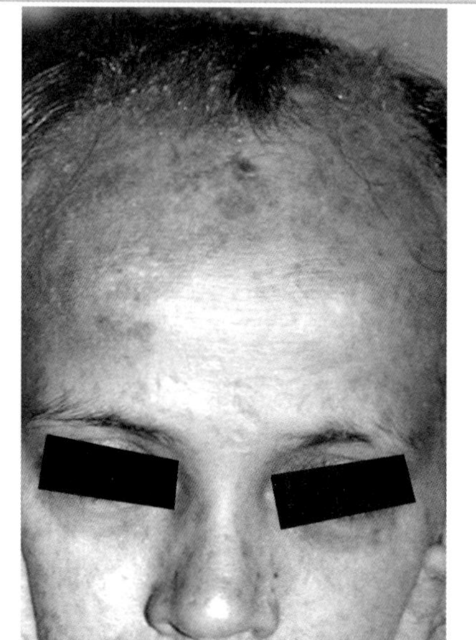

Fig. 15.5: Frontal fibrosing alopecia. Frontal hairline recession in a straight line

Pathology

The histological features are similar to those found in LPP.

Treatment

Treatment is on the same lines as for LPP.

Lupus Erythematosus

Cicatricial alopecia may be the result of lupus erythematosus (LE), a genetically predetermined autoimmune connective tissue disease characterized by the presence of circulating non-organ-specific autoantibodies to cell nuclear antigens. Three different forms of LE are described: systemic (SLE), subacute (SCLE) and discoid (DLE) lupus. Cicatrizing hair loss process is usually seen in DLE.

Clinical features

The condition usually occurs in adults, women more than men. Although lesions of DLE are often found in patients with SLE, most patients with DLE do not have systemic disease. Among patients with skin disease only, about 50% have scalp lesions.[21] The disease most commonly affects the scalp face and ears. The lesion often starts as an itchy, well-demarcated, dull red, scaly macule or papule which enlarges into a discoid alopecic patch with erythema and adherent scaling **(Figure 15.6)**. The removal of scales result

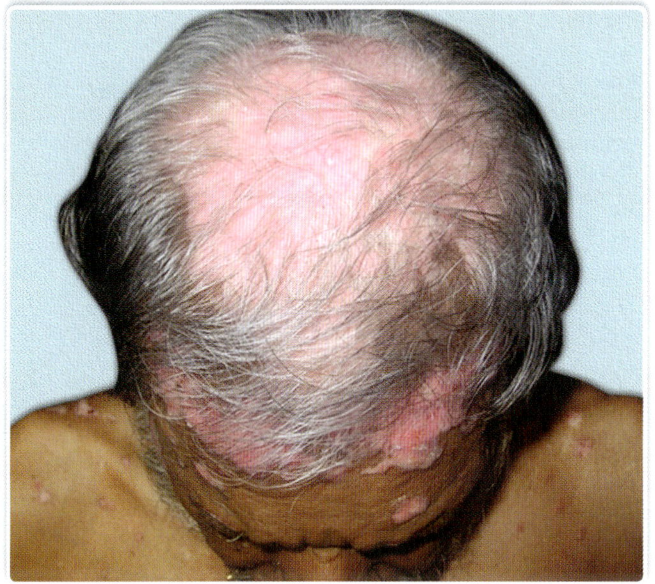

Fig. 15.6: Discoid lupus erythematosus. Cicatricial alopecia with erythematous scaly plaques (*Courtesy*: Ashique KT, Alshifa hospital, Perinthalmanna, Kerala)

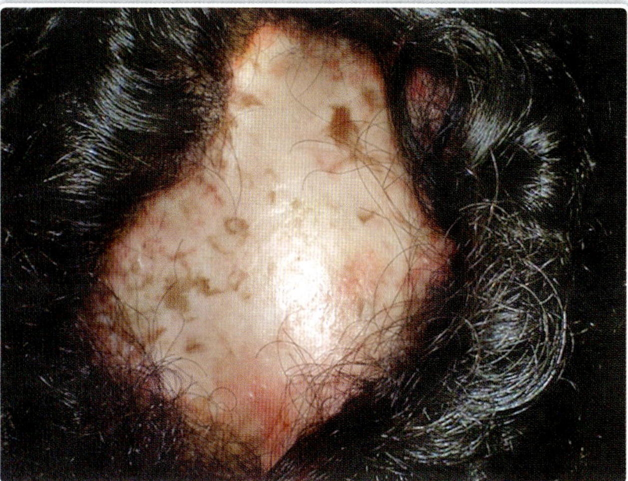

Fig. 15.7: Old inactive discoid lupus erythematosus, showing smooth, atrophic, shiny bald area with hypo- and hyperpigmentation

in slight bleeding and at times they may be lifted intact, demonstrating a carpet-tack appearance on the under surface. In most cases, there are conical plugs in the dilated follicles. Telangiectatic vessels may be seen both at the borders and in the centre of the plaques. The combination of mottled hyperpigmentation, telangiectasia and follicular plugging within the areas of scarring is highly characteristic **(Box 15.2) (Figure 15.7)**.[22] Follicular plugging in the ear is another useful sign in DLE. Long standing cases may show calcification and squamous cell carcinoma.[9]

Pathology

The epidermal changes usually develop after those in the dermis. There is relative and absolute hyperkeratosis. Thinning and flattening of the stratum malpighii predominates. Keratotic plugs are found mainly in the follicular openings which are usually funnel shaped. Focal basal cell vacuolation is an essential histologic feature **(Figure 15.8)**.

The earliest dermal changes consist of dilatation of blood and lymph vessels, edema and a slight extravasation of erythrocytes in the upper dermis. Thickening of the

Box 15.2: Clinical clues in discoid lupus erythematosus

- Discoid alopecic patch with erythema and adherent scaling
- The combination of mottled hyperpigmentation, telangiectasia and follicular plugging within the areas of scarring is highly characteristic
- Removal of scales result in slight bleeding and demonstrate a carpet-tack appearance on the under surface
- Follicular plugging in the ear

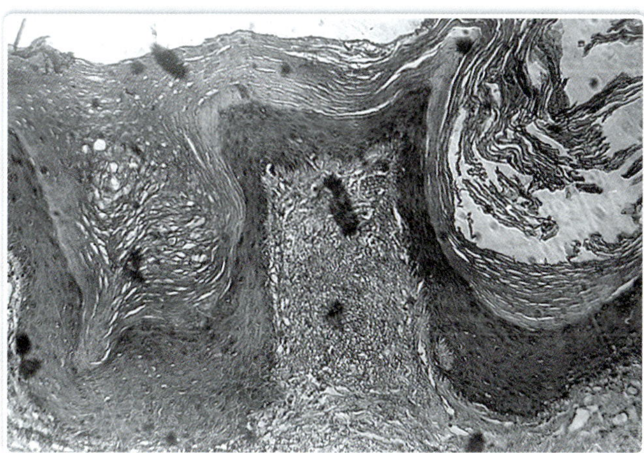

Fig. 15.8: Early active discoid lupus erythematosus of scalp showing hyperkeratosis and keratotic plugging, atrophy of stratum malphigii, hydropic degeneration of basal layer and edema of upper dermis

basement membrane zone, pigmentary incontinence, colloid bodies, increased dermal mucin and exocytosis of lymphocytes into the epidermis and follicular epithelium is often present. The infiltrate is usually distinctly patchy and is located mainly in the vicinity of the hair follicles, blood vessels, sebaceous and eccrine glands, and is composed predominantly of lymphocytes admixed with plasma cells. The infiltrate, by impinging upon the pilosebaceous structures, causes their gradual atrophy and disappearance. Frequently, hydropic changes in the basal layer of the hair follicles are seen, which may have considerable diagnostic value.[23]

The fibrous streaks left behind as traces of the vanished follicles consist of fibrotic collagenous scar tissue without elastic fibers or elastin like bodies. Elastic tissue staining usually shows widespread destruction of elastic fibers in the interfollicular dermis, and this persists as a permanent marker even if new thin elastic fibers are formed after subsidence of the inflammation.[24]

Diagnostic features on direct immunofluorescence are deposition of IgG, IgM and C3 in a granular band like pattern at the dermal interface.[23]

Treatment

Sun protection and potent topical or intralesional corticosteroids are the first choice of treatment in limited disease. Other topical agents used with variable success are tacrolimus, tazarotene and imiquimod. Antimalarials (hydroxychloroquine 200–400 mg/day for 3–6 months) are more effective in DLE than all other forms of cicatricial alopecia. Isotretinoin, dapsone, thalidomide can also be considered in refractory cases. Systemic corticosteroids, azathioprine, cyclosporine and methotrexate have also been used in rapidly progressive or more extensive disease.[9,14,17]

Pseudopelade of Brocq (Syn: Alopecia cicatrisata; Macular atrophy of the scalp; Alopecia atrophicans)

Pseudopelade was first described by Brocq in 1885. 'Pelade' is the French term for alopecia areata and the term pseudopelade emphasizes the resemblance to alopecia areata.[3] Pseudopelade of Brocq (PPB) is a rare primary lymphocyte-mediated, chronic, slowly progressive, asymptomatic, patchy cicatricial alopecia of the scalp that occurs without any evidence of inflammation. Most patients are women between the ages of 30 and 50 years. The etiology and pathogenesis is unknown.

Clinical Features

The onset of alopecia is insidious and asymptomatic. Although the vertex is primarily involved, the disease may occur anywhere on the scalp. Small, round to oval, smooth, soft, atrophic, white or ivory colored alopecic patches appear singly or in small groups. The absence of inflammatory signs is characteristic. Neighboring patches coalesce to form large irregular slightly depressed patches that are frequently compared to 'foot prints in the snow' **(Box 15.3) (Figures 15.9)**. Scattered follicles in these alopecic patches are often spared. If the alopecia is progressing, a pathognomonic hair can be plucked from the bald area by gentle traction. The hair extracted in this way is anagen hair attached to which is a succulent external root sheath, as well as keratinous debris around the shaft.[9, 23]

The course of PPB is extremely slow. Most often it is characterized by periods of quiescence and activity of varying duration. PPB usually requires 10 or more years before much alopecia appears.

Box 15.3: Footprints in snow appearance

- A characteristic clinical feature in Pseudopelade of Brocq
- Small, round to oval, smooth, soft, atrophic, white or ivory colored multiple alopecic patches which are non-inflammatory coalesce to form large irregular slightly depressed patches compared to footprints

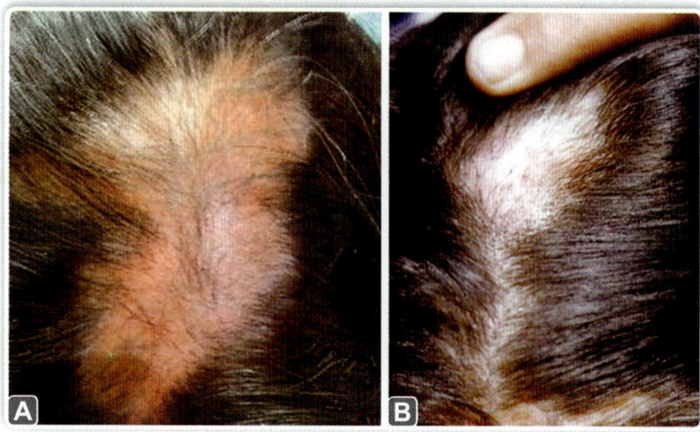

Figs 15.9A and B: Pseudopelade of Brocq. Irregular, atrophic, white, ivory colored alopecic patch with a 'footprints in the snow' appearance. (*Courtesy:* (Figure 15.9A) Department of Dermatology, BMCRI, Bengaluru)

It is still disputed whether PPB is a distinct clinical entity or an end stage of many cicatricial alopecias. However, most of the authors are of the opinion that PPB is a specific and distinct clinical disease and the term 'end stage nonspecific scarring alopecia' should be used instead of pseudopelade to describe a generic scarring alopecia, the end result of any primary cicatricial alopecias.[9,14,17] The diagnostic criteria of Braun-Falco, et al[25] **(Table 15.2)** and the histological criteria of Pinkus,[7] should be fulfilled before this specific diagnosis is made. Cases that do not fulfil these criteria should be diagnosed generically as scarring alopecia.

Table 15.2: Diagnostic criteria for pseudopelade of Brocq (After Braun-Falco, et al.)

Clinical criteria
❑ Irregularly defined and confluent patches of alopecia
❑ Moderate atrophy (late stage)
❑ Mild perifollicular erythema (early stage)
❑ Female : male ratio 3 : 1
❑ Long course (more than 2 years)
❑ Slow progression with spontaneous termination possible
Direct immunofluorescence
❑ Negative (or only weak IgM on sun-exposed skin)
Histological criteria
❑ Absence of marked inflammation
❑ Absence of widespread scarring (best seen with elastin stain)
❑ Absence of significant follicular plugging
❑ Absence, or at least a decrease of sebaceous glands
❑ Presence of normal epidermis (only occasional atrophy)
❑ Fibrotic streams into the dermis

In connection with pseudopelade, a type of patchy baldness was described by Dreuw in 1910 as alopecia parvimaculata.[26] This type of alopecia has been reported to occur in small epidemics or sporadically. The alopecia is characterized by single or multiple, asymptomatic, non-inflammed, irregular small patches. Spontaneous regrowth of hair is seen in 90% of cases, whereas atrophy may develop in 10%. Although no modern explanation for this condition has been forthcoming, the association of such cases with proved microsporum epidemics suggests an etiologic relationship.

Pathology

The histologic findings although not specific, are characteristic. There is thinning of epidermis with loss or flattening of rete pegs. In some cases, the only epidermal change is mild edema and lack of cohesion between the epidermis and cutis. In the early stage, one finds a predominantly lymphocytic infiltrate centered around the upper two-thirds of the hair follicle. It invades the walls of the follicles and the sebaceous glands. Gradually, the infiltrate destroys the hair follicles and the sebaceous glands. In the late stage, there is extensive fibrosis of the dermis with only traces of an inflammatory infiltrate. The most characteristic finding is the presence of perpendicular columns of fibrous tissue, which has replaced the follicles (follicular ghosts).[9,23] Elastic fiber stain shows abnormally increased elastic tissue both within and around the fibrous column that replaces the intradermal part of the hair follicle above the bulge **(Figures 15.10, and 15.11)**.[24,27,28]

Direct immunofluorescence is negative with occasional unspecific deposits (IgM and C3) at the basement membrane zone of the follicular infundibulum.

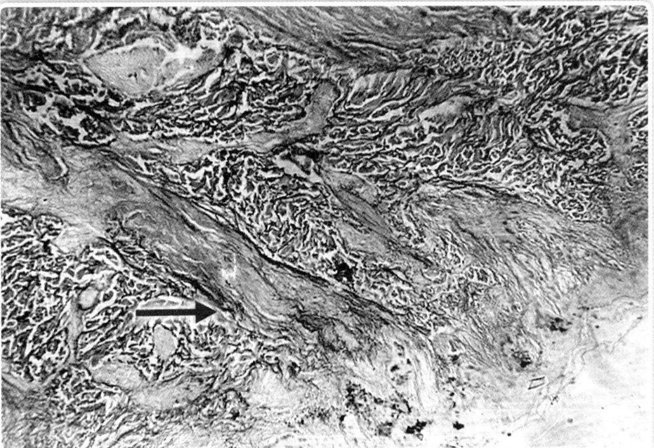

Fig. 15.11: Pseudopelade of Brocq. Elastic fibers around the fibrous remnant of hair follicle

Treatment

Treatment is almost the same as for LPP. However, response to treatment is often disappointing. The assessment of clinical activity and treatment response is difficult in PPB, as the patients often do not have overt signs and symptoms. Continued spreading of hair loss and the extent of the inflammatory infiltrate are the only two indicators of the ongoing disease activity. Hence, monitoring the size of the affected area, photographs and repeated biopsies are required to choose treatment and gauge response. A moderate to dense lymphocytic infiltrate is an indication for systemic treatment. In the burnt out stage, when the disfigurement is considerable, surgical modalities like autografting from unaffected scalp to scarred scalp or surgical 'expansion' techniques may be considered.[9,14]

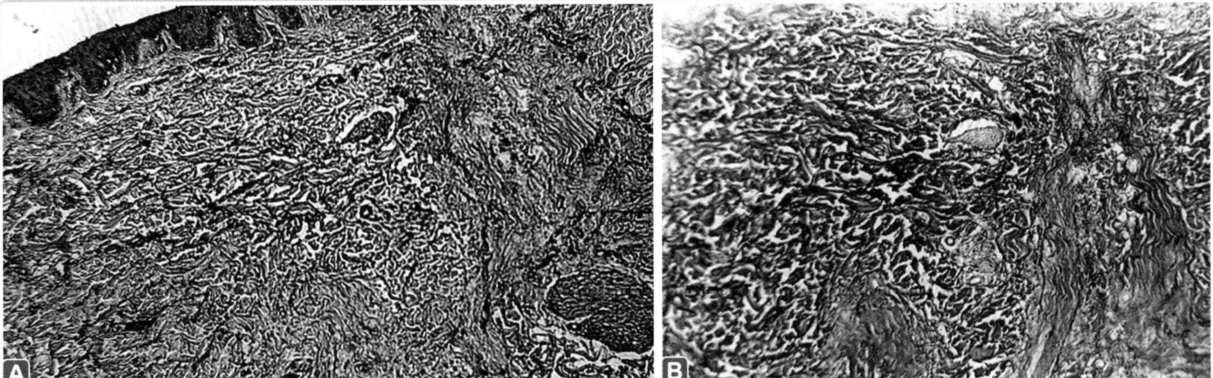

Figs 15.10A and B: Pseudopelade of Brocq. Comparison of H and E (Fig. 15.10A) and elastic tissue stains (Fig. 15.10B) shows how informative the latter is in PPB. The vertical fibrous remnant is barely discernible in Figure 15.10A, but well outlined by elastic fibers in Figure 15.10B

Central Centrifugal Cicatricial Alopecia (Syn: Follicular Degeneration Syndrome; Hot Comb Alopecia)

Central Centrifugal Cicatricial Alopecia (CCCA) is a diagnostic category adopted by the North American Hair Research Society to encompass terms such as hot comb alopecia and follicular degeneration syndrome.[29] It most often affects black females. Occurrence in men is very less compared to women. The exact cause is not known. Genetic predisposition is considered to be a likely factor. The condition has been traced to repeated trauma due to the unique grooming and hair styling practices of African women using chemical relaxers, hot combs and hair straightening agents. However, there has been no conclusive proof. Combined genetic and environmental factors may predispose to CCCA.[14]

The condition begins as a focus of cicatricial alopecia over the vertex region which gradually spreads centrifugally in a symmetrical manner affecting a large area on the top with extension to the sides of the scalp. The slow symmetrical forward progression resembles female pattern hair loss. The alopecic area shows loss of follicular ostia with usually no signs of inflammation.[9,14]

Pathology

The most distinctive histological feature of CCCA is premature desquamation of the inner root sheath (IRS) below the isthmus and eccentric thinning of the follicular epithelium. Desquamation of IRS is normally observed at the level of isthmus, whereas in CCCA, the desquamation is seen early and involves the lower half of the follicle **(Box 15.4)**. Further, premature IRS desquamation can occasionally be seen in other inflammatory and degenerative conditions of the scalp like LPP. Thus, to distinguish these diagnoses, it has been suggested that CCCA has this finding in otherwise normal hair follicles without showing lymphocytic inflammation or structural alteration and is linked to the pathogenesis of the disease.[29]

Other findings include lymphoplasmocytic inflammation, concentric lamellar fibroplasias, dermal fibrosis, loss of sebaceous gland and free hair fragments in the dermis initiating a granulomatous reaction.[23]

Box 15.4: Premature desquamation of IRS in CCA

- Premature desquamation of the inner root sheath (IRS) below the isthmus and eccentric thinning of the follicular epithelium
- Most distinctive histological feature, but not pathognomonic (also seen in LPP)

Treatment

Patients must be counselled about the probable cause of CCCA and avoidance of the same. No treatment is found to be effective. Use of topical agents like steroids, tacrolimus, minoxidil, intralesional steroids and/or oral antibiotics (tetracycline), systemic corticosteroids may be a reasonable approach in patients with active disease process. Most patients resort to wearing of wigs and hair extension.[30]

Alopecia Mucinosa (Syn: Follicular mucinosis)

Alopecia mucinosa, also known as follicular mucinosis is an uncommon disorder of unknown etiology. It can be primary or secondary to mycosis fungoides, lupus erythematosus or angiolymphoid hyperplasia.

Clinically, it presents as indolent plaques sometimes associated with mild pruritus. Dilated follicular orifices with keratin plugs can be seen over the scalp and face. Localized lesions show spontaneous remission within 2 years, often with areas of permanent hair loss. Hair shafts are usually fragile and break easily. Generally, the lesions of alopecia mucinosa confined to head and neck are entirely benign.[31]

Pathology

The histologic picture is characterized by a reticular degeneration of the epithelial cells in sebaceous glands and outer root sheaths, leading to a disruption of these cells and the formation of cystic spaces. This usually is followed by accumulation of mucin within the hair follicles and sebaceous glands. The mucin consists of acid mucopolysaccharides that stain metachromatically with giemsa stain and alcian blue. The inflammatory infiltrate in the benign form is variable, predominantly lymphocytic with an admixture of eosinophils. In patients having mycosis fungoides, the dermal infiltrate is that of mycosis fungoides, Pautrier's microabscesses may be present in the epidermis and in the upper part of the hair follicle. [32]

Keratosis Follicularis Spinulosa Decalvans (Syn: Siemens I Syndrome)

Keratosis follicularis spinulosa decalvans (KFSD), first described by Siemens in 1926 is a rare genetically heterogenous syndrome.[33] In some families, it is inherited as X-linked dominant with mutation in the spermidine/spermine N(1)acetyltransferase gene at Xp22.1 whereas in others it appears to follow an autosomal dominant pattern.[9]

KFSD begins in infancy or childhood, unlike other primary cicatricial alopecias. It is characterized by extensive keratosis pilaris and progressive cicatricial alopecia. Keratotic spiny lesions, often first appear on the scalp and later progress to involve eyebrows, eyelids and limbs. Occasionally the involvement may be almost universal. The disease tends to progress until puberty with patchy or extensive cicatricial alopecia of the scalp, eyebrows and eyelashes. There is usually associated palmoplantar keratoderma, punctate corneal epithelial defects, ophthalmitis, photophobia and facial erythema.[9, 14]

A rare variant of KFSD, folliculitis spinulosa decalvans with a more persistent pustular course has been described. The disease appears to be of autosomal dominant inheritance having symptoms of severe inflammation that goes beyond puberty.[31]

Pathology

The histologic features are that of other primary cicatricial alopecias with follicular hyperkeratosis, perifollicular and dermal inflammation, distorted follicles and fibrotic tracts.[14]

Folliculitis Decalvans (Syn: Acne Decalvans; Quinquaud's Disease)

Quinquaud in 1888 first described the disease.[34] Decalvans is a term derived from Latin meaning "making bald". Folliculitis Decalvans (FD) is a clinical pattern that is probably common to a heterogenous group of disorders characterized by clinically evident follicular inflammation which leads to destruction of the follicle and consequent scarring alopecia.[9]

The frequency is about 11% of all cicatricial alopecia cases. The disease affects both the sexes equally. The condition usually occurs between the ages of 30 and 60 years. Familial cases have also been reported.[9,35]

Etiology

The cause of the disease is unknown. Chronic bacterial folliculitis or altered host immune responses are proposed mechanisms. Coagulase positive *S.aureus* is most often recovered. Failure to confine the *S. aureus* to the infundibulum of the hair follicle and to completely eradicate it from the isthmus is postulated. This may be due to disruption by bacterial proteases of the protective barrier provided by the inner root sheath. However, recent studies report no consistent defect in cell-mediated immunity or inner root sheath keratinization.[36]

Clinical Features

Arndt in 1908 listed the following characteristics of this rare disease as the most important: (a) Inflammatory changes around the follicles of the scalp in the form of pustules followed by exudation or suppuration and crusting; (b) Peripheral extension and central healing leading to patchy cicatricial alopecia due to chronic inflammatory infiltration in the perifollicular connective tissue; (c) Almost complete lack of symptoms; (d) Chronic course; and (e) Extra-ordinary resistance to treatment with resultant unfavorable prognosis.[37]

The pustules may develop in crops. As the hairs are shed, the pustules are followed by red macules which fade to leave scars. The alopecic patches are usually round or oval in shape. Slow, intermittent extension gradually increases the size of bald areas. Center of the lesion represents the point of oldest involvement and appears as a smooth shiny, atrophic scar **(Figure 15.12)**. In some cases, the border of the alopecic area may not reveal discrete follicular papules or pustules but rather a continuous infiltrated elevated rim resulting from a deep seated inflammation in which there is fusion of the inflammatory process in adjacent follicles. Unlike dissecting cellulitis, sinus tract formation is not a feature of FD.[14]

Tufted folliculitis is a variant of FD in which tufts of hair are the cardinal and prominent feature surrounding relatively small patches of hair loss. Usually, there are only a few circumscribed areas of scalp inflammation which heal with scarring in which multiple hair tufts emerge from a single dilated follicular orifice **(Figure 15.13)**. These thick hair tufts are the 'hair bumps' that the patients describe on their scalp.[9] Some authors believe tufted folliculitis as a separate entity because of the different clinical presentation with smaller areas of hair loss and better prognosis.[38]

Pathology

Epidermis is atrophic, though edematous. In early lesions a peri- and intrafollicular infiltrate is present mainly of

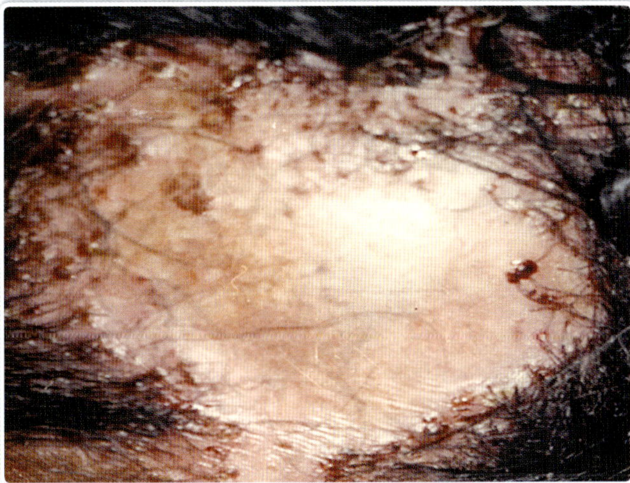

Fig. 15.12: Folliculitis decalvans. Well defined atrophic patch of alopecia with follicular pustules at the advancing margins

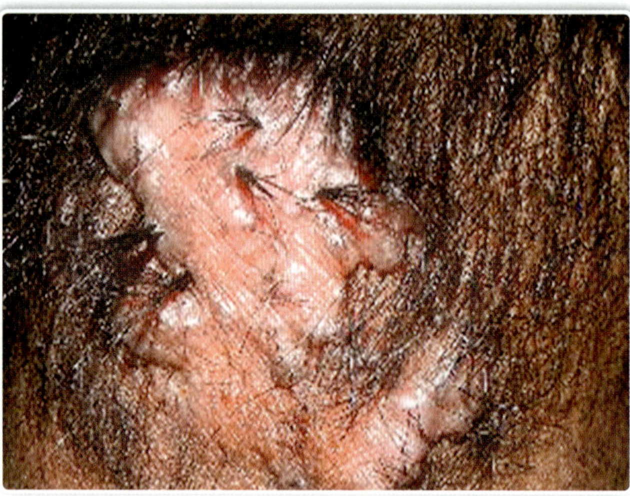

Fig. 15.13: Tufted folliculitis. Multiple hairs arising from a single orifice (*Courtesy:* Department of Dermatology, BMCRI, Bengaluru)

neutrophils but also containing lymphoid cells, histiocytes and plasma cells **(Figure 15.14)**. It is most intense around the upper portion of the follicle although the neighboring cutis and even the epidermis is somewhat infiltrated.[34] The infiltrate develops into a perifollicular abscess and often contains a good amount of plasma cells. In older lesions, chronic granulation tissue containing numerous plasma cells, lymphoid cells and fibroblasts are seen. Often, numerous foreign body giant cells are present around the remnants of hair follicles. As healing takes place, fibrosis is seen, the follicles and sebaceous glands completely disappear. Elastic fibers are usually completely lacking in the upper dermis while at the level of the sweat glands they seem normal.[4]

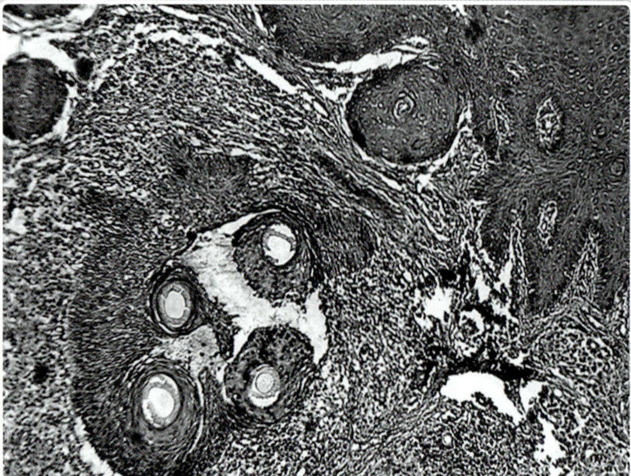

Fig. 15.14: Folliculitis decalvans. Section from pustular border showing dense inflammatory infiltrate around atrophic hair follicles and dilated blood vessels

Some authors have emphasized that the absence of inflammatory cells in the follicular lumen separates PPB from FD.[3,5]

Treatment

Antimicrobial agents are the first choice of treatment. Appropriate antimicrobials can be selected following pus culture and antibiotic sensitivity. A combination of rifampicin (300 mg bid) for 10 days with cephalexin (500 mg qid) or clindamycin (300 mg bid) or doxycycline (100 mg bid) or clarithromycin or cotrimoxazole for 10 weeks has been found to be beneficial. Topical antibiotics like clindamycin phosphate 1% solution/gel, mupirocin cream or fusidic acid 1% can be used. In case of staphylococcal carrier, topical mupirocin ointment can be applied to nostrils daily for 1 week and then once a month. Tar shampoos and topical keratolytics help to remove the scales and reduce tufting.[9,18]

Dissecting Cellulitis (Syn: Dissecting folliculitis; Perifolliculitis capitis abscedens et suffodiens; Hoffman's disease)

Dissecting cellulitis, first described by Hoffman in 1908, is a rare chronic perifolliculitis of the scalp characterized by painful suppurative nodules, interconnecting sinus tracts, foul smelling discharge and extensive scarring.[39] The term dissecting cellulitis is a misnomer because the condition is suppurative folliculitis, not a cellulitis.[21] It is seen predominantly in Black men in the second to fourth decade.

Etiology

The exact etiology is not known. Although staphylococci, streptococci, pseudomonas, propionibacterium acnes may be cultured from various lesions, no specific causative agent has been isolated. A defect in follicular keratinization results in poral obstruction, and sebaceous and keratinous material accumulate within pilosebaceous units. Ultimately, the follicles burst resulting in an intense inflammatory neutrophilic reaction with sinus tract formation. It has been suggested that the pathogenesis of dissecting cellulitis may involve an abnormal host response to bacterial antigens. However, patients with dissecting cellulitis have no evidence of immune deficiency or presence of infection at other skin sites.[40]

Clinical Features

The condition starts with painful, indurated, skin colored nodules over the vertex which later becomes soft and fluctuant **(Figure 15.15)**. Tubular ridges are formed by coalescence of confluent nodules leading to irregular cerebriform pattern, on a red edematous background. Pressure on one region of the scalp elicits discharge of pus from distant sites. Characteristically, hair is lost from the summits of these inflammatory lesions and retained in the valleys. The condition tends to be chronic with frequent acute exacerbations and ultimately leads to scarring and extensive hair loss.[9,21]

Since follicular occlusion is thought to be the initiating event, dissecting cellulitis is considered a part of follicular occlusion tetrad that includes hidradenitis suppurativa, acne conglobata and pilonidal sinus. Other reported associations include spondyloarthropathy, SAPHO syndrome, marginal keratitis and *S. aureus* osteomyelitis.[9,17]

Pathology

Histology shows moderately dense, perifollicular inflammation with a mixed infiltrate of lymphocytes, histiocytes, plasmocytes and neutrophils affecting the lower half of the dermis and subcutaneous fat. Follicular perforation results in abscess formation leading to destruction of the pilosebaceous follicles initially, and eventually the other cutaneous appendages. Keratin fragments induce a granulomatous reaction, with foreign-body giant cells, lymphoid and plasma cells. Eventually, chronic abscesses become lined with squamous epithelium and true sinus tracts are formed. When inflammation subsides, there is extensive coarse dermal fibrosis with loss of hair follicles.[17,41]

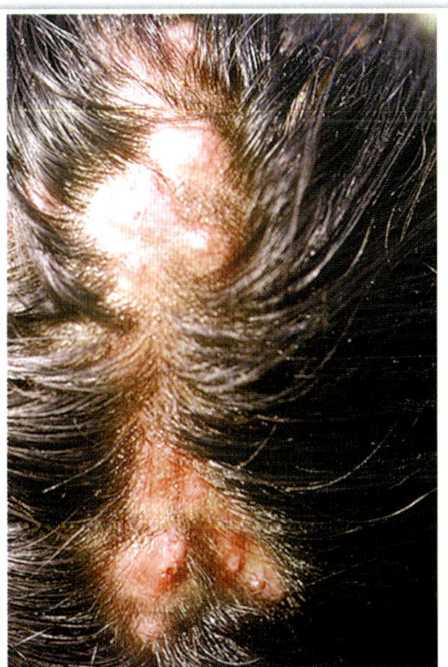

Fig. 15.15: Dissecting cellulitis showing fluctuant nodules and intercommunicating abscesses with cicatricial alopecia

Treatment

Dissecting cellulitis is a notoriously treatment-resistant disease. Isotretinoin (1–2 mg/kg/day) for 5 to 6 months may cause significant long lasting remission. Other treatment options include systemic antibiotics, corticosteroids (intralesional and/or systemic), dapsone and surgical excision with grafting.[17,21]

Folliculitis Keloidalis (Syn: Acne keloidalis; Acne keloidalis Nuchae)

The term folliculitis keloidalis (FK) is preferred over acne keloidalis and acne keloidalis nuchae because neither the disease bears any resemblance to the acne vulgaris nor the lesions are always limited to the nuchal area of the scalp.[21]

FK is a chronic inflammatory process of the hair follicles in the region of nape of the neck and occipital area of scalp leading to hypertrophic scarring. It is commonly seen in young adult Black males but is not uncommon in India. Occasionally women may also be affected. The exact etiology is not known. No specific organism has been isolated. Trauma from razor, friction from collar/helmet, frequent short haircuts and incurving hair shafts have been incriminated to be causative, but there is no convincing evidence. In predisposed individuals, follicular rupture and degenerating hair fragments may initiate an intense widespread dermal inflammatory response, granulomatous reaction and fibrosis. Some view that penetration of cut hair into the skin may initiate the process.[21,40]

Clinical Features

Early lesions are small, flesh colored, folliculocentric papules or pustules over the nuchal region and lower occiput. These lesions may be inconspicuous, and the patient may first be aware of the hard keloidal papules that follow the folliculitis. In advanced disease, the lesions coalesce to form large nodules, plaques and hypertrophic scars **(Figure 15.16)**. The condition is extremely chronic with waxing and waning for years and eventually leading to permanent scarring alopecia.[17,40]

Pathology

The histopathology of early lesions is that of folliculitis and perifolliculitis with predominant lymphocytic and plasma cell infiltrate surrounding the lower part of infundibulum and isthmus. Subsequently, there is a variable degree of inflammation around the degenerating follicles, loss of sebaceous glands, destruction of follicles and lamellar fibrosis. In advanced keloidal lesions, there are numerous "naked" hair shafts trapped within a dense fibrotic matrix

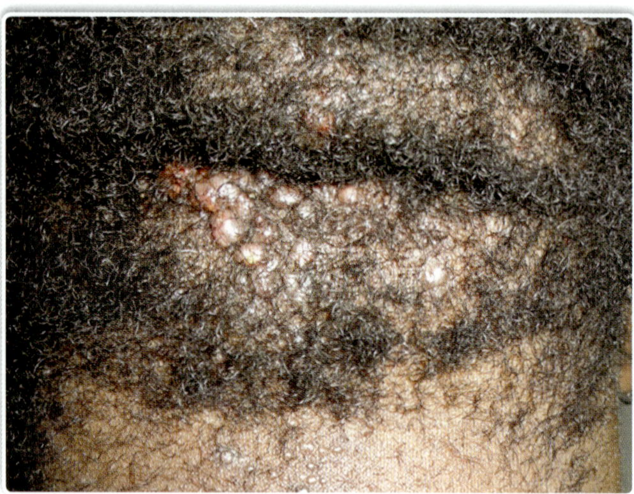

Fig. 15.16: Folliculitis keloidalis. End stage disease with large firm keloidal nodules confined to lower occiput and nape of the neck

associated with foreign body granulomatous reaction. The end result is scarring.[21,40]

Treatment

Treatment is effective if instituted in the early phase. Potent topical corticosteroids, antibiotics (topical and oral), intralesional corticosteroids are found to be effective in halting the progression of the disease. Excisional surgery may be necessary in advanced cases.[17]

Acne Necrotica

Acne necrotica is a severe form of scalp folliculitis. The exact etiology is unknown, though staphylococci are usually cultured from these patients. Papules and pustules evolve to form crusts leaving depressed scars. The condition is chronic and recurrent.

Erosive Pustular Dermatosis

Pye, et al. in 1979 first described this condition. It has no specific cause, but trauma, sun damage and destructive procedures for actinic keratoses are considered to precipitate this condition. The disease usually occurs in elderly women and presents with chronic, red, extensive, pustular, crusted and eroded plaques on the scalp. The lesions progress slowly and heal with scarring alopecia. [42]

Pathology

Histological study shows areas of epidermal erosion with non-specific changes of atrophy and chronic lymphocytic inflammation, sometimes with increased numbers of plasma cells and foreign body giant cells. Fibrosis and follicular unit loss eventually ensue.

Treatment

Potent topical corticosteroids are the mainstay of treatment. Topical tacrolimus, calcipotriol, isotretinoin (0.75 mg/kg) and oral zinc are some of the other reported treatments.[22]

End Stage Non-specific Cicatricial Alopecia[9]

The early stages of untreated primary cicatricial alopecias like LPP, FFA, PPB, CCCA and FD can usually be diagnosed based on their distinctive clinical and histopathological features. However, overtime these primary cicatricial alopecias ultimately burn out and the characteristic features are no longer present. The end stage is an irregular area of cicatricial alopecia without follicular ostia and without inflammation. One exception is DLE, which can usually be distinguished clinically from other primary cicatricial alopecias both during the acute stage and end stage by the presence of hypo- and hyperpigmentation of scalp and ears and follicular plugging in the ears.

Many authors recommend avoiding the term 'pseudopelade' to describe end stage cicatricial alopecia because of confusion with 'pseuodpelade of Brocq' which is a specific primary lymphocytic cicatricial alopecia. Instead, the preferred terminology to describe the late or burnt out stage of any cicatricial alopecia is 'end stage non-specific cicatricial alopecia.[9,14]

Pathology

The histology is variable and non-specific. The features are similar to the late stages of various primary cicatricial alopecias which include: (a) Non-specific perifollicular inflammation; (b) Mild superficial perivascular infiltrate; (c) Depletion or absence of follicles; (d) Vertical fibrous tracts as traces of vanished follicles; (e) Absence of sebaceous glands; (f) Atrophic epidermis, sclerotic dermis; and (g) Granulomatous inflammation (rare).

Treatment

Various treatment modalities have been tried, but nothing has been shown to be effective.

Note: Salient clinicohistological features of primary cicatricial alopecias are shown in **Table 15.3**.

Secondary Cicatricial Alopecia

Scleroderma

Cicatricial alopecia may occur in both general and localized (morphea) forms of scleroderma. Linear circumscribed morphea in the frontal region – 'en coup de sabre' morphea is more common **(Figure 15.17)**. It has been

Table 15.3: Salient clinco histological features of primary cicatricial alopecias

Disease	*Clinical*	*Histopathology*
Pseudopelade of Brocq	Often mistaken for alopecia areata; alopecic patches coalesce into irregular white patches resembling 'foot prints in the snow'; localized only in the scalp; few solitary hairs within the patches of atrophy	Absence of marked inflammation, scarring, and follicular plugging; perpendicular columns of fibrous tissue (follicular ghosts); abnormally increased elastic tissue around the fibrous column
Lichen planopilaris	Pruritic, spinous, hyperkeratotic, follicular papules; perifollicular erythema and scaling; center of the bald patch is smooth and atrophic with active margins	Prototypical form of lymphocyte mediated primary cicatricial alopecia; hypergranulosis within the affected infundibula; concentric lamellar fibrosis around follicles
Frontal fibrosing alopecia	Postmenopausal women; progressive frontoparietal recession; loss of eyebrows	Features similar to LPP
Lupus erythematosus	Commonly affects the scalp, face and ears; discoid, erythematous scaly plaques; telangiectasia, atrophy, dyspigmentation and follicular plugging in the center of bald patch; 'carpet tack sign'	Focal basal cell vacuolation; funnel shaped keratotic plugs; patchy dermal infiltrate; thickening of the basement membrane zone; immunopathologically deposition of IgG, IgM and C3 in a granular band like pattern at the dermal interface
Folliculitis decalvans	Crops of pustules with erythema and crusting around the rim of alopecic patches; center of the bald area shiny and atrophic	Prototypical of neutrophil-mediated primary cicatricial alopecia; intense infiltrate around the upper portion of the follicle; often, numerous foreign body giant cells around remnants of hair follicles; inflammatory cells in the follicular lumen
Dissecting cellulitis	Perifolliculitis; painful suppurative nodules; interconnecting sinus tracts, and extensive scarring; part of follicular occlusion tetrad	Mixed infiltrate; follicular perforation and abscess formation; granulomatous reaction; extensive fibrosis in dermis and subcutis
Central centrifugal cicatricial alopecia	Middle aged black women; focus of cicatricial alopecia over vertex spreading centrifugally	Premature desquamation of inner root sheath; perifollicular lymphocytic infiltrate; concentric lamellar fibroplasia
Acne keloidalis	Common in young black men; follicular papules/ pustules, keloidal plaques over the occipital scalp and neck	Mixed infiltrate at the level of isthmus and lower infundibulum; granulomatous inflammation; lamellar fibroplasias

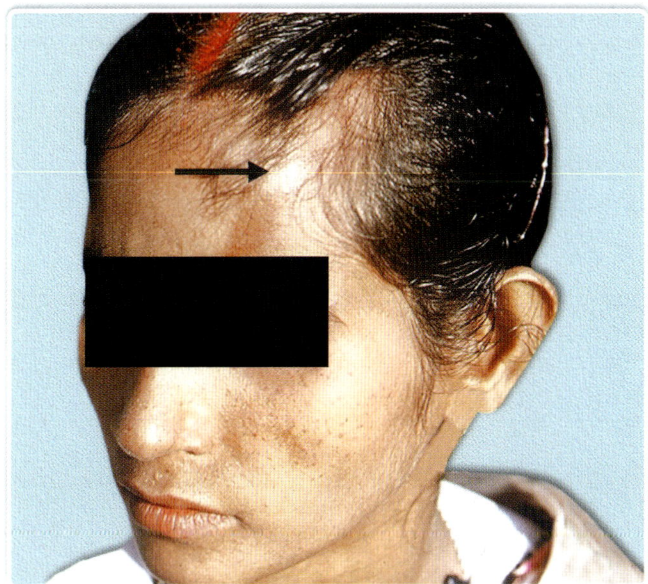

Fig. 15.17: Linear morphoea. 'En coup de sabre' with scarring alopecia

associated with hereditary deficiency of complement C2.[9] In systemic form, the condition usually manifests itself elsewhere in a characteristic fashion. Initially it presents as an erythematous, non-pitting edematous plaque. In a few weeks, the lesion develops a waxy yellowish colored center with a smooth surface and lilac colored border. The involved site becomes free of skin appendages. Histological examination in the early stage shows chronic inflammation of the upper and mid-follicle and thick collagen bundles. In the late sclerotic stage there is almost complete disappearance of the inflammatory infiltrate with atrophy of the eccrine glands and prominent fibrosis.

Sarcoidosis

Sarcoidosis has uncommonly been reported to cause cicatricial alopecia. The condition predominantly affects women. Nodular or papular lesions of sarcoidosis may produce cicatricial alopecia of the scalp. The nodules coalesce into a plaque which spreads peripherally forming an annular lesion with a depressed bald patch in the center. The histology is distinctive, with non-caseating granulomatous inflammation which may contain few irregular giant cells and inclusion bodies (Schaumann bodies, asteroid bodies). It appears that the sarcoidal infiltrates compress and/or obliterate the hair follicles[9] **(Box 15.5)**.

Box 15.5: Histopathology of sarcoidosis

- Inclusion bodies (Schaumann bodies and asteroid bodies)
- Non-caseating granulomatous inflammation
- Sarcoidal infiltrates compress and/or obliterate the hair follicles

Necrobiosis Lipoidica[9,31]

In rare instances, lesions of necrobiosis lipoidica are present in areas apart from the legs (which is a common site) particularly on the face and scalp. Lesions located in these areas are often raised and firm and have a nodular or annular appearance. The alopecic patches are glazed and yellowish, often with conspicuous telangiectasia. About three-quarters of the patients with necrobiosis lipoidica are female, and approximately two-thirds have clinical diabetes mellitus. Histologically, epidermis is often atrophic. Dermis may show two types of reactions, namely a necrobiotic and a granulomatous type. Scalp lesions show a predominantly granulomatous reaction composed of histiocytes, epitheloid cells and giant cells along with extensive fibrosis and hyalinization of the collagen. Necrobiosis and lipid deposits are not conspicuous.

Cicatricial Pemphigoid (Syn: Benign mucosal pemphigoid)[9,31]

Cicatricial pemphigoid is an immunobullous disorder predominantly affecting the elderly. Scarring alopecia is a rare occurrence in cicatricial pemphigoid. It is seen as a localized erythematous plaque with recurrent vesicles and bullae on the scalp which heals with smooth atrophic scar and permanent alopecia. Skin lesions, predominantly on the head and neck, are the major feature of the Brunsting-Perry variant. Histology shows sub-epidermal bulla. The dermal changes are not specific. In areas of scarring, bullae often show a considerable chronic inflammatory infiltrate and in the later stages, fibrosis.

Epidermolysis Bullosa[9,31]

The term epidermolysis bullosa is applied to a group of mechanobullous disorders. Cicatricial alopecia may occur in generalized atrophic benign epidermolysis bullosa and recessive dystrophic epidermolysis bullosa. The disease exhibits repeated cycles of blistering of skin and mucous membranes. The blisters heal with atrophic scarring leading to cicatricial alopecia. The bullae form through dermoepidermal separation and the underlying papillary dermis usually shows fragmentation with absent or minimal inflammatory response. In areas of healing, extensive fibrosis is seen.

Infections[9]

Fungal infections like kerion and favus of the scalp are usually followed by baldness with scarring.

Among viral infections, trigeminal herpes zoster, varicella and recurrent herpes simplex may also give rise to cicatricial alopecia. The scars are minute and few in number.

Bacterial and protozoal infections which may lead to cicatricial alopecia are lupus vulgaris, leprosy, carbuncle, deep folliculitis, syphilis (gumma), yaws and leishmaniasis.

Neoplasms[31]

Loss of hair without scarring may occur over a variety of benign and malignant tumors of the scalp, but cicatricial alopecia is unusual. The neoplastic conditions which may lead to scarring alopecia are basal (morpheic type) and squamous cell carcinomas, cutaneous T cell lymphomas, metastatic carcinomas and angiosarcoma.

Traumatic Alopecia[31]

Physical and chemical injuries from a fall, missiles, vacuum extractor, burns, irradiation, acids, etc. may account for cicatricial alopecia of the scalp. The scars following these accidents are usually severe, irregular and extensive. The linear or angular outline of bald patches is diagnostic of traumatic alopecia **(Figure 15.18)**.

Traction Alopecia

Traction alopecia is believed to be related to hair styling practices which cause sustained pulling on the hair roots **(Figure 15.19)**. It is seen worldwide. Its frequency usually

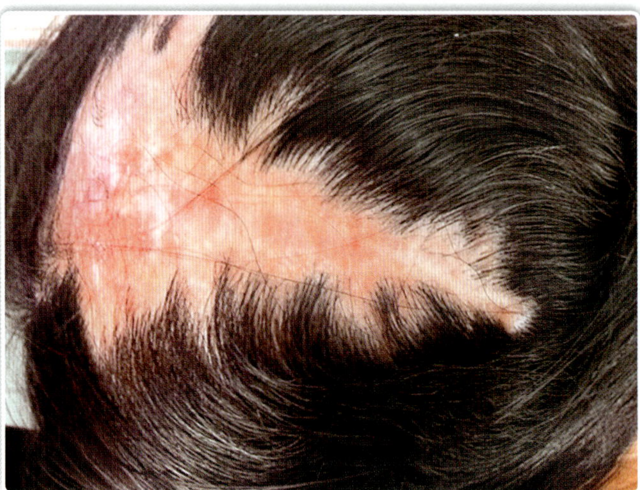

Fig. 15.18: Traumatic alopecia. Large irregular extensive cicatricial alopecia following burn injury

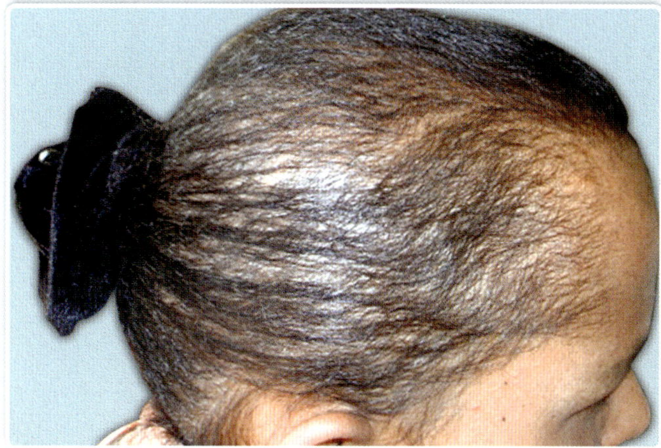

Fig. 15.19: Traction alopecia following tight hair styling practice

Box 15.6: Fringe sign

- The presence of terminal hairs outlining the original hairline seen in traction alopecia
- Helps to differentiate from alopecia areata

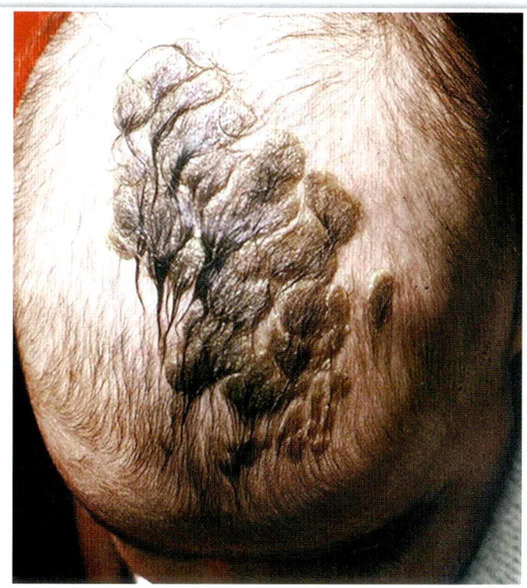

Fig. 15.20: Nevus sebaceous

depends on the cultural customs. Use of tight clips, tight braids, curling, tight head gear (nurse), twisting of uncut hair on top of head (Sikh men in India), tight pony tails and Japanese traditional hairdo are few examples of hair styling leading to cicatricial alopecia.[9]

The clinical features include perifollicular erythema, scales, pustules and reduced hair density leading to scarring alopecia. Broken hairs are common. Keratin cylinders may surround many hairs just above the scalp surface. The region affected depends upon the hair styling practice. Traction alopecia can be differentiated from alopecia areata by the "fringe sign", the presence of terminal hairs outlining the original hairline **(Box 15.6)**. Histology shows no significant perifollicular inflammation. The total number of terminal hairs is normally reduced. Distinct columns of connective tissue replace some follicles leaving obvious "blank" spaces. There is no loss of sebaceous glands, a feature which is in contrast to other cicatricial alopecias.

Congenital and Developmental Defects[9,31]

Cicatricial alopecia may also be a feature of some rare congenital and developmental defects. In aplasia cutis, there are focal areas of deficiencies, often in linear arrangement, present at birth and heal slowly to leave scars. In Conradi's disease (chondrodysplasia punctata), cicatricial alopecia of the vertex is present from early infancy. Similarly in incontinentia pigmenti, scarring alopecia may appear in about one-fourth of the cases. Epidermal nevi, particularly of sebaceous variety **(Figure 15.20)** may present with alopecia.

Other Conditions[9,31]

Some other conditions which can occasionally present with cicatricial alopecia include: (a) Trichotillomania; (b) Porokeratosis of Mibelli; **(Figure 15.21)** (c) Keratosis pilaris atrophicans; (d) Senescent alopecia; (e) Pressure alopecia (post operative); (f) Halo scalp ring; (g) Scalp necrosis after surgical embolism; (h) Pityriasis amiantacea; (i) Lumpy scalp syndrome; (j) Lipedematous alopecia; (k) Lichen sclerosus et atrophicans; (l) Polyostotic fibrous dysplasia; (m) Generalized follicular hamartoma; (n) Ectodermal dysplasia; and (o) X-linked recessive ichthyosis.

Approach to Diagnosis

There is no magic touch in making hair appear in its glory on head of the bald. Hence, the single most important consideration relevant to scarring alopecia is to establish an etiology for which specific therapy is available. Only an approach involving systematic biopsy taking and painstaking correlation of histological and clinical features can achieve this.

Below is a step by step approach that can be used in scarring alopecia.

History

An elaborate history has to be taken in every case of cicatricial alopecia with specific emphasis on onset, duration, rate of progression of alopecia, associated symptoms, previous treatments, re-growth of hair, hair care and family history.

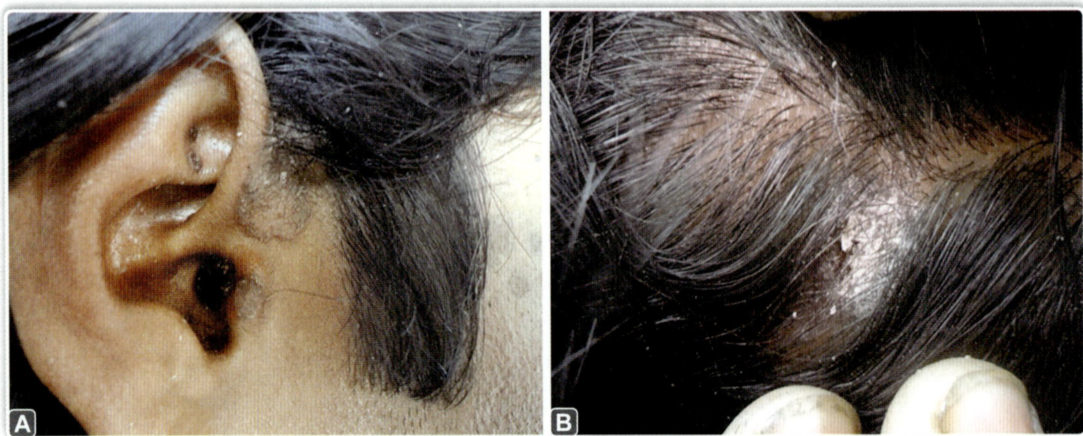

Figs 15.21A and B: Porokeratosis: (A) Showing classical lesion of porokeratosis of Mibelli, (B) Showing scalp involvement with cicatricial alopecia in the same patient

Patients of LPP, DLE, FK and acne necrotica usually present with symptoms of itching, pain, burning and photosensitivity, whereas patients of CCCA, PPB, traction alopecia, often have no symptoms and report slow onset of hair loss.

Examination

All patients of cicatricial alopecia should be examined preferably in a sitting position with good illumination using magnifying light or ideally a dermoscope. A careful evaluation of hair and scalp has to be done to assess pattern, distribution and morphology of the alopecic patches. Serial photographs and measurements of the bald area (if possible) are important to assess the ongoing activity and need for treatment, especially in conditions with no overt signs and symptoms like PPB and CCCA.

Skin Biopsy

A skin biopsy is essential to establish the diagnosis and to guide treatment in cicatricial alopecia. Usually, more than one biopsy is required for accurate diagnosis and appropriate treatment. Ideally, the site should be clinically active with a positive pull test. Scalp biopsy has been shown to be especially effective when samples are submitted for both transverse and horizontal sectioning.

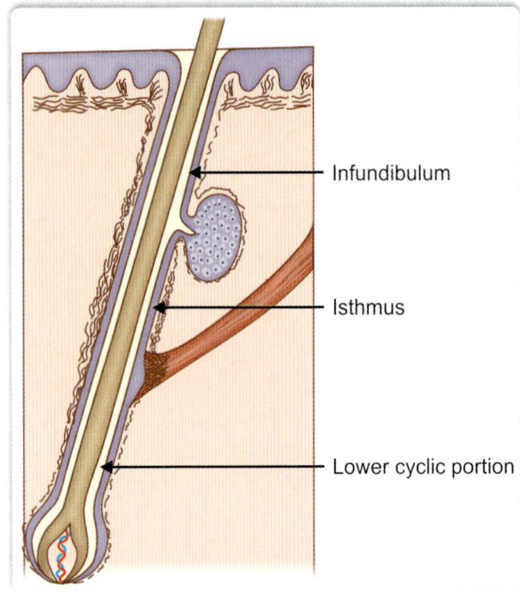

Fig. 15.22: Diagram of elastic fiber distribution on hair follicle. Loose arrangement in infundibular portion. Well organized elastic coat in isthmus portion. Elastic tendon at insertion of arrector pili muscle and elastic fibers between muscle fibers. Sparse elastic fibers on lower cyclic portion. Arao-Perkins elastin-like body in neck of dermal papilla

Elastic Tissue Staining

A routine examination for elastic fibers preferably using acid alcohol orcein and giemsa stain provides helpful information in the histologic diagnosis of cicatricial alopecia. A diagrammatic representation of elastic fiber distribution on normal hair follicle is shown in **Figure 15.22.**[24] Distinctive elastic staining patterns have been identified that may help differentiate advanced cases of PPB, LPP, and DLE.

Microarray Analysis

Currently, microarray analysis is used to identify disease associated gene expression patterns with the aims of further clarification of nosologic classifications and development of targeted therapies.

Pull Test

A hair-pull test can assist in the evaluation of all types of alopecia. An excess of loose anagen hairs can be indicative of active disease in cicatricial alopecia. Pull test is done by grasping a small bunch of hairs (about 30-50 hairs) at the margin of the bald patch close to the scalp, with the thumb and forefinger, and gently but firmly sliding the fingers along the entire length of the hair perpendicularly away from the scalp. Positive pull test (5 or more hair) indicates that the patch is active. Short fragments of pulled hair are mounted on a slide with few drops of distilled water and examined under light microscope.

Tug Test

Tug test is used to demonstrate hair fragility. It is performed by grasping a bunch of hairs with the fingers of one hand and plucking the distal ends. Fragile or damaged hair will break into small pieces. This test is of significance in diagnosis of CCCA.

Dermoscopy

Dermoscope has shown to be an important tool in the evaluation and diagnosis of cicatricial alopecia as a first step before performing a biopsy **(Figure 15.23)**. The following findings have been reported in a small series.[43]

- Discoid lupus—white patches, branching capillaries, and keratin plugs
- Lichen planopilaris—perifollicular scales and white dots
- Frontal fibrosing alopecia—perifollicular scales, perifollicular erythema and branching capillaries.

  All findings showed reduced follicular ostia as expected.

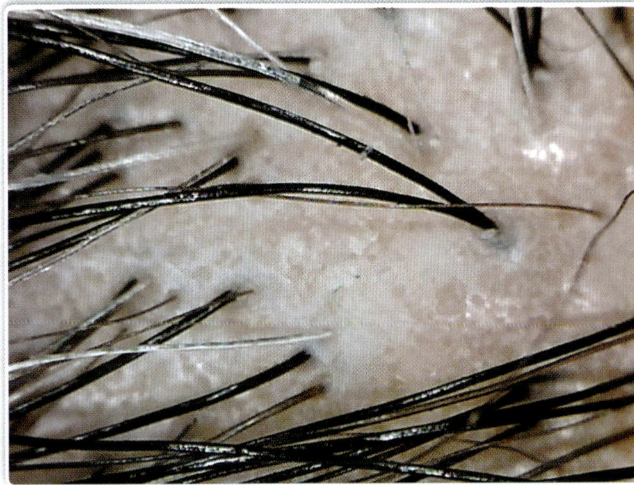

Fig. 15.23: Dermatoscopy of cicatricial alopecia (*Courtesy:* Dr Sharmila Patil, DY Patil Medical College, Mumbai)

Cicatricial alopecia: At a glance

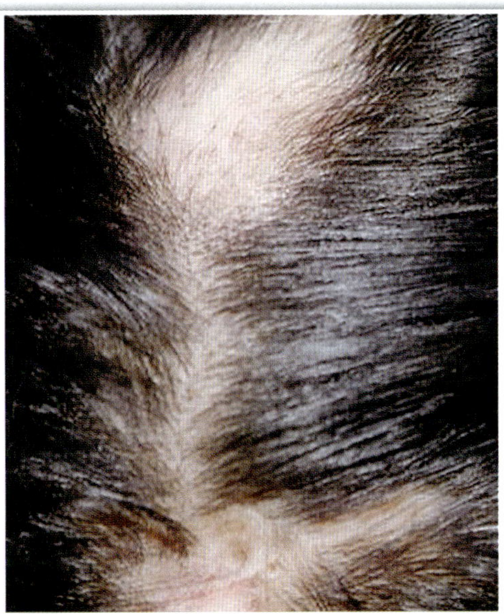

- An intractable condition and a source of considerable depression and embarrassment
- Visible loss of follicular ostia is the clinical hallmark
- Easily extracted anagen hair is an important feature of disease activity
- Scalp biopsy is the essential first step in the diagnosis
- Inflammatory infiltrate is located at the level of infundibulum and isthmus resulting in destruction of hair follicle stem cells and sebaceous gland leading to permanent hair loss
- Elastic fiber examination provides helpful information in the diagnosis
- Sebaceous gland may be central to the pathogenesis
- Hair re-growth is unlikely
- The goal of therapy is to halt further progression
- Cicatricial Alopecia Research Foundation (CARF) is entirely devoted to research and care of patients.

References

1. Somani N, Bergfeld WF. Cicatricial alopecia: classification and histopathology. Dermatologic Therapy. 2008;21:221-37.
2. Otberg N, Wu WY, McElwee KJ, Shapiro J. Skinmed: Dermatology for the clinician (Wiley-Blackwell). 2008;7:19-26.
3. Brocq L, Lenglet, Ayrignac. Recherches sur l, alopecic atrophicante variete pseudopelade. Ann de dermat et de syph. 1905;6:1-32,97-127,209-37.
4. Laymon CW. The cicatricial alopecias. J Invest Derm. 1947;8:99.
5. Degos R, Rabut R, Duperrat S, Leclorg R. L'etat pseudopeladique. Reflexions a propos de cent cas d' alopecias cicatricial les en ires, d' apparence primitive du type pseudopelade. Ann Derrm syph. 1954;81:5.

6. Gay Prieto J. Pseudopelade of Brocq: Its relationship to some forms of cicatricial alopecias and to lichen planus. J Invest Derm. 1955;24:323-35.
7. Pinkus H. Alopecia clinicopathological correlations. Int J Derm. 1980;19:245.
8. Olsen EA, Bergfeld WF, Cotsarelis G, et al. Summary of North American Hair Research Society (NAHRS)-Sponsored Workshop on Cicatricial Alopecia, Duke University Medical Center, February 10 and 11, 2001. J Am Acad Dermatol. 2003;48:103-10.
9. Sinclair RD. Disorders of Hair. In: Burns T, Breathnach S, Cox N, Griffiths C, (eds). Rook's Textbook of Dermatology, 8th edition. Oxford; Wiley-Blackwell Publishers. 2010;66.38-66.52
10. Pringle JJ. Lichen spinulosus (Vel Pilaris). Brit J Derm. 1897;9:74-6.
11. Little EG. Folliculitis decalvans et atrophicans. Brit J Derm. 1915;27:183.
12. Feldman S. Lichen planus et acuminatus atrophicans: lichen planus atrophicus lichen plan sclerux, Hallopeau: Lichen ruber planus Keloidi formis, Pawlow; Lichen planus morphoeicus, Crocker, Lichen albus. Zumbush. Arch Derm Syph. 1922;5:102-13.
13. Silver H, Chargm L, Sachs PM. Follicular lichen planus (lichen planopilaris). AMA Arch Derm Syph. 1953;67:346-54.
14. Price V, Mirmirani P. Predominantly lymphocytic group. In: Price V, Mirmirani P, (eds). Cicatricial Alopecia: An Approach to Diagnosis and Management. New York; Springer Publications. 2011;35.
15. Sevill A. The hair and scalp: A clinical study. London: Edward Arnold Ltd. 1952;137-58.
16. Altman J, Perry HO. The variations and course of lichen planus. Arch Derm. 1961;84:179.
17. Sperling LC. Alopecias. In: Bolognia JL, Jorizzo JL, Rapini RP, (eds). Dermatology, 2nd edition. Noida; Elsevier India. 2009;987-1005.
18. Price V, Mirmirani P. Medical management. In: Price V, Mirmirani P, (eds). Cicatricial Alopecia: An approach to diagnosis and management. New York; Springer publications. 2011;25-9.
19. Harries MJ, Sinclair RD, MacDonald-Hull S, Whiting DA, Griffiths CEM, Paus R. Management of primary cicatricial alopecias: Options for treatment. Brit J Derm. 2008;159:1-22.
20. Kossard S. Postmenopausal frontal fibrosing alopecia. Scarring alopecia in a pattern distribution. Arch Dermatol. 1994;130:770-4.
21. Sperling LC. Cicatricial alopecias. In: Hordinsky MK, Sawaya ME, Scher RK, (eds). Atlas of Hair and Nails. Philadelphia; Churchill Livingstone publications. 2000;129-39.
22. Habif TP. Hair diseases. In: Habif TP, (ed). Clinical Dermatology, 5th edn. New Delhi: Elsevier India. 2010;913-46.
23. Jaworsky C. Connective tissue diseases. In: Elder DE, (ed). Lever's Histopathology of the Skin, 9th ed. Philadelphia; Lippincott Williams & Wilkins. 2005;293-6.
24. Pinkus H. Differential patterns of elastic fibers in scarring and non-scarring alopecias. J Cutan Pathol. 1978;5:93-104.
25. Braun-Falco O, Imai S, Schmoeckel C, et al. Pseudopelade of Brocq. Dermatologica. 1986;172:18-23.
26. Dreuw. Uber Epidermische Alopecia. Monatash f. Prakt. Dermat. 1910;51:18-22.
27. Jaiswal AK. Cicatricial alopecias: A clinico-pathological study. Indian J Dermatol. 1983;28:31-2.
28. Panja SK, Jaiswal AK. Cicatrizing Alopecias. Indian J Dermato Venereol Leprol. 1985;51:139-43.
29. Hantash BM, Rashid RM, Schwartz RA. (2011). Scarring Alopecia. [online] Emedicine website. Available from: http://emedicine.medscape.com/article/1073559-overview#a0101 [Accessed October 2011].
30. Whiting DA, Olsen EA. Dermatologic Therapy. 2008;21: 268-78.
31. Wadhwa SL, Khopkar U, Nischal KC. Hair and Scalp Disorders. In: Valia RG, Valia AR, (eds). IADVL Textbook of Dermatology, 3rd edn. Mumbai: Bhalani Publishing House. 2008;908-18.
32. Ioffreda MD. Inflammatory diseases of Hair follicles, Sweat glands and Cartilage. In: Elder DE, (ed). Lever's Histopathology of the skin, 9th edn. Philadelphia; Lippincott Williams & Wilkins. 2005;477-8.
33. Siemens HW. Keratosis follicularis spinulosa decalvans. Arch Dermatol Syph. 1926;51:384-6.
34. Quinquaud E. Folliculite destructive des regions values. Bull. Et mem de la soc. Hop de paris. 1888;5:395-8.
35. Jaiswal AK, Vaishampayan S, Walia NS, Verma R, Baveja S. Folliculitis decalvans in a family. Indian J Dermatol Venereol Leprol. 2000;66:216-7.
36. Powell JJ, Dawber RP, Gatter K. Folliculitis decalvans including tufted folliculitis: Clinical, histological and therapeutic findings. Br J Dermatol. 1999;140:328-33.
37. Arndt G. Uber einige Foremen Narbiger Kahlheit, Ihre diagnose and therapie. Derrmat. Ztschr. 1908;15:80-91.
38. Price V, Mirmirani P. Predominantly Neutrophilic group. In: Price V, Mirmirani P, (eds). Cicatricial Alopecia: An Approach to Diagnosis and Management. New York; Springer Publications. 2011;61-7.
39. Hoffman E. Perifolliculitis capits abscedens et suffodiens. Case presentation. Derm Ztschr. 1998;15:122.
40. Price V, Mirmirani P. Mixed group. In: Price V, Mirmirani P (eds). Cicatricial Alopecia: An Approach to Diagnosis and Management. New York: Springer Publications. 2011;69-74.
41. Whiting DA. Cicatricial alopecia: Clinico-pathological findings and treatment. Clin Dermatol. 2001;19:211-25.
42. Pye RJ, Peachey RDG, Burton L. Erosive pustular dermatosis of the scalp. Brit J Derm. 1979;100:55.
43. Estrada BD, Tamler C, Sodre CT, Barcaui CB, Pereira FB. Dermoscopy patterns of cicatricial alopecia resulting from discoid lupus erythematosus and lichen planopilaris. An Bras Dermatol. Apr 2010;85:179-83.

16A

Hirsutism

KC Nischal, Urmila Nischal

"Nothing in life is to be feared, it is only to be understood."
—*Marie Curie*

Introduction

The term "Hirsutism" is of Latin origin which means excessive growth of stiff hair or hairiness, especially in women or children, with an adult male pattern of distribution.[1] Hirsutism is defined as the presence of thick terminal hair in a male pattern distribution in females. The first report of hirsutism dates back to 1921 where Archard, et al. published a report on "bearded diabetic women (*diabète des femmes à barbe*)."[2] Hirsutism is a fairly common sign and affects 5–15% of women. It should be considered as a sign rather than a disease process by itself. Most commonly, it is a manifestation of hyperandrogenism and increased action of androgens on hair follicles. There are various objective methods of assessing the extent and severity of hirsutism but the perspective and impact of excess hair growth in women is strongly influenced by the social and cultural practices.[3] It has been observed that, greater the severity of hirsutism, lower is the quality of life. Hirsutism is also associated with anxiety and depression.[4,5] As this condition has a definitive impact on the psychological well being of the affected, it is imperative to understand the pathogenesis and relevance of different treatment modalities.

Hirsutism should be distinguished from hypertrichosis. 'Hypertrichosis' is a word of Greek origin generally referring to localized or generalized excess hair. In contrast to hirsutism, hypertrichosis is excessive hair growth which is usually not terminal and occurs in areas not dependent on androgens **(Box 16A.1)**. It can be familial or induced by drugs and does not respond to anti-androgen therapy.[1]

Box 16A.1: Hirsutism vs Hypertrichosis

- Hirsutism is defined as the presence of thick terminal hair in a male pattern distribution in females
- Hypertrichosis is excessive hair growth which is usually not terminal and occurs in areas not dependent on androgens which can be localized or generalised

Epidemiology

Hirsutism is one of the distressing, demoralizing aesthetic conditions which affects women from menarche to menopause. Various studies have found the prevalence of hirsutism to vary from 5–15%, with an Indian study of Kashmiri women revealing occurrence in 10.5%.[1,6]

Etiopathogenesis

Three different types of hair can be distinguished structurally. The lanugo hair which are very fine, short non-pigmented densely covering the skin at birth. These hairs are shed subsequently in the post-partum period. Vellus hair are fine but larger than the lanugo hair, non-pigmented, < 0.03 mm in diameter and nonmedullated. Terminal hairs are thicker, longer, pigmented, coarse in texture and are medullated; they also have an associated arrector pili muscle. Terminal hairs are normally seen on the scalp, eyebrows, eyelashes, axillae and the pubic region in both the sexes. Growth hormone and thyroid hormones primarily govern the development and growth of the terminal hair and in androgen dependant areas androgens primarily govern the growth of terminal hairs. Depending on the sensitivity of the hairs to androgens, hair are classified as *sexual*, hairs become terminal on exposure to high levels of androgen viz, classical male pattern hairs (lower face, trunk, back, thighs

Box 16A.2: Types of hair (depending on the sensitivity of the hairs to androgens)

- Sexual—hairs become terminal on exposure to high levels of androgen viz., classical male pattern hairs (lower face, trunk, back, thighs and upper arms)
- Ambosexual—hair become terminal even on mild exposure to androgens (axilla, pubic, forearm, legs)
- Asexual—non-responsive to androgens (occipital scalp, eyebrows, eyelashes)

and upper arms); *ambosexual*, these hair become terminal even on mild exposure to androgens (axilla, pubic, forearm, legs) and *asexual*, non-responsive to androgens (occipital scalp, eyebrows, eyelashes) **(Box 16A.2)**.[1]

In hirsutism, the vellus hairs in the androgen dependent areas like chin, lower face, upper neck, upper arms, chest, abdomen, back and thighs get converted to terminal hairs. This happens either due to abnormal levels of androgens or abnormal sensitivity of androgen receptors in the hair bulb to androgens.

Androgens in women are derived mostly (> 50%) from adrenals and ovaries; rest is metabolized from weaker androgens (androstenedione) to testosterone in adipose tissue, liver and skin **(Table 16A.1)**. Androgens (in decreasing order of serum concentration) of relevance in women are dehydroepiandrosterone sulfate, androstenedione, testosterone and dihydrotestosterone (DHT). The most potent among these is DHT, which is produced in situ at the follicle by the conversion of testosterone to DHT by 5 alpha reductase enzyme present in dermal papilla cells. Its activity is increased by circulating androgens and local growth factors. DHT causes increased production of sebum, differentiation of vellus hair to terminal hair and prolongs the anagen phase thereby, making the hairs longer and thicker.[7] However, severity of hirsutism does not correlate with the degree of androgen excess. This could be due to ethnic variation, peripheral conversion of androgen, sensitivity of androgen receptors and other contributory factors like hyperinsulinemia.[8] 5-alpha reductase enzyme is present as two isoforms, SRD5A1 and SRD5A2 and only the former has been found to be associated with hirsutism.[9]

Table 16A.1: Source of androgens in women

Androgen	Source
Dehydroepiandrosterone sulfate (DHEAS)	Adrenal (100%)
Dehydroandrosterone	Adrenal (50%), from DHEAS (30%), ovaries (20%)
Androstenedione	Adrenal (50%), ovaries (50%)
Testosterone	Adrenal (25%), ovaries (25%), peripheral conversion of Androstenedione (50%) in fat, liver and skin
Dihydrotestosterone (DHT)	Intracellular hormone synthesized from testosterone by action of 5-alpha reductase

Various causes for hirsutism have been categorized into 5 classes by the Androgen Excess and Polycystic Ovary Syndrome Society as polycystic ovarian syndrome, idiopathic hyperandrogenism, idiopathic hirsutism, non-classical congenital adrenal hyperplasia and androgen secreting tumors **(Figure 16A.1)**.[10] Miscellaneous category includes drug induced hirsutism, postmenopausal hirsutism.

Polycystic ovarian syndrome: (Figure 16A.2) Polycystic ovarian syndrome is the most common cause of hirsutism. Nidhi, et al. have reported a prevalence of PCOS in 9.13% of the Indian adolescents in their prospective study. About 70% of PCOS women have hirsutism. The National Institute of Health (NIH) 1990 criteria for diagnosis of PCOS included hyperandrogenism, oligo/anovulation and exclusion of

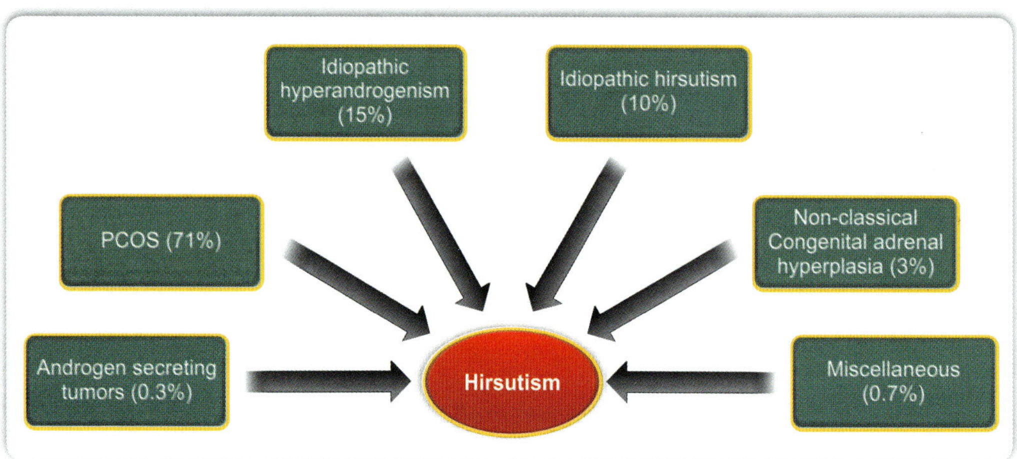

Fig. 16A.1: Classification of causes of hirsutism

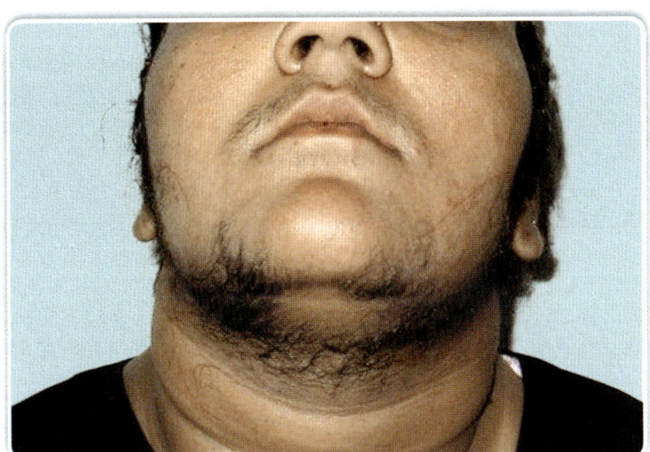

Fig. 16A.2: Severe hirsutism in a young female with polycystic ovary syndrome
(*Courtesy:* Sanjeev J Aurangabadkar, Skin and Laser Clinic, Hyderabad)

other related disorders.[11] The Rotterdam conference 2003 criteria for the diagnosis of PCOS is the presence of atleast two of the three characteristics:

1. Chronic amenorrhea (no menses in the past 6 months) or oligomenorrhea (cycles lasting longer than 35 days or a total of < 8 menses/year)
2. Clinical or laboratory evidence of hyperandrogenism
3. Transabdominal ultrasound showing presence of > 12 peripheral follicles each measuring 2–9 mm in diameter in one or both ovaries; or increased ovarian volume (> 10 mL) of one or both ovaries.

These criteria were later modified by the Androgen Excess Society (AES) 2006. It included exclusion of specific identifiable androgen excess disorders like the androgen-secreting neoplasms, hyperandrogenic insulin-resistant acanthosis nigricans syndrome, and non-classic adrenal hyperplasia (NCAH). Normal menstrual cycles do not rule out PCOS as PCOS can be anovulatory or ovulatory (15.5%).[12]

Women with PCOS have more subcutaneous fat in abdomen, waist and upper arms.[13] In their study on 224 PCOS women with hirsutism, Guzel, et al. found that body mass index correlated with the degree of hirsutism.[14] Adipokines are cytokines derived from adipocytes. Adiponectin is most important among all adipokines. Adipokines mobilize fat, acts as insulin sensitizer and lowers risk of development of type II diabetes mellitus. They are also found to reduce androgen production by suppressing the expression of various receptors and enzymes involved in androgen synthesis. There is a low expression of adipokine receptors AdipoR1 and AdipoR2 in the thecal cells of polycystic ovaries. This strengthens the link between fat cells (obesity), hyperandrogenism and PCOS.[15]

Idiopathic hyperandrogenism: Here, hirsutism is accompanied by excessive androgens but normal structure and function of ovaries. This constitutes about 15% of all cases of hirsutism.[10] Excessive androgens reduce hypothalamic feedback inhibition leading to increased GnRH pulsatility.[2] High frequency GnRH pulses stimulate LH secretion whereas low frequency GnRH pulses stimulate FSH secretion. This leads to an imbalance in LH and FSH level **(Figure 16A.3)**.

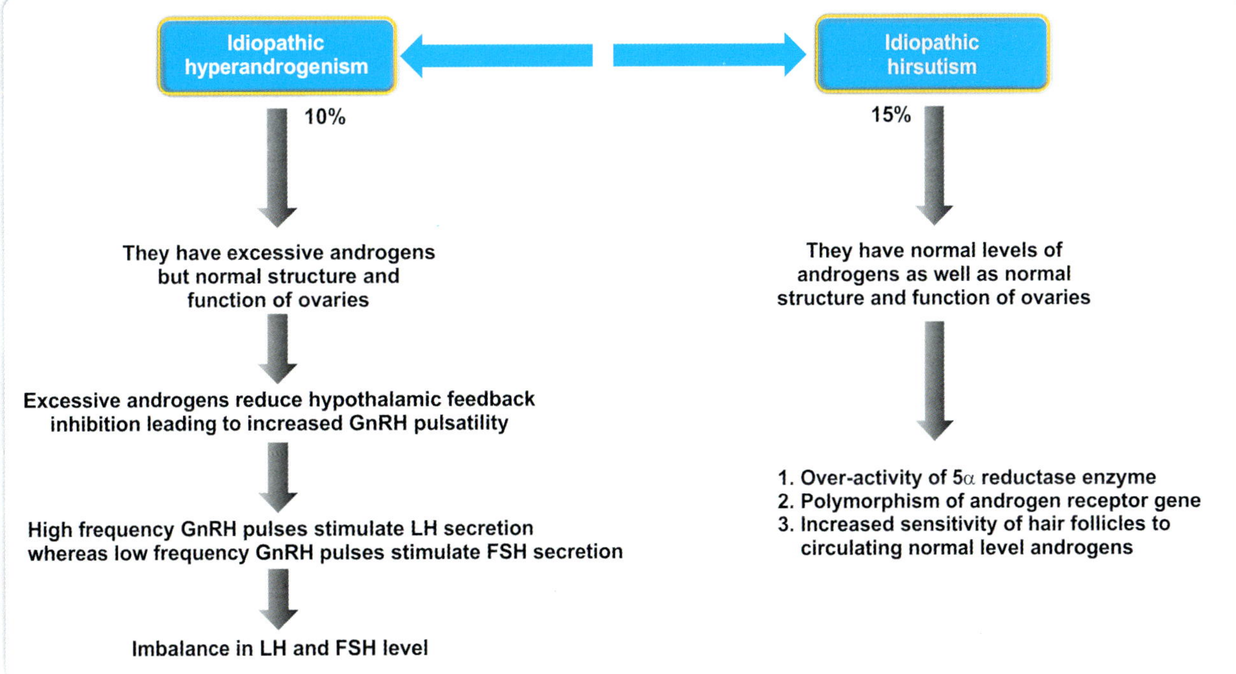

Fig. 16A.3: Schematic representation of differences between idiopathic hyperandrogenism and idiopathic hirsutism

Idiopathic hirsutism: (Figures 16A.4A and B) When hirsute women have normal levels of androgens as well as normal structure and function of ovaries, it is termed as Idiopathic hirsutism. It is a diagnosis of exclusion. Constitutes about 10% of all cases of hirsutism.[7,10] This is thought to be due to over-activity of 5α reductase enzyme, polymorphism of androgen receptor gene or increased sensitivity of hair follicles to circulating normal level androgens.[16]

Non-classic adrenal hyperplasia (NCAH): NCAH accounts for about 3% of all cases of hirsutism. However, in Hispanics and people with eastern European Jewish heritage, the NCAH constitutes upto 20% of all cases of hirsutism.[17] Unless otherwise mentioned, NCAH refers to deficiency of 21 hydroxylase enzyme. It is a homozygous recessive disorder which is characterized by deficiency of P450c21 enzyme leading to excessive accumulation of 17 hydroxyprogesterone (17-OHP) and androstenedione. Non-classic steroid β11-hydroxylase deficiency is the second most common cause of congenital adrenal hyperplasia.[18] When these 2 enzymes are blocked, the glucocorticoid and mineralocorticoid precursors are shunted towards androgens or estrogen synthesis leading to hyperandrogenic or hyperestrogenic state **(Figure 16A.5)**.

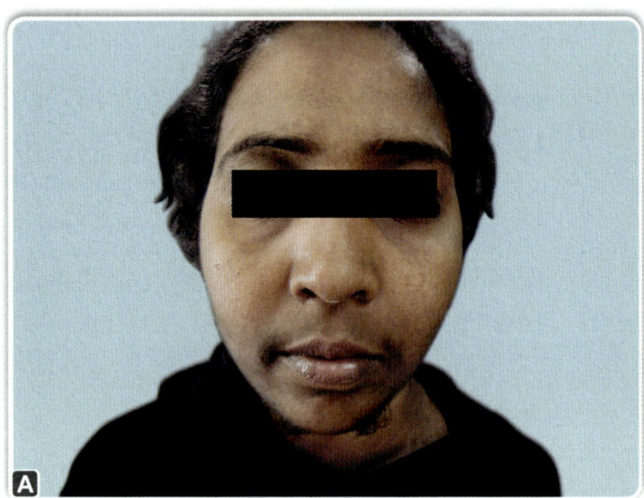

Fig. 16A.4(A): Idiopathic hirsutism
(*Courtesy:* Department of Dermatology, BMCRI, Bengaluru)

Androgen secreting tumors: These are rare but cause severe hirsutism which often progress rapidly and shows signs of virilization (clitoromegaly, loss of female body contour, deepening of voice and masculine features) **(Box 16A.3)**. Serum testosterone is much higher in these situations. These tumors can be of ovarian or adrenal origin. Ovarian androgen secreting tumors are categorized as stromal luteoma, Leydig cell tumor, and not otherwise specified steroid cell tumor. Leydig cell tumors comprise 75% of all testosterone secreting ovarian tumors.[19] Adrenal tumors often secrete cortisone, androgens, estrogens and aldosterone. Pure androgen secreting adrenal tumors are very rare and mostly benign in nature.[20] Adrenal tumors secreting a combination of hormones are suggestive of malignant neoplasms and those secreting single hormone are often benign.[21]

Miscellaneous

Drug induced: Valproic acid is the only anticonvulsant that causes elevation in plasma testosterone levels.[22] Prolactin raising antipsychotics (risperidone, paliperidone, amisulpride and zotepine) blocks the dopamine inhibition of lactotrophs in pituitary gland leading to hyperprolactinemia.[23,24] Hyperprolactinemia is also caused by opiates, monoamine oxidase inhibitors, verapamil, metoclopramide, sulpiride, estrogens and anti-androgens.[25]

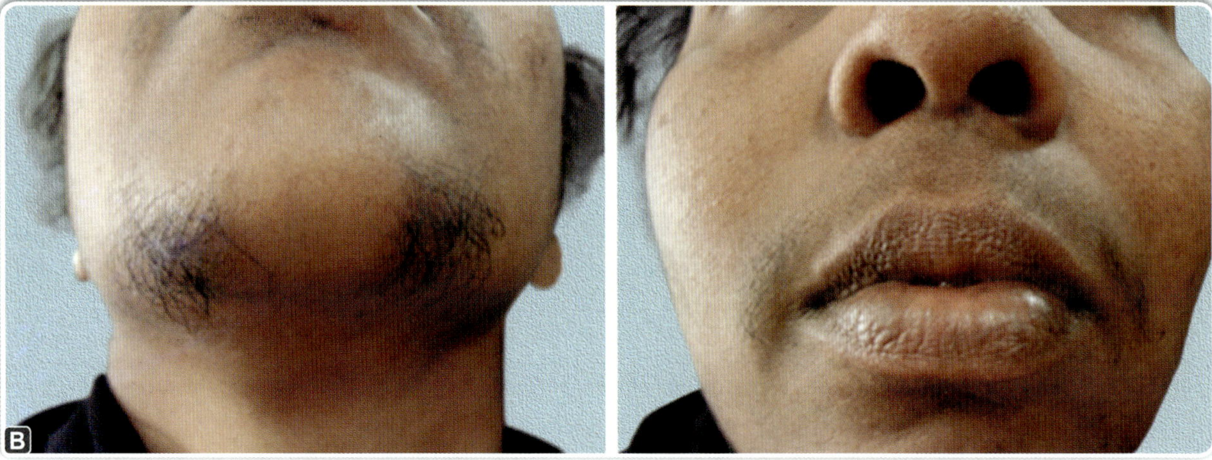

Fig. 16A.4(B): Excessive hair growth in chin and above upper lip in same patient as in Figure 16A.4(A)
(*Courtesy:* Department of Dermatology, BMCRI, Bengaluru)

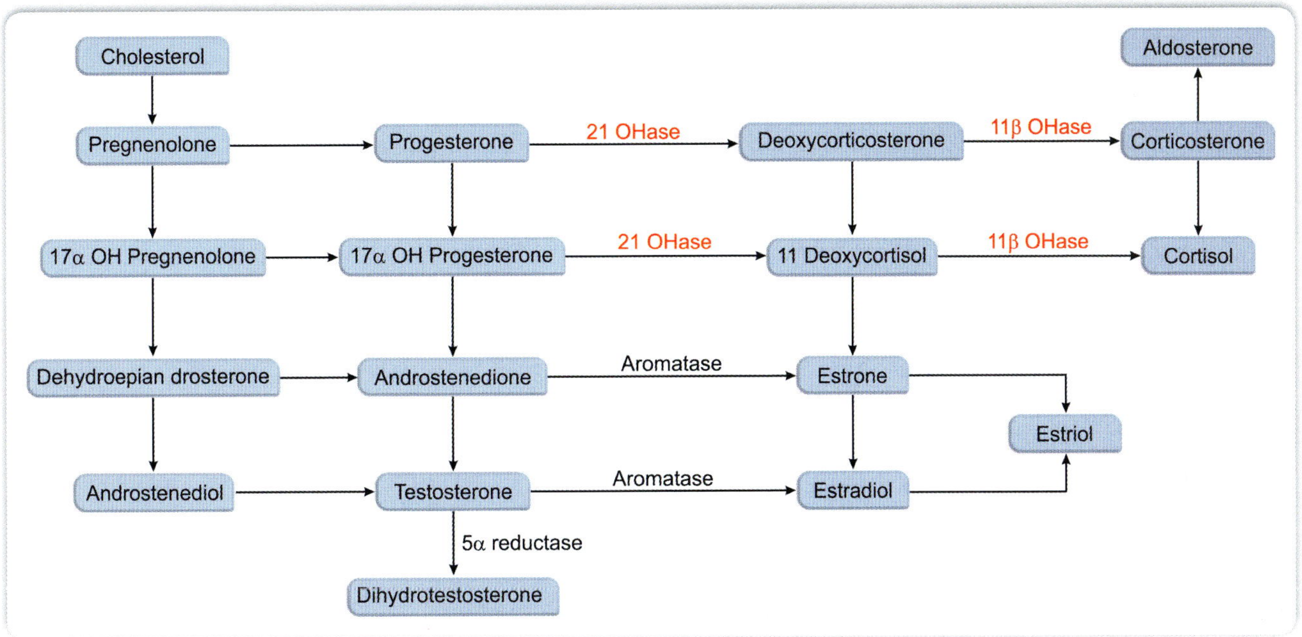

Fig. 16A.5: Adrenal hormone synthesis

Box 16A.3: Signs of virilization

- Clitoromegaly
- Loss of female body contour
- Deepening of voice
- Masculine features

Other drugs causing hirsutism include erlotinib (epidermal growth factor receptor inhibitor),[26] bimatoprost, carbamazepine, cyclosporine, corticosteroids, diazoxide, interferon alfa, isotretinoin, mycophenolate mofetil, pregabalin, tacrolimus, trazodone, estrogens, progestins and testosterone.[27]

Postmenopausal hirsutism: At menopause, estrogen secretion stops abruptly. However, androgen secretion does not stop similarly but decreases gradually. This leads to an imbalance in the estrogen-androgen milieu. Also after menopause, there is reduction in SHBG synthesis leading to increase in free androgens in circulation and an increase in gonadotropin secretion leading to increased androgen synthesis by ovaries. These events lead to unabated hyperandrogenic state which triggers thickening of hairs.[28]

Hyperthecosis: Hyperthecosis is exaggeration of structure and secretory function of ovarian stroma. Though common in premenopausal women, it can affect postmenopausal women. The mean volume of ovaries is either normal or increased (from 2.5–3.7 cm^3 to 10 cm^3). Androgen secretion by ovaries is controlled by gonadotropins. A single dose GnRH agonist administered will effectively suppress testosterone levels over 1–3 months. However, rarely adrenal tumors may also be responsive to GnRH agonists (as well as have normal androstenedione level). The increased androgen secretion as well as its association with metabolic syndrome causes hirsutism in hyperthecosis.[29,30]

Androgen receptor hypersensitivity: Shorter androgen receptor gene CAG number is associated with increased androgen responsiveness. This can also lead to increased risk of precocious pubarche (pubic hairs in age < 8 years) as well as ovarian hyperandrogenism.[31]

Hyperprolactinemia: Prolactin reduces sensitivity of LH and FSH receptors in gonads. It also decreases GnRH secretion leading to reduced pulsatile secretion of LH and FSH. This results in anovulation. This increases dehydroepiandrosterone (DHEAS) production by adrenals leading to hyperandrogenic state, thereby hirsutism.[25]

Chrousos syndrome or primary generalized glucocorticoid resistance: This is a rare sporadic or familial condition, wherein, glucocorticoids are not recognized by the target tissues. Hence, there is breakdown of negative feedback inhibition (hypothalamus-pituitary axis) of adrenal hormone secretion. The raised ACTH levels trigger excessive secretion of cortisol and other adrenal hormones leading to hypermineralocorticoidism and hyperandrogenism without features of Cushing syndrome **(Box 16A.4)**.[32]

Role of insulin resistance in hirsutism: Insulin resistance (IR) is defined as the decreased ability of insulin to stimulate glucose disposal into the target tissue or a reduced glucose response to a given amount of insulin resulting in hyperinsulinemia. Insulin resistance is characterized by increase in plasma concentration of insulin.[33]

Insulin stimulates the ovarian theca cells to overproduce androgens. Also, insulin augments CYP17 activity thereby

Box 16A.4: Chrousos syndrome (Syn:Primary generalized glucocorticoid resistance)

- Rare sporadic or familial condition, wherein, glucocorticoids are not recognized by the target tissues
- There is breakdown of negative feedback inhibition (hypothalamus-pituitary axis) of adrenal hormone secretion
- The raised ACTH levels trigger excessive secretion of cortisol and other adrenal hormones leading to hypermineralocorticoidism and hyperandrogenism without features of Cushing syndrome

increasing the androgen production. This is observed in both obese and lean polycystic ovary syndrome (PCOS). Hyperinsulinemia increases pulsatile activity of GnRH leading to an increase in LH secretion, which promotes hyperandrogenic state.[2] High serum insulin levels suppress hepatic production of sex hormone-binding globulin (SHBG), leading to increase in free serum androgens. Hyperinsulinemia causes a rise in circulating insulin like growth factor (IGF-1), which has a mitogenic effect on the pilosebaceous unit thereby causing thickening of the vellus hairs.[16] All these changes culminate into hirsutism **(Figure 16A.6)**.

Both PCOS and idiopathic hirsutism are associated with insulin resistance, former exhibiting greater resistance than latter.[16] About 64.4% of PCOS women were found to have IR. This association is irrespective of BMI or obesity; in fact, a high prevalence of IR has been found even in PCOS women who are lean.[34] Landay, et al. have demonstrated that development and progression of hirsutism correlated more with fasting insulin levels rather than total testosterone or 17-hydroxyprogesterone in women with PCOS.[35]

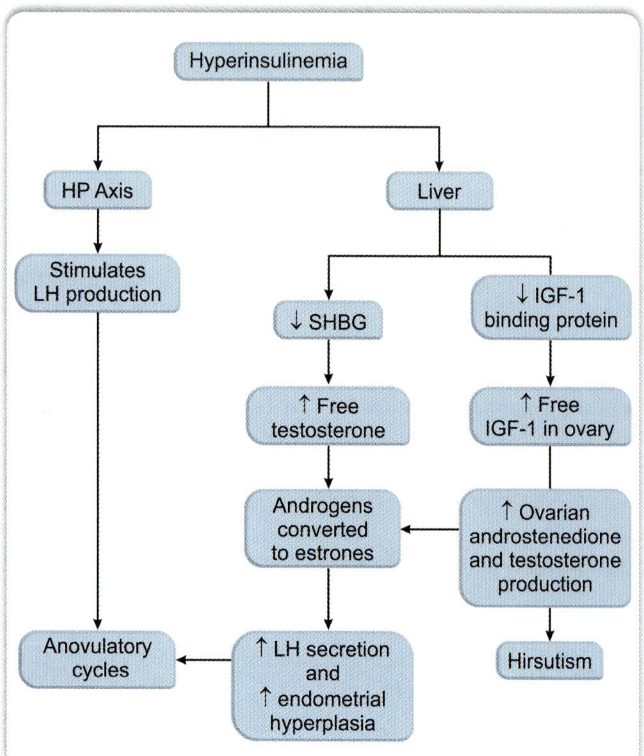

Fig. 16A.6: Role of hyperinsulinemia in hirsutism and PCOS

Role of vitamin D deficiency in PCOS and hirsutism: There is lot of interest in the role of vitamin D in hyperandrogenism, insulin resistance and PCOS **(Figure 16A.7)**. Vitamin D receptor (VDR) regulates genes that are crucial for glucose and lipid metabolism (leading to insulin resistance and metabolic syndrome). Several observational studies have pointed out the association between the hyperandrogenism markers and vitamin D levels. Levels of 25-hydroxy vitamin D were found to be lower in women with hirsutism as compared to their BMI matched controls (17 vs 29 ng/mL, respectively).[36] Similarly, the levels were lower in PCOS women with hirsutism in comparison to those without hirsutism (21·4 vs 26·8 ng/mL, respectively).[37] However, Thomson, et al. found obesity to be a confounding factor and proposed that obesity influenced hyperandrogenic state and PCOS rather than vitamin D.[38]

Meta-analysis and randomized studies have not demonstrated any beneficial effect of vitamin D supplementation on insulin resistance in PCOS women with vitamin D deficiency.[39-41] However, Belenchia, et al. have observed that, even though the BMI did not change significantly on taking vitamin D supplements, there was significant reduction in the fasting insulin and HOMA-IR score.[42] Panidis, et al. have demonstrated that parathyroid hormone levels correlated with serum testosterone and prolactin independent of age and BMI in patients with PCOS.[43] Hence at present, there is no consensus on the

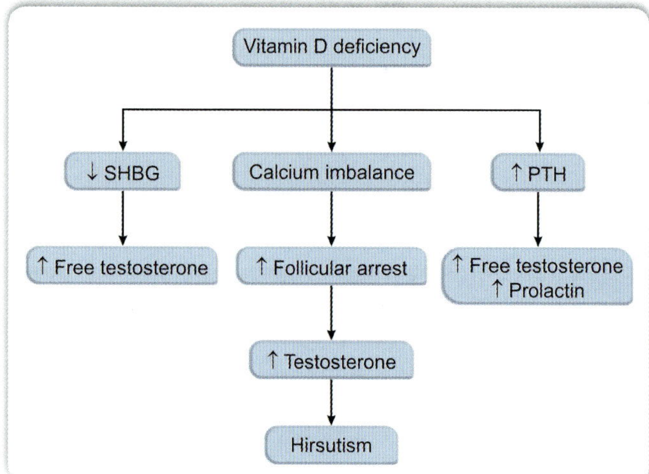

Fig. 16A.7: Role of vitamin D in hirsutism
Abbreviations: SHBG-Serum hormone binding globulin; PTH-Parathyroid hormone

role of vitamin D supplementation in hirsutism except for correction of any associated deficiency.

Clinical Features

Hirsutism is thick terminal hair growth in male pattern in a female. So, there is increased thick hair growth over lower face, upper neck, chest, abdomen, back and thighs. As hirsutism is often associated with hyperandrogensim, there can be seborrhea, acne, female pattern hair loss in these individuals. Rarely, hyperandrogenism is severe enough to cause virilization manifested as deepening of voice, clitoromegaly, loss of female body contour, atrophy of breast and masculine features. Virilization is often due to androgen secreting neoplasms. Testosterone has erythropoietic effect on bone marrow and high level of testosterone can cause polycythemia and erythrocytosis which manifests as plethora.[19,44]

Syndromes associated with hirsutism include HAIR-AN and SAHA. HAIR-AN syndrome comprises of hirsutism, insulin resistance, acanthosis nigricans. This syndrome occurs in 1–3% of hyperandrogenic women and 5% of PCOS individuals.[45] Type A HAIR-AN is primary and occurs due to insulin receptor mutations. Type B HAIR-AN syndrome is an acquired condition wherein, autoantibodies are secreted against insulin receptors in tissues. Insulin resistance is more severe in former than latter.[46] About 5% of hirsute women have acanthosis nigricans with insulin resistance[47] **(Box 16A.5)**.

SAHA syndrome comprises of seborrhea, acne, hirsutism, alopecia. This syndrome is a cutaneous manifestation of peripheral hyperandrogenism in young females. Only 20% patients reveal all four features. Seborrhea occurs in all individuals of SAHA; androgenetic alopecia occurs in 21%, acne in 10% and hirsutism in 6%. SAHA has been classified as familial, ovarian, adrenal and with polyendocrinopathy **(Figure 16A.8)**. Familial (ethnic hyperandrogenism) occurs commonly in southern Europe. This variant resembles idiopathic hirsutism as there are signs of hyperandrogenism but hormone levels are normal. Ovarian SAHA has subcapsular follicular cysts in ovaries with raised androgen levels in blood (reminiscent of PCOS). Adrenal variant reveals increased DHEAS and androstenedione levels and normal testosterone, SHBG and prolactin levels. Hyperprolactinemic SAHA shows features of hyperandrogenism with raised prolactin levels. HAIR-AN syndrome has been considered as SAHA with polyendocrinopathy.[47]

Acanthosis nigricans is a cutaneous marker of insulin resistance and is characterized by hyperpigmented, thick velvety skin change in flexures and rarely palms. Cutaneous

Box 16A.5: HAIR-AN syndrome

- Comprises of hirsutism, insulin resistance, acanthosis nigricans
- Type A HAIR-AN is primary and occurs due to insulin receptor mutations. It is a severe form
- Type B HAIR-AN syndrome is an acquired condition wherein, autoantibodies are secreted against insulin receptors in tissues

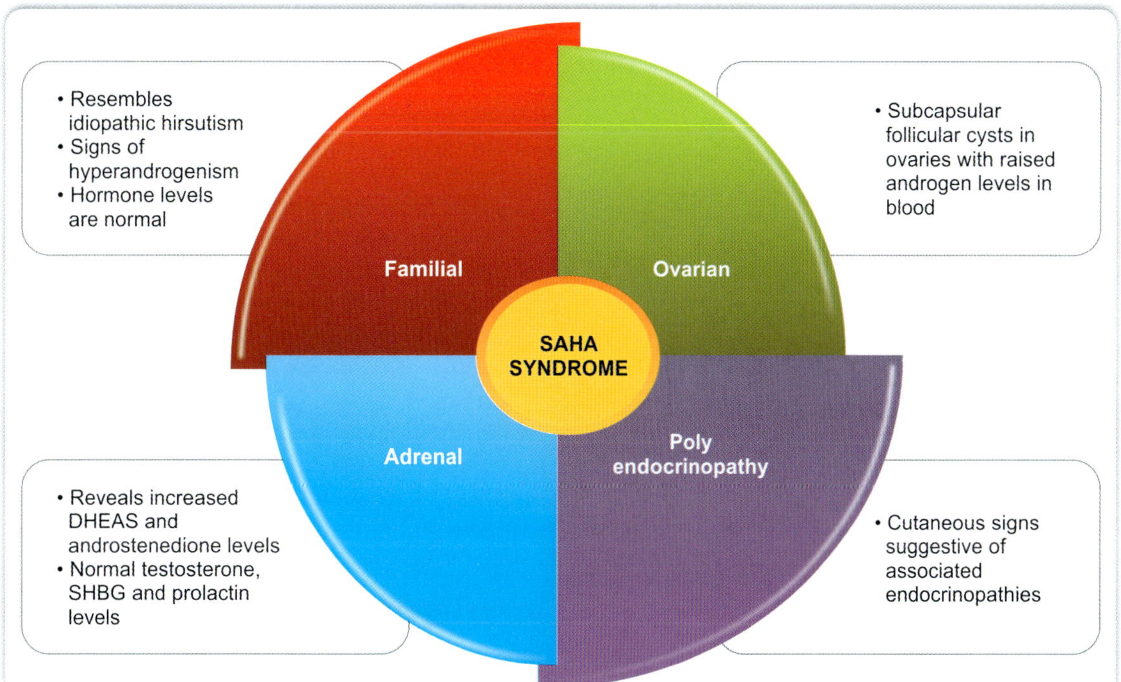

Fig. 16A.8: Variants of SAHA syndrome

signs suggestive of other endocrinopathies may be present like striae, moon facies (Cushing's syndrome); increase in the size of palms and soles, coarsening of facial features (acromegaly); exophthalmos, goiter (thyroid dysfunction); expressible or spontaneous galactorrhea (hyperprolactinemia). Menstrual irregularities can be a feature of any of these endocrinopathies per se. Hyperhomocysteinemia (homocysteinemia > 12.4 μmol/L) which has cardiovascular risk is associated with hyperandrogenism in PCOS women.[48] Hence, hirsute patients should be asked for any history of thromboembolism like transient ischemic attack, cerebrovascular accident, avascular necrosis of hip (hip pain, altered gait). The cardiovascular risk in hirsutism depends on the cause of hirsutism and reduces in the following order: anovulatory PCOS (highest), ovulatory PCOS, idiopathic hyperandrogenism and idiopathic hirsutism (lowest).[10] Rarely, adrenal mass can be palpated per abdomen.

Assessing Hirsutism

Hirsutism which is mild on objective modalities of assessment may in fact, be able to have had significant impact on the quality of life of individual. Most important way of assessing is to consider patient important hirsutism. The objective or subjective methods may not yield significant scores, but a particular woman might face significant distress due to the presence of terminal hair though localized. There are different objective and subjective methods for assessing the hair growth in hirsutism.

The objective methods are: photographic evaluations, weighing of shaved or plucked hair, determining the density of terminal hair by direct counting or by photography and microscopic examination of the hair for thickness, color etc. The rate of hair growth is measured with the help of calibrated glass capillary tubes or by photography. Ratio of vellus hairs in a sample of 100 shaved hairs is termed as the 'vellus index'. It is low in hirsute women.[1] Drawback of these methods is that they are cumbersome, expensive and time consuming **(Box 16A.6)**. As a result these methods are of seldom use in widespread clinical assessment.

The subjective methods utilize the visual scoring of the terminal hair growth in certain specific body parts. There can be significant inter-observer variation in these methods.

The most commonly used method of assessment is the modified Ferriman Gallwey (mFG) scoring system originally described by Ferriman and Gallwey in 1961. Nine body parts namely, upper lip, chin, arm, chest, upper abdomen, lower abdomen, upper back, lower back and thighs are scored **(Figure 16A.9)** on a scale of 0–4; (score 1—minimal terminal hairs seen to 4—equivalent to a hairy man, 0—if no terminal hair observed on the body part examined). A collective score of less than 8 is considered normal, score between 8 to 15 is considered as moderately severe and a score above 16 is considered as severe hirsutism **(Box 16A.7)**.

Box 16A.6: Vellus index

- Ratio of vellus hairs in a sample of 100 shaved hairs
- It is low in hirsute women
- Drawback of these methods is that they are cumbersome, expensive and time consuming

However, as the terminal body hair growth has a significant racial and ethnic variation, the cut off value of the mFG score should be ideally established for the population to which it needs to be applied. Since this method uses a visual and subjective scale, inter-observer variation is a possibility. This variation could be minimized by proper training of the physicians, asking patients to avoid laser or electrolysis for atleast three months, avoid waxing or depilation for at least four weeks and avoid shaving for at least five days before the assessment of the hair growth.[10]

Also the mFG scoring system gives an overview of the total amount of body hair, it does not take into consideration the localized distribution of the hair growth. For example, the patient might have thick growth only in the chin area giving a score of 4 maximum but this is not considered hirsutism according to the mFG scoring system. The consensus statement by Androgen Excess and Polycystic Ovary Syndrome Society recommends that the mFG scoring system using the nine body parts should be implemented in quantifying the severity of hirsutism and 95th percentile of the mFG score of the general population should be used to determine the cut off value to define hirsutism.[10] In a large scale study involving 10,120 women of reproductive age group in ten different provinces of China done by Li, et al. it was concluded that mFG score of > 4 could be considered as hirsutism in that population and also mFG score of upper lip, thighs and lower abdomen > 2 can be used to make a diagnosis of hirsutism in that community.[49] The cutoff value for Indians can be taken as ≥ 6 based on the only Indian epidemiological study by Zagar, et al. 2002.[6]

Drawbacks of Ferriman Galleway scoring is given in **Box 16A.8.** Knochenhauer, et al. and Rashidi, et al. proposed evaluation of only chin or lower abdomen for predicting hirsutism. They experienced 100% sensitivity but the specificity and positive predictive value were proportionally less. Therefore, this method of assessment is not useful in the study of population with a very low (< 5%) prevalence of hirsutism.[50,51]

Investigations

All cases of hirsutism should be investigated at baseline because, eumenorrhea does not mean normoandrogenism

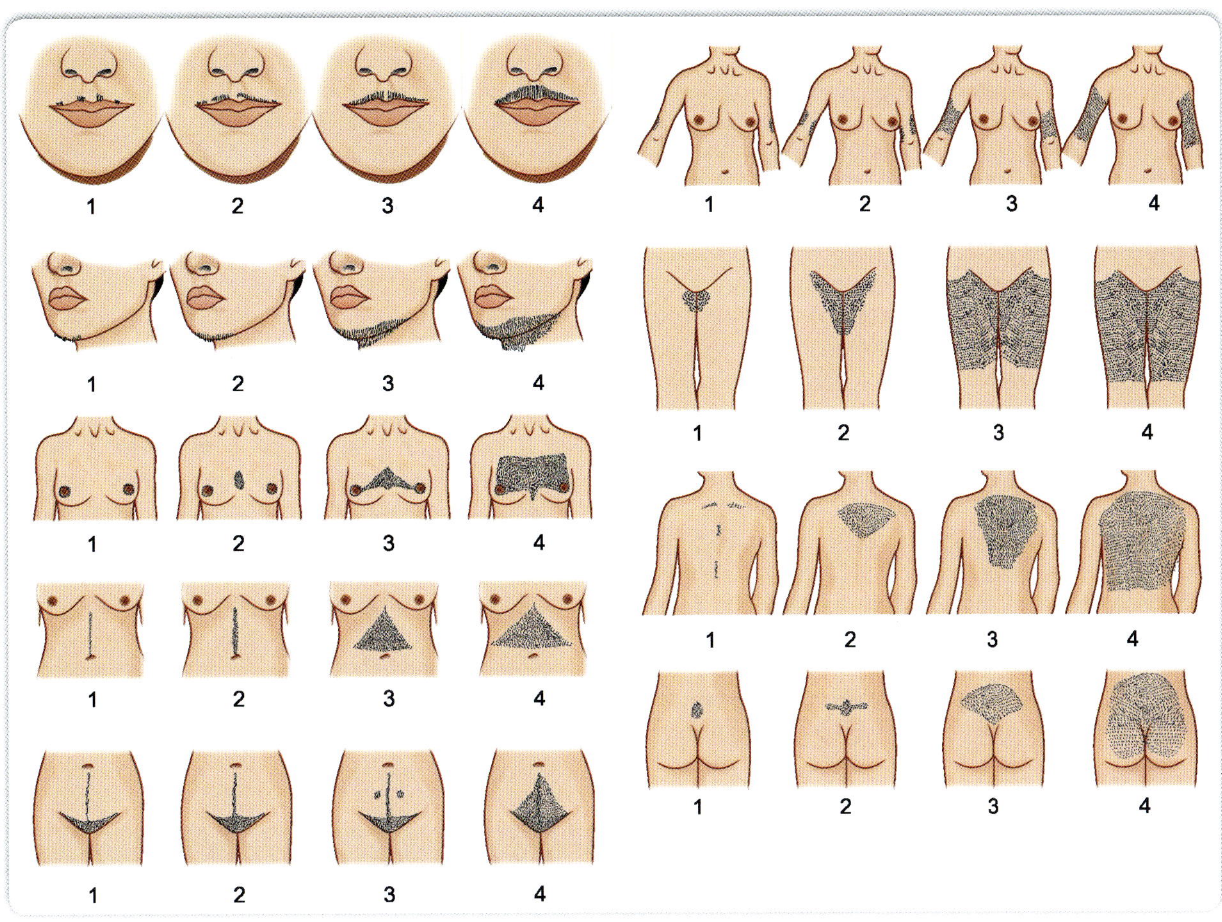

Fig. 16A.9: Modified Ferriman Gallwey score

Box 16A.7: Modified Ferriman Gallwey scoring

- A collective score of less than 8 is considered normal
- Score between 8 to 15 is considered as moderately severe
- Score above 16 is considered as severe hirsutism

Box 16A.8: Drawbacks of Ferriman Galleway scoring[27]

- Scoring is subjective, time consuming and affects privacy of the patient
- Lack of consideration of certain androgen sensitive areas like the sidelocks and buttocks
- No consideration of focal hirsutism
- Does not consider ongoing use of cosmetic measures
- Neglect of patient's perception and response to hirsutism

(22% of eumenorrheic hirsutes had androgen excess),[8] severity of hirsutism does not correlate with androgen excess (mild hirsutism may in fact have severe hormonal imbalance),[8] hirsutism is often associated with significant cardiovascular risk (hence have impact on morbidity and mortality)[52,53] and some of the conditions viz, non-classic congenital adrenal hyperplasia which cause hirsutism are heritable and need genetic counseling.[10]

Basic Vital Measurements

Blood Pressure: Raised in NCAH

Height and weight: To calculate body mass index. Obesity has a significant impact on the course and prognosis of hirsutism.

$$\text{Body mass index (BMI)} = \frac{\text{Weight in kg}}{(\text{Height in meter})^2}$$

For adolescents, if the BMI falls in the 85th–95th percentile it is considered as overweight, if the BMI is more than 95th percentile then is considered as obesity.[54] For Indian men and women above 22 years of age, BMI of more than 23 is considered obese.

Fasting blood glucose: This is used to assess insulin resistance.

Hormonal Assay

When to perform hormonal assay: Day 2–4 of menstural cycle, early morning sample, oral contraceptives (OCP) should have been stopped about 6 weeks prior. For ruling out androgen secreting neoplasm, total testosterone should be measured in early follicular phase.

In patients with prolonged amenorrhea, menses can be induced by giving medroxyprogesterone acetate 10 mg once or twice daily for five days. On discontinuing, flow is precipitated. This results in withdrawal bleeding or induced periods.[46]

Panel of hormones to be assayed: Basic investigations to be performed in all cases of hirsutism include, fasting blood glucose, fasting plasma insulin, FSH, LH, prolactin, TSH, testosterone (free and total) and SHBG. In cases with moderate to severe hirsutism (mFG score > 15) and in any degree of hirsutism with sudden onset, rapid progression, signs and symptoms suggestive of malignancy or PCOS or testosterone levels are > 5 nmol/L or twice the upper limit of normal range of the laboratory, additional tests have to be done to establish the cause for hirsutism **(Table 16A.2)**.[3]

Dexamethasone suppression test: This test is done to differentiate various causes of hypercortisol conditions **(Table 16A.3)**. Dexamethasone has a negative feedback on pituitary which leads to suppression of ACTH secretion. If hirsutism is not due to hypercorticolism, administration of low dose dexamethasone (1–2 mg) will suppress the endogenous cortisol production. High dose dexamethasone (8 mg) will decrease cortisol levels in Cushing's syndrome, but not if the hypercortisolism is due to ectopic ACTH producing cells or adrenal tumors.

Acute adrenal stimulation test: This test is performed, if 17-OH progesterone level is greater than 200 ng/dL or when diagnosis of CAH has to be definitively established. Synthetic adrenocorticotropic hormone 250 µg is injected intravenously and 17-OH progesterone levels are measured after 30–60 minutes; if the levels are greater than 1000 ng/dL, then it establishes the diagnosis of 21-OH deficient NCAH.[7] 17-OH progesterone should be measured during the follicular phase of menstrual cycle.

Determining PCOS as ovulatory or anovulatory: This is done for all hirsute women giving a history of regular menstrual cycles to know ovulatory dysfunction. Changes in basal body temperature and the serum progesterone in the luteal phase (days 20–24) of the menstrual cycle are seen in ovulatory PCOS. Luteal progesterone value less than 3–5 ng/mL is suggestive of ovulatory dysfunction.[7]

In men, testosterone synthesis and secretion is controlled by gonadotropin feedback inhibition. Eventhough SHBG alters free testosterone, because of

Table 16A.2: Hormone tests in hirsutism

Hormone	*Rationale for testing*	*Comments*
Basic investigations		
Fasting blood glucose	To assess insulin resistance (by calculating HOMA-IR)	HOMA-IR > 2.6 implies insulin resistance
Fasting insulin	To assess insulin resistance (by calculating HOMA-IR)	HOMA-IR > 2.6 implies insulin resistance
Follicle stimulating hormone and leutinizing hormone	To assess the ratio LH/FSH	LH/FSH > 2 seen in PCOS
Prolactin	To check for hyperprolactinemia	Increased in prolactinoma, hypothyroidism, Cushing's disease, medications (prolactin raising antipsychotics)
Total testosterone	To assess hyperandrogenism To calculate free androgen index	< 200 ng/dL seen in IH, PCOS > 200 ng/dL seen in ovarian tumors
Free testosterone	To assess hyperandrogenism	> 4.3 ng/dL is abnormal
TSH	Hypothyroidism can cause hirsutism	-
SHBG	To calculate free androgen index	-
Additional investigations		
DHEAS	Raised levels indicates adrenal hyperandrogenism	4000–8000 ng/dL seen in CAH > 8000 ng/dL seen in adrenal tumors
17-OH progesterone	To diagnose NCAH	< 200 ng/dL—excludes CAH 300–1000 ng/dL—requires ACTH stimulation test Post 250 µg i.v. ACTH—> 1000 ng/dL implies positive
24 hours urinary cortisol	To detect Cushing's syndrome and Chrousos syndrome	Raised in both conditions but latter lack features of Cushing's syndrome and also may demonstrate hGR gene polymorphism
Dexamethasone suppression test	To differentiate various causes for hypercortisol condition	Refer **Table 16A.3**

Table 16A.3: Interpretation of dexamethasone suppression test

Test	*Changes in cortisol levels*	*Interpretation*
Low dose dexamethasone test	Cortisol levels decrease	No impaired cortisol production
High dose dexamethasone test	Cortisol levels decrease	Cushing's syndrome
High dose dexamethasone test	Cortisol levels remain the same	Ectopic ACTH producing cells or adrenal adenoma

this feedback mechanism, serum testosterone levels are maintained. However, this does not happen in women as most of their testosterone is derived from peripheral conversion of weaker androgens and this is not controlled by gonadotropin feedback inhibition. Hence, FAI correlates with free testosterone in women but not men.

$$\text{Free androgen index (FAI)} = \frac{\text{Total Testosterone (nmol / L)} \times 100}{\text{SHBG (nmol / L)}}$$

Calculated free testosterone has been considered as the most sensitive indicator of hyperandrogenism in women.[55,56] The values for testosterone were converted from ng/mL to nmol/L using the following equation, 1 ng/mL = 3.467 nmol/L.[57]

Assessment of Insulin Resistance

Among the various indices to assess the insulin resistance, HOMA-IR and QUICKI are the best and commonly used markers.[33]

Homeostasis Model Assessment of Insulin Resistance (HOMA-IR) index is calculated as follows:

HOMA-IR = Fasting blood insulin (μU/mL) × fasting blood glucose (mmol/L)/22.5

Quantitative insulin sensitivity check index (QUICK1) is calculated as follows:

QUICKI = 1/[log(fasting insulin μU/mL) + log (fasting glucose mmol/L)]

This index has increased sensitivity to fasting measurements.

Post-glucose tests may be more sensitive than the fasting tests.[58] Till date, there is no universal test to determine IR, therefore clinicians need to use a sound clinical judgment in recognizing IR.

Fasting insulin levels more than 20mU/mL may indicate IR. Fasting glucose/fasting insulin ratio of < 4.5 is considered to be > 90% sensitive in some populations. A ratio of < 7 in young girls might predict IR.[58] Saxena, et al. observed that insulin levels 2 hours after 75 g glucose load if > 41 mU/mL was indicative of IR, so was a fasting insulin of > 25 mU/mL[59] **(Box 16A.9)**.

Box 16A.9: Indicators of Insulin resistance

- Fasting insulin levels more than 20 μU/mL
- Fasting glucose/fasting insulin ratio of <7 in young girls (< 4.5 is considered to be > 90% sensitive)
- Insulin levels 2 hours after 75 g glucose load > 41 μU/mL

Radiological Tests

Transvaginal ultrasonography should be done in all cases of hirsutism to check for polycystic ovaries and ovarian tumors. CT or MRI scan of brain to check for pituitary neoplasms like prolactinoma in cases with hyperprolactinemia or when visual defects have been diagnosed.

Other Tests

Irrespective of its cause, hirsutism has cardiovascular risk, it is prudent to check for any associated dyslipidemia and hence, lipid profile should be done in all cases of hirsutism.

Management of Hirsutism

In view of the various drawbacks of FG scoring (refer above, section on Assessing Hirsutism), for treatment purpose, it is better to consider "Patient important hirsutism". Patient important hirsutism refers to the intensity of hirsutism perceived by the women irrespective of mFG scoring or appearance.

Hirsutism does not necessarily mean excess androgen production and also the management is to a significant extent independent of the etiology. However, hirsutism might be a potential indicator of an underlying medical condition which may need specific treatment, and such a disorder might have distinct implications for fertility, medical risks, etc. Therefore, the aim of management in a case of hirsutism should be to evaluate the patient for any underlying cause and treat it accordingly.

Management of hirsutism involves assessing the severity of hirsutism, counseling, lifestyle modification, treatment of underlying factors which stimulate hair growth and finally, treating excess hair growth.

Counseling

Counseling is the most important and crucial aspect in the management of hirsutism. Following aspects have to be considered during counseling.

1. Hirsutism other than those due to hormone secreting tumors or drug induced is an ongoing process and hence continuous care is essential.
2. Hair growth does not occur simultaneously and uniformly in all androgen dependent areas. This is very important when a patient starts laser hair reduction for

one area; gradually hair growth becomes prominent in surrounding and/or other areas. This does not always mean paradoxical stimulation of hair by lasers but, a natural progression of the condition.

3. Lifestyle modifications have a significant impact over the overall results.
4. Any modality of treatment cannot remove all hairs completely but reduce it to an extent, which is aesthetically acceptable.

Lifestyle Modification

The first line of therapy in adolescents having hirsutism with PCOS should be lifestyle modification and weight loss. Insulin resistance is now an integral component in etiopathogenesis of hirsutism. It is well documented that obesity increases insulin resistance and induces anovulatory cycles thus complicating PCOS management. Weight reduction helps in improving the metabolic co-morbidities of obesity, decrease the serum insulin levels and increase the insulin sensitivity resulting in lower levels of serum LH and androgens.[2] Also, peripheral conversion of androgens reduces with loss of fat. Bariatric surgeries are also found to reduce androgen levels and there by improve hirsutism in extremely obese patients.[2]

Low caloric diet has been proved to reduce body weight and androgen levels. High protein (30% daily energy from protein) and low glycemic load food regimen significantly reduced insulin levels, HOMA-IR indices and high sensitivity C-reactive protein levels in comparison to conventional hypocaloric diet (15% daily energy from proteins) in overweight and obese women with PCOS.[60] Smoking has been associated with increased free androgen index and insulin resistance.[61] Lifestyle modification in the form of regular exercise, dietary modification, restriction on alcohol consumption and smoking, psychosocial stressors have a positive impact on long-term PCOS control and ameliorating secondary changes like hyperandrogenism.[62,63]

Treatment

Aim of the treatment in a case of hirsutism should be to address not only hirsutism but also the associated conditions like PCOS, acne, seborrhea patterned hair loss, etc.

Hair grows in nonsynchronous cycles and the anagen phase which is the growth phase varies according to different body areas. For the facial hair the anagen phase lasts for around 4 months. As a result of this long hair-growth cycle the hormonal treatment takes almost 6 months to be effective enough to show visible results. Maximum results could be appreciated by the end of 9 months.[22] Therefore, one should wait for atleast for 6 months before considering the particular therapy as a failure.

In women with irregular menses, inducing ovulation alone with clomiphene citrate, metformin or both does not alter hirsutism. Hence, OCPs or antiandrogens should be used regularly to improve hirsutism.[64]

Systemic Therapy

Treatment of hirsutism can be stratified as systemic hormonal therapy, oral contraceptive pills and anti-androgens. Adjuvant systemic therapeutics include insulin sensitizer, plant antiandrogens. Eflornithine is the only topical agent available for hair reduction.

Oral Contraceptive Pills (OCPs)

OCPs are preferred in hirsute patients who do not want to get pregnant and in women who are on antiandrogens to provide better contraception.

OCPs are the most frequently used pharmacologic treatment modality in hirsutism. They decrease LH and FSH resulting in suppression of the androgen production by the ovaries. Oral contraceptive pill contains an estrogen and a progestin. Estrogens increase SHBG leading to reduced free testosterone. The progestin in an OCP inhibits the 5α reductase activity and also acts as an antagonist of the androgen receptor. It can also cause a decrease in the SHBG, therefore an OCP with a progestin of low androgenic potential like norethindrone acetate, ethynodiol diacetate, desogestrel, gestodene, norgestimate should be preferred.[7]

When hyperandrogenic women were treated with 192 days of continuous regimen of combined oral contraceptive pill, their mFG score (by 78.5%), total testosterone, free androgen index, acne and seborrhea reduced and an increase in SHBG was seen.[65] In comparison to levonorgestrel 150 μg/ethinyl estradiol 30 μg (2nd generation OCP), desogestrel 150 μg/ethinyl estradiol 30 μg (3rd generation OCP) reduced hirsutism scores significantly without causing any significant changes in weight.[66] OCPs were found to be more efficacious when combined with either spironolactone or finasteride.[67] For any results to be appreciated, it takes around six cycles and it is better the medication be continued for further 6 months.

Although OCPs are associated with an increased risk of cardiovascular side effects like venous thrombosis or myocardial infarction, the absolute risk is minimal.[2] OCPs are better avoided in women who smoke, have history of stroke or deep vein thrombosis.

Antiandrogens

This group of medication causes feminization of male fetus and hence this medication is reserved for females who do not have any plans for expansion of family. Hence, it is better if antiandrogens are coprescribed with OCPs.

Spironolactone

Spironolactone is a potassium sparing diuretic which has antiandrogen and weak progestin action. It competitively inhibits androgen receptor at higher doses and 5-alpha reductase enzyme to lesser extent. It also increases SHBG levels (thereby decrease free testosterone) and enhances catabolism of testosterone. Hence, spironolactone shows significant improvement in hirsutism regardless of the cause. Daily dose of 100 to 200 mg is usually recommended, but in obese patients and with severe hirsutism a higher doses upto 300 mg can be given. On combining with metformin (1000 mg/day), lower doses of spironolactone (50 mg/day) gave better results and lesser side effects than when either drug was used alone in PCOS.[68] Combination of spironolactone 50 mg/day and metformin 1000 mg/day was much better in reducing mFG score, serum testosterone and insulin resistance than either drugs given alone.[68] Similarly, spironolactone along with finasteride gave better results than spironoloactone alone.[69]

Side effects include hyperkalemia, gastrointestinal disturbances, nausea, dizziness, polyuria, polydipsia.[70] Incidence of polymenorrhea reduces on combining with finasteride.[69] Hyperkalemia is common in those with renal insufficiency or on concomitant angiotensin converting enzyme inhibitors, angiotensin II receptor agonists, potassium sparing diuretics, aldosterone antagonists and potassium supplements. Such individuals should be advised to avoid bananas, tender coconut and diet soda.

Drospirenone

Drospirenone is a newer synthetic progestin, derived from spironolactone. It has antiandrogenic and antimineralocorticoid properties with no androgenic, estrogenic, glucocorticoid or anti-glucocorticoid properties. It competitively binds to the androgen receptors and also inhibits ovarian androgen production.[70] It is available as 3 mg in combination OCPs along with 20 mg or 30 mg of EE. Sidc effect profile is similar to spironolactone. When compared non-users of OCPs and users of levonorgestrel containing OCPs, women using drospirenone containing OCPs were found to have higher risk of venous thromboembolism (no evidence for arterial thrombosis). However, the overall risk as such is meager.[71]

Flutamide

Flutamide is an androgen receptor blocker. It is the only antiandrogen that specifically blocks the androgen receptors. It does not have any glucocorticoid, progestational, androgenic or estrogenic action. Flutamide inhibits the uptake and/or suppresses the nuclear binding of androgen in the target tissues forming inactive complexes with androgen receptors. Improvement is seen clinically in 3 months. Flutamide is also effective in reducing other symptoms of hyperandrogenism like acne and seborrhea.[72]

There are many studies comparing the efficacy of low dose flutamide (62.5 mg/day) to that of a high dose (375–750 mg/day). Low dose flutamide was found to be effective, safe for prolonged use and slower reversal of hirsutism as well as caused least rebound phenomenon (when compared to all antiandrogens) on stopping medications in the treatment of hirsutism.[73-75] The safety of low dose has even been studied in the treatment of female pattern hair loss as well.[76] Flutamide 125 mg/day was found to be more efficacious than finasteride 5 mg/day alone or combination therapy of finasteride 5 mg/day and flutamide 125 mg/day.[77]

The side effects of flutamide are dose related and include respiratory tract infection, nausea, vomiting, diarrhea, headache and dry skin.[75] Increase in the transaminase enzyme levels is not so common and is dose related. Regular monitoring of the liver function tests is of utmost importance during flutamide therapy. Long-term use of flutamide does not have any effects on the ovarian or adrenal androgen levels in women because of its peripheral site of action.[78]

Cyproterone Acetate (CPA)

Cyproterone acetate is a steroidal antiandrogen with progestational activity. It inhibits the production of gonadotropins leading to reduced levels of serum LH. This lowers serum testosterone and androstenedione concentration. Cyproterone acetate decreases 5α reductase activity thereby, lowering DHT synthesis.

Recommended dose is 50–100 mg/day in a cyclical pattern starting from day 1 of menstrual cycle to day 10. It is later continued with low dose OCP containing 30 μg of EE and CPA 2 mg.

Side effects include weight gain, headache, loss of libido, breast tenderness, nausea, mood changes, hepatotoxicity and fatigue.[70]

Finasteride

Finasteride is a 5-alpha reductase II enzyme inhibitor. Finasteride reduces DHT and DHEAs leading to increased total testosterone. Testosterone is converted to estradiol by aromatase enzyme. Finasteride lowered hirsutism scores by 30–60%.[79] Studies reveal that, not only low dose finasteride (2.5 mg/day) was as efficacious as high dose (5 mg/day) in the treatment of hirsutism but even twice a week dosage had same effect as daily dosing. Hair growth over thighs was found to reduce better than hairs over other body parts.[80,81] Efficacy of finasteride was found to be similar as other antiandrogens.[79]

Statistically significant reduction in hair growth was observed when radiofrequency coupled IPL was done along with twice daily application of finasteride 0.5% solution in comparison to vehicle controlled placebo solution.[82] Finasteride 5 mg/day was found to be less efficacious than flutamide 125 mg/day or the combination of flutamide 125 mg/day and finasteride 5 mg/day after 12 months of treatment in hirsute women.[77]

Bicalutamide

It is an oral nonsteroidal pure antiandrogen. It acts by blocking the androgen receptor. It also accelerates the degradation of the androgen receptor. Müderris II, et al have tried 25 mg/day of bicalutamide in 42 patients with hirsutism with significant improvement.[83] Significant reduction in hirsutism score, free androgen index as well as free and total testosterone was seen. However, it did not reduce insulin resistance.[84]

Gonadotropin Releasing Hormone Analogue

Leuprolide

Long-acting GnRH analogues like leuprolide depot 3.75 mg/month suppresses the hypothalamic-pituitary-ovarian axis and is thus found to be effective in hirsute patients with severe hyperandrogenemia and those having significant insulin resistance. For a complete suppressive effect to be appreciated the treatment needs to continued for atleast 2–3 months. GnRH analogues are given in combination with an OCP or other androgen blocking agents. Its better used as a reserve drug in patients who fail to respond to the first line of therapy. GnRH agonist leuprolide (depot preparation, 3.75 mg, intramuscular) is more efficacious than finasteride 5 mg/day.[85] Significant demineralization of the bones, atrophic vaginitis and hot flushes are the potential adverse effects which should be monitored.[7]

Insulin Sensitizers

Metformin

As hyperinsulinemia is an integral part of PCOS, obesity and hirsutism, it is imperative that all PCOS patient be treated with insulin sensitizers. In fact, it has to be more aggressively combated in hyperandrogenic teens.[86] Insulin sensitizing agents like metformin can be of use in cases of hirsutism associated with PCOS.

Metformin is a biguanide which inhibits hepatic gluconeogenesis. It suppresses fatty acid production as it inhibits the acetyl-CoA carboxylase enzyme. Metformin stimulates glucose transport and uptake in the peripheral adipose tissue. It reduces the circulating insulin levels and promotes improved insulin receptor activity. This leads to reduction in ovarian and adrenal androgen synthesis, raised SHBG levels and improved GnRH secretion; which culminate in reducing hirsutism score and improve menstrual cycles **(Box 16A.10)**.[87,88]

The beneficial effects of metformin in PCOS are independent of dosages (1000 mg/day, 1500 mg/day and 1700 mg/day) across all range of BMI. Reduction in plasma testosterone levels was more significant in individuals with higher basal BMI.[89] Meta-analysis revealed that metformin is as effective as OCP but less efficacious than spironolactone and flutamide.[87] Combination of metformin with flutamide appears to be superior to metformin alone in the treatment of hirsutism.[67] As metformin and thiazolidenediones alone are less efficacious in reducing hirsutism score, the Androgen Excess and Polycystic ovary syndrome society advises against the use of any insulin sensitizer as a therapy for hirsutism.[10] This implies that, insulin sensitizers can be used as an additional treatment modality to reduce IR in cases with hirsutism but cannot be used alone to treat hirsutism.

Metformin is occasionally associated with gastrointestinal side effects which can be minimized by slow titration of the doses over a period of one month and by taking it after meals. None of the studies have reported lactic acidosis as an adverse effect with metformin treatment. For higher doses extended release formulations can be used.

Thiazolidinediones

Thiazolidinediones are another class of insulin sensitizing agents which activate the nuclear receptor peroxisome proliferator activated receptor-gamma (PPAR-γ), causing

Box 16A.10: Mechanism of action of metformin in hirsutism

- Inhibits hepatic gluconeogenesis
- Suppresses fatty acid production as it inhibits the acetyl-CoA carboxylase enzyme
- Stimulates glucose transport and uptake in the peripheral adipose tissue
- Reduces the circulating insulin levels and promotes improved insulin receptor activity

This leads to reduction in ovarian and adrenal androgen synthesis, raised SHBG levels and improved GnRH secretion; reducing hirsutism score and improving menstrual cycles

increased production of insulin-sensitive adipocytes, increased glucose uptake in these cells and increased secretion of adiponectin.[2]

The side effect profile of thiazolidenediones needs to be considered before prescribing this class of insulin sensitizer. These are found to increase risk of fractures, congestive cardiac failure, ischemic heart disease, weight gain due to lipogenesis, infections of upper respiratory tract, cholestatic hepatitis and bladder neoplasm (pioglitazone use for more than 1 year).[90] Pioglitazone also increases fertility and hence may warrant concomitant use of oral contraceptive to prevent unwanted pregnancies. Because of these side effects, thiazolidenediones have limited usage in the treatment of hirsutism.

Alpha Lipoic Acid (ALA)

Alpha lipoic acid is an antioxidant which improves insulin sensitivity.[91] Alpha lipoic acid improves glucose uptake by muscle cells and prevents destruction of insulin receptor in adipocytes.[92] Varying doses (300–1800 mg/day) have been studied with no proper consensus.[93] It has also been found to reduce weight significantly; however, some had mild, transient urticaria and pruritus.[94] ALA contains sulphydryl group and hence causes Insulin autoimmune syndrome. Insulin autoimmune syndrome or Hirata syndrome is occurrence of spontaneous hypoglycemia with very high levels of hyperinsulinemia, autoantibodies to endogenous insulin in individuals without exposure to external insulin **(Box 16A.11)**. Though common in Japanese (HLA-DRB1*04:06 allele), cases are reported among Caucasians (HLA-DRB1*04:03 allele).[95,96]

Inositol

PCOS women exhibit peripheral insulin resistance in adipose tissue and muscles whereas, their ovaries (theca cells) are highly sensitive to insulin. Myo-inositol triggers cellular intake of glucose and D-chiro-inositol promotes glycogen synthesis.[97]

The ratio of myo-inositol/D-chiro-inositol (MI/CI) is increased in insulin resistance.[98] However, theca cells are very sensitive to insulin and hence reveal decreased MI/CI ratio (due to increased myo-inositol to chiro-inositol epimerase activity). This leads to increased chiro-inositol production. Chiro-inositol sets in chain of reactions which leads to increased non-oxidative and oxidative glucose disposal leading to increased insulin sensitivity in theca cells. Chiro-inositol glycans act as signal transduction system for testosterone production by theca cells. Insulin triggers increased testosterone production through this transduction system.

Hence, for a normal functioning, both these inositols should be balanced. Supplementation of both in a physiological ratio (MI:DCI = 550 mg:13.8 mg) i.e. 40:1, was found to reduce indicators of insulin resistance (plasma insulin, blood glucose and HOMA-IR index)[97] as well as hirsutism scores, hyperandrogenism and regularized deranged lipid profile.[99] Reduction in mFG scores was better when OCP were combined with myo-inositol than OCP alone.[100]

Box 16A.11: Hirata syndrome (Syn: Insulin autoimmune syndrome)

- Occurrence of spontaneous hypoglycemia with very high levels of hyperinsulinemia, autoantibodies to endogenous insulin in individuals without exposure to external insulin
- Common in Japanese (HLA-DRB1*04:06 allele), cases are reported among Caucasians (HLA-DRB1*04:03 allele)

Others

Vitamin E (400 mg) and omega 3 fatty acids (Eicosapentaenoic acid 180 mg + Docosahexaenoic acid 120 mg) were also found to reduce blood glucose and HbA1c.[101]

Miscellaneous Treatments

High dose of dexamethasone (about 2 mg) is administered at night to treat patients with Chrousos syndrome.[32]

Cabergoline is more effective than bromocriptine in rectifying hyperprolactinemia.[102] It is used as 0.25–1 mg twice weekly or 0.5–2 mg once weekly.[103] Radiotherapy and surgery are advised in resistant cases or those intolerant to medications.[102]

Oophorectomy is the treatment for choice for hirsutism due to ovarian androgen secreting tumors.[19]

Plant Antiandrogens

Plant antiandrogens are compounds or extracts of plants which have antiandrogenic effects and hence helpful in conditions like hirsutism, androgenetic alopecia and acne. Among various agents, spearmint is the only plant antiandrogen to have randomized clinical trials **(Table 16A.4)**.[104]

Topical Therapy

Eflornithine

Eflornithine hydrochloride 13.9% cream is the first topical preparation which was approved by US FDA for the topical treatment of facial hirsutism in 2000.[105,22] Being first synthesized as an anticancer drug in 1970, eflornithine was later used as an intravenous preparation in the treatment

Table 16A.4: Plant antiandrogens and their mechanism of action

Plant	Species name	Mechanism of action
Reishi	*Ganoderma lucidum*	Reduces 5-alpha reductase thereby inhibiting conversion of testosterone to more potent dihydrotestosterone
Licorice	*Glycyrrhiza glabra*	Has phytoestrogens Steroid glycyrrhizin and glycyrrhetic acid have weak anti-androgen properties
White peony	*Paeonia lactiflora*	Paeoniflorin inhibits testosterone production and increases aromatase activity leading to conversion of testosterone to estrogen
Green tea	*Camellia sinensis*	Epigallocatechins inhibit 5-alpha reductase
Spearmint	*Mentha spicata*	Randomized clinical trial revealed a decrease in plasma gonadotropins and androgens in hirsute PCOS patients Specifically reduces free testosterone without altering total testosterone
Chaste tree	*Vitex agnus-castus*	Reduces prolactin

Box 16A.12: Mechanism of action of eflornitine

- Irreversibly inhibits ornithine decarboxylase enzyme which is a rate limiting enzyme in the hair growth
- Reduces the hair growth and makes the hair finer
- Hair returns to the pretreatment levels after about 8 weeks of discontinuation of the cream

of African sleeping sickness. Hair loss was seen as a side effect of this therapy.

Eflornithine irreversibly inhibits ornithine decarboxylase enzyme which is a rate limiting enzyme in the hair growth. It therefore reduces the hair growth and makes the hair finer. Noticeable changes are seen after 6–8 weeks of application. It is found to significantly improve the quality of life.[22] The hair return to the pretreatment levels after about 8 weeks of discontinuation of the cream **(Box 16A.12)**.

It should be applied twice daily atleast 8 hours apart and left over for a minimum of 4 hours and needs to be continued for atleast 6–8 weeks. If results are seen it can be used indefinitely.

Ideally eflornithine should be used in conjunction with other modalities of treatment like systemic therapy, IPL or Laser. It can be used for treating the grey hair or the vellus hair which is not targeted by laser.

Side effects observed are mild like acne, burning, stinging sensation, or a folliculitis.

References

1. Yildiz BO, Bolour S, Woods K, Moore A, Azziz R. Visually scoring hirsutism. Hum Reprod Update. 2010;16(1):51-64.
2. Geller DH, Pacaud D, Gordon CM, Misra M. Drug and Therapeutics Committee of the Pediatric Endocrine Society. State of the Art Review: Emerging Therapies: The Use of Insulin Sensitizers in the Treatment of Adolescents with Polycystic Ovary Syndrome (PCOS). Int J Pediatr Endocrinol. 2011;2011(1):9-27.
3. Franks S. The investigation and management of hirsutism. J Fam Plann Reprod Health Care. 2012;38(3):182-6.
4. Ekbäck MP, Lindberg M, Benzein E, Arestedt K. Health-related quality of life, depression and anxiety correlate with the degree of hirsutism. Dermatology. 2013;227(3):278-84.
5. Altinok ML, Glintborg D, Depont RC, Hallas J, Andersen M. Prescription of antidepressants is increased in Danish patients with polycystic ovary syndrome and is associated with hyperandrogenism. A population based cohort study. Clin Endocrinol (Oxf). 2013 Nov 14. doi: 10.1111/cen.12365. [Epub ahead of print].
6. Zargar AH, Wani AI, Masoodi SR, Laway BA, Bashir MI, Salahuddin M. Epidemiologic and etiologic aspects of hirsutism in Kashmiri women in the Indian subcontinent. Fertil Steril. 2002;77(4):674-8.
7. Agrawal NK. Management of hirsutism. Indian J Endocr Metab. 2013;17:S77-82.
8. Souter I, Sanchez LA, Perez M, Bartolucci AA, Azziz R. The prevalence of androgen excess among patients with minimal unwanted hair growth. Am J Obstet Gynecol. 2004;191(6):1914-20.
9. Goodarzi MO, Shah NA, Antoine HJ, Pall M, Guo X, Azziz R. Variants in the 5alpha-reductase type 1 and type 2 genes are associated with polycystic ovary syndrome and the severity of hirsutism in affected women. J Clin Endocrinol Metab. 2006;91(10):4085-91.
10. Escobar-Morreale HF, Carmina E, Dewailly D, Gambineri A, Kelestimur F, Moghetti P, et al. Epidemiology, diagnosis and management of hirsutism: a consensus statement by the Androgen Excess and Polycystic Ovary Syndrome Society. Hum Reprod Update. 2012;18(2):146-70.
11. Ndefo UA, Eaton A, Green MR. Polycystic ovary syndrome: a review of treatment options with a focus on pharmacological approaches. P T. 2013;38(6):336-55.
12. Carmina E, Rosato F, Jannì A, Rizzo M, Longo RA. Extensive clinical experience: relative prevalence of different androgen excess disorders in 950 women referred because of clinical hyperandrogenism. J Clin Endocrinol Metab. 2006;91(1):2-6.
13. Zabuliene L, Tutkuviene J. [Body composition and polycystic ovary syndrome]. Medicina (Kaunas). 2010;46(2):142-57.
14. Guzel AI, Kuyumcuoğlu U, Celik Y. Factors affecting the degree of hirsutism in patients with polycystic ovary syndrome. Arch Gynecol Obstet. 2012;285(3):767-70.
15. Comim FV, Hardy K, Franks S. Adiponectin and Its Receptors in the Ovary: Further Evidence for a Link between Obesity and Hyperandrogenism in Polycystic Ovary Syndrome. PLoS One. 2013;8(11):e80416.

16. Talaei A, Adgi Z, Mohamadi Kelishadi M. Idiopathic hirsutism and insulin resistance. Int J Endocrinol. 2013;2013:593197.
17. Loriaux DL. An approach to the patient with hirsutism. J Clin Endocrinol Metab. 2012;97(9):2957-68.
18. Reisch N, Högler W, Parajes S, Rose IT, Dhir V, Götzinger J, et al. A diagnosis not to be missed: nonclassic steroid 11β-hydroxylase deficiency presenting with premature adrenarche and hirsutism. J Clin Endocrinol Metab. 2013;98(10):E1620-5.
19. Saraceno G, Barresi V, Trimarchi F, Cannavo S. Occult leydig cell tumour and androgen-receptor positive breast cancer in a woman with severe hyperandrogenism. J Ovarian Res. 2013;6(1):43.
20. Cordera F, Grant C, van Heerden J, Thompson G, Young W. Androgen-secreting adrenal tumors. Surgery. 2003;134(6):874-80; discussion 880.
21. Rodríguez-Gutiérrez R, Bautista-Medina MA, Teniente-Sanchez AE, Zapata-Rivera MA, Montes-Villarreal J. Pure androgen-secreting adrenal adenoma associated with resistant hypertension. Case Rep Endocrinol. 2013;2013:356086.
22. Martin KA, Chang RJ, Ehrmann DA, Ibanez L, Lobo RA, Rosenfield RL, et al. Evaluation and treatment of hirsutism in premenopausal women: an endocrine society clinical practice guideline. J Clin Endocrinol Metab. 2008;93(4):1105-20.
23. Patel A, Malek N, Haq F, Turnbow L, Raza S. Hirsutism in a female adolescent induced by long-acting injectable risperidone: a case report. Prim Care Companion CNS Disord. 2013;15(3):PCC.12l01454.
24. Carvalho MM, Góis C. [Hyperprolactinemia in mentally ill patients]. Acta Med Port. 2011;24(6):1005-12. [Article in Portuguese].
25. Ignacak A, Kasztelnik M, Sliwa T, Korbut RA, Rajda K, Guzik TJ. Prolactin--not only lactotrophin. A "new" view of the "old" hormone. J Physiol Pharmacol. 2012;63(5):435-43.
26. Munoz J, Hanbali AS. Epidermal growth factor receptor-induced hirsutism and trichomegaly. Mayo Clin Proc. 2011;86(11):e50.
27. Bode D, Seehusen DA, Baird D. Hirsutism in women. Am Fam Physician. 2012;85(4):373-80.
28. Alpañés M, González-Casbas JM, Sánchez J, Pián H, Escobar-Morreale HF. Management of postmenopausal virilization. J Clin Endocrinol Metab. 2012;97(8):2584-8.
29. Cheng V, Doshi KB, Falcone T, Faiman C. Hyperandrogenism in a postmenopausal woman: diagnostic and therapeutic challenges. Endocr Pract. 2011;17(2):e21-5.
30. Vollaard ES, van Beek AP, Verburg FA, Roos A, Land JA. Gonadotropin-releasing hormone agonist treatment in postmenopausal women with hyperandrogenism of ovarian origin. J Clin Endocrinol Metab. 2011;96(5):1197-201.
31. Ibáñez L, Ong KK, Mongan N, Jääskeläinen J, Marcos MV, Hughes IA, et al. Androgen receptor gene CAG repeat polymorphism in the development of ovarian hyperandrogenism. J Clin Endocrinol Metab. 2003;88(7):3333-8.
32. Charmandari E, Kino T. Chrousos syndrome: a seminal report, a phylogenetic enigma and the clinical implications of glucocorticoid signalling changes. Eur J Clin Invest. 2010;40(10):932-42.
33. Singh B, Saxena A. Surrogate markers of insulin resistance: A review. World J Diabetes. 2010;1(2):36-47.
34. Saxena P, Prakash A, Nigam A, Mishra A. Polycystic ovary syndrome: Is obesity a sine qua non? A clinical, hormonal, and metabolic assessment in relation to body mass index. Indian J Endocrinol Metab. 2012;16(6):996-9.
35. Landay M, Huang A, Azziz R. Degree of hyperinsulinemia, independent of androgen levels, is an important determinant of the severity of hirsutism in PCOS. Fertil Steril. 2009;92(2):643-7.
36. Glintborg D, Andersen M, Hagen C, Hermann AP. Higher bone mineral density in Caucasian, hirsute patients of reproductive age. Positive correlation of testosterone levels with bone mineral density in hirsutism. Clin Endocrinol (Oxf). 2005;62(6):683-91.
37. Wehr E, Pilz S, Schweighofer N, Giuliani A, Kopera D, Pieber TR, Obermayer-Pietsch B. Association of hypovitaminosis D with metabolic disturbances in polycystic ovary syndrome. Eur J Endocrinol. 2009;161(4):575-82.
38. Thomson RL, Spedding S, Buckley JD. Vitamin D in the aetiology and management of polycystic ovary syndrome. Clin Endocrinol (Oxf). 2012;77(3):343-50.
39. George PS, Pearson ER, Witham MD. Effect of vitamin D supplementation on glycaemic control and insulin resistance: a systematic review and meta-analysis. Diabet Med. 2012;29(8):e142-50.
40. Ardabili HR, Gargari BP, Farzadi L. Vitamin D supplementation has no effect on insulin resistance assessment in women with polycystic ovary syndrome and vitamin D deficiency. Nutr Res. 2012;32(3):195-201.
41. Strobel F, Reusch J, Penna-Martinez M, Ramos-Lopez E, Klahold E, Klepzig C, et al. Effect of a Randomised Controlled Vitamin D Trial on Insulin Resistance and Glucose Metabolism in Patients with Type 2 Diabetes Mellitus. Horm Metab Res. 2013. [Epub ahead of print].
42. Belenchia AM, Tosh AK, Hillman LS, Peterson CA. Correcting vitamin D insufficiency improves insulin sensitivity in obese adolescents: a randomized controlled trial. Am J Clin Nutr. 2013;97(4):774-81.
43. Panidis D, Balaris C, Farmakiotis D, Rousso D, Kourtis A, Balaris V, et al. Serum parathyroid hormone concentrations are increased in women with polycystic ovary syndrome. Clin Chem. 2005;51(9):1691-7.
44. Yetkin DO, Demirsoy ET, Kadioglu P. Pure leydig cell tumour of the ovary in a post-menopausal patient with severe hyperandrogenism and erythrocytosis. Gynecol Endocrinol. 2011;27(4):237-40.
45. Unluhizarci K, Kaltsas G, Kelestimur F. Non polycystic ovary syndrome-related endocrine disorders associated with hirsutism. Eur J Clin Invest. 2012;42(1):86-94.
46. Lakshmi C. Hormone therapy in acne. Indian J Dermatol Venereol Leprol. 2013;79:322-37.
47. Orfanos CE, Adler YD, Zouboulis CC. The SAHA syndrome. Horm Res. 2000;54(5-6):251-8.
48. Lin YH, Huang SY, Hsu MI, Chang YC, Cheng CY, Hsu CS, et al. Hyperhomocysteinaemia is associated with biochemical hyperandrogenaemia in women with reproductive age.

Eur J Obstet Gynecol Reprod Biol. 2013 Oct 10. pii: S0301-2115(13)00499-5.
49. Li R, Qiao J, Yang D, Li S, Lu S, Wu X, et al. Epidemiology of hirsutism among women of reproductive age in the community: a simplified scoring system. Eur J Obstet Gynecol Reprod Biol. 2012;163(2):165-9.
50. Knochenhauer ES, Hines G, Conway-Myers BA, Azziz R. Examination of the chin or lower abdomen only for the prediction of hirsutism. Fertil Steril. 2000;74(5):980-3.
51. Rashidi H, Parizi ZT, Mohammadi M. Evaluation of only the chin or lower abdomen for predicting hirsutism. Indian J Endocrinol Metab. 2013;17(5):896-8.
52. Scicchitano P, Dentamaro I, Carbonara R, Bulzis G, Dachille A, Caputo P, Riccardi R, Locorotondo M, Mandurino C, Matteo Ciccone M. Cardiovascular Risk in Women With PCOS. Int J Endocrinol Metab. 2012;10(4):611-8.
53. Wild RA, Carmina E, Diamanti-Kandarakis E, Dokras A, Escobar-Morreale HF, Futterweit W, et al. Assessment of cardiovascular risk and prevention of cardiovascular disease in women with the polycystic ovary syndrome: a consensus statement by the Androgen Excess and Polycystic Ovary Syndrome (AE-PCOS) Society. J Clin Endocrinol Metab. 2010;95(5):2038-49.
54. Orsino A, Van Eyk N, Hamilton J. Clinical features, investigations and management of adolescents with polycystic ovary syndrome. Paediatr Child Health. 2005;10(10):602-8.
55. Al Kindi MK, Al Essry FS, Al Essry FS, Mula-Abed WA. Validity of serum testosterone, free androgen index, and calculated free testosterone in women with suspected hyperandrogenism. Oman Med J. 2012;27(6):471-4.
56. Rosner W, Auchus RJ, Azziz R, Sluss PM, Raff H. Position statement: Utility, limitations, and pitfalls in measuring testosterone: an Endocrine Society position statement. J Clin Endocrinol Metab. 2007;92(2):405-13.
57. Hwang KR, Choi YM, Kim JJ, Chae SJ, Park KE, Jeon HW, et al. Effects of insulin-sensitizing agents and insulin resistance in women with polycystic ovary syndrome. Clin Exp Reprod Med. 2013;40(2):100-5.
58. Traub ML. Assessing and treating insulin resistance in women with polycystic ovarian syndrome. World J Diabetes. 2011;2(3):33-40.
59. Saxena P, Prakash A, Nigam A, Mishra A. Polycystic ovary syndrome: Is obesity a sine qua non? A clinical, hormonal, and metabolic assessment in relation to body mass index. Indian J Endocrinol Metab. 2012;16(6):996-9.
60. Mehrabani HH, Salehpour S, Amiri Z, Farahani SJ, Meyer BJ, Tahbaz F. Beneficial effects of a high-protein, low-glycemic-load hypocaloric diet in overweight and obese women with polycystic ovary syndrome: a randomized controlled intervention study. J Am Coll Nutr. 2012;31(2):117-25.
61. Cupisti S, Häberle L, Dittrich R, Oppelt PG, Reissmann C, Kronawitter D, et al. Smoking is associated with increased free testosterone and fasting insulin levels in women with polycystic ovary syndrome, resulting in aggravated insulin resistance. Fertil Steril. 2010;94(2):673-7.
62. Norman RJ, Davies MJ, Lord J, Moran LJ. The role of lifestyle modification in polycystic ovary syndrome. Trends Endocrinol Metab. 2002;13(6):251-7.
63. Thomson RL, Buckley JD, Brinkworth GD. Exercise for the treatment and management of overweight women with polycystic ovary syndrome: a review of the literature. Obes Rev. 2011;12(5):e202-10.
64. Roth LW, Huang H, Legro RS, Diamond MP, Coutifaris C, Carson SA, et al. Reproductive Medicine Network. Altering hirsutism through ovulation induction in women with polycystic ovary syndrome. Obstet Gynecol. 2012;119(6): 1151-6.
65. Caruso S, Cianci S, Malandrino C, Cicero C, Presti LL, Cianci A. Hyperandrogenic women treated with a continuous-regimen oral contraceptive. Eur J Obstet Gynecol Reprod Biol. 2013;171(2):307-10.
66. Sanam M, Ziba O. Desogestrel+ethinylestradiol versus levonorgestrel+ethinylestradiol. Which one has better affect on acne,hirsutism, and weight change. Saudi Med J. 2011;32(1):23-6.
67. Swiglo BA, Cosma M, Flynn DN, Kurtz DM, Labella ML, Mullan RJ, et al. Clinical review: Antiandrogens for the treatment of hirsutism: a systematic review and metaanalyses of randomized controlled trials. J Clin Endocrinol Metab. 2008;93(4):1153-60.
68. Ganie MA, Khurana ML, Nisar S, Shah PA, Shah ZA, Kulshrestha B, et al. Improved efficacy of low-dose spironolactone and metformin combination than either drug alone in the management of women with polycystic ovary syndrome (PCOS): a six-month, open-label randomized study. J Clin Endocrinol Metab. 2013;98(9):3599-607.
69. Keleştimur F, Everest H, Unlühizarci K, Bayram F, Sahin Y. A comparison between spironolactone and spironolactone plus finasteride in the treatment of hirsutism. Eur J Endocrinol. 2004;150(3):351-4.
70. Unluhizarci K, Karaca Z, Kelestimur F. Hirsutism - from diagnosis to use of antiandrogens. Front Horm Res. 2013;40:103-14.
71. Wu CQ, Grandi SM, Filion KB, Abenhaim HA, Joseph L, Eisenberg MJ. Drospirenone-containing oral contraceptive pills and the risk of venous and arterial thrombosis: a systematic review. BJOG. 2013;120(7):801-10.
72. Calaf J, López E, Millet A, Alcañiz J, Fortuny A, Vidal O, et al. Spanish Working Group for Hirsutism. Long-term efficacy and tolerability of flutamide combined with oral contraception in moderate to severe hirsutism: a 12-month, double-blind, parallel clinical trial. J Clin Endocrinol Metab. 2007;92(9):3446-52.
73. Somani VK, Sucharita V, Sharma VK, Sita V, Razvi F, Bang R. The efficacy of flutamide, an antiandrogen in idiopathic hirsutism. Indian J Dermatol Venereol Leprol. 1998;64(1):17-22.
74. Ibáñez L, Jaramillo A, Ferrer A, de Zegher F. Absence of hepatotoxicity after long-term, low-dose flutamide in hyperandrogenic girls and young women. Hum Reprod. 2005;20(7):1833-6.
75. Paradisi R, Venturoli S. Retrospective observational study on the effects and tolerability of flutamide in a large population of patients with various kinds of hirsutism over a 15-year period. Eur J Endocrinol. 2010;163(1):139-47.
76. Paradisi R, Porcu E, Fabbri R, Seracchioli R, Battaglia C, Venturoli S. Prospective cohort study on the effects and

tolerability of flutamide in patients with female pattern hair loss. Ann Pharmacother. 2011;45(4):469-75.

77. Unluhizarci K, Ozel D, Tanriverdi F, Karaca Z, Kelestimur F. A comparison between finasteride, flutamide, and finasteride plus flutamide combination in the treatment of hirsutism. J Endocrinol Invest. 2009;32(1):37-40.
78. Cusan L, Dupont A, Bélanger A, Tremblay RR, Manhes G, Labrie F. Treatment of hirsutism with the pure antiandrogen flutamide. J Am Acad Dermatol. 1990;23(3 Pt 1):462-9.
79. Townsend KA, Marlowe KF. Relative safety and efficacy of finasteride for treatment of hirsutism. Ann Pharmacother. 2004;38(6):1070-3.
80. Bayram F, Müderris II, Güven M, Keleştimur F. Comparison of high-dose finasteride (5 mg/day) versus low-dose finasteride (2.5 mg/day) in the treatment of hirsutism. Eur J Endocrinol. 2002;147(4):467-71.
81. Tartagni M, Schonauer MM, Cicinelli E, Petruzzelli F, De Pergola G, De Salvia MA, et al. Intermittent low-dose finasteride is as effective as daily administration for the treatment of hirsute women. Fertil Steril. 2004;82(3):752-5.
82. Farshi S, Mansouri P, Rafie F. A randomized double blind, vehicle controlled bilateral comparison study of the efficacy and safety of finasteride0.5% solution in combination with intense pulsed light in the treatment of facial hirsutism. J Cosmet Laser Ther. 2012;14(4):193-9.
83. Müderris II, Bayram F, Ozçelik B, Güven M. New alternative treatment in hirsutism: bicalutamide 25 mg/day. Gynecol Endocrinol. 2002;16(1):63-6.
84. Bahceci M, Tuzcu A, Canoruc N, Tuzun Y, Kidir V, Aslan C. Serum C-reactive protein (CRP) levels and insulin resistance in non-obese women with polycystic ovarian syndrome, and effect of bicalutamide on hirsutism, CRP levels and insulin resistance. Horm Res. 2004;62(6):283-7.
85. Bayhan G, Bahçeci M, Demirkol T, Ertem M, Yalinkaya A, Erden AC. A comparative study of a gonadotropin-releasing hormone agonist and finasteride on idiopathic hirsutism. Clin Exp Obstet Gynecol. 2000;27(3-4):203-6.
86. Marshall JC, Dunaif A. Should all women with PCOS be treated for insulin resistance? Fertil Steril. 2012;97(1):18-22.
87. Cosma M, Swiglo BA, Flynn DN, Kurtz DM, Labella ML, Mullan RJ, et al. Clinical review: Insulin sensitizers for the treatment of hirsutism: a systematic review and metaanalyses of randomized controlled trials. J Clin Endocrinol Metab. 2008;93(4):1135-42.
88. Velija-Ašimi Z. Evaluation of endocrine changes in women with the polycystic ovary syndrome during metformin treatment. Bosn J Basic Med Sci. 2013;13(3):180-5.
89. Fulghesu AM, Romualdi D, Di Florio C, Sanna S, Tagliaferri V, Gambineri A, et al. Is there a dose-response relationship of metformin treatment in patients with polycystic ovary syndrome? Results from a multicentric study. Hum Reprod. 2012;27(10):3057-66.
90. Lincoff AM, Wolski K, Nicholls SJ, Nissen SE. Pioglitazone and risk of cardiovascular events in patients with type 2 diabetes mellitus: a meta-analysis of randomized trials. JAMA. 2007;298(10):1180-8.
91. Udupa AS, Nahar PS, Shah SH, Kshirsagar MJ, Ghongane BB. Study of comparative effects of antioxidants on insulin sensitivity in type 2 diabetes mellitus. J Clin Diagn Res. 2012;6(9):1469-73.
92. Bajaj S, Khan A. Antioxidants and diabetes. Indian J Endocrinol Metab. 2012;16(Suppl 2):S267-71.
93. Jacob S, Ruus P, Hermann R, Tritschler HJ, Maerker E, Renn W, et al. Oral administration of RAC-alpha-lipoic acid modulates insulin sensitivity in patients with type-2 diabetes mellitus: a placebo-controlled pilot trial. Free Radic Biol Med. 1999;27(3-4):309-14.
94. Koh EH, Lee WJ, Lee SA, Kim EH, Cho EH, Jeong E, et al. Effects of alpha-lipoic Acid on body weight in obese subjects. Am J Med. 2011;124(1):85.e1-8.
95. Uchigata Y. The novel agent, alpha lipoic acid, can cause the development of insulin autoimmune syndrome. Intern Med. 2007;46(17):1321-2.
96. Gullo D, Evans JL, Sortino G, Goldfine ID, Vigneri R. Insulin autoimmune syndrome (Hirata Disease) in European Caucasians taking α-lipoic acid. Clin Endocrinol (Oxf). 2013. doi: 10.1111/cen.12334. [Epub ahead of print].
97. Minozzi M, Nordio M, Pajalich R. The Combined therapy myo-inositol plus D-Chiro-inositol, in a physiological ratio, reduces the cardiovascular risk by improving the lipid profile in PCOS patients. Eur Rev Med Pharmacol Sci. 2013;17(4):537-40.
98. Heimark D, McAllister J, Larner J. Decreased myo-inositol to chiro-inositol (m/c) ratios and increased m/c epimerase activity in pcos theca cells demonstrate increased insulin sensitivity compared to controls. Endocr J. 2013. [Epub ahead of print].
99. Minozzi M, D'Andrea G, Unfer V. Treatment of hirsutism with myo-inositol: a prospective clinical study. Reprod Biomed Online. 2008;17(4):579-82.
100. Minozzi M, Costantino D, Guaraldi C, Unfer V. The effect of a combination therapy with myo-inositol and a combined oral contraceptive pill versus a combined oral contraceptive pill alone on metabolic, endocrine, and clinical parameters in polycystic ovary syndrome. Gynecol Endocrinol. 2011;27(11):920-4.
101. Udupa A, Nahar P, Shah S, Kshirsagar M, Ghongane B. A comparative study of effects of omega-3 Fatty acids, alpha lipoic Acid and vitamin e in type 2 diabetes mellitus. Ann Med Health Sci Res. 2013;3(3):442-6.
102. Wang AT, Mullan RJ, Lane MA, Hazem A, Prasad C, Gathaiya NW, et al. Treatment of hyperprolactinemia: a systematic review and meta-analysis. Syst Rev. 2012;1:33.
103. Huang W, Molitch ME. Evaluation and management of galactorrhea. Am Fam Physician. 2012;85(11):1073-80.
104. Grant P, Ramasamy S. An Update on Plant Derived Anti-Androgens. Int J Endocrinol Metab. 2012;10(2):497-502.
105. Jobanputra KS, Rajpal AV, Nagpur NG. Eflornithine. Indian J Dermatol Venereol Leprol. 2007;73(5):365-6.

16B

Hypertrichosis

S Sacchidanand, Divya Gorur

"Everything in excess is opposite to nature"

—*Hippocrates*

Definition

Hypertrichosis is defined as excessive hair growth for a particular site of the body or age of a patient that is not hormone-dependent.[1]

Hypertrichosis and hirsutism need to be differentiated as the latter occurs in response to androgens and thus selectively affects the androgen-dependent hair. Hirsutism may be defined as the occurrence in women or children of growth of coarse terminal hair in a male sexual pattern. However, hypertrichosis can also be excess of either the vellus or the lanugo type **(Table 16B.1)**.[2]

It can be classified as follows

- Based on the age of onset as congenital or acquired

Table 16B.1: Differences between hypertrichosis and hirsutism

Hypertrichosis	*Hirsutism*
Excessive hair growth on face and body	Excessive hair growth in androgen dependent areas
Congenital/acquired	Due to androgen excess states
Both males and females affected	Females
Generalized or localized in distribution. Commonly seen over face and trunk	Seen over androgen dependent areas
Type of hair involved can be lanugo, vellus or terminal	Vellus hairs transformed to terminal hair
Congenital forms show poor response to medical line of treatment	Good response when underlying cause is treated
Physical methods of management preferred	Can be managed medically

Table 16B.2: Congenital causes of hypertrichosis

- Hypertrichosis of lanugo hairs: Congenital hypertrichosis lanuginosa
- Hypertrichosis of vellus hairs: Ambras syndrome

Hypertrichosis of terminal hairs

a. Localized
   - Anterior cervical hypertrichosis
   - Posterior cervical hypertrichosis
   - Hypertrichosis cubiti
   - Hypertrichosis with gingival fibromatosis
   - Lumbosacral hypertrichosis

   Associated with other cutaneous abnormalities
   - Congenital nevocellular nevi
   - Becker's nevi
   - Linear epidermal nevi
   - Congenital smooth muscle hamartomas
   - Familial hypertrichosis of palms and soles

b. Generalized
   - Hypertrichosis universalis congenita
   - X-linked dominant hypertrichosis

   Associated with other genetic diseases
   - Congenital porphyrias
   - Leprechaunism (Donohue syndrome)
   - Cornelia de Lange syndrome
   - Mucopolysaccharidosis
   - Barber–Say syndrome
   - CAHMR syndrome
   - Cantu syndrome

- Based on distribution as localized and generalized
- Based on type of hair affected—lanugo, vellus and terminal (**Table 16B.2 and 16B.3**).

Hypertrichosis of Lanugo Hair

Congenital Hypertrichosis Lanuginosa

This is a rare autosomal dominantly transmitted disorder characterized by the persistence of fetal lanugo hair indefinitely instead of its usual replacement by vellus hair.

Table 16B.3: Acquired causes

- Hypertrichosis of lanugo hairs : Paraneoplastic
- Hypertrichosis of vellus hairs : Drug induced—bimatoprost

Hypertrichosis of terminal hair:

Localized

- Idiopathic **(Figure 16B.1)**
- Topical drugs
  - Corticosteroids
  - Methoxypsoralen
  - Minoxidil
- Trauma
- Chronic inflammation
- Pretibial myxedema
- Peripheral neuropathy
- Irradiation
  - X-rays
  - Ultraviolet light

Generalized

- Systemic drugs
  - Minoxidil
  - Diaxozide
  - Androgenic hormones
  - Phenytoin sodium
  - Cyclosporine
- Dermatomyositis
- Acquired porphyrias
- Thyroid abnormalities
- Malnutrition

The child is usually noticed to be excessively hairy at birth. The hair gradually lengthens until by early childhood the entire skin, apart from the palms and soles, is covered by silky hair, which may be 10 cm or more in length. The long eyelashes, eyebrows, and facial hair have led to this condition being termend as 'dog faced' and 'monkey faced'.

Onset later in childhood and recessive inheritance is also known. Once established, the hypertrichosis is permanent, but some diminution of hairiness of trunk and limbs may be noted in later childhood. At puberty, axillary, pubic and beard hairs retain their downy character. Teeth, bone, and ear defects may be associated.

The condition should be distinguished from the normal lanugo hair of the premature infant that are shed in a few weeks. Treatment of children with long-pulsed ruby laser can result in a significant reduction of hair, although the benefits tend to wane over 6–12 months.[3,4]

Acquired

Hypertrichosis Lanuginosa Acquisita (HLA)

HLA may occur in metabolic and endocrine diseases, e.g. porphyria and hypo- or hyperthyroidism, or may be induced by drugs such as cyclosporine, penicillamine, psoralens, glucocorticosteroids, diazoxide, interferon, minoxidil, phenytoin or cetuximab. It can also be associated with various malignancies **(Box 16B.1)**.

Box 16B.1: Drugs causing hypertrichosis lanuginosa acquisita

- Cyclosporin
- Penicillamine
- Psoralens
- Glucocorticosteroids
- Diazoxide
- Interferon
- Minoxidil
- Phenytoin
- Cetuximab

Hypertrichosis Lanuginosa Acquisita Associated with Malignancy

Etiology: This condition is associated with a variety of internal malignancies, especially carcinoma of the lung, colon or breast and lymphoreticular malignancy. Acquired hypertrichosis lanuginosa can precede the diagnosis of the neoplasm, and it may also be associated with abnormalities of the tongue (e.g. burning pain) and other paraneoplastic dermatoses such as acanthosis nigricans, palmoplantar keratoderma, sign of Leser Trélat and acquired ichthyosis.

A hormone-like substance secreted by the tumor is thought to alter the growth rate and anagen/telogen durations of the follicles and reverts them back to the lanugo type.

Clinical features: Rapid onset of hypertrichosis resulting in a striking simian appearance, because of the growth of dense, long, fine, white or red-black, lanugo hair all over the body except palms, soles, penis, and the surfaces covered with terminal hair. Such hair may grow even on previously bald scalp. The rate of growth of this hair is fast, up to 2.5 cm per week, and they may grow up to 15 cm long. In the milder form the hypertrichosis may be restricted to the face (Malignant Down).[4] The condition needs to be differentiated from drug-induced hypertrichosis.

Patients with hypertrichosis lanuginosa acquisita usually have metastatic disease at the time of diagnosis and, therefore, a poor prognosis. However, successful antitumor therapy is associated with regression of hair growth.[4,5]

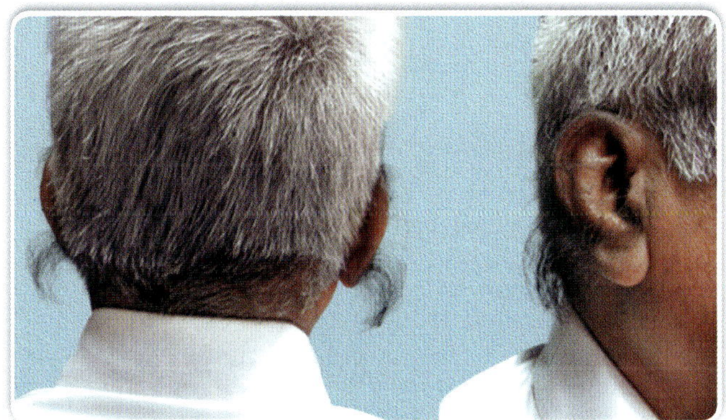

Fig. 16B.1: Hypertrichosis over pinna

Hypertrichosis of Vellus Hairs

Vellus hair hypertrichosis is rare. It has been described in Ambras syndrome[6] (a congenital cause) and following use of ocular bimatoprost (an acquired cause).[7]

Ambras Syndrome

Ambras syndrome (AS) was first described by Baumeister et al. in 1993. Baumeister postulates that AS is associated with a relative decrease of the telogen phase of the hair growth cycle.

Etiology: Inherited autosomal dominantly with specific genetic alteration of pericentric inversion.

Clinical features: Fine, long silky hair more than 10 cm long, uniformly distributed on face including nose, ears and shoulders which persists for life. It may be associated with minor facial dysmorphism, dental anomalies, and supernumerary nipples. It has to be differentiated from congenital hypertrichosis universalis characterized by hair accentuation in the frontal, temporal and peri-auricular regions, hair whorl forms at the spine **(Box 16B.2)**.[8]

Box 16B.2: Ambras syndrome

- Congenital hypertrichosis of vellus hair
- Inherited autosomal dominantly with specific genetic alteration of pericentric inversion
- Associated with minor facial dysmorphism, dental anomalies, supernumerary nipples
- To be differentiated from congenital hypertrichosis universalis, which is characterized by hair accentuation in the frontal, temporal and peri-auricular regions, hair whorl forms at the spine

Hypertrichosis of Terminal Hairs

Congenital

Localized

Genetic

Hairy elbows/hypertrichosis cubiti: Hypertrichosis cubiti is an uncommon variety of congenital, circumscribed hypertrichosis. Beighton first reported this syndrome in 1970 in Amish patients. It usually appears in a sporadic form, but familial occurrence with autosomal dominant inheritance are reported.[9]

Clinical features: It affects both sexes, onset is at birth or during early childhood, and tends to regress spontaneously at puberty. Abnormal long hair is present bilateral and symmetrically, from mid-humerus to mid- forearm, in an otherwise normal hairy person. The hairs are thin, lanuginous, downy, and progressively they become coarser and more pigmented, evolve into medullated vellus hair and attain a considerable length of several centimeters. May be associated with short stature.[9]

Anterior cervical hypertrichosis: This autosomal recessive condition is characterized by patchy hypertrichosis occurring just proximal to the laryngeal prominence. A patch of hair is present in the cervical midline, located at the lower anterior part of the neck just above the sternal notch. A few patients have peripheral sensory and motor neuropathy. The mode of inheritance is variable, either autosomal or X-linked dominant inheritance or can occur sporadically.[10]

Other associated conditions are developmental and mental retardation, learning disturbance, peripheral neuropathy, microcephaly, halux valgus, back hypertrichosis, optic atrophy, chorioretinitis, strabismus, Turner's syndrome. Since, the lesions are on visible parts of body such as face and neck, it may lead to social stigmata and psychological impact on patients.

Currently available hair removal methods include bleaching, trimming, tweezing, shaving, waxing, chemical depilatories, electrolysis, intense pulsed light therapy, and lasers, such as diode, Nd: YAG and Alexandrite.[11]

Posterior cervical hypertrichosis: This autosomal dominant or X-linked inherited disorder is characterized by localized hypertrichosis occurring over the spine in the lumbo-thoracic or cervical area and usually overlying a spinal or neural defect.[12] It is commonly associated with kyphoscoliosis and is distinct from hypertrichosis occurring over the sacral area, which is known as "faun tail".

Hypertrichosis with gingival fibromatosis: This condition is autosomal dominantly inherited.

Clinical feature: Onset is at puberty. There is hypertrichosis of the terminal hair with bushy eyebrows and synophrys, which is more prominent in males than in females.

Gingival hyperplasia gives rise to an "orange peel" like stippling of the gingiva and impedes teeth eruption leading to periodontal abscesses. The hyperplasia interferes with speech and chewing, necessitating repeated surgical debulking.[13] The condition may or may not be associated with seizures and/or mental retardation.

Developmental

Nevus/nevoid hypertrichosis: Nevoid hypertrichosis (NH) is an uncommon disorder consisting of a solitary, circumscribed area of terminal hair growth present at or soon after birth. The involved hair may be normal or hypopigmented, with or without any associated cutaneous and extra-cutaneous abnormalities.

Etiology: Autosomal dominant mode of inheritance has been proposed in giant NH. Lopez-Barrantes, et al. concluded that NH may occur in a mosaic pattern and may be associated with other cutaneous diseases that may show a segmental pattern as a twin spotting phenomenon with severe mental, ocular or myoskeletal anomalies or without any associated abnormalities.

Clinical features: The skin lesions are usually present at or soon after birth and are typically solitary, though cases of multiple patches developing after puberty have been reported. A few cases of multiple NH in which patches are either round, in a checker board or linear pattern, along Blaschko's lines have also been documented. The color of the terminal hair may be the same as the color of the scalp hair, rarely gray or white. The histopathology usually shows a normal epidermis with increased number of morphologically normal hair follicles in the dermis, but is needed to rule out any underlying nevus.

Differential diagnosis includes other congenital disorders in which localized hypertrichosis occur like Becker's nevus, congenital melanocytic nevi **(Figure 16B.2)** and smooth muscle hamartoma.

The cutaneous lesions may persist for life, however, spontaneous resolution has also been reported. Hair reduction lasers Nd: YAG laser can be used to reduce the lesional hair growth.

NH may be associated with ocular, cerebral, mental, myoskeletal, neurological, gastrointestinal, pulmonary abnormalities, facial dysmorphia and hypertrichosis cubiti. Patients with NH must be investigated to rule out any systemic involvement associated with the skin lesions.[14]

Faun tail or sacral hirsutism: Faun tail nevus is a posterior midline cutaneous marker for underlying spinal abnormalities like spinal dysraphism.

Abnormal lumbar hypertrichosis may present as "Silky down" or a "Faun tail". When this occurs away from the spine, it is known as simple nevoid hypertrichosis. Silky down presents as soft nonterminal hair, while a faun tail is a wide patch of coarse terminal hair, several inches long.

It is more common in females **(Box 16B.3 and Figure 16B.2)**.

Midline lumbosacral hypertrichosis is more common in females and may overlie bony and spinal cord defects (spinal dysraphism). Spinal dysraphism is a generic term describing pathologic conditions related to improper closure of the caudal neuropore. It encompasses all the conditions associated with spina bifida. Other cutaneous markers of spinal dysraphism are dimples, dermal sinuses, subcutaneous lipomas, port wine stain, acrochordons, hemangiomas, aplasia cutis and telangiectasia, capillary malformation **(Box 16B.4)**.

Box 16B.3: Faun tail

- Posterior midline cutaneous marker for underlying spinal abnormalities presenting as abnormal lumbar hypertrichosis
- Silky down presents as soft nonterminal hair, while a faun tail is a wide patch of coarse terminal hair, several inches long

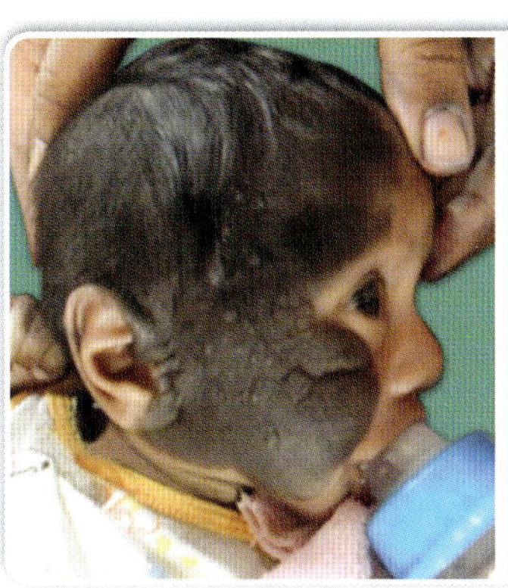
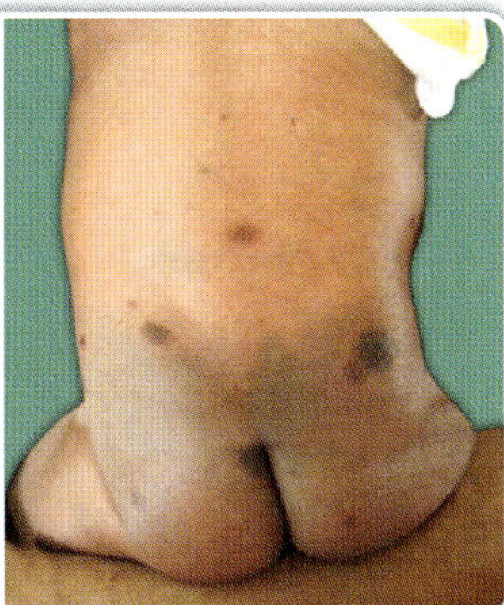

Fig. 16B.2: Congenital melanocytic nevi

Box 16B.4: Cutaneous markers of spinal dysraphism

- Dimples, dermal sinuses, subcutaneous lipomas, port wine stain, acrochordons, hemangiomas, aplasia cutis, telengiectasia and capillary malformation

Traction on the spinal cord transfixed with a bony spicule may lead to progressive sensory-motor affection of the lower limbs with or without sphincter involvement. Imaging techniques are needed to establish the diagnosis before surgical correction. In occult cases of dysraphism, except for cosmetic disfigurement, treatment is rarely required for tethered cord or spinal instability. A good cosmetic result can be achieved with intense pulsed light lasers (IPL).[15]

Generalized

Hypertrichosis Universalis

This is the commonly seen, dominantly transmitted trait in which the body hair is longer and coarser than normal. It is common in the Middle East, the Mediterranean, and some parts of the Indian subcontinent. It is essential to differentiate this condition from Ambras syndrome. The latter is associated with generalized vellus hypertrichosis with involvement of the nose and eyelids and various dysmorphic features. Characteristic curls of hair protruding from the external auditory canal are a diagnostic clue.

Associated with Syndromes (Table 16B.4)

1. *Hurler's syndrome and other mucopolysaccharidoses:* Hypertrichosis is usually present from early infancy

Table 16B.4: Congenital generalized hypertrichosis associated with other syndromes[18]

Dysmorphic syndromes
❑ Cornelia de Lange syndrome
❑ Rubinstein–Taybi syndrome
Lipodystrophic syndromes
❑ Berardinelli Seip syndrome
❑ Leprechaunism
Metabolic
❑ Hurler's and other mucopolysaccharidoses
Sclerodermoid
❑ Winchester syndrome
❑ POEMS
Associated facial dysmorphism, skeletal defects, gingival hyperplasia
❑ Cantu syndrome
❑ Zimmermann–Laband syndrome
❑ Adducted thumb syndrome
❑ Coffin Siris syndrome
❑ Barber Say syndrome
❑ CAHMR syndrome (cataract, hypertrichosis, mental retardation)
Teratogenic syndromes
❑ Fetal alcohol syndrome
❑ Fetal hydantoin syndrome
❑ Fetal valproate syndrome

or early childhood on the face, trunk and limbs. The eyebrows are often bushy and confluent. In abortive forms, the hair growth may first appear after puberty and be more limited in extent.

2. *Congenital macrogingivae:* Exuberant overgrowth of the gingivae as an isolated congenital defect is not uncommon. The association with profuse hypertrichosis of trunk, limbs and lower face has been reported . Some patients have marked acromegaloid features or thyroid disease.[3]
3. *Cornelia de Lange syndrome:* These mildly microcephalic, mentally defective children have a low hairline and profuse overgrowth of the eyebrows. The forehead is covered with long fine hair. Hypertrichosis is also conspicuous on the lower back, or may be generalized.
4. *Winchester syndrome:* A rare hereditary disorder characterized by dwarfism, joint destruction and corneal opacities. The skin in many parts of the body becomes thickened, hyperpigmented and hypertrichotic.
5. *Berardinelli syndrome:* In early life, growth and maturation are accelerated and later there is lipodystrophy with muscular hypertrophy. Enlargement of the liver and hyperlipidemia, coarse skin and hypertrichosis are other features.
6. *Trisomy 18:* Generalized hypertrichosis of variable degree is present in these patients. Hypertrichosis has been reported in the rare hereditary globoid leukodystrophy, Krabbe's disease. However, most patients die during infancy.

Teratogenic Syndromes

Fetal alcohol syndrome: This develops in a high proportion of infants born of alcoholic mothers. The infant is small and microcephalic with retarded milestones, heart, and joint defects. Hypertrichosis and capillary angiomatosis accompany a distinctive facies (short palpebral fissures, prominent nose, and maxillary hypoplasia).[16]

Fetal hydantoin syndrome: Hypertrichosis, low posterior hairline, short webbed neck, depressed nasal bridge, ocular hypertelorism and psychomotor retardation are some of the numerous congenital defects that can result from maternal consumption of phenytoin.[17]

Acquired

Localized

Chronic inflammatory conditions and repeated trauma can induce a growth of coarse long hair **(Figure 16B.4)**.

Trauma: Occupational trauma of carrying weights on the shoulders, habitual trauma of biting in the mentally challenged individuals can lead to hypertrichosis of the concerned region.

Chronic inflammatory conditions leading to hypertrichosis are chronic venous stasis, inflamed joints or bones, thrombophlebitis and other inflammatory conditions like lupus panniculitis,[19] subsiding psoriatic plaque,[20] post-laser epilation,[21] postfriction.[22] The skin over a plaque of linear melorheostotic scleroderma may be similarly affected.

Hypertrichosis may also occur around a scar of vaccination, surgery including those of dystrophic epidermolysis bullosa. Application of a plaster of Paris cast in children can lead to hypertrichosis that is rapidly reversible.

Hypertrichosis has also been described at sites of neoplasms (tufted angioma, fibromatous hamartoma of infancy[23]), wart,[24] and following use of topical tacrolimus.[25]

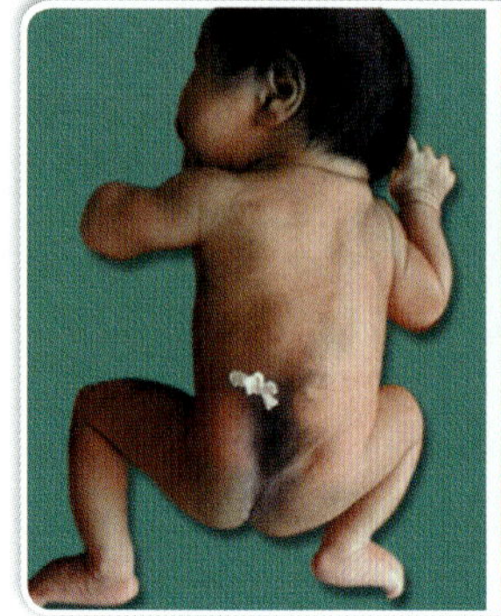
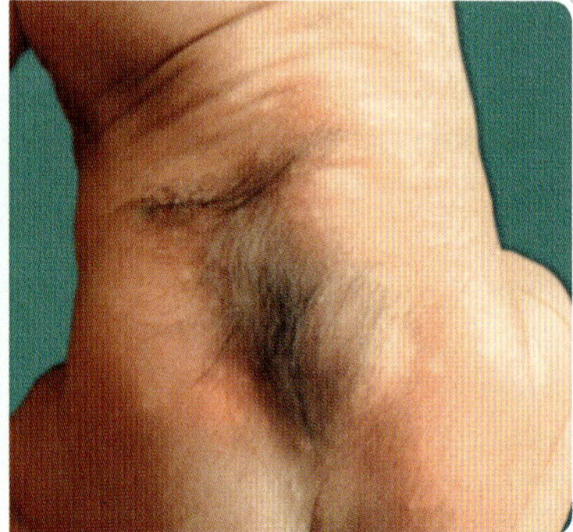

Fig. 16B.3: Faun tail

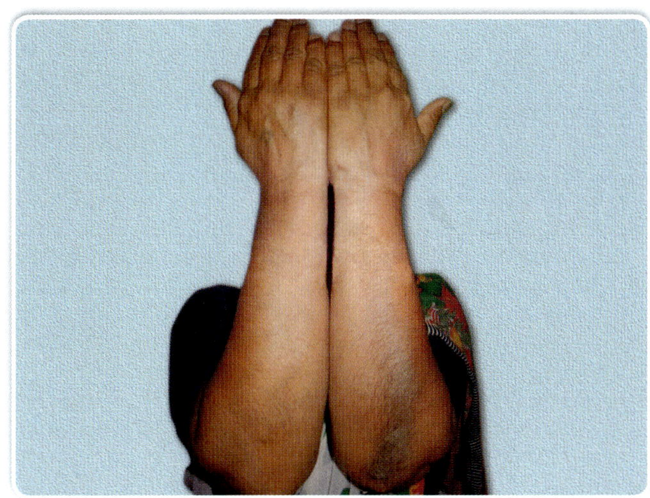

Fig. 16B.4: Hypertrichosis of left forearm due to friction

Long-pulsed Alexandrite laser and intense pulse light have been found to be associated with post laser hypertrichosis.

The IPL may induce the release of certain mediators and cytokines, which may have a stimulatory effect on hair growth and metabolism. The cytokine release may stimulate the follicular stem cells and/or the remaining germinative cells, leading to increased hair growth in the treated and surrounding areas.[26]

Acquired Generalized Hypertrichosis

Endocrine Disturbances

Hypothyroidism: Congenital as well as juvenile hypothyroidism may be accompanied by hypertrichosis.

Cushing's syndrome may cause hirsutism as well as hypertrichosis.

Hyperthyroidism: Pretibial myxedematous plaques may be covered with coarse hair.

Pituitary mechanism: Severe, generalized hypertrichosis has been reported in young children after encephalitis and after mumps followed by the sudden onset of obesity. A diencephalic disturbance is postulated. Generalized hypertrichosis occurred in a girl after traumatic shock and remitted in 6 months.

There are many reports of hypertrichosis after head injuries, especially in children. The hair growth is first noticed 4–12 weeks after the injury and appears as fine silky hair on the forehead, cheeks, back, arms and legs, and may be asymmetrical. It is sometimes shed after a few months, but may persist.

Other Conditions

Malnutrition[3]: Gross malnutrition, which may be primary or secondary as in celiac disease/other malabsorption states or in severe infections, may cause profuse generalized hypertrichosis in children.[3]

Table 16B.5: Drugs causing hypertrichosis

Drug	Remarks
Phenytoin	Preferentially in females
Diazoxide	Affects children more frequently
Psoralens and benoxaprofen	May induce hypertrichosis of the sun-exposed areas
Minoxidil	May disappear even when the drug is continued, forehead is affected when applied to scalp
Cyclosporine	Associated with sebaceous hyperplasia
Therapy with streptomycin, penicillamine, danazol, IFN-α,[84] and gefitinib[85] may also result in hypertrichosis	

Anorexia nervosa[3]: An increased growth of fine, downy hair on the face, trunk and arms, sometimes of severe degree, has been reported in 20–77% of adult cases, and is also seen in children. The prevalence of hypertrichosis in bulimia is reported to be half of that in anorexia, and both are associated with approximately 60% prevalence of scalp alopecia.

Porphyrias: Hypertrichosis involving the exposed areas is a characteristic sign of the porphyrias in erythropoietic porphyria, variegate porphyria, erythropoietic protoporphyria, and porphyria cutanea tarda, in order of frequency. An extreme degree of hypertrichosis is seen in children with hepatic porphyria induced by hexachlorobenzene or other chemicals. The hypertrichosis is striking and has led to them being labeled as "monkey children".

Dermatomyositis[3]: Excessive hair growth has been noted mainly in children and principally on the forearms, legs and temples, but it may be more extensive.

Epidermolysis bullosa: Although rare, gross hypertrichosis of the face and limbs has occurred in association with epidermolysis bullosa of the dystrophic type. Hypertrichosis is seen affecting the extensor surface of the arm in a sporadic or familial form in children, resolving in adolescence.

Drugs (Table 16B.5)

The existing vellus hair increase in length and diameter but are rarely more than 3 cm long. The condition is usually noticed over the extensors of extremities but only after precipitating drug has been taken for a few months.[3]

References

1. Fantauzzo KA1, Kurban M, Levy B, Christiano AM. Trps1 and its target gene Sox9 regulate epithelial proliferation in the developing hair follicle and are associated with hypertrichosis, PLoS Genet. 2012;8(11):e1003002. doi: 10.1371/journal.pgen.1003002. Epub 2012 Nov 1.

2. Dawber RPR, Ebling FJG, Wojnarowska FT. Disorders of hair. In: Champion RH, Burton JL, Ebling FJG, editors. Textbook of Dermatology. 5th edn. Oxford: Blackwell Scientific. 1991;pp.2533-638.
3. Dawber RPR, Ebling FJG, Wojnarowska FT. Disorders of hair. In: Champion RH, Burton JL, Ebling FJG, editors. Textbook of Dermatology. 5th edn. Oxford: Blackwell Scientific. 1991;pp.2533-638.
4. Messenger AG, Berker DAR, Sinclair RD. Disorder of Hair. In: Burns T, Breathnach S, Cox N, Griffiths C, eds. Rook Textbook of Dermatology. 8th edn. Oxford: Blackwell Science. 2010;p.66.77-9.
5. Slee PH, van der Waal RI, Schagen van Leeuwen JH, Tupker RA, Timmer R, Seldenrijk CA, et al. Paraneoplastic hypertrichosis lanuginosa acquisita: uncommon or overlooked?Br J Dermatol. 2007;157(6):1087-92. Epub 2007 Oct 17.
6. McKusick VA. Ambras syndrome. Online Mendelian Inheritance in Man. [created on 1993 November 3; last updated 2004 October 4]. Available from: http://www.ncbi.nlm.nih.gov/entrez/dispomim.cgi?id=145701.
7. Hart J, Shafranov G. Hypertrichosis of vellus hairs of the malar region after unilateral treatment with bimatoprost. Am J Ophthalmol. 2004;137:756-7.
8. Rashid RM1, White LE. A hairy development in hypertrichosis: A brief review of Ambras syndrome. Dermatol Online J. 2007;13(3):8.
9. Beighton PH. Familial hypertrichosis cubiti: Hairy elbows syndrome. J Med Genet. Pediatric Dermatology Vol. 27 No. 3 2010. 1970;7:158-60.
10. Heitink MV1, Quaedvlieg PJ, van Neer FJ, Frank J. Sporadic nonsyndromal anterior cervical hypertrichosis: Case report and review of the literature. Int J Dermatol. 2007;46 Suppl 3:9-12.
11. Kacar SD. Laser treatment of anterior cervical hypertrichosis, Eur J Pediat Dermatol. 2013;23:89-92.
12. Reed OM, Mellette JR Jr, Fitzpatrick JE. Familial cervical hypertrichosis with underlying kyphoscoliosis. J Am Acad Dermatol. 1989;20:1069-72.
13. Stratigos AJ, Baden HP. Unraveling the molecular mechanisms of hair and nail genodermatoses. Arch Dermatol. 2001;137:1465-71.
14. Gupta L, Gautam RK, Bharadwaj M, Gupta L, Gautam RK, Bharadwaj M. Nevoid Hypertrichosis: Case Report with Review of the Literature. Int J Trichology. 2011;3(2):115-7. doi: 10.4103/0974-7753.90829.
15. Yamini M1, Sridevi KS, Babu NP, Chetty NG.Faun tail nevus. Indian Dermatol Online J. 2011;2(1):23-4. doi: 10.4103/2229-5178.79865.
16. Hanson JW, Jones KL, Smith DW. Fetal alcohol syndrome: Experience with 41 patients. J Am Med Ass. 1976;235:1458-60.
17. The fetal hydantoin syndrome. J Pediatrics. 1975;87:285-90.
18. Camacho-Martínez FM, Hypertrichosis and Hirsutism, In: Bolognia JL, Jorizzo JL, Rapini RP, eds. Bolognia Textbook of Dermatology. 2nd edn. Elsevier. 2008.
19. Garcia-Doval I, Roson E, Abalde M, et al. Coexistence of acquired localized hypertrichosis and lipoatrophy after lupus panniculitis. J Am Acad Dermatol. 2004;50:799-800.
20. Kumar B, Sandhu K, Kaur I. Localized hypertrichosis in subsiding psoriatic plaques. J Dermatol. 2004;31:693-5.
21. Lolis MS, Marmur ES. Paradoxical effects of hair removal systems: A review. J Cosmet Dermatol. 2006;5:274-6.
22. Biolcati G, Berlutti G, Bagarone A, et al. Dermatological marks in athletes of artistic and rhythmic gymnastics. Int J Sports Med. 2004;25:638-40.
23. Yoon TY, Kim JW. Fibrous hamartoma of infancy manifesting as multiple nodules with hypertrichosis. J Dermatol. 2006;33:427-9.
24. Egawa K, Honda Y, Miyawaki Y. Local hypertrichosis associated with a human papillomavirus type 1-induced wart. Br J Dermatol. 2005;153:1224-5.
25. Prats Caelles I, Herranz Pinto P, de Ayala Casado EL, et al. Focal hypertrichosis during topical tacrolimus therapy for childhood vitiligo. Pediatr Dermatol. 2005;22:86-7.
26. Radmanesh. Cutaneous surgery and oncology paradoxical hypertrichosis and terminal hair change after intense pulsed light hair removal therapy. Journal of Dermatological Treatment. 2009;20:1; 52–54ISSN 0954-6634 print/ ISSN 1471-1753 online © 2009 Informa UK Ltd. DOI: 10.1080/09546630802178224.

17

Hair and Nutrition

Shashikumar BM

"Let food be thy medicine and medicine be thy food."

—*Hippocrates*

Introduction

The integrity of normal skin and hair function relies largely on an adequate and balanced nutritional intake. Dietary imbalance, whether in the form of an overall deficiency, specific shortage or excess of one component over another, can disturb this equilibrium. Hair follicle cells have a high turnover. Their active metabolism requires a good supply of nutrients and energy. Dietary imbalance of proteins, vitamins, essential fatty acids, and minerals can lead to structural abnormalities, pigmentary changes, or hair loss.[1] Thus hair analysis is often marketed as a tool to diagnose deficiencies and intoxications.

Dietary supplements have traditionally been used unspecifically to improve hair growth, a few of which have been studied systematically in animals and humans. Recommended dietary allowance (RDA) are given in **Table 17.1**[2,3] along with the rich sources of the particular nutrient.

Protein-energy Malnutrition (PEM)

In humans, the association of nutrition with hair changes emanates primarily from studies on protein-energy malnutrition.[4,5] Hair is composed almost entirely of proteins, so a reduction of hair growth denotes a reduction of protein synthesis by hair follicles. PEM is a spectrum of conditions ranging from growth failure to overt marasmus or Kwashiorkor. Malnutrition influences the structure of the hair shaft and sometimes, the color of the hair. Hair root

Table 17.1: Recommended dietary allowance of important nutrients essential for hair

	RDA		*Source*
	Male	*Female*	
Protein (g)	60	55	Milk, meat, egg, cheese, pulses, cereals, nuts
Niacin (mg)	18	14	Liver, kidney, meat, poultry, fish, legumes, groundnuts
Biotin (µg)	30	30	Swiss chard, raw egg yolk, liver, Saskatoon berries, and leafy green vegetables
Vitamin B_{12} (µg)	1	1	Liver, kidney, meat, fish, eggs, milk, cheese
Ascorbic acid (mg)	40	40	Fresh fruits and green leafy vegetables, germinating pulses, amla
Vitamin A (retinol) (µg)	600	600	Liver, egg, butter, meat, green and yellow fruits, vegetables
Essential fatty acids			Oils like safflower, corn, sunflower, soybean, meat, egg, fish oil
Iron (mg)	17	21	Hem iron—liver, meat, poultry, fish Non-hem iron—cereals, green leafy vegetables, legumes, nuts, jaggery
Copper (µg)	900	900	Seafood, liver, whole grains, legumes, chocolate
Selenium (µg)	55	55	Nuts, cereals, meat, mushrooms, fish, eggs
Zinc (mg)	12	10	Animal foods—meat, milk, fish, legumes, whole grains, dairy

response to protein malnutrition has been studied widely in children with kwashiorkor and marasmus.[6]

Marasmus is a form of severe malnutrition due to inadequate energy intake in all forms, including protein. The hairs in marasmus are thin, fragile and texture changes leading to lack of pliability, giving rise to rough, lusterless, straight hair that cannot be easily groomed. The diameter of the hair bulbs is reduced to a third of normal and almost all follicles are in telogen.[7, 8] These changes are secondary to protein and glycogen deficiency leading to reduced cell mitosis. In contrary, lanugo body hair may be increased. Similar hair changes may be seen in persons on crash diet but less pronounced.

Kwashiorkor is an acute form of childhood protein-energy malnutrition primarily due to protein deficiency. The hair becomes "dyspigmented," often assuming a reddish color which is common in African children, and falls out readily. The easy pluckability of hair is a common feature of the disease. Morphological changes in scalp hair include reduction in the diameter of the hair shaft, bulb, and medulla; the medulla may even be absent.[9] The hair is sparse, thin, brittle, wavy, and silky or shows a mixed picture with rough and standing hair as in marasmus. In older children, the "flag" sign may be observed; when the hair is held up away from the scalp, stripes of normal color and of depigmentation may be noted, presumably signifying periods of dietary improvement and inadequacy, respectively. Sometimes either the peripheral fringe of scalp or cranium alone is involved, giving a halo effect.[8,10] In children with curly hair, the newly growing straight hair give the appearance of trees with straight trunks and a canopy (forest sign). Unlike the scalp hair, the eyelashes are usually long and luxuriant. Lanugo hair may also be excessive.[11] Other features are similar to marasmus but with more anagen follicles although most are atrophic. Factors responsible for these changes in the hair have not been elucidated. It has been postulated that deficiencies of sulfur-containing amino acids or of B complex vitamins may be responsible **(Figures 17.1 and 17.2, Box 17.1)**.

Box 17.1: Hair changes in protein-energy malnutrition

Marasmus
- Thin
- Fragile
- Lack of pliability
- Rough, lustreless
- Straight hair that cannot be easily groomed
- More follicles in telogen
- Lanugo body hair increased

Kwashiorkor
- Dyspigmented
- Easy pluckability
- Thin hair with absent medulla
- Sparse, wavy and silky
- Flag sign
- Forest sign
- Eyelashes are usually long and luxuriant
- Lanugo hair may also be excessive
- Hair in anagen phase

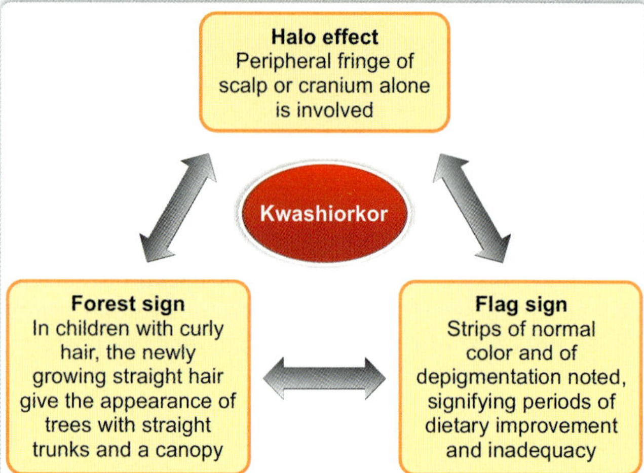

Fig. 17.1: Hair changes in Kwashiorkor

Deficiency of Vitamins

Niacin Deficiency

Niacin encompasses two compounds:
a. Nicotinamide
b. Nicotinic acid.

These are part of coenzymes nicotinamide adenine dinucleotide (NAD) and nicotinamide adenine dinucleotide phosphate (NADP) which are essential in oxidative release of energy. Tryptophan is the precursor amino acid through which nicotinic acid can be synthesized in the body. Deficiency of nicotinic acid is usually accompanied by deficiency of several vitamins. Early signs are diffuse hair loss, weakness, irritability, glossitis and stomatitis.[12]

Vitamin H (Biotin)

Biotin is a water-soluble vitamin that acts as an essential cofactor for four carboxylases, each of which catalyzes an essential step in intermediary metabolism. Biotin deficiency is rare because it is also produced by intestinal bacteria. It has been seen in congenital or acquired biotinidase or carboxylase deficiency,[13] parenteral alimentation, impaired gastrointestinal flora caused by antibiotics, and after excessive ingestion of raw egg whites due to binding by avidin **(Box 17.2)**. Mental changes (depression, hallucinations), paresthesia, anorexia, and nausea are the features of biotin deficiency in adults. In infants, biotin deficiency presents

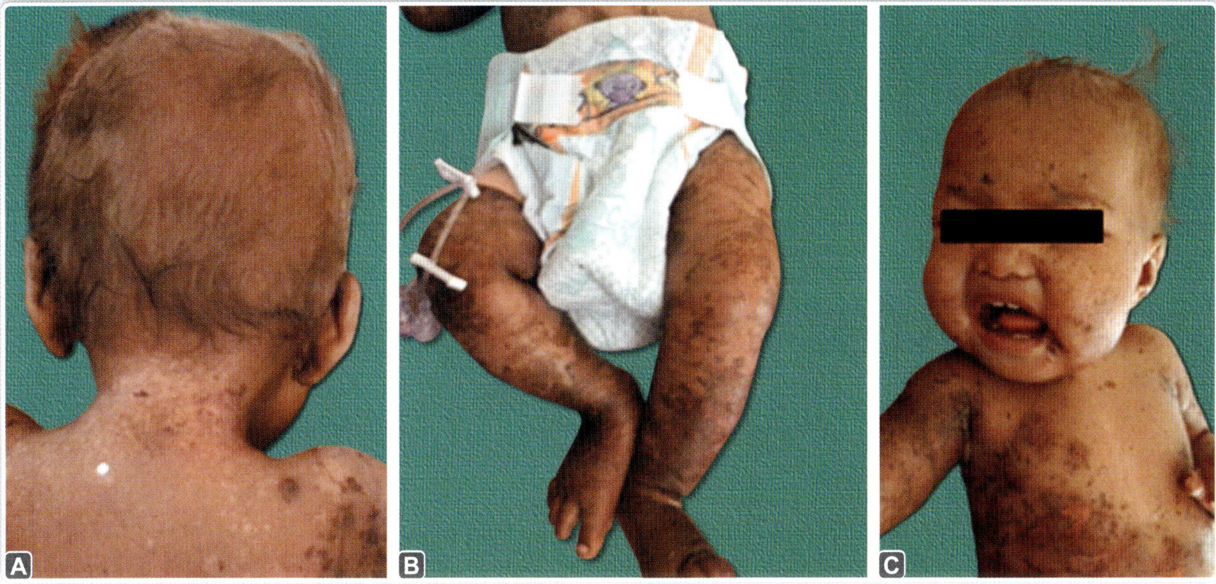

Figs 17.2A to C: Child with protein energy malnutrition: (A) Diffuse hair loss; (B) Flaky paint dermatosis; (C) Irritable child. (*Courtesy:* Department of Dermatology, STD and Leprosy, BMCRI, Bengaluru)

Box 17.2: Conditions associated with biotin deficiency

1. Congenital or acquired biotinidase or carboxylase deficiency
2. Parenteral alimentation
3. Impaired gastrointestinal flora caused by antibiotics
4. After excessive ingestion of raw egg whites due to binding by avidin

as hypotonia, lethargy and apathy. In infants, children, and adults, deficiency of biotin causes alopecia and perioral dermatitis.[14] Hair changes include alopecia and trichorrhexis nodosa and other structural anomalies.[15] The reference daily intake for adults is 30 mg. Antiepileptic drugs can reduce biotin levels; a prophylactic supplementation can therefore be recommended. The laboratory diagnosis of biotin deficiency can be established based on a decreased urinary concentration. Treatment requires pharmacologic doses of biotin, using up to 10 mg/d.

It has not been sufficiently shown that additional supplementation of biotin in patients with normal blood levels can improve hair loss, although an effect on hair and nail structure is possible.[12]

Vitamin B_{12}

Vitamin B_{12} is a complex organo-metallic compound with a cobalt atom. A deficiency of cyanocobalamin is seen in vegetarians and various gastrointestinal disorders. Vitamin B_{12} deficiency is a common cause of megaloblastic anemia and pancytopenia. It has been implicated as a cause of peripheral neuropathy, subacute combined degeneration of the spinal cord, ataxia, optic atrophy, psychosis, depression, and dementia.[16] It is a possible risk factor for thrombosis, myocardial infarction and stroke. Cutaneous changes include hyperpigmentation, vitiligo and recurrent angular stomatitis. Premature greying and hair loss was associated with deficiency states.

Vitamin C

Vitamin C (ascorbic acid) is a water soluble vitamin necessary for collagen synthesis. It is a potent antioxidant necessary for absorption of non-heme iron, carnitine biosynthesis, and the conversion of dopamine to nor epinephrine. Vitamin C is a component of many drug metabolizing enzyme systems, particularly the mixed-function oxidase systems.

Deficiency is seen in elderly and chronic alcoholics. Incidence is more in chronic smokers, those on hemodialysis, and in episodes of stress (e.g. infection, trauma).

Deficiency causes scurvy which manifests as bleeding into skin (petechiae, ecchymoses, perifollicular hemorrhages), joints, peritoneal cavity, pericardium, adrenal glands and gums. There is impaired bone growth. Follicular hyperkeratosis with perifollicular hemorrhages are characteristic cutaneous lesions in scurvy.[11] Vitamin C deficiency leads to corkscrew hairs due to reduced disulfide bonds, perifollicular hyperkeratosis and hemorrhage, follicular plugging, and curling due to perifollicular fibroses.

Laboratory confirmation of vitamin C deficiency is made on the basis of low plasma or leukocyte levels. Treatments include administration of vitamin C in a dose of >200 mg/dL, which improves scurvy symptoms over several days.

Vitamin A

Excessive consumption of vitamin A gives rise to a variable syndrome in which the principal features are dryness, irritability and sometimes pigmentation of the skin. Hair changes in hypervitaminosis A includes slowly progressive thinning of scalp and body hairs, eyebrows and eyelashes. The mode of action of vitamin A on hair is unknown. Systemic features like loss of weight, fatigue, anemia and bone pain are frequent, and sometimes liver and spleen are enlarged. The symptoms develop insidiously after doses in excess of 50,000 units daily ingested for many months **(Table 17.2)**.

Essential Fatty Acids (EFA)

The essential fatty acids are a group of naturally occurring fatty acids. Linolenic acid (ώ-6 fatty acid) and α-linolenic acid are the two fundamental essential fatty acids. They have a role in the normal structure and function of the epidermal barrier. EFAs are important for maintaining the function and integrity of cellular and subcellular membranes.[11]

EFA deficiency is rare and seen in gastrointestinal anomalies or inflammatory bowel disease, pancreatic failure, chronic alcoholism, fat malabsorption, intestinal surgery, and prolonged total parenteral nutrition devoid of lipid supplements. Deficiency leads to growth retardation, fatty liver, anaemia, thrombocytopenia, poor wound healing, increased susceptibility to infection, and diarrhea. Cutaneous manifestations include generalized xerosis, eczematous dermatitis, intertriginal and periorificial dermatitis. Loss of the scalp hairs and eyebrows with premature graying are the noted hair changes.[11]

Deficiency of Micronutrients

Iron

Iron deficiency is the most common nutritional deficiency. Iron is required for the formation of hemoglobin, the transport of oxygen, and for the various oxidation reduction reactions in the tissues. It is essential for several cellular processes including synthesis of DNA, RNA and proteins. Common causes of iron deficiencies are inadequate dietary intake, increased need in growing children and pregnant women, chronic blood loss and hookworm parasitic infestations. Cutaneous manifestations include chronic generalized pruritus, koilonychias, angular stomatitis, cheilosis, glossitis, atrophy of the filiform papillae of the tongue and increased susceptibility to bacterial and fungal infections, particularly *Candida albicans.*

Table 17.2: Hair changes due to abnormal level of vitamins

Niacin	Diffuse hair loss
Biotin	Alopecia and trichorrhexis nodosa
Vitamin B_{12}	Premature greying and hair loss
Vitamin C	Corkscrew hairs, perifollicular hyperkeratosis, follicular plugging, curling due to perifollicular fibrosis
Hypervitaminosis A	Thinning of scalp and body hairs, eyebrows and eyelashes

Hair follicle matrix cells are among the rapidly dividing cells in the body and may be exquisitely sensitive even to a minor decrease in iron availability, thus resulting in diminished hair growth in the presence of iron deficiency.[17,18] Also iron deficiency even in the absence of iron deficiency anemia is associated with certain kinds of hair loss.[19] Thus iron deficiency is related to many hair changes like alopecia areata, androgenetic alopecia, telogen effluvium and diffuse hair loss. Many studies have demonstrated iron deficiency as a reason for the chronic telogen effluvium especially in females whom the iron deficiency is common but few studies have shown no association between low serum ferritin and chronic diffuse telogen hair loss.[19] The impaired keratin production secondary to iron deficiency can lead to thinner anagen hairs. Also band-like colour changes have been reported among iron deficient Africans.

Blood cell count (complete hemogram including leukocyte count, hemoglobin concentration, hematocrit, and platelet count), red blood cell indices (including mean corpuscular volume), serum ferritin, total iron binding capacity (TIBC), serum iron, and transferrin saturation are among the important investigations in evaluation of iron deficiency.

Copper

Copper is an integral part of numerous enzyme systems, including amine oxidases, ferroxidase (ceruloplasmin), cytochrome-c oxidase, superoxide dismutase, and dopamine hydroxylase. Copper plays a role in iron absorption and metabolism, melanin synthesis, energy production, neurotransmitter synthesis, and CNS function; the synthesis and cross-linking of elastin and collagen; and the scavenging of superoxide radicals. Copper deficiency is rare and seen in Menkes' kinky hair syndrome, aceruloplasminemia, infants with malabsorption, Wilson's disease, patients with chronic high doses of oral zinc[20] and in nephrotic syndrome[11] **(Box 17.3)**. Hair changes are not much reported in acquired copper deficiency but alteration of keratinization and pigmentation of hair is associated with Menkes' kinky hair syndrome, a rare X-linked metabolic disturbance of copper metabolism characterized by mental retardation, hypocupremia, and decreased circulating ceruloplasmin. The hair is normal at birth but after the

Box 17.3: Conditions associated with copper deficiency

1. Menkes' kinky hair syndrome
2. Aceruloplasminemia
3. Infants with malabsorption
4. Wilson's disease
5. Patients on chronic high doses of oral zinc
6. Nephrotic syndrome

shedding of the first hair in infancy the new hairs that grow are hypopigmented, fragile and twisted like a "steel wire". Hair shaft examination reveals pilitorti,[21] irregular twisting, trichorrhexis nodosa, trichoclasis, and irregularities in thickness of hair. Unlike classic pili torti the adjacent hair twists may be in opposing directions.

Selenium

Selenium is a component of selenoproteins that include oxidoreductases such as glutathione peroxidase, which catalyses the reduction of hydrogen peroxide and lipid hydroperoxide, and protects cells from oxidative damage.[22] Deficiency of selenium is seen more commonly in areas like Scandinavia, China, and New Zealand where there is low soil selenium content and in patients on parenteral nutrition. Whitening of finger nail beds, loss of pigment of the hair and skin, thinning and curling of hair (pseudoalbinism) have been reported in deficiency states.[23] The mechanism of hypopigmentation is unclear but selenium is intimately associated with sulfur and amino acid metabolism and, elevated glutathione levels in selenium deficiency may be interfering with pigment synthesis in melanocytes. Also, chronic ingestion of high amounts of selenium leads to selenosis, characterized by hair and nail brittleness.

Zinc

Zinc is an integral component of many metalloenzymes in the body. It is involved in the synthesis and stabilization of proteins, DNA, and RNA, structural component of ribosomes, protection against free radical damage, male sex hormones, fetal development, brain development and its function and vitamin A metabolism.[24, 25] Zinc deficiency may be genetic or acquired, acute or chronic. Acrodermatitis enteropathica, an autosomal recessive condition characterized by malabsorption of zinc is the common genetic cause and acquired causes includes diabetes mellitus, HIV/AIDS, cirrhosis, alcoholism, inflammatory bowel disease, malabsorption syndromes, and sickle cell disease. Acute zinc deficiency leads to diffuse progressive thinning of scalp hair leading to total alopecia, whereas more structural abnormalities is seen in chronic zinc deficiency and acrodermatitis enteropathica **(Figure 17.3)**. Hair changes in chronic zinc deficiency include dry and unruly hair with poor growth. Hair may show broken spear head-like endings, transverse striations of the shafts, pseudomonilethrix, longitudinal splits, and bayonet hairs.[11] These changes are better visualized under polarized light **(Table 17.3)**.

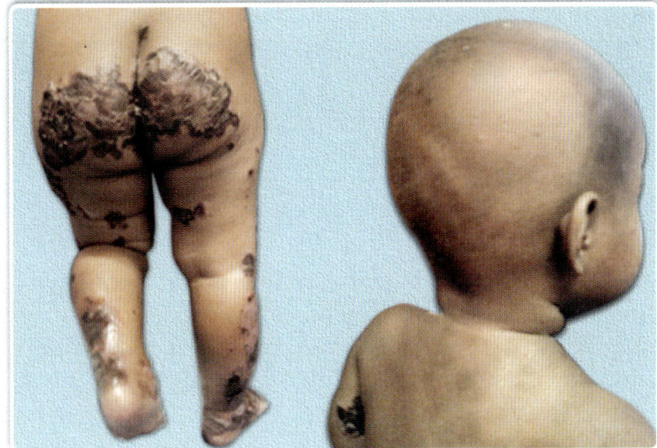

Fig. 17.3: Acrodermatitis enteropathica (*Courtesy:* Department of Dermatology, STD and Leprosy, BMCRI, Bengaluru)

Table 17.3: Hair changes due to deficiency of micronutrients

Iron	Alopecia areata, androgenetic alopecia, telogen effluvium, diffuse hair loss, band-like color changes
Copper	Menkes kinky hair syndrome—hypopigmented, fragile, twisted like a "steel wire", pili torti, trichorrhexis nodosa, trichoclasis, irregularities in thickness of hair
Selenium deficiency	Loss of pigment of the hair, thinning and curling of hair
Selenosis	Hair brittleness
Zinc (Acute deficiency)	Diffuse progressive thinning of scalp hair leading to total alopecia
Chronic zinc deficiency and acrodermatitis enteropathica	Dry and unruly hair with poor growth. Hair may show broken spear head-like endings, transverse striations of the shafts, pseudomonilethrix, longitudinal splits, and bayonet hairs

Treatment

Nutritional Supplements[12]

Although many nutritional supplements have been used traditionally to treat hair disorders, there is limited evidence of their use in non-deficient patients. Long-term effects of antioxidants on hair ageing may be possible, but are difficult to assess. L-cysteine has showed significant effect in the treatment of diffuse telogen effluvium. In a randomized, placebo-controlled study in 30 women, a supplement of L-cysteine in combination with medicinal yeast and

Table 17.4: Role of nutritional supplements

Supplement	*Indication*
Antioxidants	Hair ageing
L-cystiene	Diffuse telogen effluvium
Orthosilicic acid	Hair tensile strength
Soybeans	Hair growth

pantothenic acid led to a normalization of the rate of anagen after 6 months, whereas a placebo did not.[26] Clinically, this supplement of L-cystiene would correspond to avoiding a temporary loss of several thousands of long hairs. Further studies are needed to increase the evidence on nutritional supplements on hair.

The amino acids taurin and L-carnitine has been shown to promote follicle cell survival in vitro. Components derived from soybeans may also have an effect on hair growth through anti-inflammatory and estrogen-dependent mechanisms, but studies in vivo are lacking and an increase of angioma rubi has been reported. Orthosilicic acid, increased hair tensile strength and thickness in a controlled study after 6 months and decreased hair brittleness in a study after 20 weeks **(Table 17.4)**.

References

1. Rushton DH. Nutritional factors and hair loss. Clin Exp Dermatol. 2002;27:396-404.
2. Park K. Nutrition and health. Park's Textbook of Preventive and Social Medicine, 22nd edn. Jabalpur: Banarsidas Bhanot. 2013;563-619.
3. Stark C. Guidelines for food and nutrient intake. In: Stipanuk MH (ed). Biochemical, Physiological, Molecular Aspects of Human Nutrition. 2nd ed. Philadelphia: Saunders Elsevier. 2006;47-63.
4. Jelliffe DB. Protein-calorie malnutrition in tropical pre-school children. J Pediatr. 1959;54:227-56.
5. Golden BE. Primary protein-energy malnutrition. In: Gar-row JS, James WPT, (eds). Human Nutrition, Dietetics, 9th edn. Edinburgh: Churchill Livingstone. 1993:440-55.
6. Bradfield RB, Bailey MA. Hair root response to protein undernutrition. In: Montagna W, Dobson RL, (eds). Biology of Skin, Hair Growth, Vol.IX; VII. Oxford: Pergamon Press. 1969:109-19.
7. Ruiz-Maldonado R, Beecerril-Chihu G. Skin manifestations of malnutrition. In: Harper J, Oranje A, Prose N, (eds). Textbook of Pediatric Dermatology, 1st edn. Paris: Blackwell Science. 2000;499-505.
8. Desai SC, Sheth RA, Udani PM. Nutrition and hair anomalies. In: Orfanos CE, Montagna W, Stuttgen G, (eds). Hair research. Berlin: Springer. 1981.
9. Viswesera Rao K, Bhatia RYP, Pralhad Rao N. Morphological changes in scalp hair in mild and moderate forms of protein-calorie malnutrition. Indian J Med Res. 1978;68:631-40.
10. Phadke MA, Khedkar VA, Pashankar D, et al. Serum amino acids and genesis of protein-energy malnutrition. Indian Pediatrics. 1995;32:301-6.
11. Patnaik R, Chowdary TN, Sesikeran B, Satyanath RV, Uday Kumar P. Nutrition and the Skin. In: Valia RG, Valia AR, (eds). Textbook and Atlas of Dermatology, 3rd edn. Mumbai: Bhalani Publishing House. 2008;1267-97.
12. Finner AM. Nutrition and hair deficiencies and supplements. Dermatol Clin. 2013;31:167-72.
13. Williams ML, Packman S, Cowan MJ. Alopecia and periorificial dermatitis in biotin-responsive multiple carboxylase deficiency. J Am Acad Dermatol. 1983;9:97-103.
14. Longo DL, Fauci AS, Kasper DL, Hauser SL, Jameson JL, Loscalzo J (eds). Harrison's Principles of Internal Medicine. 18th edn. New York: McGraw Hill. 2011;1554-59.
15. Fiedler VC, Gray AC. Diffuse alopecia: telogen hair loss. In: Olsen EA, (ed). Disorders of Hair Growth: Diagnosis and Treatment, 2nd edn. New York, NY: McGraw-Hill Publishing. 2003;303-20.
16. Oh R, Brown DL. Vitamin B12 deficiency. Am Fam Physician. 2003;67:979-86.
17. Kantor J, Kessler LJ, Brooks DG, Cotsarelis G. Decreased serum ferritin is associated with alopecia in women. J Invest Dermatol. 2003;121:985-8.
18. Fiedler VC, Gray AC. Diffuse alopecia: telogen hair loss. In: Olsen EA, (ed). Disorders of Hair Growth: Diagnosis and Treatment, 2nd edn. New York: McGraw-Hill. 2003;303-20.
19. Trost LB, Bergfeld WF, Calogeras E.The diagnosis and treatment of iron deficiency and its potential relationship to hair loss. J Am Acad Dermatol. 2006;54:824-44.
20. Olivares M, Uauy R. Copper as an essential nutrient. Am J Clin Nutr. 1996;63:791S-6S.
21. Aguilar MJ, Chadwick DL, Okuyama K, Kamoshita S. Kinky hair disease. I. Clinical and pathological features. J Neuropathol Exp Neurol. 1966;25:507-22.
22. Rotruck JT, Pope AL, Ganther HE et al. Selenium: Biochemical role as a component of glutathione peroxidase. Science. 1973;179:588-90.
23. Vinton NE, Dahlstrom KA, Strobel CT, Ament ME. Macrocytosis and pseudoalbinism: manifestations of selenium deficiency. J Pediatr. 1987;111:711-7.
24. MacDonald RS. The role of zinc in growth and cell proliferation. J Nutr. 2000;130(5S Suppl):S1500-S1508.
25. King JC, Cousins RJ. Zinc. In: Shils ME, Shilke M, Ross CA, Caballero B, Cousins RJ, (eds). Modern Nutrition in Health and Disease, 10th edn. Philadelphia: Lippincott Williams and Wilkins. 2005;271-85.
26. Lengg N, Heidecker B, Seifert B, et al. Dietary supplement increases anagen rate in women with telogen effluvium: results of a randomized, placebo controlled study. Therapy. 2007;4:59-65.

18

Cultural Influence on Hair Disorders

D Dinesh Kumar, Anoosha P

"A cheerful intelligent face is the end of culture, and success enough. For it indicates the purpose of nature and wisdom attained."

—*Ralph Waldo Emerson*

Introduction

Hair, the crowning glory of the human race is of utmost aesthetic significance in this era. Hair is an appendage of the skin that is characteristic of all mammals. Having lost its original purpose/function—protection; hair has gained aesthetic significance over the years. Too much or too little hair can have a major impact on one's psychological status and quality of life.

"Culture" (Latin - Cultura) has been used to depict a range of activities over the centuries. However, Hoebel describes culture as an integrated system of learned behavior patterns which are characteristic of members of a society and which are not a result of biological inheritance.[1]

Cultural practices in different groups tend to influence health and disease. In specific, the various hair care practices, grooming patterns and aesthetic practices have been the cause for a host of hair and scalp disorders of late.

This chapter aims to put forth the various hair care practices in different cultural groups and the impact that they have on hair and scalp.

A lot of devastating psychological issues can arise as a result of hair problems in men and women. Although all ethnic groups face hair loss, there is a considerable variation in aetiology between the different groups. The extent can range from a bare patch to an extensive diffuse pattern of hair loss.

A well-groomed head of hair always serves as a visual marker for social affiliation and personal identity for any individual. The prevailing cultural trends at a given place always have a dominant influence on the styling practices even though these practices are determined by individual hair characteristics and preferences.

The whole idea of identifying the various cultural styling/hair care practices is to guide and educate the patients about the impact that these practices can have on their hair and to motivate them to change certain of these practices in order to avoid permanent damage to their hair which can have a major effect on their personality and confidence.

Structural Evaluation

Although no biochemical variations have been found among the different ethnic groups, certain morphological differences have been evident **(Table 18.1)**.[2]

Although the hair density was found to be low among the Blacks, the predominant number of hairs per follicular unit (FU) was 3/FU, while the Caucasians and Asians had a normal density, they had 2 hairs/FU.

The increased dryness in the hair of Blacks could be responsible for the various styling and grooming practices in order to set the hair well.

Table 18.1: Biochemical variations among different ethnic groups[3]

	Shape	*Breakage*	*Density*	*Dryness*
Blacks	Curly Elliptical on C/S HF—Curved	Prone to breakage	Low	Dry
Caucasians	Straight—Wavy Round-oval on C/S HF—Straight	Not easily prone	Normal	Normal
Asians	Straight Round on C/S HF—Straight	Not easily prone	Normal	Lustrous

Abbreviation: C/S – Cross section; HF – Hair follicle

Hair Care Practices Among Different Cultures (Box 18.1)

There is a significant variation among hair styles and hair care practices of different ethnic populations. Multiple factors affect hairstyles and hair care practices, including current and historical trends and convenience.[2] It is well accepted that distinctive hair care practices among various cultures have been implicated as risk factors for several scalp and hair disorders/dermatoses.[4-14]

It has been suggested that hair wash frequency, and possibly other hair care practices, are dependent on social or cultural norms (race, gender, and age group) rather than hair attributes (hair type, texture, length, and scalp type) itself.[5]

The following hair care practices are practiced by people of various ethnic origins:

Heat Styling (Figure 18.1)

Heat restructuring was a common hair-care practice used by African-Americans in the past. One of the first ever methods used for straightening hair temporarily was hot combing. This works by temporarily manipulating the hydrogen/disulfide bonds **(Box 18.2)**. This practice began in the early twentieth century and required the use of an ointment-based lubricant.[15] This process uses a hot comb and a heating element (e.g. a regular stovetop or a specially designed heating stove that fits around the comb). The hot comb is pulled through the hair from the scalp to the tip. It is a temporary process, because the hair reverts to its original state with the application of water.[2]

Box 18.1: Cultural hair care practices

1. Heat styling
2. Chemical relaxers
3. Hair extension and weaves
4. Hair oils
5. Henna
6. Hair dyes
7. Tonsuring
8. Patterns of hair settings with traction on hair

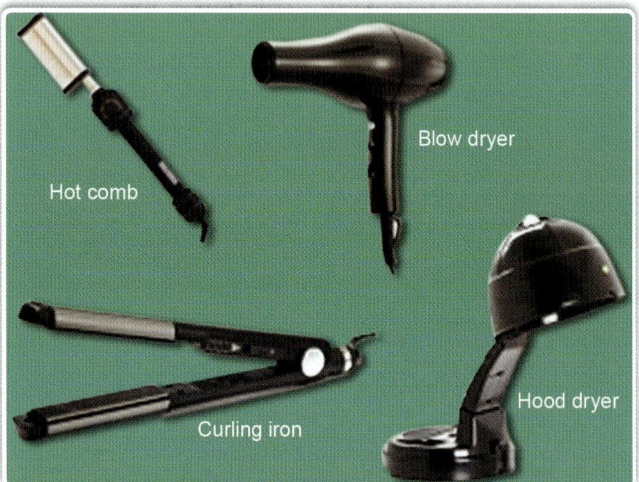

Fig. 18.1: Various equipments used in hair styling

Curling irons commonly used increase the likelihood of scalp and hair damage. Curling irons and other heating elements have been used on native or untreated hair as well. Other hair-care practices commonly used by African-American patients, particularly women, include other heat sources like blow-dryers and hood dryers.

Chemical Relaxers

With the availability of chemical relaxers, hot combing lost its fame. In the early twentieth century, crude forerunners of chemical relaxers became available and these crude chemicals were used primarily by African-American men to straighten their hair. Some of the early chemicals used included lye, hog lard, and boiled eggs.[16]

In the 1960s, the emergence of more elegantly formulated chemical relaxers increased their use by women. These relaxers primarily contained sodium, potassium, lithium, and guanine hydroxides; other products contained sulfites and thioglycolates. These products break the hydrogen/disulfide bonds and reset the hair in a straighter form **(Figure 18.2)**. The effects of the chemical relaxers last

Box 18.2: Principle of hot combing

- Hot comb and a heating element is used
- Temporarily manipulates the hydrogen/disulfide bonds causing straightening of hairs
- Hair reverts to its original state with the application of water

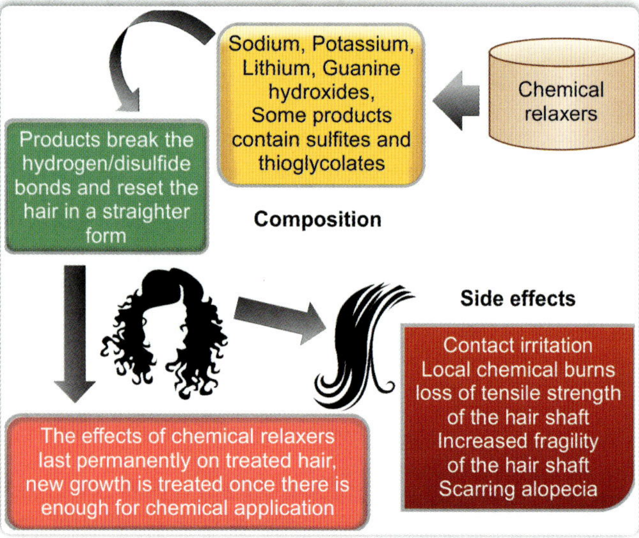

Fig. 18.2: Schematic representation of mechanism of action of Chemical relaxers and their side effects

permanently on treated hair, and new growth is treated once there is enough for chemical application. This has become an easy way for African-American women and men to control the kinkiness and curliness of their hair. Little knowledge of potential problems of this chemical method of straightening the hair has been reported until recently.[2]

Patterns of Hair Setting Associated with Traction on Hair

People especially women with long scalp hair use various styling methods to tie or set their hair. Generally, these practices are associated with varying degrees of traction on the hair. The patterns are:

1. Ponytail/Pigtail—Hair divided into one or more sections and pulled together by a hair accessory (elastic band, clip)
2. Braids—2 or more pieces of hair woven together in various numbers and sections
3. Cornrows—Similar to braids, but lay flat or close to the scalp resembling "rows of corn".[17]

Hair Extensions/Weaves

Hair extensions or weaves constitute human or synthetic hair that is clipped, pinned, cornrowed or braided into hair for added length or body.[15] The extensions may be attached, which are hair pieces that extend the length of the hair and accentuate style. Weaves are human or synthetically manufactured hair (tracks) that can be glued onto hair or sewn onto hair that is cornrowed.[17]

Hair Oils

The use of hair oil is a common South Asian cultural practice which may cause dermatological problems. The main reason for such extensive hair oil usage in this region is due to a belief that hair oil promotes hair growth. Hair oils are not only used to condition and soften hair but they also help inhibit dermatophyte growth. It is thought that the saturated and unsaturated fatty acids in hair oil contribute to their toxicity against dermatophytes **(Box 18.3)**. The toxicity of different types of hair oils varies and this may explain why hair oils may be not be inhibitory to dermatophytes in various populations using them.[18]

Box 18.3: Myths of hair oils massage

"Effects to side effects"

- *Effects:* Hair oil promotes hair growth and softens hair
  They inhibit dermatophyte growth as saturated and unsaturated fatty acids in hair oil contribute to their toxicity against dermatophytes
- *Side effects:* Essential oils (peppermint and cinnamon oil) cause contact dermatitis, occupational exposure to mineral oils, petroleum, and greases cause folliculitis, pomade oil causes pomade acne

Box 18.4: Henna

- Natural dye extracted from Lawsonia inermis leaves, natural conditioning agent used to dye skin, hair, leather, and fur
- "Black henna," a mixture that contains paraphenylenediamine (PPD), for quicker drying and darker color
- Side effects: Allergic contact dermatitis to PPD, papulovesicular eruptions, bulla formation, and erythema multiforme-like reactions, Type I hypersensitivity leading to angioedema, acute renal failure

Henna

Henna is a natural dye extracted from *Lawsonia inermis* leaves, native to South Asia and North Africa as a natural hair dye as well as a natural conditioning agent by many people. It is frequently used to dye skin, hair, leather, and fur. Pure henna stains red brown and is generally very hypoallergenic with only two reported cases of contact dermatitis (both confirmed by patch testing)**(Box 18.4)**.[18]

Hair Dyes

It is a very common practice all over the world to color the hair with different hair dyes. Some do it as a method to cover gray hair which occurs due to aging while, others do it just for a change from the routine hair color. A significant amount of hair and scalp disorders are associated with hair dye usage.

Tonsuring

This is a practice followed in South Asia for religious purposes wherein the entire scalp hair is shaved with a razor. Most often tonsuring is done by a barber in not so hygienic setting and on large number people in quick succession. The razor blade is not changed very often and also the common

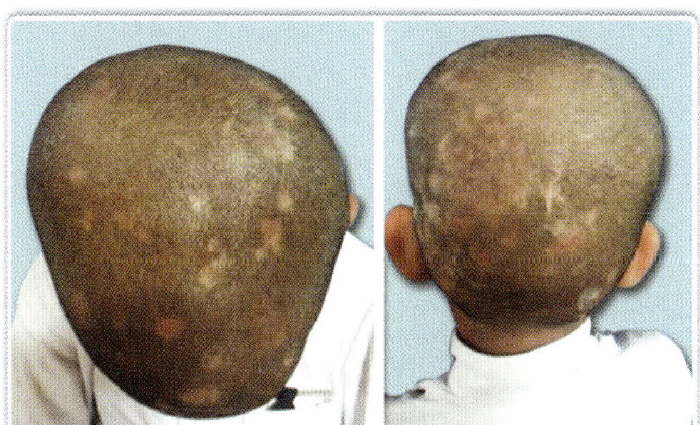

Fig. 18.3: Tinea capitis post-tonsuring.
(*Courtesy:* Department of Dermatology, BMCRI, Bengaluru)

towels used to wipe the tonsured head leads on to a lot of scalp infections like tinea capitis **(Figure 18.3)**.

Association of Hair and Scalp Disorders with the Prevailing Cultural Trends

A range of hair and scalp disorders are caused by the various hair care practices of various cultures **(Box 18.5)**.[19,20]

Seborrheic Dermatitis (SD)

SD is a chronic papulosquamous disorder affecting sebaceous-rich areas like the scalp and face caused by an inflammatory response to yeast, *Malassezia furfur* (*Pityrosporum ovale*). The incidence varies from 2–5% of the total population. Although no racial or ethnic predisposition has been reported in the literature, the incidence may be higher in Black women due to the frequency of hair washing. While males with short natural haircuts wash their hair daily, many Black females wash their hair less frequently, from once per week to every four weeks, depending upon their hairstyle. Thus, an overgrowth of yeast occurs and may place this population at a higher incidence of scalp dermatoses.

Traction Alopecia

Traction alopecia refers to hair loss occurring in the fronto-temporal areas due to mechanical loosening of the hair from the follicle. The hair root when subjected to prolonged tension/traction due to certain hairstyles lead to traction alopecia, which can over time result in irreversible cicatricial alopecia.[21,22]

Central Centrifugal Cicatricial Alopecia (Hot Comb Alopecia)

This condition is characterized by hair loss affecting the crown and vertex of the scalp, resultant of scarring. In 1968, LoPresti, et al. described hot-comb alopecia,[23] in which the fragility of the hair shaft was increased and burns on the scalp could occur. The scarring process was believed to have occurred when the lubricants placed on the hair during the hot-combing process dripped down the hair shaft onto the scalp, with particular involvement of the frontal and vertex scalp. This was never confirmed causally in this scientific description.

Hair straighteners (chemical relaxers) and hair dyes may cause allergic/irritant contact dermatitis, chemical burns, scarring alopecia, and increased hair breakage.[8,10-13] Sewn-in weaves and artificial hair extensions have been associated with central centrifugal cicatricial alopecia.[24]

Box 18.5: Scalp disorders in cultural trends

1. Seborrheic dermatitis
2. Traction alopecia
3. Central centrifugal cicatricial alopecia
4. Tinea capitis
5. Allergic/Irritant contact dermatitis
6. Folliculitis
7. Hair shaft damage
8. Plica polonica
9. Pediculosis capitis
10. Mudichood

Tinea Capitis

The exact role of hair care practices in scalp dermatoses like tinea capitis is unclear although tinea capitis has a high prevalence in African-American children.[25,26] Their hair grooming practices have been speculated to play a role in the acquisition of fungus to the hair and scalp.[26-28] Due to some hair styles, patients may restrict styling time to once or twice per week.[2] These restrictions may be detrimental to the health of the hair and scalp, predisposing to tinea capitis and seborrheic dermatitis.

Allergic Contact Dermatitis/Irritant Contact Dermatitis/Folliculitis

There has also been concern about allergic contact reactions of the skin to some of the extension materials used[29], for example, some of the glues used to bond the hair extensions to the scalp contain latex.

There are several reports of contact anaphylaxis to the latex-based glue products.[29,30] One particular report demonstrated a positive radioallergosorbent test for hair-bonding glue and latex in a patient with systemic anaphylaxis on repeated exposure to hair-bonding glue.[8] Her sera reacted to latex antigens as well. Assays of the glue revealed antigen patterns resembling ammoniated latex.

Essential oils, such as peppermint and cinnamon oil, may cause contact dermatitis, but there have been no formal reports of contact dermatitis secondary to hair oils in the medical literature. Oils may be occlusive, and occupational exposure to mineral oils, petroleum, and greases has been shown to cause folliculitis. However, there are no reported cases of folliculitis secondary to commercial hair oils specifically designated for cosmetic use.

Henna has shown to cause immediate hypersensitivity (characterized by rhinitis, conjunctivitis, urticaria, and wheezing), which was subsequently confirmed by prick testing. However, many henna tattoos use "black henna," a mixture that contains paraphenylenediamine (PPD), for quicker drying and darker color. There are many reports of allergic contact dermatitis to PPD, sometimes with papulovesicular eruptions, bulla formation, and erythema multiforme-like reactions.[18] Henna and PPD have also been reported to cause type I hypersensitivity leading to angioedema and in a few cases, acute renal failure.[18]

Potential problems with the usage of chemical relaxers include local contact irritation, local chemical burns, loss of tensile strength of the hair shaft, increased fragility of the hair shaft and possibly, scarring alopecia.[30]

Hair Shaft Damage

Blow-dryers and hood dryers can become extremely hot and cause fragility of hair and damage to the tensile strength of the hair shaft leading to hair breakage. Curling irons too result in hair shaft damage. The other potential hazards associated with these heat sources include over drying of the hair cuticle and scalp damage that can result from local burns to the scalp.[20] Extensions may be heavy and attached to a few very fragile hair shafts; this may cause damage similar to that observed with the use of ponytails, in which increased traction has been noted.[8]

Plica Polonica (Plica Neuropathica)[31,32]

Plica polonica refers to an acquired matting of hair which is not so uncommon condition in South Asia. The condition is characterized by irreversible tangling of scalp hair. In Indian cultures as a religious practice, people who are considered to be holy do not comb/groom/wash their hair; as a result, the hair gets matted to form thick uncombable/unmanageable locks **(Figure 18.4)**. This condition is also seen in women with long hair who have the habit of piling of long hair on the top of the head while shampooing. Vigorously combing the wet hair, excessive perming of hair, excessive usage of harsh shampoos are predisposing factors to plica polonica. The treatment involves cutting off the affected hair.

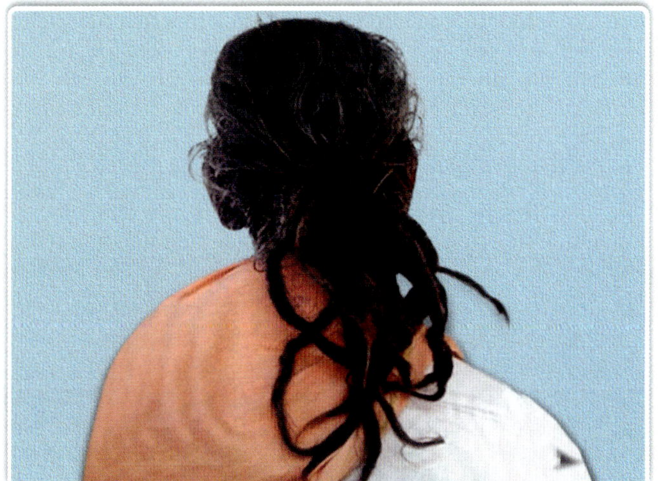

Fig. 18.4: Plica polonica.
(*Courtesy:* Department of Dermatology, BMCRI, Bengaluru)

Pediculosis Capitis[33]

Pediculosis capitis is a condition wherein there is infestation of the scalp hair with head louse acquired by head to head direct contact. The condition is more commonly seen in communities where there is poor hygiene along with over crowding. In Indian subcontinent, pediculosis capitis is common. Among the American Blacks the infestation rates are low whereas among the African Blacks the infestation rates are high. The low infestation rates among American blacks could be due to the fact that use of pomades by them could make the environment unsuitable for the louse. The modification of the legs of the louse to grasp hair of different cross-sectional shape is thought to influence transmission between ethnic groups.

Mudichood[34] (Figure 18.5)

Mudichood disease, described by Sugathan, et al. It is a distinct clinical entity seen nearly exclusively in young women in Kerala State, India. The term Mudichood is derived from Malayalam (Mudi- Hair, Chood-Heat), literally means heat of the hair. In Kerala, application of hair oils either before or after bathing either alone or in a preparation with leaves, flowers seeds, roots, etc. are used in the belief of promoting hair growth. This coupled with the habit of not braiding the hair but letting it fall loose over the back, results in the oily wet hair rubbing the exposed part of the back. In places with high day temperature and humidity this combination of the oily wet hair, sweating and friction results in a follicular vesico-pustule which soon crusts and starts slowly expanding peripherally. This condition presents as skin colored or slightly hyperpigmented, well-

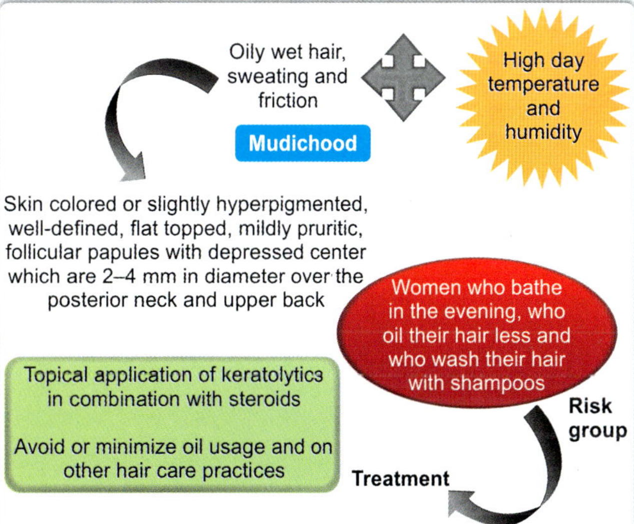

Fig. 18.5: Schematic representation of causes and treatment of mudichood

defined, flat topped, mildly pruritic, follicular papules which are 2-4 mm in diameter over the posterior neck and upper back. A typical papule has a very thin keratinous rim with a slightly depressed center. Long-standing cases may show confluence of papules. This condition was found to be common among young girls, particularly teenagers and described to occur seldom in women who bathe in the evening, who oil their hair less and who wash their hair with shampoos. Treatment consists of the topical application of keratolytics in combination with steroids. The patients are advised to avoid or minimize oil usage and other hair care practices.

Conclusion

In this era, wherein people are easily influenced by the prevailing cultural trends, the number of hair and scalp disorders is on a constant rise. Hence, dermatologists need to familiarize and update themselves with the range of local cultural hair care practices in different ethnic strata. This would not only help the clinician to identify the cause for the disorder, but also counsel and educate the patients to change some of their practices for a better lifestyle.

References

1. E Adamson Hoebel. Anthropology: A Study of man. Mc Graw Hill Book Company. Newyork, 1966.
2. McMichael A, Ethnic hair update: Past and present; J Am Acad Dermatol. 2003;48S:127-33.
3. Callender VD, et al. Hair and scalp disorders in ethnic populations, J Drugs Dermatol. 2013;12(4):420.
4. Quinn C, Quinn T, Kelly A. Hair care practices in African-American women. Cutis. 2003;72:280-2, 285-9.
5. Chappell J, Hair care practices in different populations: What makes the difference? J Am Acad Dermatol. 2010;P2107: AB76.
6. McMichael A. Hair and scalp disorders in ethnic populations. Dermatol Clin. 2003;21:629-44.
7. Bulengo-Ransby S, Bergfeld W. Chemical and traumatic alopecia from thioglycolate in a black woman: a case report with unusual clinical and histologic findings. Cutis. 1992;49:99-103.
8. Nicholson A, Harland C, Bull R, Mortimer P, Cook M. Chemically induced cosmetic alopecia. Br J Dermatol. 1993;128:537-41.
9. Khumalo N, Jessop S, Ehrlich R. Hairdressing and the prevalence of scalp disease in African adults. Br J Dermatol. 2007;157:981-8.
10. Khumalo N, Jessop S, Ehrlich R. Prevalence of cutaneous adverse effects of hairdressing. Arch Dermatol. 2006;142:377-83.
11. Swee W, Klontz KC, Lambert L. A nationwide outbreak of alopecia associated with the use of a hair-relaxing formulation. Arch Dermatol. 2000;136:1104-8.
12. Khumalo N, Pillay K, Ngwanay R. Acute 'relaxer'-associated scarring alopecia: a report of five cases. Br J Dermatol. 2007;156:1394-6.
13. Nnoruka N. Hair loss: is there a relationship with hair care practices in Nigeria? Int J Dermatol. 2005;44S:13-7.
14. Gathers R, Jankowski M, Eide M, Lim H. Hair grooming practices and central centrifugal cicatricial alopecia. J Am Acad Dermatol. 2008;60:574-8.
15. Syed AN. Ethnic hair care: history, trends and formulation. Cosmet Toil. 1993;108:99-107.
16. Harris RT. Hair relaxing. Cosmet Toil. 1979;94:51-6.
17. Wright DR, et al. Hair care practices and their association with scalp and hair disorders in African American girls, J Am Acad Dermatol. 2011;64(2):254-62.
18. Lilly E, Kundu RV. Dermatoses secondary to Asian cultural practices, Int J Dermatol. 2012;51(4):379-82.
19. Alexis A, Sergay A, Taylor S. Common dermatologic disorders in skin of color: A comparative practice survey. Cutis. 2007;80:387-94.
20. Halder R, Grimes P. Incidence of common dermatoses in a predominantly black dermatologic practice. Cutis. 1983;32:388-90.
21. Hantash B, Schwartz R. Traction alopecia in children. Cutis. 2003;71:18-20.
22. Sharma V, Silverberg N, Howard R, Tran C, Laude T, Frieden I. Do hair care practices affect the acquisition of tinea capitis? Arch Pediatr Adolesc Med. 2001;155:818-21.
23. LoPresti P, Papa CM, Kligman AM. Hot comb alopecia. Arch Dermatol. 1968;98:234-8.
24. Nnoruka NE, et al. Hair loss: is there a relationship with hair care practices in Nigeria? Int J Dermatol. 2005;44(S1):13-7.
25. Bocobo F, Eadie G, Miedler L. Epidemiologic study of tinea capitis caused by T tonsurans and M audouinii. Public Health Rep. 1965;80:891-8.
26. Sharma V, Hall J, Knapp J, Sarai S, Galloway D, Babel D. Scalp colonization by Trichophyton tonsurans in an urban pediatric clinic. Arch Dermatol. 1988;124:1511-3.
27. Frieden I, Howard R. Tinea capitis: epidemiology, diagnosis, treatment and control. J Am Acad Dermatol. 1994;31(S):42-6.
28. Callender V, McMichael A, Cohen G. Medical and surgical therapies for alopecia in black women. Dermatol Ther. 2004;17:164-76.
29. Wakelin SH. Contact anaphylaxis from natural rubber latex used as an adhesive for hair extension. Br J Dermatol. 14;146(2):340-1.
30. Cogen FC, Beezhold DH. Hair glue anaphylaxis: a hidden latex allergy. Ann Allergy Asthma Immunol. 2002; 88:61-3.
31. Sarkar R, et al. Plica neuropathica: matting of hair. Dermatology. 2000;201:184.
32. Suresh Kumar PN, Anthony B, Chakravarthy A, Koyamu KA. Plica neuropathica (polonica) in schizophrenia: A case report and review of literature. Indian J Psychol. 2001;43:281-3.
33. Burns DA. Diseases caused by arthropods and other noxious animals. Burns TS, Breathnach S, Cox N, Griffiths C (Ed). Rook's Textbook of Dermatology. 2010;2(8th Ed):38.17-21.
34. Sugathan P, Nair MB. Mudi-chood - A New Dermatosis. Marshall J (Ed). In Essays on Tropical Dermatology. Excerpta Medica Amsterdam. 1972;2:183-8.

19

Canities

Asha GS, Lakshmi DV

"It is not by the gray of the hair that one knows the age of the heart."

—*Edward G Bulwer Lytton*

Synonyms: Hypomelanosis of hair, graying of hair, canities seritis.

Introduction

Hair is the fastest growing tissue in the human body only next to bone marrow. Canities refers to graying of hair. It must be regarded as a physiological condition, a manifestation of ageing process and is due to progressive reduction in melanocyte function in hair buds **(Box 19.1)**. Canities is a process of chronologic ageing and occurs regardless of gender or race.[1] It may be genetically programed to occur as early as adolescence, reflecting the intense biological activity in the hair bulb, which may in some follicles produce melanocyte 'senescence' by the second decade of life.[2] Premature canities/pediatric canities needs to be differentited from various genetic hypomelanotic hair disorders. This chapter deals with varous conditions in which canities occurs and also conditions where in pigmentary abnormalities of hair occurs, which are the close differentials for canities.

In general, graying of hair is progressive and permanent. There is a gradual dilution of pigment in graying hairs along a individual hair and also from hair to hair. Loss of hair shaft color is associated with a decrease and eventual cessation of tyrosinase activity in the lower bulb.[3,4]

Box 19.1: Canities: Definition

- It is a genetically programed phenomenon that leads to early melanocyte senescence due to intense biological activity in the hair bulb causing permanent and progressive graying of hair

Epidemiology

The usual age of onset is in the fourth decade and appears to be hereditary. The average age for Caucasians is 34 ± 9.6 years, and for Africans 43.9 ± 10.3 years.[5] It is said that by 50 years of age, 50% of people have 50% gray hair.[5]

Pathophysiology (Figure 19.1)

Follicular melanogenesis is linked to follicular cycling with melanin synthesis occurring only in the anagen phase. This pigmentary unit recycling occurs effectively only upto first 40 hair cycles, which scale upto 40 years of age in an

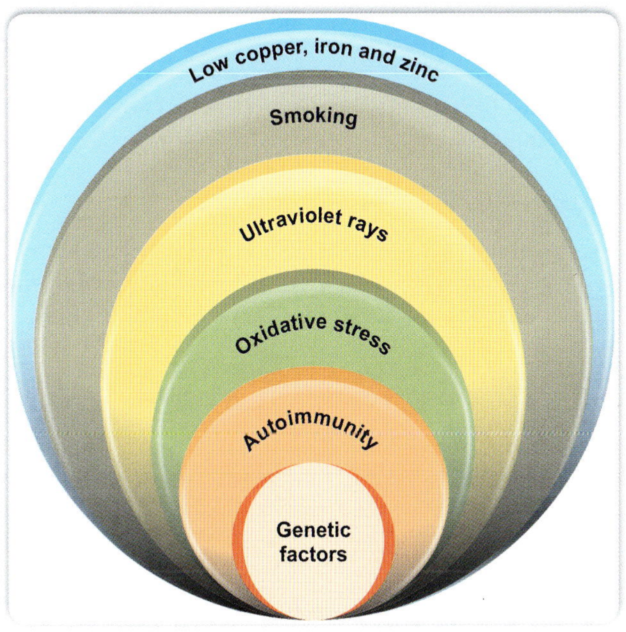

Fig. 19.1: Factors involved in causation of canities

individual. The hairbulb tyrosinase activity gradually peaks at middle age. With progressing age, reduced melanocyte activity occurs, which leads to graying of hair.

Electron microscopy of gray hair shows that number of melanocytes are normal in structure but with incompletely melanized melanosomes. In completely white hairs melanocytes are decreased or absent. True gray hair shows reduced DOPA reaction (indicator of tyrosinase activity) while white hair bulbs are negative for the same. The various pathways causing melanin depletion leading to gray hair are shown in **Box 19.2**.

Genetic Factors

Hair follicles are subjected to intrinsic and extrinsic ageing. Intrinsic factors are related to individual genetic and epigenetic mechanisms with inter-individual variation.[5] Extrinsic factors related to the environmental factors includes ultraviolet radiation, air pollution, smoking, nutrition, and lifestyle changes.

Gene PAX3 and MITF is found to play an important role in melanocytic stem cell maintenance and differentiation.[6] Bone morphogenetic proteins receptor type 2 (BMPR2), a known receptor for bone morphogenetic proteins (BMPS), and activin receptor type-2A (ACVR2A), a known receptor for BMPS and activins, are together essential for multiple follicular traits. Animal studies have shown that reduced BMPR2/ACVR2A function in melanocytes in mutant mice was shown to result in gray hair due to aberrant hair shaft and melanosomes differentiation.[7] Stem cell factor (SCF) and its receptor (KIT) also play an important role in signaling in the maintenance of human hair follicle melanogenesis during the anagen cycle and in physiological ageing of the hair follicle pigmentary unit.[8] Notch 1 and Notch 2 signaling pathways are required for the maintenance of melanoblasts and melanocyte stem cells and are essential for proper hair pigmentation in mice.[9]

Autoimmunity

It has been suggested that autoimmunity also plays a part in the pathogenesis of graying. Association of canities with other autoimmune conditions also supports possible etiology.

Box 19.2: Pathogenesis of canities

- Exhaustion of enzymes involved in melanogenesis
- Melanocyte degeneration causing defective melanosomal transfer to the cortical keratinocytes
- Loss of telomerase and impaired DNA repair
- Antioxidant mechanisms
- Antiapoptotic signals
- Autophagolysosomal degradation of melanosomes within the melanocytes itself, followed by the degeneration of the melanocyte

Oxidative Stress in Ageing of Hair

With age the production of free radicals increases, while endogenous defense mechanism decreases. This imbalance leads to progressive damage of cellular and molecular structure, presumably resulting in the ageing phenotype.

Melanocytes in graying hair bulbs are found to be frequently highly vacuolated, a common cellular response to increased oxidative stress.[4] The melanogenic activity of pigmented bulbar melanocytes, generates large amounts of reactive oxygen species through the hydroxylation of tyrosine and the oxidation of DOPA to melanin. If not adequately removed by an efficient antioxidant system, an accumulation of these reactive oxidative species will generate significant oxidative stress. It leads to damage to the melanocyte itself from its own melanogenesis-related oxidative stress. Mutations occur at a higher rate in tissue exposed to high levels of oxidative stress, and these accumulate with age, the induction of replicative senescence with apoptosis is likely to be an important protective mechanism against cell transformation.[4]

Ultraviolet Rays[10]

The effect of UV light on hair has received less attention. While it has been recognized that at least 50% UV rays induced damage to skin is attributed to UV rays induced free radicals. Photochemical impairment of hair includes degradation of hair pigment. UVB is responsible for loss of hair protein, UVA is responsible for color change. Photosensitive amino acids of hair and their photochemical degradation produces free radicals. These free radicals have adverse effect on hair protein especially keratin.

Effect of Smoking

Mosleby and Gibler were the first to indicate a relationship between smoking, graying of hair and alopecia in men. The mechanism by which smoking causes graying of hair are multifactorial, probably effect of cigarette smoke on microvasculature of dermal hair papillae, smoke induced imbalance in follicular protease/anti-protease system controling tissue remodeling during hair growth cycle. Pro-oxidative effect of smoking leads to release of pro-inflammatory cytokines resulting in follicular micro-inflammation and perifollicular fibrosis.[11]

Role of Serum Iron, Copper, Zinc Concentration in Premature Graying of Hair

Studies have shown that among copper, zinc and iron, a low serum copper concentration may play a role in premature graying of hair. Studies have also showed significant reduction in levels of serum Ca, serum ferritin and vitamin D_3.[12]

Pattern of Graying

The wave of graying progresses from temporal to vertex and finally ends in the occipital area. Beard and body hair are affected later. Graying of hair appears in different shades from dirty gray to silvery white color. Onset of graying of hair occurs earlier in males while compared to females.[13]

Characteristics of Gray Hair (Box 19.3)

Gray hair is coarser and stiffer than pigmented hair. It is thicker and larger than terminal hair. In ageing hair follicles matrix, keratinocytes are programed to increase production of medullary rather than cortical keratinocytes resulting in an enlarged and collapsed medulla, forming a central cavity in gray and white hair which provides enhanced UV protection unlike pigmented hair which has melanin. White hair have increased sensitivity to weathering, increased cysteic acid residues and decreased cystine, and increased fiber reactivity to reducing and oxidizing agents. The white color of canities is an optical effect, that is, the reflection/refraction of incident light masks the intrinsic pale yellow color of hair keratin.

Classification (Figure 19.2)

Canities can be broadly classified depending on possible underlying causes for better understanding as

1. Diffuse: Primary diffuse, premature canities, acquired diffuse reversible pigmentation
2. Localized
3. Alteration of hair color due to exogenous agents.

Box 19.3: Features of gray hair

- Coarser, stiffer and thicker
- Collapsed medulla, forming a central cavity
- Increased cysteic acid residues and decreased cystine
- Increased fiber reactivity to reducing and oxidizing agents
- Less susceptible to UV radiation effects

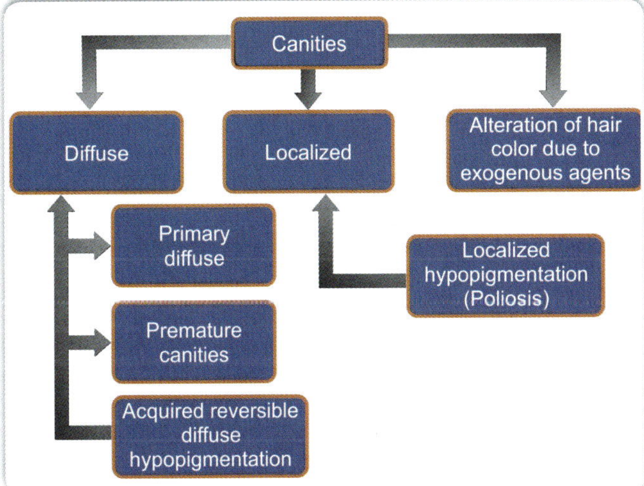

Fig. 19.2: Schematic representation of classification of canities

Primary Diffuse Hypopigmentation of Hair

Primary diffuse hypopigmentation of hair is present from birth, particularly seen in certain genetic conditions. It can be completely depigmented, simply fairer than expected or may have a silvery aspect. Conditions associated with primary diffuse hypopigmentation are as shown in **Table 19.1**.[14]

Albinism[15]

It comprises of a group of inherited disorders of melanin synthesis characterized by decrease of pigmentation in skin, hair and eyes. It occurs in two forms: oculocutaneous albinism and ocular albinism. Oculocutaneous albinism (OCA) is characterized by varying degrees of unpatterned reduction of pigment in skin and hair and associated symptoms. **Table 19.2** shows the various subtypes of OCA and characteristic features. In OCA 1A, there is complete absence of hair pigmentation while in OCA1B different

Table 19.1: Conditions with a primary absence or reduction of hair color

Conditions	*Disorders*	*Hair color changes*
Oculocutaneous albinism	1. Tyrosinase negative albinism 2. Tyrosinase positive albinism	Hair has no color Hair color is diluted, often yellowish
Silvery hair syndromes	1. Griscelli syndrome 2. Elejalde syndrome 3. Chediak–Higashi syndrome	Silvery color
Metabolic disorders	1. Phenylketonuria 2. Homocystinuria 3. Oast House disease	Alternating light and darker when on and off treatment Light hair Very light, almost white hair
Hair shaft disorders	1. Isolated Pili torti 2. Menkes syndrome	Fairer than expected
Other syndromes	1. Cross McKusick Breen syndrome 2. Hermansky Pudlak syndrome 3. Ziprowsky Margolis syndrome	Hair color varies from yellowish white to cream yellow White hair

Table 19.2: Subtypes of oculocutaneous albinism with associated features in each subtype

Type	Mutation	Characteristics
OCA1A	Tyrosinase (absent)	White skin and hair, blue irides, photophobia, nystagmus, strabismus, blindness
OCA1B	Tyrosinase (decreased)	Yellow mutant–yellow hair Platinum–metallic tinge Minimal pigment–eyes darken Temperature sensitive–melanin at acral sites
OCA2	Tyrosinase positive absence of P (pink-eyed dilution protein)	Slight to moderate decrease in pigmentation of skin, hair, eyes, lentigines, nevi at sun-exposed sites
OCA3	Tyrosinase-related protein 1 (absence)	Reddish-bronze color of skin, ginger-red hair blue/brown irides
OCA4	Mutations in gene encoding membrane-associated transporter protein (MATP)	Rare; slight decrease in pigmentation of skin, hair, eyes

phenotypic subtypes are present. In yellow mutant form, hair color turns yellow within the first few years and golden blond to light brown by end of second year. In platinum OCA, hair has a metallic tinge in late childhood while skin appears normal. In OCA 2 type there is slight decrease in hair color while in Rufous OCA, i.e OCA 3 hair color is reddish bronze. MATP mutation also causes slight decrease in hair color.

Management

Genetic counseling is important. Avoidance of sun exposure, strict sun protection, regular ophthalmological evaluation are advised. Early actinic changes, premalignant lesions like actinic keratoses, and basal cell tumors, squamous cell carcinomas are increased in these individuals. Hence clinical examination for cutaneous malignancies annually is done. Prenatal diagnosis from fetal cells obtained from amniocentesis is feasible.[15]

Silvery Hair Syndromes

It includes Chediak-Higashi, Griscelli and Elejalde syndrome. These are autosomal recessive disorders characterized by an early silvery sheen to the hair, and relative pigmentary dilution of skin with a grayish coloration.

Griscelli Syndrome

They present with silver colored gray hair and skin color, recurrent episodes of fever with or without infection, increasing hepatosplenomegaly due to lymphohistiocytic infiltration, and progressive neurological deterioration. It is caused due to mutations in chromosome 15q21, Rab27A and Myosin Va.

Three subsets of patients with Griscelli syndrome have been described, based on clinical manifestations and underlying gene defects as shown in **Table 19.3.** Myosin Va encodes a protein that binds organelles such as melanosomes to actin while, Rab 27A is a GTP binding protein involved in the movement of melanosomes. Melanocytes are unable to transfer melanosomes to epidermal cells and ultrastructural examination of skin biopsy reveals accumulation of melanosomes in melanocytes **(Figures 19.3A and B).**

Silvery hair is more prominent in type 3 subtype wherein mutation in melanophilin is present.

Blood smears show pancytopenia but, in contrast to the patients with Chediak-Higashi syndrome, no leukocyte inclusions are seen. Microscopic examination of the hair shows clumping of pigment in the hair shaft with larger, more irregularly spaced macromelanosomes.

Elejalde Syndrome

(Neuroectodermal melanolysosomal disease)

Elejalde syndrome is a silvery hair disorder characterized by severe neurologic dysfunction (seizures, severe hypotonia, ocular abnormalities, and mental retardation), but no immunodeficiency or hemophagocytosis. Elejalde syndrome is now thought to be allelic to Griscelli syndrome type, resulting from mutations in Myosin Va.

Hair shaft examination shows large, irregularly distributed melanosomes in hair similar to that seen in Griscelli syndrome.

Chediak–Higashi Syndrome (CHS) (Box 19.4)

It is a autosomal recessive condition characterized by silvery sheen to hair, grayish discoloration of skin, decreased iris pigmentation, immunodeficiency, lymphohistiocytic infiltration and neurological deterioration. Mutation in LYST gene, a lysosomal transport protein leads to inability of melanosmal fusion and transfer to keratinocytes.

Table 19.3: Subtypes of Griscelli syndrome

Subset	Mutation	Features
Type 1	Mutation in myosin Va	Neurological problems with no immunodeficiency or hemophagocytosis
Type 2	Mutation in Rab27A	Immunodeficiency and hemophagocytosis No neurological problems
Type 3	Mutation in melanophilin	Silvery hair and light colored skin No immunodeficiency, hemophagocytosis or neurological problems

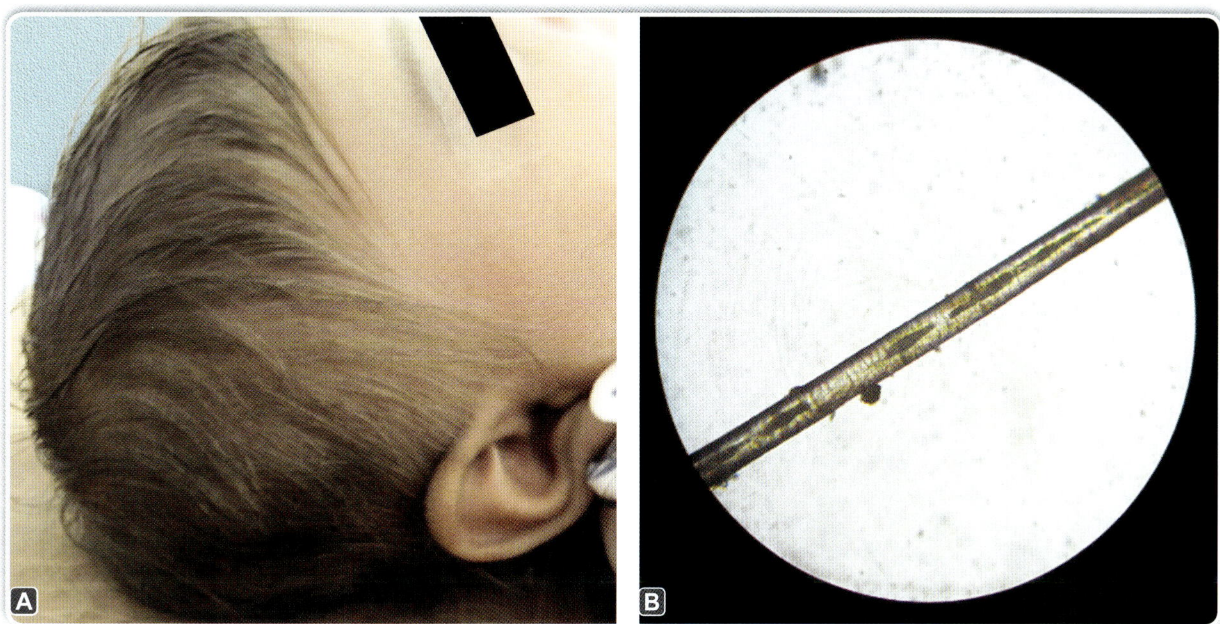

Figs 19.3A and B: (A) Griscelli syndrome; silvery white hairs (B) Light microscopy of hair shaft of the same child showed numerous irregularly arranged clumps of melanosomes along the hair shaft

Box 19.4: Chediak Higashi syndrome

- Mutation in LYST gene, a lysosomal transport protein leads to inability of melanosmal fusion and transfer to keratinocytes
- The hallmark of CHS are giant abnormal granules or melanosomes found in circulating leukocytes, melanocytes of skin and hair, renal tubular epithelial cells, central nervous system (CNS) neurons, and other tissues
- In the hair shaft, these giant melanosomes are smaller than those of Griscelli syndrome and regularly spaced
- Immunodeficiency with silvery hair, decreased iris pigmentation, lymphohistiocytic infiltration

The hallmark of CHS are giant abnormal granules found in circulating leukocytes, melanocytes of skin and hair, renal tubular epithelial cells, central nervous system (CNS) neurons, and other tissues. In the hair shaft, these giant melanosomes are smaller than those of Griscelli syndrome and regularly spaced.

Neutropenia is common, and neutrophils are deficient in chemotactic and bactericidal capability with selective deficiency of natural killer (NK) cells. These immune abnormalities leads to increased susceptibility to infections. The mean age of death for patients with CHS without immune reconstitution is 6 years of age.

Management

For all silvery hair syndromes, early bone marrow transplant or stem cell transplant is the treatment of choice. It reverses the immunodeficiency, prevents fatal accelerated phase but has no effect on pigmentation or neurological deterioration.

Supportive treatment includes antibiotics to control recurrent infections. Immunoglobulins or immunosuppressive agents to control hemophagocytic or lymphohistiocytic phase. Splenectomy is done in patients with accelerated phase unresponsive to other forms of therapy.

Metabolic Disorders

In phenylketonuria, an autosomal recessive disorder, tissues are unable to metabolize phenylalanine to tyrosine because of phenylalanine hydroxylase deficiency. Mental retardation, convulsions and decreased pigmentation of skin, eyes and hair occur with eczema and dermographism. Black hair may become brown while older, 'institutionalized' phenylketonurias may have pale blond or gray hair. Tyrosine treatment causes darkening towards normal color within 1–2 months.

In homocystinuria, error in methionine metabolism causes the hair to appear lighter due to defective keratinization. In Oast-house disease, light almost white hair and recurrent edema are the manifestations.

Hair Shaft Disorders

Isolated Pili Torti

It is seen at birth or in the early months of life. The hair is usually fairer than expected and is spangled, dry, and brittle, breaking at different lengths. It may stand out from the scalp and tends to be short, especially in areas subject to trauma.

Menkes Syndrome (Refer Chapter 4)

It is an X-linked recessively transmitted disorder caused by mutations in *ATP7A* gene located on chromosome Xq12–q13. *ATP7A* gene encodes for MNK protein, a copper transporting p-type adenosine triphosphate. This enzyme is expressed ubiquitously except in the liver. A copper metabolism defect results in the alteration of keratinization as well as pigmentation of hair, as copper is required in the formation of melanin as well as cystine synthesis.

The hair is normal at birth but after the shedding of first hair in infancy the new hair that grow are light colored, twisted, and fragile with a "steel wire" appearance. The infant is mentally and physically retarded, shows progressive psychomotor retardation and hypotonia from the third month.

The plasma copper and ceruloplasmin levels are reduced as well as the hair copper content. If treatment with copper histidine is started within the first month of life, progression of neural changes is retarded and this substantially improves the life span.

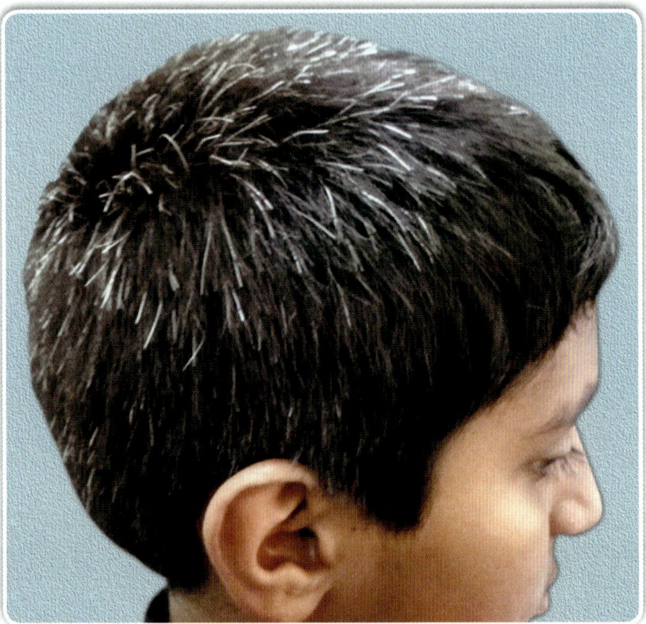

Fig. 19.4: Premature canities—diffuse

Other Syndromes

Cross-McKusick-Breen syndrome is characterized by generalized dilution of pigment in skin, hair, eyes, microphthalmia, small corneas, jerky nystagmus, delayed physical and mental development, writhing motions of arms and legs, weak high pitched cry and spasticity.

Hermansky-Pudlak syndrome is characterized by dilution of pigment of skin, eyes, hair and reddish-brown pigmentation of skin may be present. Hemorrhagic diathesis due to storage pool platelet defect- ecchymoses in skin, epistaxis, hematuria, hematemesis are seen. Ceroid like material deposition in reticuloendothelial system, oral mucosa, lungs occurs.

Ziprowsky-Margolis syndrome is characterized by total absence of skin and hair pigmentation, heterochromia of the irides, and deaf-mutism.

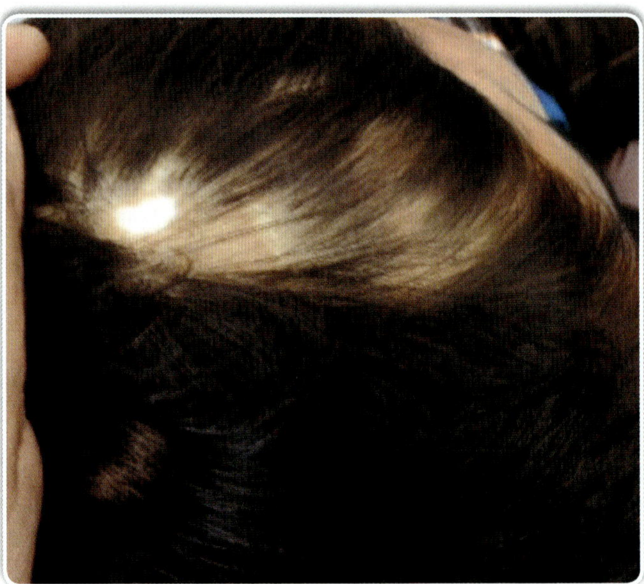

Fig. 19.5: Co-localization of vitiligenous and alopecic patch

Premature Canities

Premature canities refers to a diffuse loss of color, especially of scalp hair, at an age earlier than that generally accepted as physiologic, before the age of 20 in Whites and before age 30 in Blacks **(Figure 19.4)**.[5] It can be an isolated autosomal dominant condition. It is also found to be associated with certain organ-specific autoimmune diseases like alopecia areata, vitiligo[16] **(Figures 19.5 and 19.6)** and may be an early sign of pernicious anemia, hyperthyroidism and, less commonly, hypothyroidism. In a controlled study of the integumentary associations of pernicious anemia, 11% of patients had premature graying.[17] The various causes are enumerated in **Table 19.4**.

Syndromes Associated with Premature Canities

Premature ageing syndromes like progeria and Werners syndrome show early graying of hairs.[6] Patients progressively develop additional signs of premature ageing, including alopecia of the scalp, eyebrows and lashes, early skin wrinkling, osteopenia with fractures,[18,19] and atherosclerosis. In Böök's syndrome, an autosomal dominant trait, premature graying, is associated with premolar hypodontia

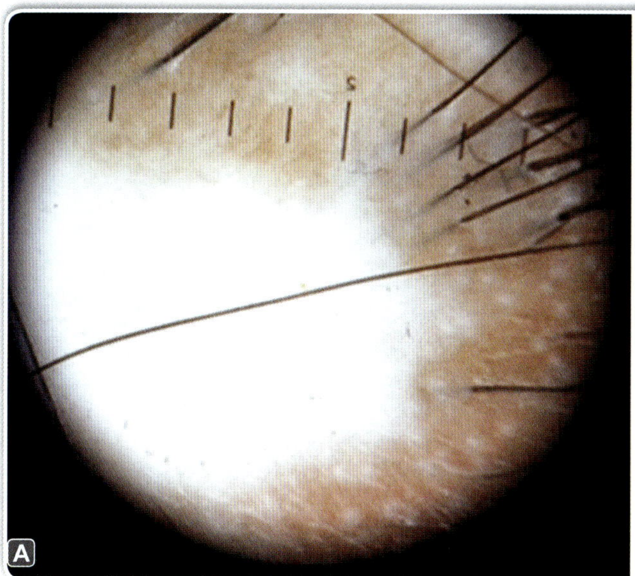

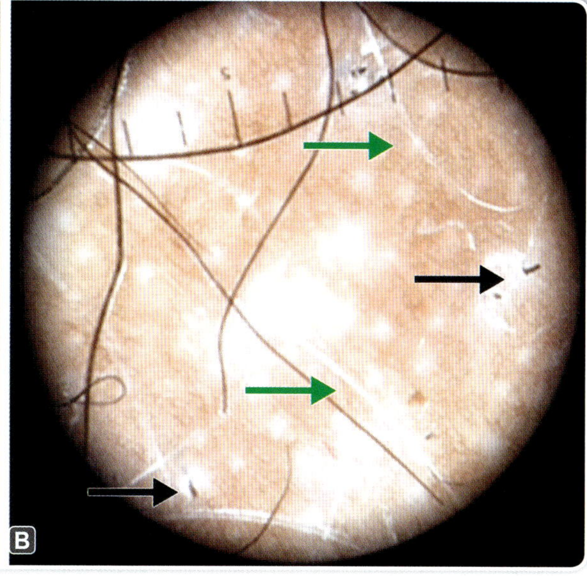

Figs 19.6A and B: (A) Dermoscopy showing vitiligo patch of same child seen in Figure 19.5; (B) Poliosis (green arrows) and few broken hairs (black arrows)

Table 19.4 : Causes of premature canities

Disorders		*Conditions*
1. Genetic disorders	1. Consistent associations	Progeria, Werner syndrome, myotonic dystrophy, Book syndrome, Fisch syndrome
	2. Inconsistent associations	Rothmund-Thompson syndrome, ataxia telangiectasia, Seckel syndrome, Cri du chat syndrome, prolidase deficiency, dyskeratosis congenita
2. Autoimmune disorders	1. Cutaneous	Generalized vitiligo Widespread alopecia areata
	2. Systemic	Pernicious anemia Hypothyroidism Hyperthyroidism Addison disease
3. Drugs		Chloroquine Triparanol Fluorobutyrophenone Mephenesin Dixyrazine IFN α
4. Infection		HIV infection
5. Miscellaneous		Facial hemiatrophy

and palmoplantar hyperhidrosis. Premature canities is an inconstant feature of the Rothmund-Thomson syndrome; when present, it typically commences in adolescence. One-third of patients with chromosome 5p-syndrome (Cri-du-chat syndrome) have premature gray hair. In dystrophic myotonica, the onset of gray hair may precede the myotonia and muscle wasting.

Acquired Reversible Diffuse Hypopigmentation

Various deficiency states may lead to acquired reversible diffuse hypopigmentation of hair. In protein malnutrition, or kwashiorkor, the hair is lighter than expected. If periods of malnutrition alternate with periods of adequate diet, alternating lighter and darker bands may occur, the so-called flag sign *(signe de la bandera)* **(Figures 19.7A and B)**.[20]

Lightening of hair is also an occasional feature of severe iron deficiency[21], vitamin B_{12} deficiency.[22,23]

Poliosis

Poliosis is defined as a localized patch of white hair due to the absence or deficiency of melanin in a group of neighboring follicles. The individual hair follicles can indeed exhibit pigment dilution or suboptimal melanocyte-cortical keratinocyte interactions leading to poliosis. **Table 19.5** shows conditions associated with localized poliosis and **Table 19.6** shows patterns of poliosis.

Piebaldism

It is a autosomal dominant condition characterized by congenital patchy areas of white skin and hair, mostly around the forehead (Forelock – **Figure 19.8**), ventral chest, abdomen, upper arms, and lower legs. It is caused by different mutations in the c-KIT gene necessary for melanocyte proliferation. Lesions typically grow proportionally with the child and are stable. No extracutaneous abnormalities

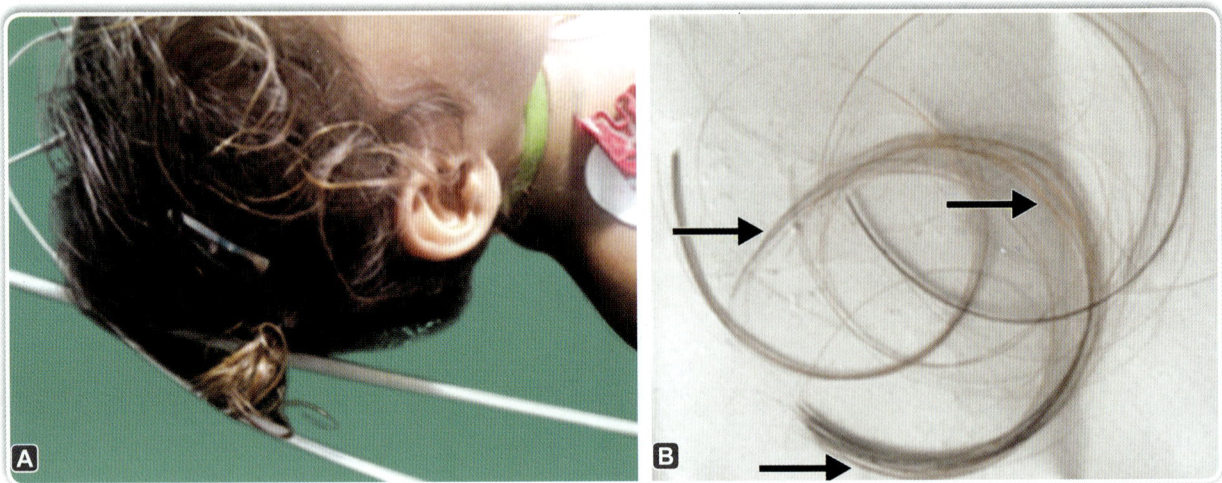

Figs 19.7A and B: Protein malnutrition: (A) Discoloration of hair; (B) Dark and light bands

Table 19.5: Conditions associated with localized poliosis

Conditions	Disorders
1. Genetic disorders	Piebaldism, Waardenburg syndrome, Woolf syndrome, tuberous sclerosis
2. Autoimmune disorders	Vitiligo, alopecia areata, Vogt-Koyanagi-Harada syndrome
3. Exogenous causes	Hydroquinone, monobenzyl ether of hydroquinone, hydrogen peroxide, topical prostaglandin F 2α analog

Table 19.6: Patterns of poliosis

Condition	Pattern of Poliosis
Piebaldism	White forelock
Waardenburg syndrome	White forelock
Vogt-Koyanagi-Harada syndrome	Patchy/vitiligo
Alezzandrini syndrome	Patchy/vitiligo
Vitiligo	Patchy
Alopecia areata	Regrowing hair shows heterochromia

seen. Melanocytes are decreased in number, but are morphologically abnormal and contain normal non-melanized premelanosomes, and also premelanosomes and melanosomes of abnormal appearance. White Forelock, Piebaldism, and deafness occur in Woolf's syndrome.

Waardenburg Syndrome

It is an autosomal dominant disorder, characterized by pigmentary anomalies of skin and hair similar to Piebaldism, pigmentary abnormalities of the iris (heterochromia irides), lateral displacement of the inner canthi of the eyes and lower lacrimal puncta (dystopia canthorum) and sensorineural deafness.

Tietze Syndrome

It is a rare autosomal dominant generalized form of piebaldism (like albinism) characterized by loss of pigment in hair, total deaf mutism, hypoplastic eyebrows, but normal eye color.

Vogt-Koyanagi-Harada Syndrome

It consists of a post-febrile illness comprising of bilateral uveitis, labyrinthine deafness, tinnitus, vitiligo, poliosis, alopecia areata and meningitis.

Vitiligo

Well defined depigmented macules to patches which show variable number of depigmented hair without any change in skin texture can be seen.[16] White hair is of diagnostic and prognostic significance **(Figure 19.9)**.

Alezzandrini's syndrome combines unilateral facial vitiligo, retinitis and poliosis of eyebrows and eyelashes; perceptive deafness is rarely associated.

Alopecia areata

In alopecia areata, regrowing hair is frequently white particularly in cases of late onset **(Figure 19.10)**. Though absent hair pigment is only evident at this stage of resolution, melanocytes are lost from the hair bulb quite early and migrate to the dermal papilla.With regrowth of hair, initially it is gray hair which eventually pigments. Selective loss of pigmented hair as a manifestation of diffuse alopecia areata

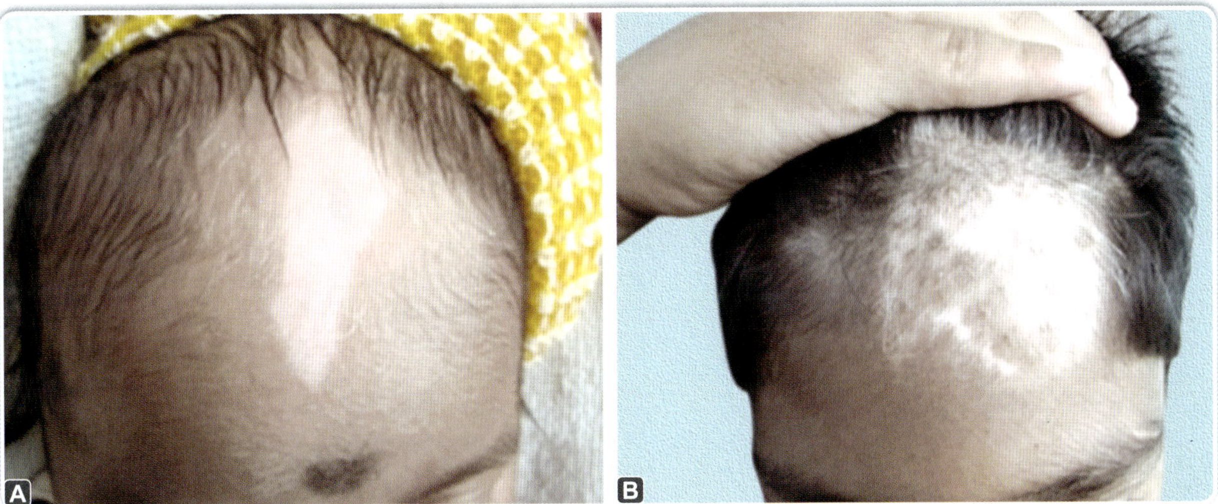

Figs 19.8A and B: Piebaldism

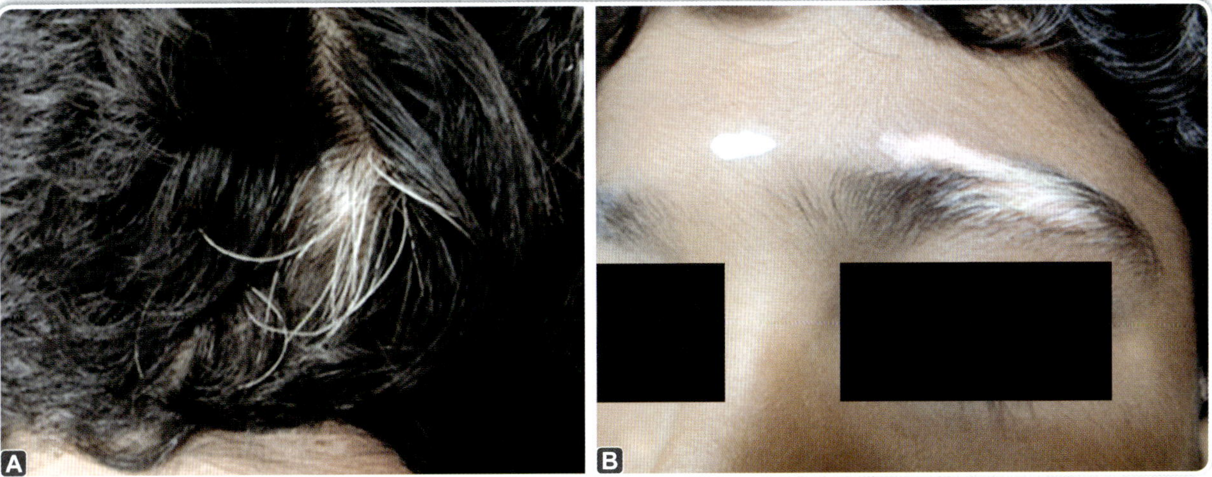

Figs 19.9A and B: Vitiligo patch over the (A) Scalp; (B) eyebrow with poliosis

referred to as canities subita can occur. Patient presents with sudden overnight graying of hair **(Box 19.5)**.

Alteration of Hair Color Due to Exogenous Agents

Various drugs can lead to reversible alterations in hair color. Chloroquine, triparanol, fluorobutyrophenone, mephenesin, prostaglandin F2α,[24] dixyrazine,[25] IFN-α[26] can cause premature canities.

Chloroquine interferes with pheomelanin synthesis causing progressive lightening and silvery coloration. Alpha-interferon and etretinate therapy can also cause poliosis. Mephenesin, a glycerol ester used extensively in the past for diseases with muscle spasms, causes pigmentary loss in dark haired people. Triparanol, an anti-cholesterolemic drug, and fluorobutyrophenone, an antipsychotic drug, both interfere with keratinization and cause hypopigmented and sparse hair.

Management

Canities is permanent and progressive in nature yet, needs evaluation due it its autoimmune associations. Patient counseling is vital in managing a case of canities as acceptance of nature of condition is the sole modality of treatment for the patient.

1. *Reassurance:* The response of canities to present modalities of treatments available is poor. In conditions like piebaldism and associated syndromes being autosomal dominant in nature, future generations shall also be affected. Thus counseling of patient is important.

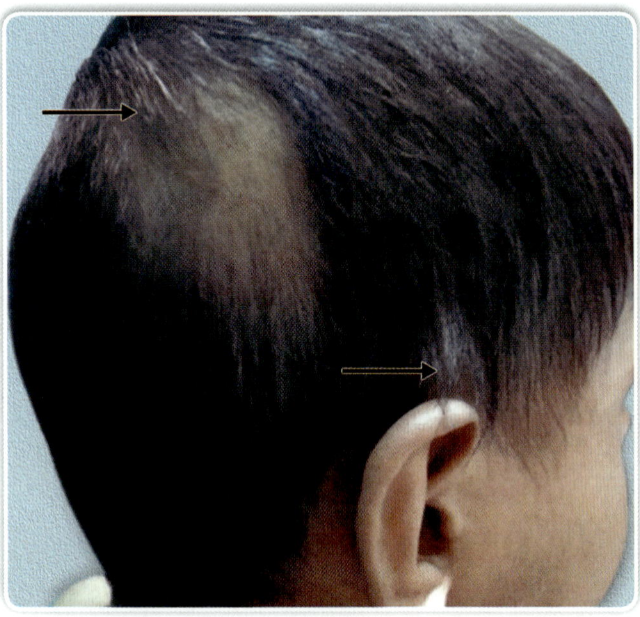

Fig. 19.10: Alopecia areata patch with localized poliosis

Box 19.5: Canities subita (over night graying)

- Selective loss of pigmented hair as a manifestation of diffuse alopecia areata
- An acute episode of alopecia areata may present with very sudden overnight graying due to preferential targeting of pigmented hair by the autoimmune pathology

2. *Elimination of causes:* The acquired causes of poliosis secondary to iron deficiency states and malnutrition are completely treatable. Protein supplementation and iron supplementation will reverse the phenomenon of canities. Administration of iron, zinc, calcium pantothenate, biotin, amino acids have also been tried with partial response.
   Always evaluate for thyroid, hematological disorders and autoimmune disorders and closely follow up the cases for the same.
3. *Para-amino benzoic acid:* Sieve et al have studied the efficacy of large doses of PABA in graying of hair, 100 mg three times daily and noted a response in 82% within 2–4 months of starting treatment.[27] But, the hairs turned gray after stopping the treatment in 2–4 weeks. The mechanism of action has remained unclear. Other studies also have shown moderate response to para amino benzoic acid.[28]
4. *Calcium pantothenate:* Pasricha, et al. have shown that high dose of calcium pantothenate causes repigmentation of gray hair.[29,30] On a follow-up of 29 days and 13 months, respectively, 300 and 1069 gray hairs were counted to have got converted into black hair. Hair with a proximal black portion and a distal gray part were termed as converted hair.[30] In another study, they combined calcium pantothenate with gray hair avulsion; at every 3-monthly follow-up, any converted hair was snipped at the gray-black junction, and all gray hair were avulsed. They found the combination of gray hair avulsion and calcium pantothenate to be more effective than calcium pantothenate used alone. On the contrary, Brandaleone, et al. used 200 mg of PABA with 100 mg of calcium pantothenate (vitamin B_5) and 50 g of brewer's yeast for 8 months to patients with gray hair without any success.[31]
5. *Prostaglandins:*[32] Prostaglandins are potent stimulators of melanocyte growth and melanogenesis. Prolonged use of latanoprost, a PGF2 alpha eye drops has shown repigmentation of gray hair from the root and proximal portion of hairs, and then gradual increase over the entire length of hair. Darkening of hair has also been reported as an incidental finding with other drugs such as defibrotide, cyclosporine, corticosteroid, etretinate, L-thyroxine, verapamil, tamoxifen, levodopa, cisplatin, acitretin, triiodothyronine, and lenalidomide.
6. *Puvasol:* Psoralens trigger melanin synthesis and can also be tried in poliosis. Pavithran, et al. reported PUVASOL to be effective in almost two-thirds of patients with premature graying.[33]
7. Dyeing is often the only effective method of changing the color of gray hair. In the absence of a natural way to reverse hair graying, hair colorants are the mainstay of recovering lost hair color. The major types of hair colors used are: Temporary (textile dyes), natural coloring (henna), semipermanent (low molecular weight direct dyes), and permanent (aromatic amines). Commonly used dyes are henna, metallic dye, chemical dye.
8. *Surgical modalities:* Stable vitiligo, segmental vitiligo and Piebaldism can be treated by surgical methods.The response is seen as perifollicular pigmentation which eventually spreads to surrounding areas.
9. *Miscellaneous:* Topical anti-aging compounds like green tea polyphenols, selenium, copper, phytoestrogens, melatonin are also tried. Use of hormonal anti-aging protocols containing recombinant human growth hormone have shown improvement of hair thickness and also darkening of hair. L-methionine suppresses methionine oxidation and restores the methionine-sulfoxide repair mechanism, and thus preventing graying of hair.[34] This needs further evaluation. A new type of compounds SkQs comprising plastoquinone (an antioxidant moiety), a penetrating cation, and a decane or pentane linker have been synthesized that specifically target mitochondria and act as rechargeable antioxidants.[35] These have been shown to inhibit

development of age-related diseases and traits such as cataract, retinopathy, glaucoma, balding, canities, and osteoporosis in animals.

Conclusion

Graying of hair is physiological/pathological but progressive and can't be reversed. The scalp hair is subjected to intrinsic or physiologic ageing, and extrinsic or premature ageing due to external factors. But if graying occurs at birth or in early childhood, we should carefully evaluate the patient for any underlying causes such as albinism, piebaldism, vitiligo. Premature graying of hair is a bothersome condition and cumbersome for patients to readily accept consequences, hence there is a need for identifying effective treatment options. Developing natural, or semi-synthetic hair repigmentation techniques for delivering coloring agents directly to the hair follicle is needed. Targeting the pathophysiology of hair graying will be promising in near future.

References

1. Courtois M, Loussouarn G, Hourseau C, et al. Aging and hair cycles. Br J Dermatol. 1995;132:86-93.
2. Commo S, Gaillard O, Bernard BA. Human hair greying is linked to a specific depletion of hair follicle melanocytes affectıng both the bulb and the outer root sheath. Br J Dermatol. 2004;150:435-43.
3. van Neste D, Tobin DJ. Hair cycle and hair pigmentation: dynamic interactions and changes associated with aging. Micron. 2004;35:193-200.
4. Tobin DJ, Paus R. Graying: Gerontobiology of the hair follicle pigmentary unit. Exp Gerontol. 2001;36:29-54.
5. Trueb RM. Pharmacologic interventions in aging hair. Clin Interv Aging. 2006;1(2):121-9.
6. Mosher DB, Fitzpatrick TB, Ortonne JP, et al. Disorders of pigmentation. In: Fitzpatrick TB, Eisen AZ, Wolff K, Frredberg IM, Austen KF, editors. Dermatology in general medicine, 3rd edn. New York: McGraw-Hill. pp.794-876.
7. Han R, B eppu H, Lee YK, Georgopoulos K, Larue L, Li E, et al. A pair of transmembrane receptors essential for the retention and pigmentation of hair. Genesis. 2012;50:783-800.
8. Hachiya A, Sriwiriyanont P, Kobayashi T, Nagasawa A, Yoshida H, Ohuchi A, et al. Stem cell factor-KIT signalling plays a pivotal role in regulating pigmentation in mammalian hair. J Pathol. 2009;218:30-9.
9. Schouwey K, Delmas V, Larue L, Zimber-Strobl U, Strobl LJ, Radtke F, et al. Notch 1 and Notch 2 receptors influence progressive hair graying in a dose-dependent manner. Dev Dyn. 2007;236:282-9.
10. Gao T, Bedell A. Ultraviolet damage on natural gray hair and its photoprotection. J Cosmet Sci. 2001;52:103-18.
11. Trüeb RM. Aging of hair. J Cosmet Dermatol. 2005;4(2): 60-72.
12. Fatemi NF, Ebrahimi B, Vakilian HR, Shahmoradi Z. Serum iron, zinc and copper concentration in premature graying of hair. Boil Trace Elem Res. 2012;146(1):30-4.
13. van Neste D. Thickness, medullation and growth rate of female scalp hair are subject to significant variation according to pigmentation of scalp location during aging. Eur J Dermatol. 2004;14:28-32.
14. Li Chuen W. Abnormalities of hair colour. In: Lawrence AB, Ronald CH editors. Paediatric Dermatology, 4th edn. Morby Elsiever. 2011;pp.767-8.
15. Tomita Y. The molecular genetics of albinism and piebaldism, Arch Dermatol. 1994;130:355-8.
16. Lerner AB. On the etiology of vitiligo and gray hair. American Journal of Medicine. 1971;51(2):141-8.
17. Dawber RPR. Integumentary association of pernicious anemia. Br J Dermatol. 1970;82:221-6.
18. Orr-Walker BJ, et al. Pemature hair graying and bone mineral density. J Clin Endocrinol Metab. 1997;82:3580-5.
19. Morton DJ, et al. Premature graying, balding, and low bone mineral density in older women and men: The Rancho Bernardo study.J Aging Health. 2007;19(2):275-85.
20. Narsinga Rao BS, Gopalan C. Some aspects of hair changes in kwashiorkor. Ind J Med Res. 1957;45:85-93.
21. Sato S, Jitsukawa K, Sato H, et al. Segmented heterochromia in black scalp hair associated with iron-deficiency anemia. Canities segmentata sideropaenica. Arch Dermatol. 1989;125:531-5.
22. Noppakun N, et al. Reversible hyperpigmentation of skin and nails with white hair due to vitamin B_{12} deficiency. Arch Dermatol. 1986;122(8):896-9.
23. Carmel R. Hair and fingernail changes in acquired and congenital pernicious anemia. Arch Int Med. 1985;145:484-5.
24. Chen CS, Wells J, Craig JE. Topical prostaglandin F (2alpha) analog induced poliosis. Am J Ophthalmol. 2004;137:965-6.
25. Poulsen J. Hair loss, depigmentation of hair, ichthyosis, blepharoconjunctivitis produced by dixyrazine. Acta Derm Venereol (Stockh). 1981;61:85-8.
26. Bernstein D, Reddy KR, Jeffers L, et al. Canities and vitiligo complicating interferon therapy for hepatitis C. Am J Gastroenterol. 1995;90:1176-7.
27. Sieve BF. Darkening of hair following para-aminobenzoic acid. Science. 1941;94:257-8.
28. Zarafonetis C. Darkening of gray hair during para-aminobenzoic acid therapy. J Invest Dermatol. 1950;15: 399-491.
29. Pasricha JS. Successful treatment of gray hairs with high dose calcium pantothenate. Indian J Dermatol Venereol Leprol. 1981;47:311-3.
30. Pasricha JS. Effect of gray hair evulsion on the response to calcium pantothenate on premature gray hairs. Indian J Dermatol Venereol Leprol. 1986;52:74-8.
31. Brandaleone H, Main E, Steele JM. The effect of calcium pantothenate and para-aminobenzoic acid on gray hair in man.A Study on a group of younger and older individuals. Am J Med Sci. 1944;208:315-20.

32. Bellandi S, Amato L, Cipollini EM, Antiga E, Brandini L, Fabbri P. Repigmentation of hair after latanoprost therapy. J Eur Acad Dermatol Venereol. 2011;25:1485-7.
33. Pavithran K. PUVASOL therapy in premature graying. Indian J Dermatol Venereol Leprol. 1986;52:54-8.
34. Wood JM, Decker H, Hartmann H, Chavan B, Rokos H, Spencer JD, et al. Senile hair graying: H2O2-mediated oxidative stress affects human hair color by blunting methionine sulfoxide repair. FASEB J. 2009;23:2065-75.
35. Skulachev VP, Anisimov VN, Antonenko YN, Bakeeva LE, Chernyak BV, Erichev VP, et al. An attempt to prevent senescence: A mitochondrial approach. Biochim Biophys Acta. 2009;1787:437-61.

20

Follicular Tumors

Rajiv Sharad Joshi

"Live as if you were to die tomorrow. Learn as if you were to live forever."

—*Mahatma Gandhi*

Introduction

The hair follicle is an extremely complex structure and in the fetus develops along with the sebaceous gland and apocrine glands (at certain body areas) from a common anlage termed the 'folliculo-sebaceous-apocrine' germ at about 12–14th week of intrauterine life. The main function of the hair follicle is to produce the hair and protect it physically and recapitulate the process of hair formation in postnatal life in every cycle of anagen-catagen-telogen.

Neoplasms (commonly benign) are known to develop from hair follicles as are cysts designated as follicular cysts, which develop due to blockage of the hair follicle at various levels. The classification of follicular tumors is extremely complex and will not be covered in this essay but several instructive articles and books are available for readers interested in this field.[1-3]

In general follicular tumors are classified based on tenets of embryology, findings of combinations and associations between neoplasms, anatomic distribution and morphologic (microscopic) details of the constituent part of the neoplasm. It is important to recognize the part of the hair follicle that the neoplasm differentiates towards and therefore, before discussing the common follicular tumors it behooves the reader to be familiar with the anatomy and keratinization patterns of the hair follicle.

Functional Anatomy of the Hair Follicle (Figures 20.1A to C)

The hair follicle may be considered to be made up of a series of concentric cylinders that surround a central hair shaft, which is made up of inner medulla and outer cortex surrounded by a cuticle. The hair bulb is made up of rapidly proliferating matrical (germinative) cells admixed with melanocytes and gives rise to the hair shaft, the inner root sheath and the outer root sheath. The inner root sheath is

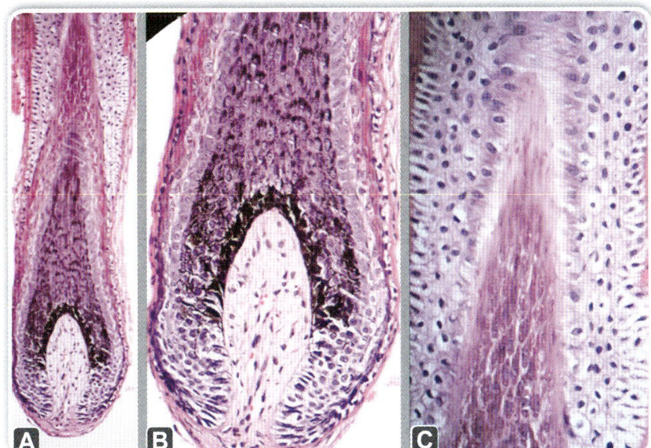

Figs 20.1A to C: (A) Vertical section of hair follicle showing follicular bulb, papilla and stem with inner and outer root sheath. H and E, 100x; (B) Close up vertical section of lower part of hair follicle showing pigmented folllcular bulb, mesenchymal papilla and inner root sheath and lower part of outer root sheath. H and E, 400x; (C) Transverse section of lower part of stem of hair follicle showing pale cells of outer root sheath and bright pink trichohyaline granules of inner root sheath. H and E, 400x

immediately outside the hair and extends from the bulb upto the lower part of the isthmus. It is formed of three layers, from outside in, layer of Henle, Huxley and the cuticle of the inner root sheath that interdigitates with the cuticle of the hair shaft. It forms a rigid funnel like sleeve that covers and protects the growing hair. Interdigitating with the cuticle of the hair shaft, it ascends together with the hair and is essential for the proper moulding, adherence and keratinization of the hair.

The outer root sheath forms the outer cylinder and is many layers thick. It is limited externally by a thick hyaline basement membrane. The outer sheath keratocytes appear pale with abundant and almost clear cytoplasm. The outer sheath extends from the lower part of the bulb to the upper part of the isthmus where it desquamates. It varies in thickness from a few layers thick at the lower bulb to many layers at the isthmus. Traditionally considered to be just a protective layer not contributing to the development of the hair shaft, it is now thought to function as a sensory organ and immunological sentinel of the skin. The outer sheath is now known to contain nestin expressing undifferentiated progenitor cells which can be used as a source of keratinocytes that may be expanded in tissue culture as a source of stem cells.

Connective tissue (perifollicular fibrous sheath) surrounds the outer root sheath and is separated from it by the glassy basement membrane and terminates at the lower level of the infundibulum. The perifollicular fibrous sheath has two components, an outer layer of collagen bundles arranged longitudinally and an inner layer that has collagen bundles that encircle the follicle.[4]

Keratinization of Various Follicular Structures

The different components of the hair follicle undergo keratinization at different levels and with differing mechanisms. Recognition of these varied expressions of keratinization helps in classification of follicular tumors and cysts. The main patterns of follicular keratinization are as follows:

1. *Formation of hair shaft:* The hair shaft proximally is nucleated and at the keratogenous zone (Adamson's fringe) loses the nuclei to become anucleate hard keratin.
2. *Inner root sheath (IRS):* IRS starts keratinization at the level of Adamsons's fringe in the lower part of the stem of the follicle and the hard pale blue-grey keratin is formed half way up the stem with loss of the bright pink tricho-hyalin granules.
3. *Outer root sheath (ORS):* ORS keratinizes at the level of the follicular isthmus and does so without formation of either trichohyaline or keratohyaline granules. This type of keratinization is known as 'trichilemmal' keratinization.
4. *Infundibulum:* It forms basket weave keratin similar to that formed by the epidermis with formation of dark blue keratohyalin granules.

Hamartomas of Follicular Origin

Hamartomas are benign proliferations of varied cellular and stromal elements that are normal in a given site, albeit present in abnormal proportions or aberrant structures. The following are common hamartomas associated with hair follicles **(Box 20.1)**.

Hair Follicle Nevus

Hair follicle nevus also known as vellus hamartoma, is a rare hamartoma that clinically presents as a small asymptomatic papule usually on the face and histologically shows numerous small fully formed vellus hair follicles oriented in various directions with few small sebaceous glands. No stromal changes are seen unlike trichofolliculoma. Dermoscopy shows numerous uniform hair follicles and interfollicular pseudopigment network.

Ackerman considered the hair follicle nevus to be the peripheral part of a trichofolliculoma,[5] however other observations suggest that hair follicle nevus is a rare entity distinct from trichofolliculoma and can be classified as a hair follicle hamartoma.[6]

Nevus Comedonicus

Nevus comedonicus is considered as a hamartoma wherein improper stimulation of the epithelial component of the folliculosebaceous unit by its associated dermal mesenchymal cells leads to poor development of the follicle, albeit with continued production of keratin that accumulates in distorted and dilated follicular infundibula forming comedo like structures. A contrary view considers nevus comedonicus to be an epidermal nevus involving the terminal parts of the hair follicle and eccrine ducts. It is usually a sporadic occurrence but it has been described in twins[7] and it is believed to result from genetic mosaicism.

Nevus comedonicus was first described by Koffman[8] in 1895, who believed it to be an unusual form of acne. Thiberge was the first to use the term nevus comedonicus.[9] Nevus comedonicus presents clinically as groups of black

Box 20.1: Hamartomas of follicular origin

- Hair follicle nevus
- Nevus comedonicus
- Nevus sebaceous of Jadassohn
- Trichofolliculoma

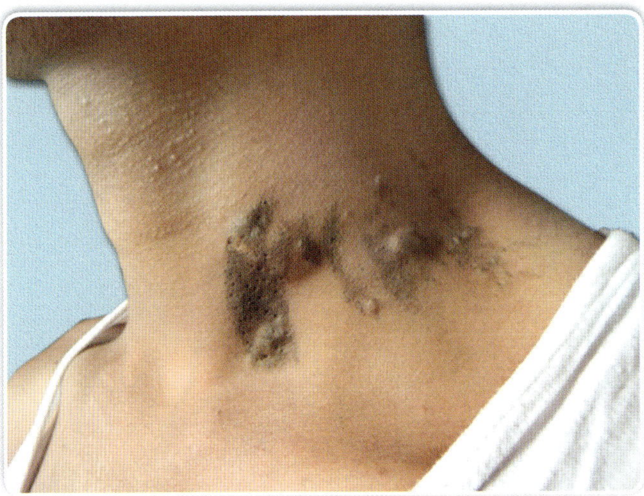

Fig. 20.2: Nevus comedonicus (*Courtesy:* Department of Dermatology, STD and Leprosy, BMCRI, Bengaluru)

pits, which are discrete dilated follicular ostia plugged with dark keratin resembling comedones **(Figure 20.2)**. Nevus comedonicus presents either at birth or in early childhood but cases developing much later in life, usually following some trauma have also been described.[10] No racial or gender predilection is seen. Nevus comedonicus has been described at almost all sites including palms and soles and even on the glans penis[11] and may be localized, linear, segmental and has also been described to follow Blaschko's lines. Most cases are asymptomatic and cause only cosmetic disfigurement, uncommonly, however, the lesions are repeatedly inflamed and infected and may lead to development of painful cysts, abscesses and even fistulas with scarring.

Biopsy shows marked dilatation of contiguous follicular infundibula which are packed with orthokeratin. The infundibular walls are thin and attenuated and may show budding with the sebaceous glands and other follicular structures being absent or poorly developed. Epidermolytic hyperkeratosis of the follicular epithelium has been reported in nevus comedonicus.[12]

Nevus comedonicus syndrome is association of nevus comedonicus with systemic abnormalities that may affect the CNS, skin, skeletal system, eyes and teeth.

Nevus Sebaceous of Jadassohn

Organoid nevus is a generic term used for complex hamartomatous changes that affect not only the pilosebaceous follicle but also the epidermis and other adnexal structures. While nevus sebaceous is the prototype organoid nevus, other conditions like nevus comedonicus, porokeratotic eccrine nevus, Becker's nevus, trichilemmal cyst nevus and phacomatosis pigmentokeratotica have also been considered to be organoid nevi **(Box 20.2)**.

Box 20.2: Organoid nevi

- Nevus sebaceous
- Nevus comedonicus
- Porokeratotic eccrine nevus
- Becker's nevus
- Trichilemmal cyst nevus
- Phacomatosis pigmentokeratotica

Jadassohn in 1895 first described nevus sebaceous as a verrucous lesion that had circumscribed proliferation of sebaceous glands. Post-zygotic mutations are thought to cause various expressions of mosaicism with mutations of pluripotent cells giving rise to hamartomas involving different structures. HPV DNA has been demonstrated in many lesions of nevus sebaceous[13] and the high frequency of oncogenic HPV types has been suggested to implicate maternal transmission of HPV and infection of an ectodermal stem cell leading to epigenetic mosaic and altered skin development along Blaschko's lines.

Typically three clinical stages are seen in the development of nevus sebaceous:

1. *Infantile stage:* Usually presents at birth or soon after as a linear or rounded slightly elevated tan colored or slightly orange-yellow colored plaque with a smooth or velvety surface. A biopsy at this stage shows papillomatous epidermal hyperplasia that resembles an epidermal nevus. The sebaceous glands at this stage are not prominent. Apocrine glands are usually seen in the mid and deep dermis with a marked absence of follicular structures. Sometimes rudimentary follicular buds and distorted follicles may be present, but in general the absence of follicles underlying the papillomatous epidermal proliferation, which on the scalp contrasts with the large normal follicles in the adjacent dermis on the scalp is typical of infantile nevus sebaceous **(Figure 20.3)**.
2. *Adolescent stage:* At the onset of puberty there is growth of sebaceous glands and the surface too becomes more verrucous and thickened in appearance. Histology shows numerous large mature sebaceous glands in the upper dermis just beneath the verrucous epidermis with a paucity of accompanying hair follicles. The sebaceous glands may open directly onto the skin surface **(Figures 20.4 and 20.5)**.
3. *Adult stage:* In most individuals the lesion remains the same or shows minimal thickening in later life, remaining alopecic throughout. At times an appendageal tumor develops causing focal nodule formation in the verrucous plaque with or without crusting and ulceration. The commonest tumors arising within a nevus sebaceous are syringocystadenoma papilliferum and trichoblastoma. Less commonly other tumors like hidradenoma, apocrine cystadenoma, spiradenoma,

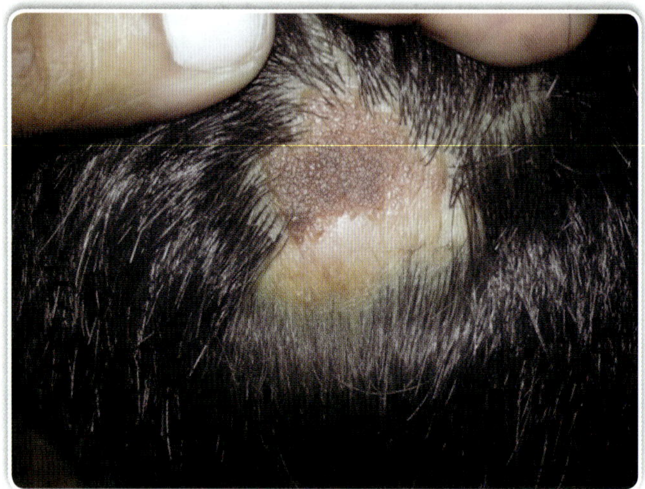

Fig. 20.3: Infantile stage of nevus sebaceous (*Courtesy:* Department of Dermatology, STD and Leprosy, BMCRI, Bengaluru)

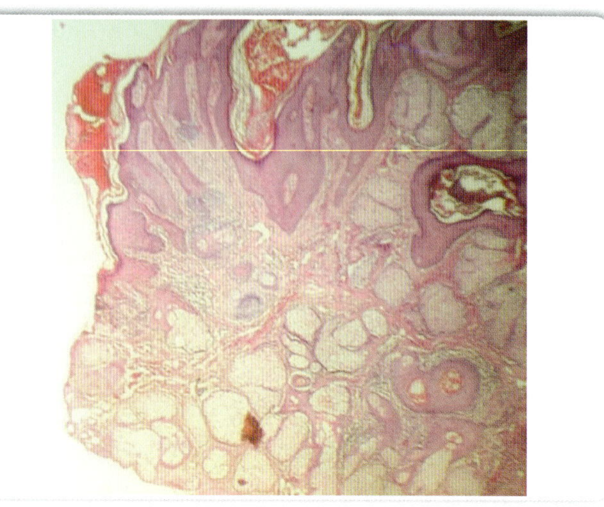

Fig. 20.5: Nevus sebaceous showing papillomatous and verrucous epidermal hyperplasia with numerous large mature sebaceous glands in the upper dermis. H and E, 40x

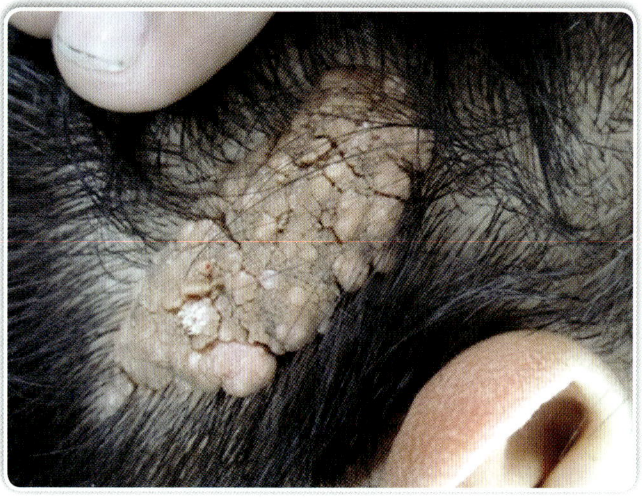

Fig. 20.4: Nevus sebaceous- Adolescent phase (*Courtesy:* Department of Dermatology, STD and Leprosy, BMCRI, Bengaluru)

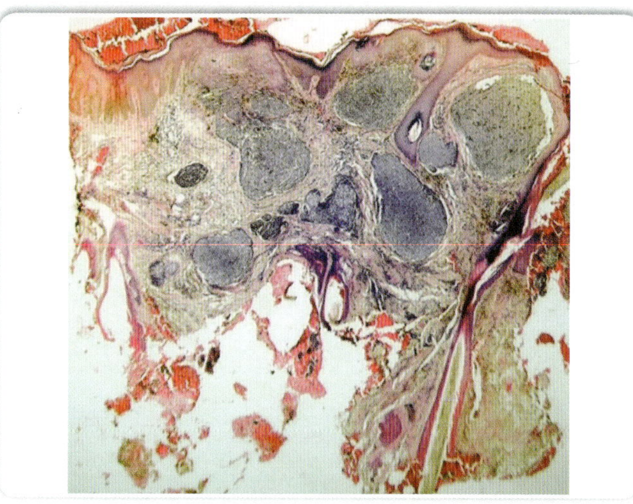

Fig. 20.6: Trichoblastoma within a nevus sebaceous. Large nodules of basaloid follicular germinative cells. H and E, 40x

follicular cysts, basal cell carcinoma (BCC), sebaceous epithelioma and eccrine carcinoma may be seen. In the past basal cell carcinoma was considered to be a very common tumor associated with nevus sebaceous, however, several studies have shown that the basaloid tumors developing in a nevus sebaceous are mostly benign trichoblastomas and not basal cell carcinoma **(Figures 20.6 and 20.7)**.[14,15] Also associated with nevus sebaceous are various epithelial hyperplasias that may be associated with HPV infection **(Box 20.3)**.

Nevus sebaceous may rarely be associated with multiple internal abnormalities similar to those seen in the epidermal nevus syndrome and may involve the CNS, bone and eye. Common abnormalities seen are epilepsy, mental retardation, vitamin D resistant rickets, ocular abnormalities like ptosis, nystagmus and poor development of the optic nerve **(Box 20.4)**.

The medical importance of nevus sebaceous is the likelihood, albeit in a small percentage of patients of development of malignant tumors. The risk of malignancy is difficult to establish in a given patient and many authorities recommend complete surgical excision. The surgery is done usually before puberty, before the pubertal growth phase starts and also because the risk of developing a malignancy increases with increasing age. A recent study[16] concluded that prophylactic excision of all sebaceous nevi is not warranted and should be done only when tumors are clinically suspected or for cosmetic reasons.

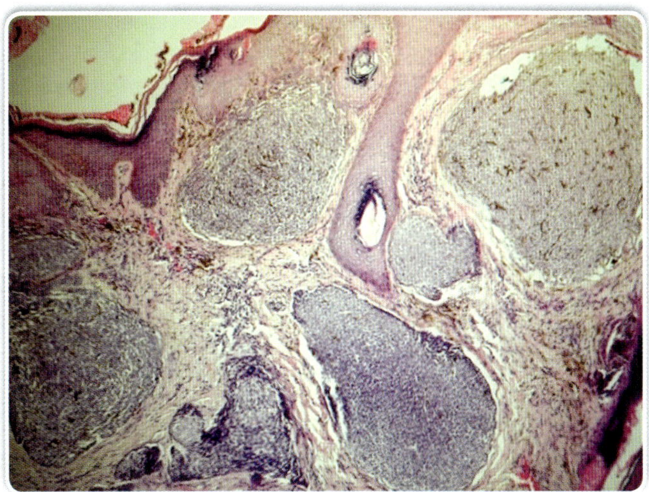

Fig. 20.7: Trichoblastoma in nevus sebaceous. Basaloid nodules with prominent pigment and dendritic melanocytes. H and E, 100x

Box 20.3: Tumors arising within a nevus sebaceous

- Syringocystadenoma papilliferum
- Trichoblastoma
- Hidradenoma
- Apocrine cystadenoma
- Spiradenoma
- Follicular cysts
- Basal cell carcinoma
- Sebaceous epithelioma
- Eccrine carcinoma

Box 20.4: Abnormalities associated with nevus sebaceous

- Epilepsy
- Mental retardation
- Vitamin D resistant rickets
- Ocular abnormalities
  - Ptosis
  - Nystagmus
  - Poor development of the optic nerve

Trichofolliculoma

Trichofolliculoma is a generic term for a group of follicular hamartomas in which follicular structures (usually fully formed but also incomplete and aberrant) radiate outwards from a central cystically dilated structure that is similar to the follicular infundibulum.

Clinically, it presents as a papule or small nodule commonly on the face, less often on the scalp or upper trunk. A small central depression is noted through which may be seen emanating a small tuft of tiny vellus hair.

Histologically there is a large central, at times cystic cavity that is lined by epidermis like epithelium and contains laminated and basketweave orthokeratin like the infundibulum of the follicle, with few hair shafts. Emanating from the central infundibular structure from all directions are seen near normal vellus follicles that radiate outwards, and show a bulb and papilla with development of both inner and outer root sheaths. At the base of the follicles abortive follicles with follicular germs but no well developed follicular structures may be seen. As the lesion is large, many of the radiating follicles are cut tangentially and a varied morphological picture may be seen depending on which part of the lesion the sections under scrutiny represents. The entire lesion is enveloped by a fibrocytic stroma.

Sections taken away from the central cystic infundibulum may show only well developed vellus hair follicles and may be misinterpreted as a hair follicle nevus. At times sebaceous lobules are very prominent in a trichofolliculoma and it is then referred to as a sebaceous trichofolliculoma. Clinically however it is similar to a trichofolliculoma without prominent sebaceous glands. The term folliculosebaceous cystic hamartoma has been used to describe large nodular and cystic lesions which histologically may resemble a trichofolliculoma. Some authors believe that it represents a trichofolliculoma in its late stage **(Table 20.1)**.[17]

Table 20.1: Hair follicle hamartomas

Sl.No.	Hamartoma	Clinical features	Histopathology
1.	Hair follicle nevus	Small asymptomatic papule usually on the face	Numerous small fully formed vellus hair follicles with few small sebaceous glands. No stromal changes
2.	Nevus comedonicus	Groups of black pits which are discrete dilated follicular ostia plugged with dark keratin resembling comedones	Marked dilatation of contiguous follicular infundibula which are packed with orthokeratin
3.	Nevus sebaceous of jadassohn		
	Infantile stage	Presents at birth or soon after, slightly elevated tan colored or slightly orange-yellow colored plaque with a smooth or velvety surface	Papillomatous epidermal hyperplasia, sebaceous glands are not prominent
	Adolescent stage	At the onset of puberty, surface becomes more verrucous and thickened	Large mature sebaceous glands in the upper dermis just beneath the verrucous epidermis with a paucity of accompanying hair follicles
	Adult stage	May remain same, may develop appendageal tumors	Same as above, with appendageal tumors
4.	Trichofolliculoma	Papule or small nodule commonly on the face, with small central depression	Large central or cystic cavity lined by epidermis like epithelium and contains laminated and basket weave orthokeratin with few hair shafts, entire lesion is enveloped by a fibrocytic stroma

Neoplasms with Follicular Germinative Differentiation

These lesions are composed of proliferations of follicular germinative cells along with variable proliferation of the perifollicular fibrous tissue giving rise to a fibrocyte rich stroma which along with the presence of papillary mesenchymal bodies (embryonic mesenchymal cells that accompany and stimulate the follicular bulb) are indicators of the benign nature of these tumors.

The proliferating germinative cells are grouped together in nodular aggregates that form various patterns (cribriform, racemiform, retiform) and are associated with varying numbers of cystic structures that indicate a higher degree of differentiation.

Trichoblastoma is the generic term used for these tumors of which trichoepithelioma is well known as a distinct clinicopathological entity and is considered to be a superficial expression of trichoblastoma **(Box 20.5)**.

Trichoepithelioma (TE)

Trichoepithelioma is a common clinically distinct follicular tumor that has predilection for the central face, nasolabial folds, upper lip and forehead. It may occur as a solitary lesion, but more commonly is seen as part of multiple trichoepitheliomas, which is a familial trait and is associated with abnormalities of a gene located on chromosome 9p21. Other cases of multiple trichoepitheliomas may be associated with mutations of the cylindromatosis oncogene (CYLD) which is on chromosome 16q12-q13 and a study has suggested that abnormalities in this gene may result in any one of 3 syndromes, viz. Brooke-Spiegler syndrome, familial cylindromatosis and multiple familial trichoepitheliomas **(Box 20.6)**.[18]

Clinically the lesions of trichoepithelioma are multiple skin colored firm juicy papules and nodules, 2–10 mm in size, located mainly on the central part of the face. Lesions may also occur on the scalp and neck and upper trunk. Rare involvement of the vulva has been reported.[19] Dermatomal distribution has been reported and association with other cutaneous tumors like cylindroma, spiroadenoma is not uncommon. Solitary giant lesions of trichoepithelioma have been described on the lower trunk and buttocks.

Tendency for developing multiple trichoepitheliomas is an autosomal dominant trait but due to variable penetrance and decreased expressivity in men, most patients are women. The lesions begin in childhood and adolescence and increase in number with age.

Histologically trichoepitheliomas show the silhouette of a benign neoplasm, namely, a small symmetrical well circumscribed neoplasm without cytological atypia. There is predominance of follicular germinative (basaloid) cells, which are seen to form nodules in the upper and mid dermis. There is often arrangement of the basaloid cells into reticulate or cribriform pattern with strands of basaloid cells separated by stroma. Advanced differentiation toward the follicular bulb is indicated by the presence of papillary mesenchymal bodies that represent the embryonic follicular mesenchymal cells that stimulate the growth of the follicular bulb in the hair cycle and the presence of melanocytes within the neoplasm. The stroma is characteristically fibrocytic and envelops entirely the aggregates of basaloid cells. Peripheral palisading of cells like in basal cell carcinoma is not seen and clefts if seen are within the fibrocytic stroma and not between the epithelium and the stroma as typically seen in BCC and serves to help in differentiating the two entities **(Figures 20.8 to 20.10)**.

Apart from the proliferating nodules of follicular germinative epithelium, trichoepithelioma (unlike other forms of trichoblastoma) also shows differentiation towards upper follicular structures with small cystic spaces surrounded by keratinocytes that have pink squamoid appearance which indicates isthmic and

Box 20.5: Neoplasms with follicular germinative differentiation

- Trichoepithelioma
- Desmoplastic trichoepithelioma
- Trichoblastoma

Box 20.6: Syndromes associated with mutations of the cylindromatosis oncogene

- Brooke-Spiegler syndrome
- Familial cylindromatosis
- Multiple familial trichoepitheliomas

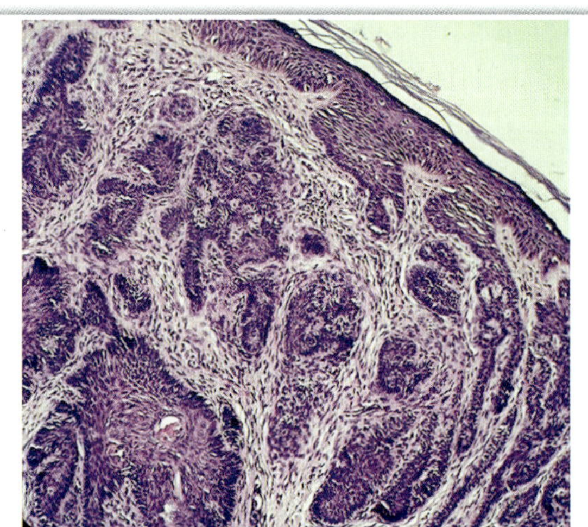

Fig. 20.8: Trichoepithelioma showing aggregates of basaloid cells in the upper dermis with surrounding stroma that is fibrocytic. H and E, 40x

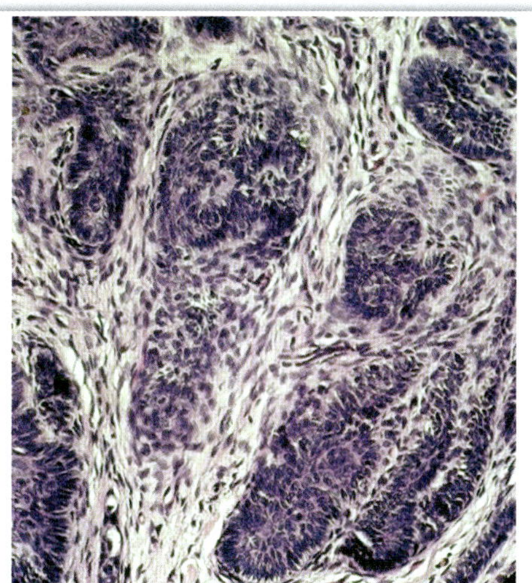

Fig. 20.9: Trichoepithelioma showing a papillary mesenchymal body resembling a normal hair germ. H and E, 100x

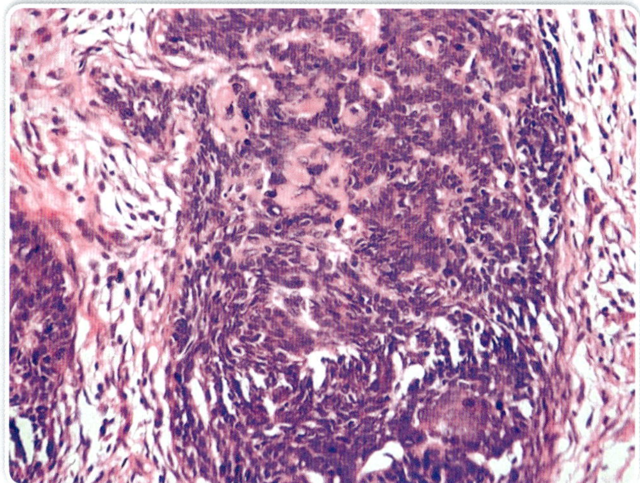

Fig. 20.10: Trichoepithelioma, nodule with cribriform arrangement of basaloid cells. H and E, 400x

infundibular differentiation. Calcification with foreign body granulomatous reaction and cholesterol clefts is common in trichoepitheliomas while mucin deposits are distinctly uncommon. Immunohistochemical studies show outer root sheath associated keratins (cytokeratin 5,6,8,17) and bcl-2 expression in the nodular proliferations. The surrounding stromal cells are CD 34 and CD 10 positive and serve to differentiate from BCC where these antigens are usually absent.[20]

Treatment of multiple trichoepitheliomas is primarily surgical and includes removal of lesions by cold steel surgery, cryotherapy, electrodessication, radiation and laser treatment. All these have propensity for scarring with a high rate of recurrence. A recent report has described satisfactory clearance of lesions of trichoepithelioma with topical imiquimod and tretinoin.[21]

Desmoplastic Trichoepithelioma

Described earlier as sclerosing epithelial hamartoma, this is a variant of trichoepithelioma which is most often mistaken for the morphea-like sclerosing form of BCC. It presents clinically as a firm annular skin colored plaque with a central dell, located usually on the cheek in women. Histologically the lesion is made up of extensive stromal sclerosis (desmoplasia) in which are seen splayed interstitially strands of basaloid cells, usually just two or three cells thick. Small foci of infundibular or isthmic differentiation with small microcysts may be seen. Findings that favor desmoplastic TE over BCC include compact collagen around strands and groups of basaloid cells, lack of cellular atypia, lack of apoptotic and dyskeratotic keratinocytes and presence of calcification in the small keratinous cysts with foreign body type of granulomatous inflammation. Unlike BCC fibroblasts surrounding trichoepithelioma do not express matrix metalloproteinase stromelysin-3 **(Table 20.2)**.[22,23]

Trichoblastoma

Trichoblastoma designates tumors that are made up of nodular proliferations of mainly follicular germinative cells with follicular bulbar differentiation and is a generic term which includes trichoepithelioma, which is considered as a superficial expression of trichoblastoma.[24] Some authors have described trichoblastoma as 'immature trichoepithelioma.'[25]

Trichoblastoma may be considered to be the benign counterpart of BCC which conceptually is a trichoblastic carcinoma and it is now known that most lesions arising in a nevus sebaceous which in the past were considered to be BCC's are in fact trichoblastomas and benign in nature and in biological behavior.

Trichoblastomas clinically are larger tumors than trichoepitheliomas and are located deep in the dermis and may even involve the subcutis. They are made up of nodular aggregates of crowded hyperchromatic follicular germinative cells admixed with variable numbers of melanocytes. The proliferating cells may be arranged in various patterns and Ackerman[24] has described small and large nodules, racemiform, retiform and cribriform pattern for trichoblastomas. While the nodular aggregates of follicular germinative cells is the striking feature morphologically, an equally important finding in trichoblastomas is the proliferation of the surrounding stroma elements which show numerous fibrocytes surrounding every nodule of the tumor forming individual perinodular fibrous compartments. Clefts if seen are within the fibrous tissue and not between the epithelium and the stroma as seen in BCC and serves to differentiate trichoblastomas from BCC.

Differential staining pattern for CD 10 (stromal in trichoblastomas and staining of basaloid cells in BCC) helps in differentiating trichoblastoma from BCC.[25]

Neoplasms with Matrical Differentiation

Matrical differentiation or cornification refers to the hair shaft keratinization in which the follicular germinative cells of the follicular bulb lose their nuclei at the keratogenous zone ie. Adamson's fringe, and get transformed into hard anucleate keratin of the shaft. The loss of nuclei is a graded event with formation of intermediate shadow cells which show pale or salmon pink cytoplasm and central clear spaces which denote sites of lost nuclei. The presence of shadow cells within benign and malignant epithelial neoplasms has been thought to represent faulty attempts at hair shaft formation. Several neoplasms are characterized by matrical differentiation and the most common and well known of them is pilomatricoma also known as 'calcifying epithelioma of Malherbe' **(Box 20.7)**.

Pilomatricoma

Pilomatricoma was first described by Mahlerbe [26] and Chenantais in 1880 and it was Lever[27] in 1949 who noted that the proliferating cells of the neoplasm were similar to hair matrix cells and hence the initial name of pilomatrixoma which now is more appropriately known as pilomatricoma. Pilomatricomas are common tumors that are seen mostly in children and young adults and are considered to be the most common solid skin tumor in persons below 20 years of age.

Clinically they present as a single firm to hard, skin colored nodule on the face, head and neck region, less commonly on the proximal arms and lower extremity and morphologically do not show any characteristic features **(Figure 20.11)**.

Stretching of the overlying skin may give an angulated appearance known as the 'tent sign', which is due to calcification within the lesion. Unusual morphological variants of pilomatricoma are given in **Box 20.8**.

Many patients with pilomatricomas have shown mutations in the gene CTNNB1, indicating that beta-catenin/LEF misregulation is the major cause of hair matrix tumorigenesis in humans and results in the development of pilomatricomas.[28]

Histologically findings of an early pilomatricoma are those of a cyst which shows matrical cornification. The cyst wall and surrounding dermis has hyperchromatic basaloid follicular matrical cells which show transition to pale pink shadow or ghost cells which have lost the nuclei but leave behind outlines of the nuclear space. Sometimes pink trichohyalin granules may be seen suggesting matrical and inner root sheath cornification. In old lesions the cystic

Table 20.2: Histopathological differences between desmoplastic trichoepithelioma and basal cell carcinoma

	Desmoplastic TE	*Basal cell carcinoma*
Compact collagen	Present	Absent
Cellular atypia	Absent	Present
Apoptotic keratinocytes	Absent	Present
Dyskeratotic keratinocytes	Absent	Present
Calcification in the small keratinous cysts	Present	Absent
Stromelysin-3 expression	Absent	Present

Box 20.7: Neoplasms with matrical differentiation

- Pilomatricoma
- Matricoma
- Melanocytic matricoma
- Pilomatrical carcinoma

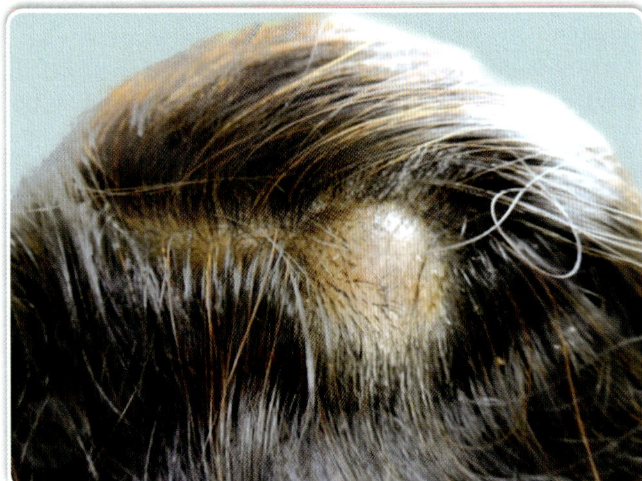

Fig. 20.11: Skin colored nodule of the scalp- pilomatricoma (*Courtesy:* Department of Dermatology, STD and Leprosy, BMCRI, Bengaluru)

Box 20.8: Unusual variants of pilomatricoma

- Perforating lesions
- Bullous
- Lymphangiectactic
- Keratoacanthoma
- Cutaneous horn like lesions
- Anetoderma of overlying skin

nature of the neoplasm is lost and seen are nodules of dark matrical cells with varying proportions of pink shadow cells. A well developed lesion shows dark blue nodules that have at their centres pale pink areas of shadow cells. In long standing lesions prominent fibrosis and foreign body type of granulomatous inflammation is seen along with foci of calcification which may predominate the histological picture. Because the matrical cells show many mitotic figures due to their high proliferative capacity, a misdiagnosis of a carcinoma may be made. Long standing lesions may show no matrical cells but show only the pink shadow cells with varying degrees of calcification and granulomatous inflammation **(Figures 20.12 to 20.16)**.

Kaddu, et al[29] have categorized pilomatricomas into four chronologically distinct stages viz early, fully developed, early regressive and late regressive and proposed that pilomatricoma begins as an infundibular-matrix cyst and ends up as a calcified and ossified nodule with no viable

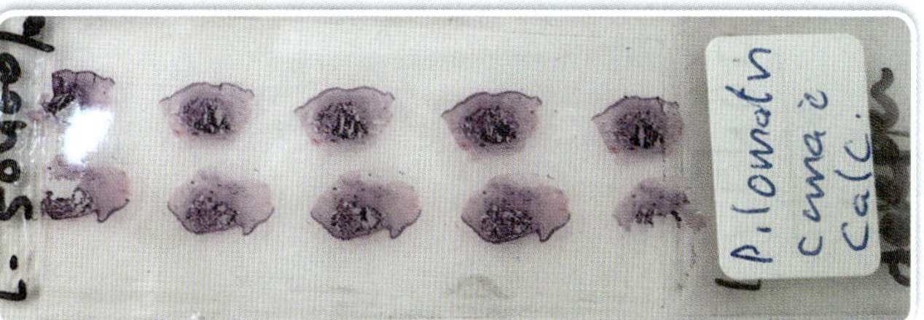

Fig. 20.14: Pilomatricoma, late calcified lesion. H and E, 20x

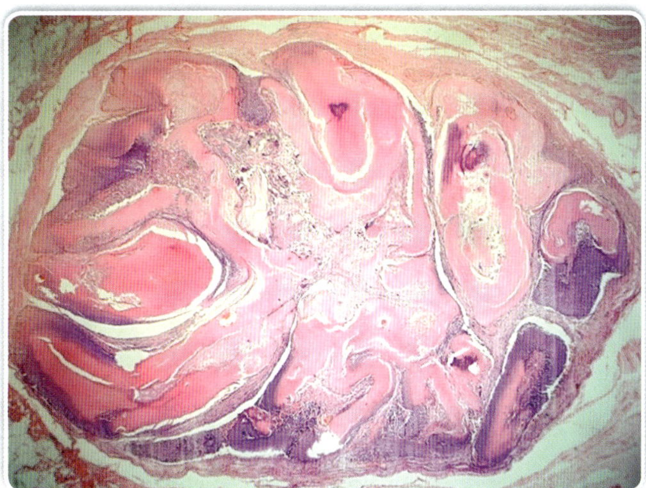

Fig. 20.12: Pilomatricoma showing nodules of blue matrical cells surrounding pink areas of shadow cells. H and E, 40x

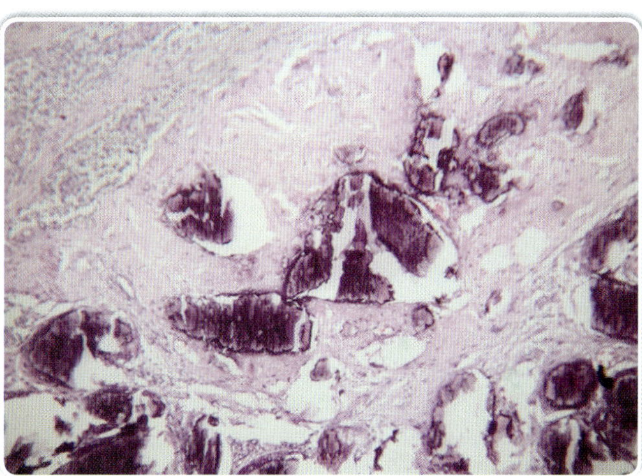

Fig. 20.15: Calcified pilomatricoma, no matrical cells seen, only calcification of shadow cells is seen. H and E, 100x

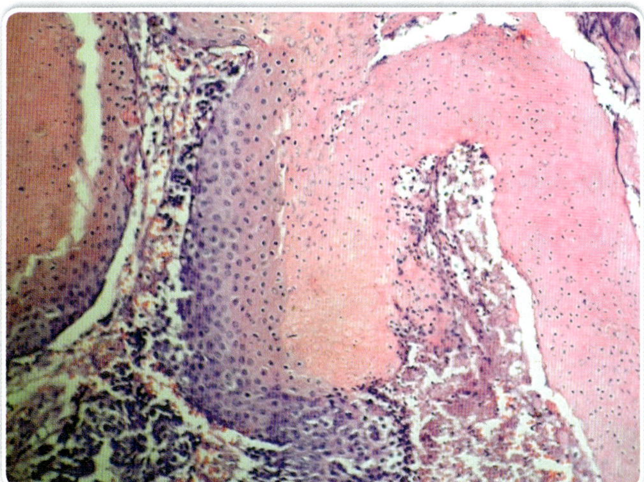

Fig. 20.13: Pilomatricoma showing a nodule with basophilic matrical cells on the left and pink shadow cells on the right with intervening transitional area of gradual nuclear loss. H and E, 100x

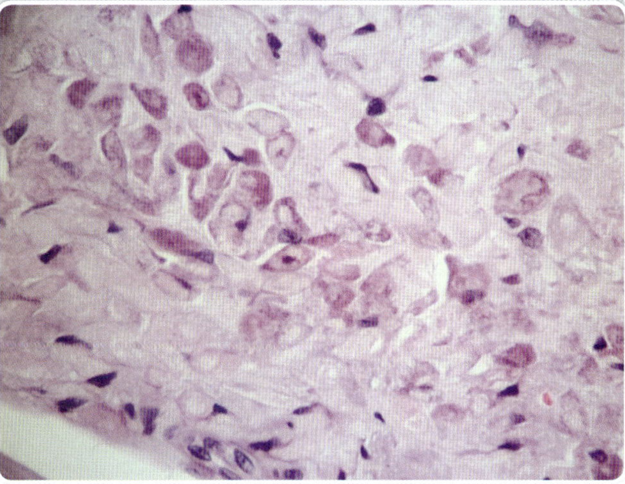

Fig. 20.16: Pilomatricoma, calcification of individual shadow cells. H and E, 400x

epithelial component with intervening stages of variable proportions of basophilic matrical cells and pink shadow cells surrounded by stromal changes of granulomatous inflammation, calcification and ossification.

Matricoma and Melanocytic Matricoma

Matricomas, like pilomatricomas are epithelial neoplasms that derive from hair matrix and have in common matrical cells and shadow cells. Matricomas show a predominantly solid basaloid proliferation with only focal zones of shadow cells.

Melanocytic matricoma is a recently described entity which shows prominent melanocytic proliferation and pigmentation and may be a pigmented variant of matricoma.[30]

Pilomatrical Carcinoma

Pilomatrical carcinoma is an uncommon carcinoma that shows matrical differentiation similar to a pilomatricoma. Pilomatrical carcinomas develop in adults on severely sun damaged skin and histologically show dark basaloid matrical cells and pink shadow cells. The basaloid cells show cytologic atypia and are arranged in infiltrative pattern in the dermis. Parts of the tumor may show similarities with a squamous cell carcinoma.

Finding of cytologic atypia in a pilomatricoma like lesion makes the diagnosis easy with the only differential being basal cell carcinoma with matrical differentiation, in which a conventional BCC shows foci of matrical differentiation with presence of shadow cells.[31]

Neoplasms with Trichilemmal (Outer Root Sheath) Differentiation

Trichilemmal differentiation is suggested by proliferation of cells that resemble those that constitute the bulk of the outer root sheath and appear histologically as large pale cells with central nuclei and clear cytoplasm **(Box 20.9)**.

Trichilemmomas

Trichilemmomas may be solitary or multiple. Solitary trichilemmomas are small skin colored verrucous and keratotic papules that clinically resemble viral warts and it has been averred by some authorities[32] that they are clinically and histologically viral warts with trichilemmal differentiation. The lesions mostly occur on the nose and face but may occur in any other part of the body including the genital mucosa.

Box 20.9: Neoplasms with trichilemmal differentiation

- Trichilemmomas
- Desmoplastic trichilemmomas

Multiple trichilemmomas are most often associated with Cowden's syndrome, which also shows sclerotic fibromas and acrokeratosis verruciformis as associated skin findings. Cowden's syndrome is associated with adenocarcinomas affecting the breast, thyroid and gastrointestinal tract.

Trichilemmomas were first described by Headington[33] and histologically show nodular aggregates of pale outer root sheath cells with palisading of the outer layer of cells which rest on a thickened PAS positive basement membrane. Squamous eddies are frequent and there are broad connections to overlying epidermis or preexisting follicular infundibula. The surface may show verrucous hyperplasia with hypergranulosis resembling a viral wart **(Figures 20.17 to 20.19)**.

Desmoplastic Trichilemmomas

Desmoplastic trichilemmomas were described by Hunt, et al.[34] and usually occur as secondary tumors in nevus

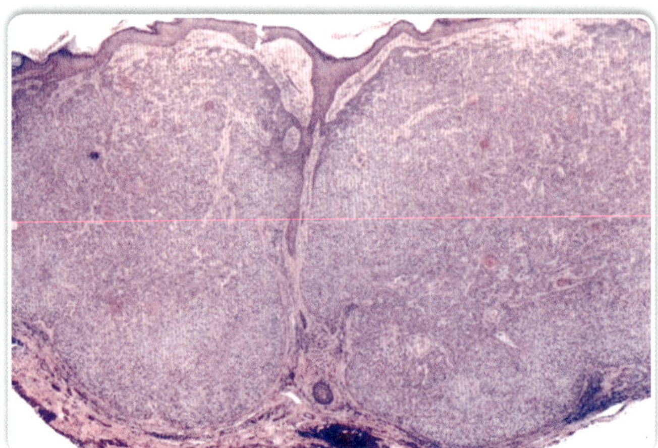

Fig. 20.17: Trichilemmoma showing nodular proliferation of pale cells arising from pre-existing hair follicle. H and E, 40x

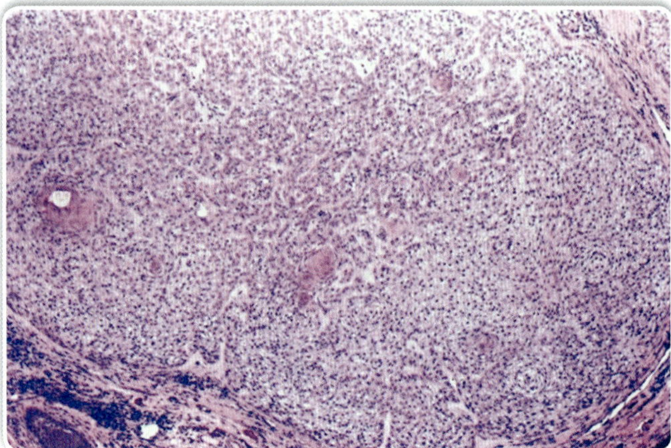

Fig. 20.18: Trichilemmoma, showing few ductal structures amidst pale outer root sheath cell. H and E, 100x

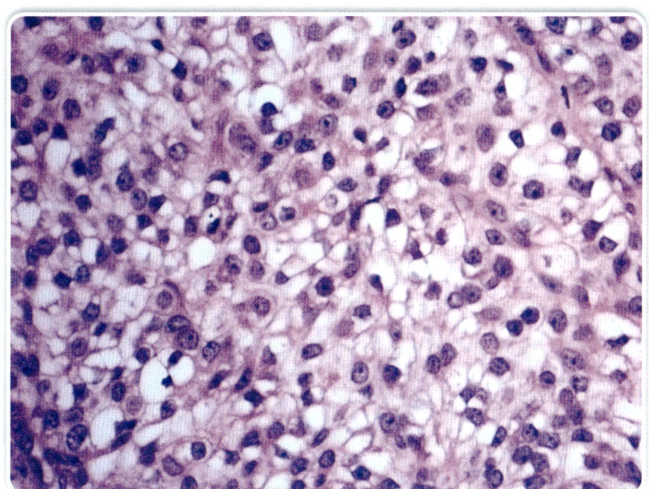

Fig. 20.19: Trichilemmoma with typical pale cells of outer root sheath differentiation. H and E, 400x

sebaceous. They histologically show the basic features of typical trichilemmomas, namely, pale cells that show peripheral palisading resting on a thickened basement membrane, however, in addition they also show marked fibrosis (desmoplasia) of the stroma that may insinuate between the cells causing strands of epithelial cells to be trapped by dense fibrous stroma. This may simulate malignant tumors especially squamous cell carcinoma. Absence of cytological atypia and mitotic activity and presence of typical clear outer root sheath like cells are the clues to a desmoplastic trichilemmoma.

Neoplasms with Upper Follicular Segment (Infundibulum and Isthmus) Differentiation (Box 20.10)

Isthmicoma [Tumor of Follicular Infundibulum (TFI) or Infundibuloma]

This tumor shows differentiation towards follicular isthmus and presents clinically as a flat or atrophic skin colored or hypopigmented plaque. Lesions are seen most often in elderly individuals and clinically two presentations have been described. Solitary lesions have no characteristic features and are usually incidental diagnoses where the biopsy was done to rule out a cutaneous malignancy. Multiple lesions have been described and may resemble pityriasis versicolor or superficial porokeratosis clinically.[35] The terms infundibulomas and infundibulomatosis have been used for the multiple eruptive presentation. An association with Cowden's syndrome has been reported.[36]

Box 20.10: Neoplasms with upper follicular segment differentiation

- Isthmicoma
- Trichoadenoma
- Proliferating trichilemmal cyst

Histologically the lesion was first described by Mehregan[37] and shows a plate like proliferation of pink keratinocytes arranged in a reticulate pattern in the upper dermis with connections to the overlying epidermis. The keratinocytes forming this entity are similar to the keratinocytes of the isthmus, of follicles in catagen and the cells of a isthmic-catagen cyst and have a pale pink cytoplasm and may show trichilemmal changes with pale cells resting on a thickened basement membrane. Deep sections often show connections between the pale staining, glycogen containing cells and the external root sheath of adjacent hair follicles **(Figures 20.20 to 20.22)**.

Other histological features described in TFI are eosinophilic cuticle, ductal differentiation, cornoid lamellae and desmoplasia.[38] Some authors consider TFI to be a

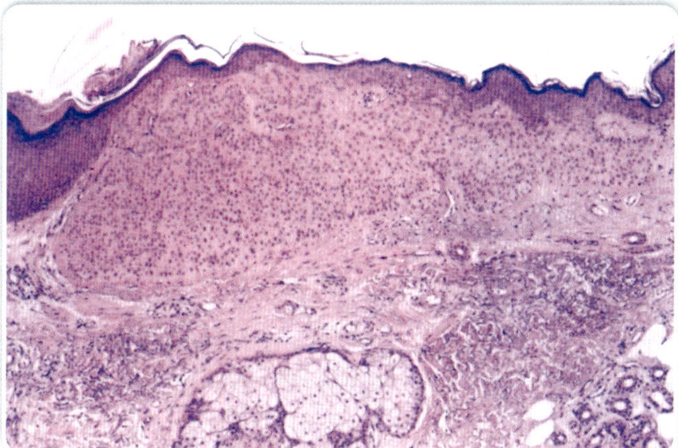

Fig. 20.20: Tumor of follicular infundibulum (TFI) with broad plate like proliferation of pale pink epithelium just beneath the epidermis. H and E, 10x

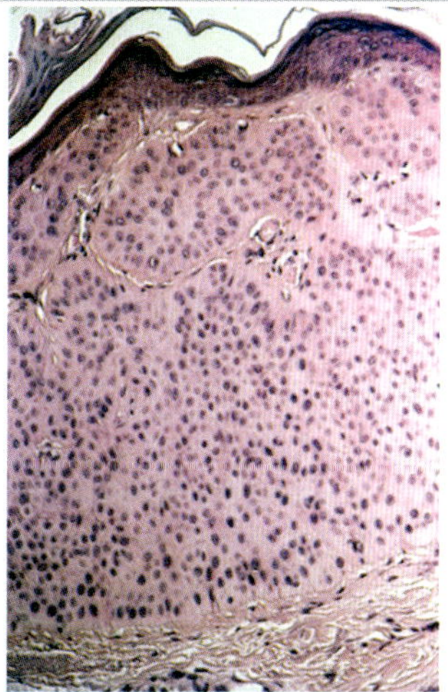

Fig. 20.21: Tumor of follicular infundibulum with epithelium connecting to overlying epidermis. H and E, 100x

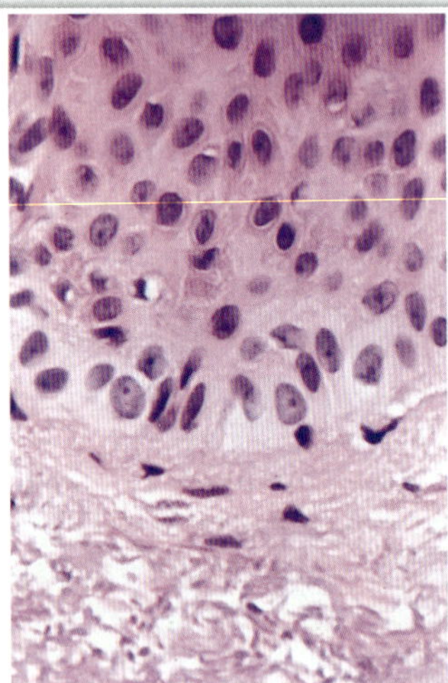

Fig. 20.22: Tumor of follicular infundibulum showing pale pink isthmic epithelial cells. H and E, 400x

variant expression of BCC rather than being a common association in skin biopsies.[39]

Trichoadenoma

Trichoadenoma of Nikolowski is a benign follicular neoplasm that consists of small cysts with infundibular and sometimes isthmic differentiation surrounded by stroma that is moderately sclerotic. The lesion usually occupies the upper dermis. Like in desmoplastic trichoepithelioma, strands of basaloid cells are seen traversing the sclerotic stroma and at times differentiation between the two entities may be difficult. In trichoadenoma, the cystic component predominates, and it has been suggested that it represents a cystic variant of desmoplastic trichoepithelioma.

Trichoadenoma is considered to be less mature than trichofolliculoma and more differentiated than a trichoepithelioma.[40]

Proliferating Trichilemmal Cyst (Tumor) PTC: (Proliferating Follicular-cystic Neoplasm)

Proliferating trichilemmal tumor has features of typical trichilemmal (pilar) cyst but also shows extensive irregular epithelial proliferations with variable cytologic atypia and high mitotic activity and in some cases has an aggressive biologic behavior. Malignant PTT may be considered when there is a combination of non-scalp location, history of recent rapid growth, size greater than 5 cms and infiltrative growth pattern with cytological atypia and high mitotic activity.[41]

Ackerman proposed the term proliferating follicular cystic neoplasm (PFCN) for what earlier was known as proliferating pilar cyst. This term encompasses a group of nodular and cystic tumors which show trichilemmal keratinization and occur most commonly on the scalp. It was suggested that a benign PFCN should be known as proliferating follicular-cystic acanthoma while a malignant PFCN should be called a proliferating follicular-cystic squamous cell carcinoma.[42]

Although considered to be benign, PFCN is known to simulate squamous cell carcinoma microscopically and local destructive behavior has been documented in several case reports.[43,44]

Clinically PFCN presents most commonly as a large nodule which may exceed 20 cms in diameter. The most common site is the scalp and it is seen more often in elderly women.

Histologically PFCN shows nodular and cystic areas in the deep dermis and subcutis. The cystic areas show isthmic keratinization with abrupt formation of laminated keratin without formation of keratohyaline granules. The keratinocytes have dense eosinophilic cytoplasm and few dyskeratotic cells may be seen. Other patterns of follicular keratinization like shadow cells of matrical differentiation may be seen. Focal calcification is often present and the stroma is sclerotic and may show foci of granulomatous inflammation.

Changes suggestive of malignant potential are lack of circumscription, prominent cytological atypia, extensive necrosis and numerous mitotic figures. This tumor is often a source of controversy because several authors affirm that all PTC are low grade squamous cell carcinomas.[45,46]

Tumors of the Perifollicular Fibrous Sheath (Box 20.11)

Fibrofolliculoma and Trichodiscoma are tumors that present clinically as small 1-3 mm skin colored papules mainly on the face or neck and may have a central hair. Lesions may be few or multiple and develop in middle age and persist.

Multiple lesions may be associated with the Birt-Hogg-Dube syndrome which is an autosomal dominant genodermatosis caused by mutations in the FLCN gene on chromosome 17p11, coding for the protein folliculin. Patients with this syndrome present with multiple fibrofolliculomas and run an increased risk for developing pneumothorax, renal tumors, colonic polyps and neural tumors.

Both fibrofolliculoma and trichodiscoma are believed to be different stages in the development of a single entity[3] and are hamartomas that may be related to the hair disc (Haarsheibe) as first proposed by Pinkus.[47] The Haarsheibe is a slowly adapting mechano-receptor in the perifollicular fibrous sheath.

Histological findings are of two types with combinations of the two in any given lesion.

Box 20.11: Tumors of the perifollicular fibrous sheath

- Fibrofolliculoma
- Trichodiscoma

At one end of the spectrum, *Fibrofolliculoma* presents with cords and strands of epithelial cells that radiate outwards from an infundibulum like structure. The epithelial cords may anastomose with each other and often show few sebocytes, a finding that prompted Ackerman to coin the term *Mantleoma* as he believed that the epithelial strands originated from mantles of atrophic sebaceous glands. The epithelial component is surrounded by proliferation of connective tissue of the perifollicular fibrous sheath along with some mucin.

The *Trichodiscoma* presents as a well demarcated, non-encapsulated tumor made up of mainly fascicles of fine fibrillary or slightly thick connective tissue with intervening mucinous ground substance. Fibrocytes are increased in numbers along with dilated and telangiectatic vessels. Located at the periphery may be epithelial structures resembling a fibrofolliculoma **(Figures 20.23 and 20.24)**.

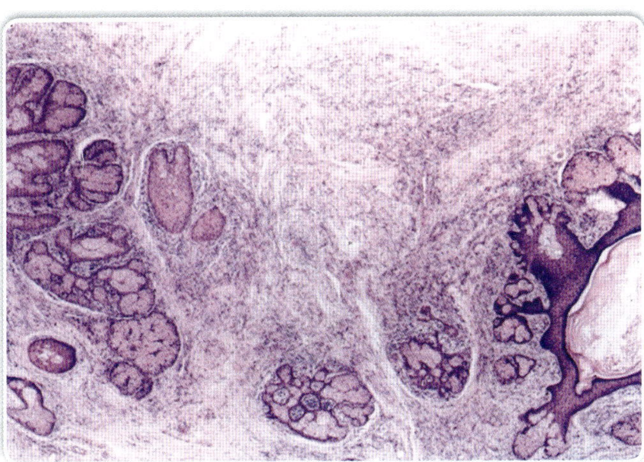

Fig. 20.23: Trichodiscoma, showing prominent connective tissue elements in the centre and fibro-folliculoma like structures at the periphery of the sections. H and E, 40x

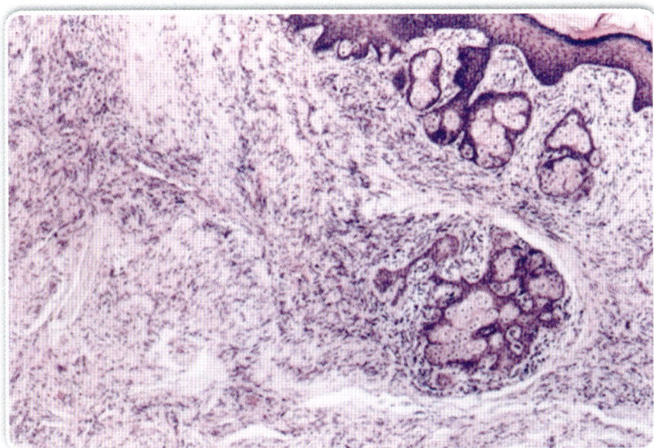

Fig. 20.24: Trichodiscoma showing closer view of the connective tissue proliferation. H and E, 100x

References

1. Headington JT. Tumors of the hair follicle: A review. Am J Pathol. 1976;85:479-514.
2. Rosen LB. A review and proposed new classification of benign acquired neoplasms with hair follicle differentiation. Am J Dermatopathol. 1990;12:496-516.
3. Ackerman AB, Reddy VB, Soyer HP. Neoplasms with follicular differentiation, 2nd edn. Ardor Scribendi, New York, 2001.
4. Ackerman AB, Boer A, Bennin B, Gottlieb G. Histologic diagnosis of inflammatory skin diseases: An algorithmic method based on pattern analysis, 3rd edn. 2005, New York, Ardor Scribendi. p 26.
5. Ackerman AB, De Viragh PA, Chongchitnant N. Hamartomas. In: Neoplasms with Follicular Differentiation. Philadelphia, Lea & Febiger publishers. 1993;169-204.
6. Labandeira J, Peteiro C, Toribio J. Hair follicle nevus: a case report and review of literature. Am J Dermatopathol. 1996;18:90-3.
7. Giam YC, Ong BH, Rajan VS. Nevus comedonicus in homozygous twins. Dermatologica. 1981;162:249-53.
8. Kofmann S. A case of rare localization and spreading of comedones. Arch Dermatol Syphilol. 1895;32:177-8.
9. Thibierge G. Naevus acneique unitateral en bandes et en plaques (naevus a comedons). Ann Dermatol Syphilol. 1896;7:1298.
10. Grimalt R, Caputo R. Post traumatic nevus comedonicus. J Am Acad Dermatol. 1993;28:273-4.
11. Abdel Al H, Abdel Aziz A. M. Nevus comedonicus. Report of three cases localized on glans penis. Acta Derm Venereol. 1975;55:78-80.
12. Schecter AK, Lester B, Pan TD, Robinson-Bostom L. Linear nevus comedonicus with epidermolytic hyperkeratosis. J Cutan Pathol. 2004;31:502-5.
13. Carlson JA, Cribier B, Nuovo G, Rohwedder A. Epidermodysplasia verruciformis-associated and genital-mucosal high risk human papillomavirus DNA are prevalent in nevus sebaceous of Jadassohn. J Am Acad Dermatol. 2008;59:279 94.
14. Jaqueti G, Requena L, Sanchez Yus E. Trichoblastoma is the most common neoplasm in nevus sebaceous of Jadassohn: a clinic-pathologic study of a series of 155 cases. Am J Dermatopathol. 2000;22:108-18.
15. Cribier B, Scrivener Y, Grosshans E. Tumors arising in nevus sebaceous: A study of 596 cases. J Am Acad Dermatol. 2000;42:263-8.
16. Barkhan MC, White N, Brundler MA, Richard B, Moss C. Should nevus sebaceous be excised prophylactically? A clinical audit. J Plast Reconstr Aesthet Surg. 2007;60:1269-70.
17. Schulz T, Hartschuh W. Folliculo-sebaceous cystic hamartoma is a trichofolliculoma at its very late stage. J Cutan Pathol. 1998;25:354-64.
18. Young AL, Kellermayer R, Szigeti R, Teszas A, Azmi S, Celebi J. T: CYLD mutations underlie Brooke-Spiegler, familial cylindromatosis and multiple familial trichoepithelioma syndromes. Clin Genet. 2006;70:246-9.
19. Heller J, Roche N, Hameed M.: Trichoepithelioma of the vulva: report of a case and review of the literature. J Low Genit Tract Dis. 2009;13:186-7.

20. Pham TT, Selim MA, Burchette JL Jr, Madden J, Turner J, Herman C. CD 10 expression in trichoepithelioma and basal cell carcinoma. J Cutan Pathol. 2006;33:123-8.
21. Urquhart JL, Weston WL. Treatment of multiple trichoepitheliomas with topical imiquimod and tretinoin. Pediatr Dermatol. 2005;22:67-70.
22. Takei Y, Fukushiro S, Ackerman AB. Criteria for histologic differentiation of desmoplastic trichoepithelioma (sclerosing epithelial hamartoma) from morphea-like basal cell carcinoma. Am J Dermatopathol. 1985;7:207-21.
23. Thewes M, Worret WI, Engst R, Ring J. Stromelysin-3: a potent marker for histopathologic differentiation between desmoplastic trichoepithelioma and morphea like basal cell carcinoma. Am J Dermatopathol. 1998;20:140-2.
24. Ackerman AB, Reddy VB, Soyer HP. Neoplasms with follicular differentiation, 2nd edn. 2001, New York: Ardor Scribendi.
25. Zaim MT. Immature trichoepithelioma. J Cutan Pathol. 1989;16:287-9.
26. Malherbe A, Chenantis J. Note sur l'epitheliomecalcifie des glandes sebacees. Prog Med. 1880;8:826-8.
27. Lever W, Griesemer RD. Calcifying epithelioma of Malherbe: report of 15 cases with comments on its differentiation from calcified epidermal cyst and on its histogenesis. Arch Dermatol. 1949;59:506-18.
28. Lazar AJ, Calonje E, Grayson W, et al . Pilomatrix carcinomas contain mutations in CTNNB1, the gene encoding beta-catenin. J Cutan Pathol. 2005;32:148-57.
29. Kaddu S, Soyer PH, Hodl S, Kerl H. Morphological stages of pilomatricoma. Am J Dermatopathol. 1996;18:333-8.
30. Tallon B, Cerroni L. Where pigmented pilomatricoma and melanocytic matricoma collide. Am J Dermatopathol. 2010;32:769-73.
31. Ambrojo P, Aguilar A, Simon P, Requena L, Sanchez Yus E. Basal cell carcinoma with matrical differentiation. Am J Dermatopathol. 1992;14:293-7.
32. Ackerman AB, Reddy VB, Soyer PH. Neoplasms with follicular differentiation. 2nd edn. 2001, New York: Ardor Scribendi. Pg 1109.
33. Headington JT, French AJ. Primary neoplasms of the hair follicle: histogenesis and classification. Arch Dermatol. 1962;86:430-1.
34. Hunt SJ, Kilzer B, Santa Cruz DJ. Desmoplastic trichilemmoma: histologic variant resembling invasive carcinoma. J Cutan Pathol. 1990;17:45-52.
35. Kossard S, Finley AG, Poyzer K, Kocsard E. Eruptive infundibulomas: A distinctive presentation of the tumour of follicular infundibulum. J Am Acad Dermatol. 1989;21:361-6.
36. Cribier B, Grosshans E. Tumour of the follicular infundibulum: A clinicopathologic study. J Am Acad Dermatol. 1995;33: 979-84.
37. Mehregan AH, Butler JD. A tumour of follicular infundibulum. Report of a case. Arch Dermatol. 1961;83:924-7.
38. Abbas O, Mahalingam M. Tumor of the follicular infundibulum: an epidermal reaction pattern? Am J Dermatopathol. 2009;31:626-33.
39. Weyers W, Horster S, Diaz-Cascajo C. Tumor of the follicular infundibulum is Basal cell carcinoma. Am J Dermatopathol. 2009;31:634-41.
40. Rahbari H, Mehregan A, Pinkus H. Trichoadenoma of Nikolowski. J Cutan Pathol. 1977;4:90-8.
41. Folpe AL, Reisenauer AK, Mentzel T, Rutten A, Solomon AR. Proliferating trichilemmal tumors: clinicopathologic evaluation is a guide to biologic behavior. J Cutan Pathol. 2003;30:492-8.
42. Ackerman AB, Reddy VB, Soyer HP. Neoplasma with follicular differentiation, 2nd edn. 2001; New York: Ardor Scribendi 1109.
43. Brownstein MH, Arluk DJ. Proliferating trichilemmal cyst: a stimulant of squamous cell carcinoma. Cancer. 1981;48:1207-14.
44. Lopez-Rios F, Fernando MD, Rodriguez-Peralto, Jose Luis, Aguilar A, Hernandez L, Gallego M. Proliferating trichilemmal cyst with focal invasion: report of a case and review of literature. Am J Dermatopathol. 2000;22:183-7.
45. Noto G, Pravata G, Arico M. Proliferating tricholemmal cyst should always be considered as a low grade carcinoma. Dermatology. 1997;194:374-5.
46. Mones JM, Ackerman AB. Proliferating trichilemmal cyst is squamous cell carcinoma. Dermatopathol Pract and Concept. 1998;4:295-310.
47. Pinkus H, Coskey R, Burgess G.H. Trichodiscoma: A benign tumor related to Haarscheibe (Hair disk). J Invest Dermatol. 1974;63:212-18.

21

Psychosomatic Hair Disorders

Smitha Prabhu, Sudhir Nayak UK, Shrutakirthi D Shenoi

"Biology gives you a brain, Life turns it into a mind."

—*Jeffery Eugenides*

Introduction

"Skin is the index of the mind", is an old adage. The skin and the brain have a common embryological origin from the neuroectoderm. The relation between skin and psyche is bidirectional. Acne, hirsutism, urticaria, pruritus, alopecia and herpes infection are some of the primary skin diseases with a high incidence of psychiatric comorbidity. Hair is one of the main appendages of the skin and the manifestations of the mind can be expressed in it too. On the other hand, loss of scalp hair leading to baldness can severely impact the psyche of the patient.

Psychotrichology is a sub-specialty of psychodermatology that deals with the relation between hair and psyche.

An arbitrary classification of psychotrichological disorders is given in **Table 21.1**.

Primary Psychotrichological Conditions

Scalp Dysesthesia

Scalp dysesthesia is a mucocutaneous pain syndrome characterized by altered sensation over the scalp in the absence of any primary cutaneous disorder or systemic illness and objective findings.

Trichoesthesia is a feeling that one's hair has been touched, caused by the stimulation of the hair follicle receptor.[1]

Trichodynia refers to the dysesthesia perceived in hair (root of hair) especially subsequent to touch of hair, whereas scalp dysesthesia is perceived on the scalp skin.

Table 21.1: Classification of psychotrichological disorders

Primary psychotrichological	Scalp dysesthesia Trichoesthesia Trichodynia Trichotillomania Trichotemnomania Trichoteiromania Trichophobia Pseudoeffluvium
Primary trichological with secondary psychological impact	Androgenetic alopecia Telogen effluvium
Multifactorial/miscellaneous diseases affecting the scalp	Alopecia areata Scalp psoriasis Lichen planus Seborrheic dermatitis Discoid lupus erythematosus Vitiligo Prurigo/lichen simplex chronicus

It is believed that the dysesthesia occurs on the scalp which then subsequently appears projected on the hairs.[2,3]

The exact etiology is unknown and is considered to be multifactorial. Significant association between telogen effluvium and androgenetic alopecia has been seen.[4]

Scalp dysesthesias are common in females and may be associated with somatoform pain disorder, generalized anxiety disorder, depression and conversion disorder.[5]

Substance P and other neuropeptides have been implicated in the causation of scalp dysesthesia.[5]

Patients with diffuse hair fall with psychological stress may also report trichodynia.

Differential Diagnosis (Box 21.1)

Investigations: Dermatoscopy shows irregular arrangement of telangiectatic vessels.[6] Patch testing with standard series and psychological assessment may be done.

Box 21.1: Differential diagnosis for scalp dysesthesia

- Giant cell arteritis
- Migraine
- Post-herpetic neuralgia
- Tension headache
- Contact dermatitis to topical applications

Treatment: Treatment of any underlying primary psychiatric problem is the corner stone of treatment. In the absence of any underlying primary cause various drugs like gabapentin, amitriptyline, doxepin, imipramine, fluoxetine may be tried. Doxepin may be tried for itchy scalp.

Trichotillomania

Trichotillomania is the best example of dermatitis parae artefacta syndrome or impulse control disorder.[7] It may also be viewed as an anxiety disorder.

Definition: This is an impulse control disorder characterized by an irresistible urge to pull hair, which subsides subsequent to the action of pulling the hair.

The revised DSM-IV criteria for the diagnosis of trichotillomania are

1. Recurrent pulling out of one's own hair resulting in hair loss
2. An increasing sense of tension immediately before pulling out the hair or when attempting to resist the behavior
3. Pleasure, gratification or relief when pulling out the hair
4. The disturbance is not better accounted for by any other mental disorder
5. The disturbance provokes clinically marked distress and/or impairment in occupational, social or other areas of functioning.

Dysfunction in the dopaminergic and serotonergic functions, disorganization of white matter tracts involved in motor habit generation and suppression have been implicated in trichotillomania.[8]

Clinical features: Two peaks of age are noticed in trichotillomania, the first in childhood (5–12 years) and the other in adults. The childhood phase tends to involve boys whereas the adult phase, females.[9] It usually presents with patchy alopecia over scalp predominantly on the dominant hand side. Involvement of eyebrows, upper eyelashes, pubis, torso and extremities may also be seen.[10] Children generally admit to hair pulling, whereas adults tend to conceal **(Figure 21.1 and Table 21.2).**

Clinically 3 zones may be seen:

- Zone-1: Long normal or unaffected hair in the periphery
- Zone-2: Alopecia with scattered hemorrhages
- Zone-3: Short regrowing hairs which are too short to be grasped and pulled. Trichogram shows a reduced proportion of telogen hairs.[7]

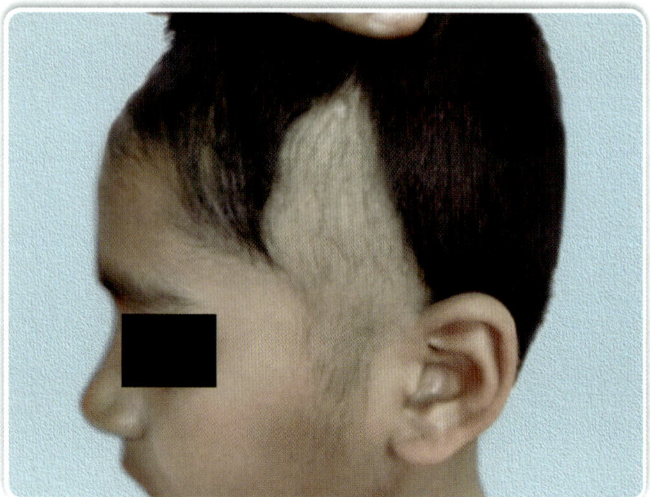

Fig. 21.1: Trichotillomania
(*Courtesy:* Department of Dermatology, STD and Leprosy, BMCRI, Bengaluru)

Table 21.2: Differences between childhood and adult trichotillomania

Childhood	Adult
Onset at 5–12 years	Onset in adults
More common in boys	Common in females
Children generally admit to hair pulling	Adults tend to conceal
Associated with nail biting, thumb sucking, skin and nose picking, anxiety, dysthymia, learning disability and iron deficiency	Associated with anxiety, sexual and physical abuse, body image changes, school difficulties, parental disturbance, depression, anxiety, obsessive-compulsive disorder
Responsive to psychotherapy alone	Needs to be treated both with psychotherapy and pharmacotherapy

Trichotemnomania: This is a type of malingering in which the hair is deliberately cut to simulate hair damage.

Trichoteiromania is a terminology which is used to describe the condition of alopecia which occurs secondary to rubbing of hair rather than pulling. Patient tends to produce pseudo-alopecia by scratching or rubbing the scalp. Clinically alopecia can be seen and the hair tips are whitish with split ends. Hair shafts are of different lengths.[11] Light microscopic examination of the hair reveals trichoptilosis or brush like hair breaks. Trichogram tends to show dystrophic hairs sometimes with reduced proportion of telogen hairs.[7] Dermatoscopy shows coiled fractured short hairs and trichomalacia and this is considered to be diagnostic.[11]

Trichoteiromania is usually associated with sensory disorders of the scalp.[12]

Trichopathophobia (trichophobia): It is a fear of hair.[13] Trichophobia is a delusion and the term used to describe the plucking of hair with the purpose of removing something from the root.[12]

Trichomalacia is a terminology used when the injured follicles tend to produce soft twisted hair instead of the usual coarse hair.[14]

In some patients trichotillomania may be accompanied by trichophagia, which is a form of a pica characterized by a habit of eating hair. This may lead to the formation of trichobezoar which is the presence of balls of hair in the stomach or intestines.[15]

Associations: Childhood trichotillomania is often associated with nail biting, thumb sucking, skin and nose picking, anxiety, dysthymia, learning disability and iron deficiency. The adult trichotillomania is associated with anxiety, sexual and physical abuse, body image changes, school difficulties, parental disturbance, depression, anxiety, obsessive-compulsive disorder.[9] Other conditions which have been associated include lip biting, nose picking, acne excoriee and cheek chewing. Panic attacks and substance abuse have also been demonstrated.[10]

Complications (Box 21.2)

Differential diagnosis: Alopecia areata, non-inflammatory tinea capitis. Myxedematous alopecia, alopecia mucinosa, traumatic alopecia, alopecia syphilitica.[10] Benign hair pulling is associated with thumb sucking and hair pulling in children.[16]

Investigations: The diagnosis is primarily clinical. Scalp biopsy can be done which tends to show normally growing hair along with empty follicles without any signs of inflammation.[17] The empty follicles may contain soft keratin or deformed hair. Perifollicular hemorrhages can also be sometimes seen. The biopsy may help in convincing parents of children who refuse to believe that their ward suffers from trichotillomania.[14] Follicular plugging and keratin debris may be seen. Trichoscopy shows broken hairs of varying lengths **(Figure 21.2)**. Dermoscopic trichogram shows absence of telogen hair and presence of catagen and anagen hairs with ruptured hair root sheaths.[17] In trichobezoars, barium contrast meals, CT scans and gastric endoscopy may be done.[9]

Box 21.2: Complications of trichotillomania

- Common
  - Secondary folliculitis
  - Psychosocial problems
- Rare
  - Intestinal obstruction
  - Death due to trichobezoar
  - Shoulder and back pain due to abnormal hair pulling postures[10]
  - Carpal tunnel syndrome due to action of repeated pulling of hair[14]
  - Blepharitis
  - Avoidance of health care due to shame[10]

Treatment: Complete response to any treatment modality is often not seen. Both pharmacological and nonpharmacological measures have found benefit in the treatment of trichotillomania. Children are usually responsive to psychotherapy alone. Adults on the other hand need to be treated both with psychotherapy and pharmacotherapy. Patients with comorbid disorders are better treated with drugs which tend to address both the conditions. The

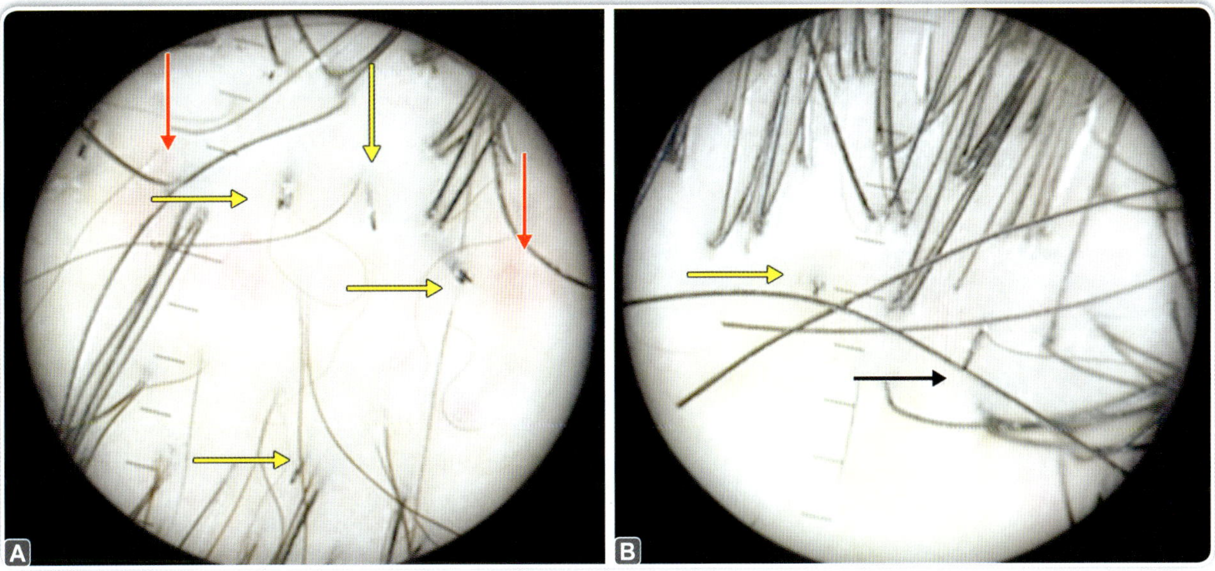

Figs 21.2A and B: (A) Dermoscopic appearance of trichotillomania of child in Fig. 21.2A. Broken hair shaft (yellow arrows) and perifollicular erythema (Red arrows) (B) Broken hairs (yellow arrows) and terminal hair follicles without anisometry of hair shafts. (*Courtesy:* Department of Dermatology, BMCRI, Bengaluru)

various pharmacological drugs which have found benefit in the management of trichotillomania are clomipramine, desipramine, fluoxetine, naltrexone and olanzapine. Other drugs which have found benefit in the management include buspirone, clonazepam, pimozide (in combination with SSRIs), lithium and trazodone,[18] dronabinol, aripiprazole[8] and mirtazapine.[10] Pharmacologic pain sensitizers like capsaicin have been also used. This tends to increase the usually perceived sensation; thereby the patient becomes aware whenever he/she tries to play with hair.[16]

The various psychotherapy procedures of benefit in the management include habit reversal, stimulus control, self-monitoring, awareness training, competing response training, covert sensitization, aversion, negative practice, relaxation techniques, overcorrection and biofeedback.[18] Dialectical behavior therapy- enhanced habit reversal therapy (DBT-HRT) has shown long term results in trichotillomania.[8] Hypnotherapy can be tried as adjuvant treatment **(Table 21.3)**.[10]

Table 21.3: Treatment of trichotillomania

Pharmacotherapy	*Psychotherapy*
Clomipramine	Habit reversal
Desipramine	Stimulus control
Fluoxetine	Self-monitoring
Naltrexone	Awareness training
Olanzapine	Competing response training
Buspirone	Covert sensitization
Clonazepam	Aversion
Pimozide	Negative practice
Lithium	Relaxation techniques
Trazodone	Biofeedback
Dronabinol	Dialectical behavior therapy
Aripiprazole	Hypnotherapy
Mirtazapine	

Primary Trichological Condition with Secondary Psychological Impact

Pseudoeffluvium (Alopecia Phobia)[19]

Psychogenic pseudoeffluvium is the terminology which is used to describe the fear or conviction of hair loss or baldness occurring in patients in whom no objective evidence of hair loss is seen.[12] Alopecia per se is associated with loss of self-esteem, depression, introversion and neuroticism.

This can be a manifestation of either depression or delusion.[12]

Pseudoeffluvium is commonly reported in the females. This is especially more common among students (personal observation). However, an increase in incidence in single young men is reported.[2] In women pseudoeffluvium is often associated with a belief of developing severe baldness resembling male pattern baldness.

Psychotherapy and treatment of any underlying psychiatric condition (if any) is required.[5]

Androgenetic Alopecia (AGA)

Hair loss in either males or females is associated with low self-esteem, feeling of unattractiveness, helplessness, introversion, neuroticism (excessive emotional lability, nervousness, hypersensitivity, anxiety and excitability) and occasionally depression.[2] These are especially seen when pronounced alopecia occurs at a younger age. Hair plays a vital role in socio-sexual communication. Balding scalp and hirsute face play a major role in the psyche of an individual.

AGA or pattern baldness is a progressive non-cicatricial alopecia which occurs in genetically predisposed men and women. The four factors that determine AGA are susceptibility to AGA, age of onset, pattern of progression and rate of progression.[20]

In 90% of males, by the age of 20 years, the pre-pubertal straight hairline is replaced by some degree of recession.[20] The earliest sign of AGA is recession of the frontal hairline and recession of hair at the temples. This is followed by progressive backward recession and thinning at the vertex. Earlier onset and faster rate of progression is often associated with peer criticism which in some individuals can lead to social withdrawal and depression. Early onset AGA tends to progress by one to two stages each decade, whereas late onset AGA may progress by a single stage in two decades.[20] Sometimes a pattern of diffuse hair loss with preservation of hairline is encountered in some men simulating Ludwig's classification of hair loss.[21]

Female pattern AGA is graded by the 3 point Ludwig scale, 5 point Sinclair scale, Olsen scale and occasionally the Hamilton-Norwood scale.[21]

Hair follicle miniaturization and progressive replacement of terminal hair by the vellus hair due to shortening of the anagen phase and elongation of the telogen phase summarizes the pathogenesis of AGA. Miniaturization of the entire follicle unit only leads to the appearance of baldness.[22]

The psychological effect of baldness is often noticed in individuals with early onset, faster rate of progression, later stages of Hamilton-Norwood scale and those who perceive it to be socially noticeable.[20] There are studies examining the social impact of baldness in men. The number of life time sexual partners was less in bald men than non-bald men with identical libido. Digitally altered photographs for job application to create baldness resulted in lesser interview calls in the altered photographs in comparison to the non-altered. Decreased attractiveness of bald men was noted among women and non-bald men, more so among women.[20] AGA can sometimes affect the quality of life of an individual.[23] The quality of life in females with AGA was less than women without hair loss.[22] Baldness in women as a result of AGA is occasionally considered as a sign of loss of feminity.

Sketches of bald men have been variously described as weak, inactive, unkind, bad, ugly, hard, less potent, stable as well as intelligent. Peer teasing was reported by 45% and 79% of men with moderate and extensive hair loss respectively. Loss of hair in men is associated with belief of decreased chance of romance but not employability.[23]

Women with AGA have lower self-esteem, psychological adjustment issues and poorer social adequacy than women without AGA or men with AGA. Women with AGA also tend to have more emotional stress due to hair loss, negative body image, social anxiety, externalization and take more efforts to adjust with AGA. Psychological well-being and self-esteem and satisfaction are also low.[23]

Hair loss is often blamed for other social inadequacies and lack of contentment. Individuals with AGA tend to avoid situations which tend to make baldness more evident like wet, windy climates and brightly lit environment. Individuals with baldness tend to resort to compensatory mechanisms like growing of facial hair or paradoxically shaving the scalp bald.[23]

Treatment: Individuals with AGA seeking treatment are often more distressed than those AGA patients not seeking treatment.[23] The most important step in the management of AGA is counseling. A patient not only has to be counseled about the disease, but also about the various treatment modalities available. Various medical, surgical and cosmetic approaches exist in the management of AGA. The medical line of management includes topical minoxidil which is the cornerstone of therapy. Other topical agents which have been incorporated along with minoxidil for better efficacy include azelaic acid, tretinoin, finasteride and occasionally steroids. Ketoconazole shampoos have also been used as an adjuvant in view of the antiandrogen effect of ketoconazole. Oral medications include finasteride and dutasteride (in men and post-menopausal women), cyproterone acetate, oral contraceptive pills, spironolactone and flutamide (in women). Cosmetic therapy includes alteration of hair style so as to cover or mask the baldness, tinted hair sprays and hair pieces, extensions and wigs. The surgical management for AGA is usually reserved for the advanced stages and these include scalp reduction, hair weaving, and follicular unit hair transplantation. The most important factor in the medical line of approach lies in the compliance with treatment. Patients need to be counseled on the importance of compliance with treatment. Regular application of topical preparations and consumption of oral medicines on an everyday basis is difficult on a long-term basis. The initial improvement with regular medication is often associated with cessation of treatment or irregularity in treatment.

Compliance and adherence to therapy is probably the most important psychological management of AGA. Further psychological interventions in AGA are usually reserved for those who present with severe distress in view of the baldness or those who tend to exaggerate their condition. The role of psychology in the treatment of AGA is best exemplified by the mention in the editorial review in the international journal of trichology.[24] Improvement of the alopecia by medical, surgical and sometimes even the cosmetic approach can help in improving the mood and quality of life in patients with AGA.

Telogen Effluvium

Telogen effluvium is the loss of telogen hair and is usually noticed 3–4 months after a stressful event and regrowth tends to occur in 6–7 months. Sometimes this can occur as chronic pattern with fluctuations over years.[14]

It presents with generalized and diffuse loss of scalp hair, but not sufficient enough to cause visible baldness.[20] Examination of hair by atomic emission spectrometer and mass spectral spectrometer have shown deficiencies of magnesium, phosphorus, sulfur, calcium, chromium, molybdenum, manganese, copper, zinc and selenium.

No specific therapy exists for telogen effluvium. In acute telogen effluvium the recovery is usually complete in 6–7 months. However chronic telogen effluvium tends to have a prolonged course and the main approach to treatment in these patients would be reassurance to the fact that one will never be bald.[14] Reduction of stress is an important step in the management of telogen effluvium.

Multifactorial Diseases Affecting the Scalp

Alopecia Areata (Syn: Pelade, Area Celsi)[25-27]

Alopecia areata (AA) is a common disorder of immunological pathogenesis mediated by T cells, wherein there is a rapid onset of patchy rounded or oval shaped hair loss in single or multiple foci.

Clinical features: The patches are 1–5 cm in diameter, non-inflammatory and non-atrophic in nature, and a few resting hair may be found within the patches. Paresthesia and erythema may be initially present. Gray hair may be spared **(Refer to Chapter 10)**.

Exclamation point hair: These are characteristically seen at the periphery of the patches. These hair have a small, non-pigmented bulb and a tapering shaft which is fractured and flattened towards the extremity. This is because of the inflammation of the hair matrix causing tapering of hair shaft and fracture to anagen hair. As the hair converts from anagen to telogen, the lower portion rises up in the scalp, finally resulting in the exclamation point appearance.

Coudability sign: In AA, a normal looking hair kinks at about 5–10 mm above the surface if bent or pressed inwards. This is because the seemingly unaffected terminal hair within a patch have one or more constrictions in their shaft.

In 10%, especially in chronic cases, the nails are involved and characteristic uniform pits are formed arranged transversely and longitudinally, the so called *Glen Plaid or Scotch Plaid pattern*. The other nail changes include trachyonychia, onychomadesis and red or spotted lunulae.

Clinical Classification

Ikeda's classification **(Box 21.3)**:

a. *Common type (81%):* Fast progressing form affecting adults without any predisposing factors. Spontaneous regrowth in upto 3 years' time is the norm.
b. *Atopic type (10%):* Starts in childhood and slowly progresses. Seen in atopics. Ophiatic and reticular patterns common.
c. *Autoimmune type (5%):* Affects adults, may be associated with other autoimmune disorders like diabetes mellitus.
d. *Prehypertensive type (4%):* Occurs in adolescents or young adults who have hypertensive parents. Fast progress may lead to total alopecia. Reticular pattern is common.

Course

White hairs are usually spared, so also nevoid conditions like melanocytic nevi or hemangiomatous areas. During regrowth, the new hair are usually depigmented and fine, and gradually become thicker and darker. Regrowth first occurs at the center, then at periphery. Sometimes areas of hair loss and regrowth may coexist.

Other Associations

Alopecia areata is associated with a higher incidence of other autoimmune diseases like thyroiditis, diabetes mellitus, SLE, vitiligo, myasthenia gravis, pernicious anemia, atopic dermatitis, Down syndrome and lichen planus **(Box 21.4)**.

Box 21.3: Ikeda's classification of alopecia areata

- Common (71%)
- Atopic (10%)
- Autoimmune (5%)
- Prehypertensive (4%)

Box 21.4: Autoimmune associations in alopecia areata

- Endocrine: Hashimoto's thyroiditis, Addison's disease, diabetes mellitus
- Dermatological conditions: Vitiligo, lichen planus, morphea, lichen sclerosus et atrophicus
- Autoimmune disorders: Systemic lupus erythematosus, Sjögren's syndrome, autoimmune hemolytic anemia
- Inflammatory bowel disorders: Ulcerative colitis
- Pernicious anemia
- Myasthenia gravis
- Chronic mucocutaneous candidiasis with endocrinopathy

***Differential diagnosis*:** Common type should be differentiated from other causes of patchy hair loss like traumatic alopecia, pseudopelade, congenital triangular alopecia, hamartomas, etc. Diffuse and total alopecia areata has to be differentiated from conditions like androgenetic alopecia, telogen effluvium, anagen effluvium, and folliculitis decalvans **(Refer to Table 10.2)**.

Trichogram reveals raised telogen count without dystrophic hair and anagen hair of varying thickness.

Psychosocial Aspects of AA

This condition does not discriminate between the sexes or ages and may be a cause for considerable anguish. The affected person, especially a female may not be able to cope with the drastic changes, especially if the patches are multiple, large and are enlarging day by day. Though hair on any part of the body may be affected, and even nails develop a peculiar pattern of stippling, scalp hair loss and to some extent beard and moustache area loss in males are the chief causes for mental distress, not only to the patient, but also to other close family members in many instances. It may adversely affect the performance in school and at work place, though the patient is in no way physically impaired. The reaction to the disease may vary from person to person and the National Alopecia Areata Foundation, USA has described reactions to the disease under various headings **(Table 21.4)**.[28] If such feelings are especially intense or overwhelming and are negatively impacting the patient's life, psychological counseling should be sought. Counseling will go a long way in focusing on the problem in a positive way and alopecia areata support foundations help in providing chances for interaction with others who suffer from the same problem and thereby provide a conducive environment for mental healing. The negative psychosocial impact of alopecia areata can be alleviated to some extent by interaction with therapists, work groups, psychologists, or support groups leading to group or individual therapy. Studies on the benefits of hypnosis in alopecia areata in patients with refractory disease showed that it could significantly ameliorate alexithymia, anxiety,

Table 21.4: Psychological reactions to alopecia areata in self or family member

- Withdrawal, isolation and loneliness
- Loss and grief
- Fear of others finding about the disease or attempts to hide it by wearing wigs and toupees
- Sadness and depression
- Hopelessness
- Anger
- Embarrassment
- Guilt or self-blame that one has somehow brought upon the disease on oneself, and guilt related to how one's disease is affecting other family members
- Frantic and extreme search for an answer or cure
- For parents, guilt that they may have genetically contributed to their child's disease and helplessness of not able to stop the disease progression or allay their child's fear and anxiety
- For siblings and other close relatives, shame and anger that the disease has affected their lives too

depression and provide mental well-being; these effects were maintained upto 6 months post hypnotherapy.[29,30] Further, as Paus and Arck have concluded, stress can precipitate alopecia areata via the neuroendocrine stress response pathway involving Substance P, nerve growth factor and mast cells which lead to perifollicular neurogenic inflammation causing premature induction of catagen phase in murine models, which they say can be extrapolated to humans.[31] An observational study done in India has revealed that socioeconomic factors and stress play a pivotal role in initiation as well as persistence of the lesions.[32]

Treatment

Though many cases of alopecia areata heal spontaneously, treatment is desirable as an early regrowth can minimalize the psychosocial problems in the sufferer. There are variable treatment modalities, most leading to unpredictable outcomes. Treatment should be chosen based on the merits and demerits of individual case taking into consideration age of the patient and type of the disease.

Topical modalities include immunosuppressants and immunomodulators like topical steroids, tacrolimus, contact sensitizers like diphencyprone, SADBE, irritants like dithranol, phenol, salicylic acid, cantharidin, and topical retinoids.

Phototherapy using psoralens have been tried. Excimer laser therapy and pulsed infrared diode laser therapy are newer modalities.

Systemic agents include immunosuppressants and modulators like systemic corticosteroids, sulfasalazine.

In patients with psychosocial problems supportive therapy including psychotherapy and psychiatric evaluation is a must. A holistic approach using mind relaxing methods like progressive muscle relaxation, yoga and hypnosis may help.

Scalp Psoriasis[33]

More than 50% of psoriasis patients have lesions on the scalp, which vary in intensity. Severe and long standing scalp psoriasis can lead to considerable amount of hair loss, which can lead to mental anguish. The factors leading to hair loss are given in **Box 21.5**.

Clinically, thick erythematous scaly coalescent plaques as well as diffuse scaling are seen. The plaques may extend beyond the scalp margins giving rise to 'Corona psoriatica'.

It has to be differentiated from severe seborrheic dermatitis of the scalp, where yellow greasy scales are more prominent; tinea amiantacea, where cement like crusting entrapping the hair occurs due to various scaling disorders of the scalp which are neglected and; non-inflammatory tinea capitis like gray patch and black dot variants. Scrapings from the scalp or plucked hair from the involved area may reveal fungal filaments on KOH examination in tinea capitis, whereas in psoriasis of the scalp, examination of other parts of the body may show characteristic psoriatic plaques.

Psoriasis, especially if there are lesions in visible body sites like scalp, is associated with various psychological morbidities like anxiety, depression, poor self-esteem and suicidal tendencies in 5% patients.[34] There is a definite decrease in health related quality of life with negative impact on psychological, occupational and social behavior.[35] The impaired quality of life in psoriatics is supposed to be equal to or worse than in other chronic diseases like ischemic heart disease and diabetes.[36]

There is a feeling of stigmatization in psoriatics which includes 'anticipation of rejection, feeling flawed, sensitivity to others' attitudes, guilt, shame and secretiveness'.[37] Various Indian studies on clinical severity, psychosocial morbidity and stress revealed that psoriasis had adverse impact on daily activities and employment and that sufferers often felt self-conscious, inconvenienced by the shedding of scales, tended to avoid social interaction and lived in fear of relapse.[38]

Decreased work efficiency and impairment in interpersonal relationships in upto 67% cases was also seen.[39] One study has found 24.7% psychiatric morbidity in the form of adjustment disorder, dysthymia and depression **(Box 21.6)**.[40]

Treatment: Scalp treatment must be diligently undertaken until the disease is controlled, which may be as long as 8–12 weeks. Patient should be reassured that hair loss is only temporary, and hair will regrow after proper control of the

Box 21.5: Causes for hair loss in psoriasis

- Forceful removal of scales
- Harsh topical treatment
- Frequent scratching
- Mental stress—causes hair to enter telogen stage quickly and prolongs the telogen phase

Box 21.6: Psychological morbidity associated with psoriasis

- Adjustment disorder
- Anticipation of rejection
- Anxiety
- Avoid social interaction
- Decreased work efficiency
- Depression
- Dysthymia
- Fear of relapse
- Feeling flawed
- Guilt, shame
- Impairment in interpersonal relationships
- Inconvenienced by the shedding of scales
- Poor self esteem
- Self-conscious
- Sensitivity to others' attitudes
- Suicidal tendencies

disease. Adjuvants like multivitamin pills, iron capsules and antidandruff shampoos may be tried in the meanwhile.

Regular shampooing with salicylic acid-coal tar shampoos, topical steroid salicylic acid combination lotion, topical coal tar, pomade, topical anthralin in varying concentrations and contact periods, topical calcipotriene and tazarotene may be used singly or in combinations. For thick scales, scale softeners like salicylic acid, lactic acid, urea and phenol may have to be applied overnight and shampooed off the next morning. Oils and creams applied overnight also act as good scale softeners. Scales can then be removed using fine toothed combs or brushes used in a circular motion. Vigorous removal of scales may lead to secondary infection or even worsening of psoriasis via Koebner response.

Other modalities include topical or systemic PUVA (Psoralen with UVA light), narrow band UVB light therapy and use of systemic agents like methotrexate and biologicals when warranted. Secondary bacterial and fungal infections should be treated with respective oral antimicrobials.

Hair loss due to scalp psoriasis will improve once the disease is controlled. However, protein and multivitamin supplements, mild exfoliating shampoos and hair oil may be used as adjuvants.

In patients with significant depression or anxiety, psychological or psychiatric intervention is necessary for overall improvement.

Lichen Planus (LP)[41,42]

Lichen planus may involve the scalp hair, as in case of lichen planopilaris (LPP) and Graham Little Piccardi syndrome.

Lichen planopilaris (follicular LP) presents as tiny erythematous to pigmented spiny follicular papules affecting a group of hair follicles which may cause permanent scarring alopecia. Rarely, if the inflammation is severe, blistering may occur. In some cases, there is no follicular papules, but a slowly progressive, irregularly shaped scarring alopecia may occur which gives to a clinical impression of 'footprints in snow'. If the cause is not known, this is called as pseudopelade of Brocq.

Graham Little Piccardi Lasseur syndrome consists of a triad of multifocal cicatricial alopecia of the scalp, non-scarring alopecia of axilla and groin and a follicular LP eruption on the body with or without scalp involvement.[41]

Frontal fibrosing alopecia, which leads to scarring alopecia of the frontal region, and which is more common in African races, is also considered to be a type of LPP.

Differential diagnoses includes DLE lesions of the scalp, wherein depigmented scaly atrophic plaques with the characteristic carpet tack sign and peripheral hyperpigmentation are seen, along with DLE lesions at other characteristic sites like malar area, pinna and chest. Pseudopelade, an end stage scarring alopecia due to varying unknown causes is another important differential diagnosis, which clinically reveals alopecia resembling 'foot prints in the snow'.

Since scalp is a cosmetologically prominent area, this condition can have major psychological repercussions in the patient.

Treatment: Follicular LP eruptions usually respond well to medical treatment, but cicatricial alopecia of scalp is permanent and progressive, may lead to considerable mental anguish. Such patients may be advised methods like hair bonding.

Seborrheic Dermatitis

Seborrheic dermatitis is a common endogenous eczema seen in the pubertal and adult age groups, in both sexes and presents as asymptomatic to itchy, flaky scaling of scalp in mild to moderate cases and with thick greasy yellowish crusted scales in severe cases. It is supposed to be a hypersensitivity reaction to the presence of the fungus *Pityrosporum ovale* on the scalp. The associated inflammation and scratching may lead to temporary hair loss.

It has to be differentiated from scalp psoriasis **(Refer to Table 9.3**).

Though a relatively common disease, there are studies which prove that psychological stressors precipitate as well as perpetuate the condition. Depression and anxiety are common in such people.[43,44]

Treatment is by eliminating the fungal colonization and reducing inflammation.

In mild to moderate cases, topical treatment will suffice. Topical medications used in seborrheic dermatitis, either alone or in combinations are given in **Table 21.5**.

The topical shampoos are to be lathered and left on the scalp for 5–10 minutes at a time, on daily or alternate day basis till the disease is controlled and then the frequency

Table 21.5: Topical medications for seborrheic dermatitis

1	Antifungal agents in shampoo or lotion base	a. Azoles – clotrimazole, fluconazole, ketoconazole, oxiconazole, bifonazole b. Cyclopiroxolamine c. Terbinafine d. Miscellaneous – selenium sulfide 2.5%, zinc pyrithione 1%
2	Antiproliferative agents	a. Salicylic acid 3-6% b. Coal tar
3	Anti-inflammatory agents	Topical steroids – flucinolone, betamethasone dipropionate, desonide, mometasone furoate, clobetasol propionate, fluticasone dipropionate

may be reduced to once or twice a week. The lotions may be left on the scalp overnight.

In severe cases, a course of oral antifungals or even a short course of oral steroids are tried. In recurrent and unresponsive cases oral isotretinoin, a potent sebum inhibitor may be given at the dosage of 0.25–0.5 mg/kg body weight/day for 6 months.

The hair loss associated with seborrheic dermatitis recovers spontaneously once the inflammation has subsided. However adjuvants like multivitamin preparations including biotin, calcium pantothenate and zinc, adding iron supplements in patients with anemia may help to some extent.

Discoid Lupus Erythematosus (DLE)

DLE is the chronic subtype of lupus erythematosus, a connective tissue disease, and can lead to scarring alopecia as it affects the lower portion of the hair follicles. The lesions commonly involve scalp, face, upper extremities and sun exposed areas **(Figures 21.3 and 21.4)**.

Clinically, DLE presents as a scaly erythematous to pigmented plaque with follicular plugging and central atrophy with peripheral hyperpigmentation. Large, coalescing patches can be quite disfiguring leading to considerable psychosocial embarrassment.

Differential diagnoses include other causes for scarring alopecia like follicular lichen planus, trauma or tick bite alopecia. Presence of typical lesions in other parts of the body, especially in the pinnae are a clue to diagnosis in atypical cases.

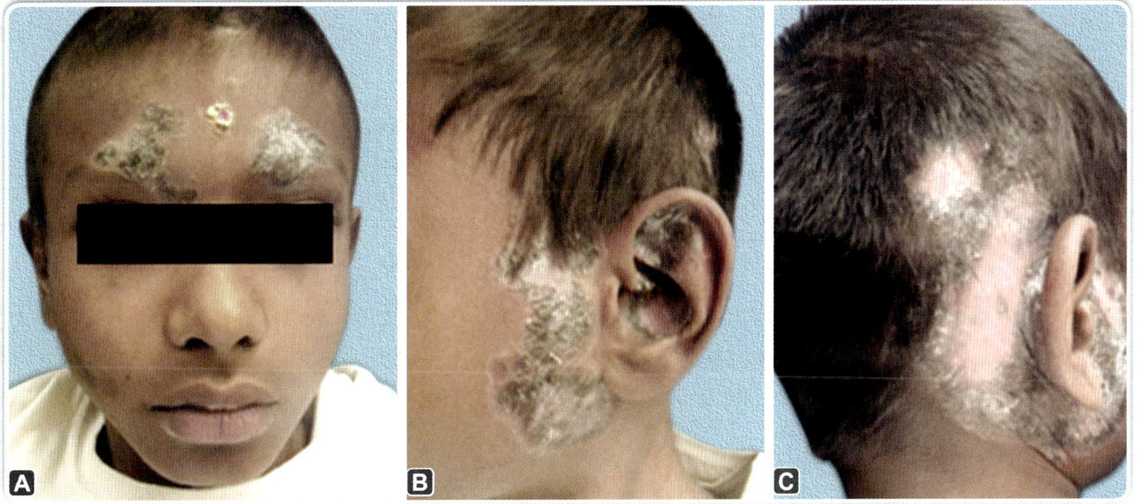

Figs 21.3A to C: Discoid lupus erythematosus in a young child (*Courtesy:* Department of Dermatology, BMCRI, Bengaluru)

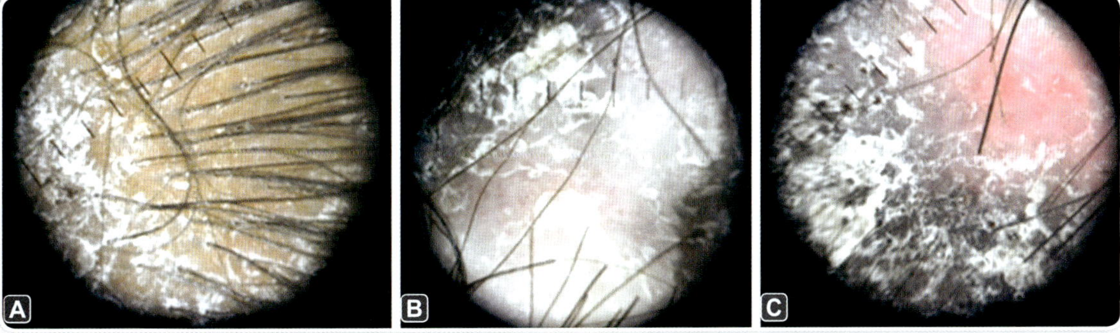

Figs 21.4A to C: Dermoscopic features in above child (A) Perifollicular plugging (B) Thick adherent scales with underlying dilated vessels (C) Removal of scales showing erythema (*Courtesy:* Department of Dermatology, STD and Leprosy, BMCRI, Bengaluru)

Treatment is by topical or systemic steroids depending on the intensity of the lesions along with hydroxychloroquine sulfate 200 mg once or twice daily. Though active lesions respond to treatment, the scarring alopecia persists.

Vitiligo[45]

Vitiligo is an acquired disorder of depigmentation wherein there is autoimmune destruction of melanocytes. It is a disfiguring and psychologically incapacitating condition, more so when it affects the face and scalp. Scalp lesions may be associated with leukotrichia which is an additional disfigurement, especially in young people with dark colored hair. It has to be differentiated from congenital disorders of depigmentation given in **Box 21.7**.

The various modalities of treatment used include topical or systemic steroids, other immunomodulators like levamisole, topical pimecrolimus, narrow band UVB light therapy, oral or topical psoralens with UVA light exposure and surgical modalities like autologous skin grafts in stable cases. Treatment is usually prolonged and unsatisfactory, leading to partial improvement, if at all, in most cases.

Psychological morbidity of vitiligo varies from 25% to 75% in various studies. Indian studies have shown 56–75% prevalence of psychological morbidity.[46,47] Such patients need extensive psychological counseling and should be taught coping strategies like cognitive behavioral therapy, positive mind body imaging, mindfulness, meditation, progressive muscle relaxing exercises. Bessel and Moss have compared various studies evaluating the effectiveness of alternative methods in patients with visible differences including vitiligo.[48]

Prurigo Simplex/Lichen Simplex Chronicus (LSC)

These are chronic lesions which may either arise de novo or as a hypersensitivity response to initially itchy stimuli like insect bite, which later become perpetuated by repeated and habitual scratching. Prurigo simplex and LSC usually affect exposed, accessible areas of the body like arms and legs. Nape of neck and posterior scalp are common sites. Lichenified excoriated papules, nodules or plaques are seen, which may be extremely itchy with paroxysms of itch which subside only after elicitation of pain. The common differentials are given in **Box 21.8**.

Box 21.7: Congenital causes for depigmentation of hair

- Poliosis
- Albinism
- Vogt-Koyanagi-Harada
- Alezzandrini syndrome
- Waardenberg syndrome

Box 21.8: Differential diagnosis of lichen simplex chronicus

- Chronic folliculitis of the scalp
- Acne keloidalis nuchae
- Scalp psoriasis
- Seborrheic dermatitis

Treatment: Potent topical steroids combined with keratolytics like salicylic acid, and other immunomodulatory agents like topical tacrolimus may be tried. In severe cases intralesional steroids like triamcinolone acetonide 5 mg/mL may help in amelioration of the lesions. Adjuvants like sedative antihistaminics and antiseptic antifungal shampoos may be given.

The severe itch can be a source of extreme psychosocial distress, which in turn leads to increase in itching thus perpetuating a vicious cycle. It is seen that the itching increases during periods of emotional stress and can be reduced by psychotherapy and cognitive behavior therapy.

Conclusion

Psychosomatic hair disorders are a diverse group of diseases with diverse pathophysiologies affecting the scalp and hair which have in common, the ability to affect the psychosocial well-being of the individual thereby adversely affecting their wholesome functioning in the society. In addition to specific treatment, psychological counseling and behavioral modification play an important role in the optimal management of such disorders.

Glossary

Psychotrichology	Sub-speciality of psychodermatology that deals with the relation between hair and psyche
Scalp dysesthesia	Mucocutaneous pain syndrome characterized by altered sensation over the scalp in the absence of any primary cutaneous disorder
Trichobezoar	Presence of balls of hair which can be found in the stomach or intestines
Trichodynia	Dysesthesia perceived in hair (root of hair) especially subsequent to touch of hair
Trichoesthesia	Feeling that one's hair has been touched, caused by the stimulation of the hair follicle receptor
Trichomalacia	The injured follicles tend to produce soft twisted hair
Trichopathophobia	Fear of hair, plucking of hair with the purpose of removing something from the root
Trichophagia	Habit of eating hair
Trichoteiromania	Alopecia which occurs secondary to the rubbing of hair
Trichotemnomania	Hair is deliberately cut to simulate hair damage
Trichotillomania	Irresistible urge to pull hair which subsides subsequent to the action of pulling the hair

References

1. Dorland's illustrated medical dictionary, 31st edn. Philadelphia: Saunders Elsevier. Trichoesthesia. 2007;p.1989.
2. Harth W, Gieler U, Kusnir D, Tausk FA (eds). Clinical Management in psychodermatology. Berlin: Springer. 2009;p.50-2.
3. Durusoy C, Ozenli Y, Adiguzel A, Budakoglu IY, Tugal O, Arikan S, et al. The role of psychological factors and serum zinc, folate and vitamin B12 levels in the aetiology of trichodynia: a case-control study. Clin Exper Dermatol. 2009;34:789-92.
4. Kivanç-Altunay I, Sava C, Gökdemir G, Köşlü A, Ayaydin EB. The presence of trichodynia in patients with telogen effluvium and androgenetic alopecia. Int J Dermatol. 2003;42:691-3.
5. Blume-Peytavi U, Tosti A, Whiting DA, Trüeb R. Hair Growth and Disorders. Berlin: Springer. 2008;pp.422-5.
6. Zalaudek I, Argenziano G, Di Stefani A, Ferrara G, Marghoob AA, Hofmann-Wellenhof R, et al. Dermoscopy in General Dermatology. Dermatology. 2006;212:7-18.
7. Harth W, Gieler U, Kusnir D, Tausk FA (eds). Clinical Management in Psychodermatology. Berlin: Springer. 2009;pp.21-3.
8. Gude D. Comprehending trichotillomania. Int J Trichol. 2012;4:100-1.
9. Millard LG, Millard J. Psychocutaneous disorders. In: Burns T, Breathnach S, Cox N, Griffiths C (eds). Rook's Textbook of Dermatology, 8th edn. Singapore: Wiley- Blackwell. 2010;p.64.30-2.
10. Siddappa K. Trichotillomania. Ind J Dermatol Venereol Leprol. 2003;69:63-8.
11. Traction alopecia. In. Diagnosis and Treatment of Hair Disorders: An evidence based Atlas. Tosti A, Piraccini BM, (eds). Oxon: Taylor and Francis. 2006;106-8.
12. Trueb RM, Tobin DJ. Aging Hair. Berlin: Springer. 2010;p.157-8.
13. Campbell's psychiatric dictionary, 8th edn. New York: Oxford University press. Trichopathophobia. 2004;p.673.
14. Wadhwa SL, Khopkar U, Nischal KC. Hair and scalp disorders. In: Valia RG, Valia AR (eds). IADVL Textbook of Dermatology, 3rd edn. Mumbai: Bhalani Publishing House. 2008; pp.896-917.
15. Dorland's Illustrated Medical Dictionary, 31st edn. Philadelphia: Saunders Elsevier. Trichobezoar. 2007;p.1989.
16. Singh G, Singh G, Kaur V. Psychocutaneous disorders. In: Valia RG, Valia AR (eds). IADVL Textbook of Dermatology, 3rd edn. Mumbai: Bhalani Publishing House. 2008;p.1423-4.
17. Mathew J. Trichoscopy as an aid in the diagnosis of trichotillomania. Int J Trichol. 2012;4:101-2.
18. Impulse Control disorders not elsewhere classified. In: Sadock BJ, Sadock VA (eds). Kaplan and Sadock's Concise Textbook of Clinical Psychiatry, 3rd edn. Derived from Kaplan and Sadock's Synopsis of Psychiatry, 10th edn. New Delhi: Wolters Kluwer India Pvt Ltd. 2008;pp.367-9.
19. Trüeb RM. Telogen effluvium and trichodynia. Dermatology. 199;196:374-5.
20. Messenger AG, de Berker DAR, Sinclair RD. Disorders of hair. In: Burns T, Breathnach S, Cox N, Griffiths C (eds). Rook's Textbook of Dermatology, 8th edn. Singapore: Wiley-Blackwell. 2010;p.66.16-22.
21. Blume-Peytavi, BlumeyerA,Tosti A, Finner A, MarmolV, Trakatelli M, et al. The European Consensus Group. S1 guideline for diagnostic evaluation in androgenetic alopecia in men, women and adolescents. Br J Dermatol. 2011;164:5-15.
22. Sinclair R, Patel M, Dawson Jr TL, Yazdabadi A, Yip L, Perez A, et al. Hair loss in women: medical and cosmetic approaches to increase scalp hair fullness. Br J Dermatol. 2011;165 (Suppl 3):12-8.
23. Cash TF. The psychosocial consequences of androgenetic alopecia: a review of the research literature. Br J Dermatol. 1999;141:398-405.
24. Yesudian P. Mind the hair. Int J Trichol. 2012;4:61.
25. Wells PA, Willmoth T, Russell RJ. Does fortune favour the bald? Psychological correlates of hair loss in males. Br J Psychol. 1995;86:337-44.
26. Diseases of the skin appendages. In: James WD, Berger TG, Elston DM (eds). Andrews' Diseases of the Skin: Clinical Dermatology, 10th edn. Canada: Saunders Elsevier. 2006; pp.749-57.
27. Paus R, Olsen EA, Messenger AG. Hair growth disorders. In: Wolff K, Goldsmith LA, Katz SI, Gilchrest BA, Paller AS, Leffell DJ (eds). Fitzpatricks' Dermatology in General Medicine, 7th edn. USA: McGraw Hill. 2008;pp.753-70.
28. Wadhwa SL, Khopkar U, Nischal KC. Hair and scalp disorders. In: Valia RG, Valia AR (eds). IADVL Textbook of Dermatology, 3rd edn. Bhalani Publishing House, Mumbai, India.
29. Living with alopecia areata. National alopecia areata foundation. [Internet] [cited 2012 May 14] Available from http://www.naaf.org/site/PageServer?pagename=living_with_alopecia.
30. Willemsen R, Haentiens P, Roseeuw D, Vanderlinden J. Hypnosis and alopecia areata: Long-term beneficial effects on psychological well-being. Acta Derm Venereol. 2011;9:35-9.
31. Willemsen R, Haentjens P, Roseeuw D, Vanderlinden J. Hypnosis in refractory alopecia areata significantly improves depression, anxiety, and life quality but not hair regrowth. J Am Acad Dermatol. 2010;62(3):517-8.
32. Paus R, Arck P. Neuroendocrine perspectives in alopecia areata: does stress play a role? J Investigative Dermatol. 2009;129:1324-6.
33. Sehgal VN, Srivastava G, Aggarwal A, Sethi G, Adhikari T. Alopecia Areata in the Indian Subcontinent. Skinmed. 2007;6:63-9.
34. Scalp psoriasis. Natinal psoriasis foundation. [Internet] [cited 2012, June 5] Available from: http://www.psoriasis.org/document.doc?id=155.
35. Gupta MA, Schork NJ, Gupta AK. Suicidal ideation in psoriasis. Int J Dermatol. 1993;32:188-90.
36. Relevance of psychiatry in dermatology: present concepts. Basavaraj KH, Navya MA, Rashmi R. Ind J Psychiatry. 2010;52:270-5.
37. Finlay AY, Kelly SE. Psoriasis—an index of disability. Clin Exp Dermatol. 1987;12:8-11.

38. Ginsburg IH, Link BG. Feelings of stigmatization in patients with psoriasis. J Am Acad Dermatol. 1989;20:53-63.
39. Rakhesh SV, D'Souza M, Sahai A. Quality of life in psoriasis: a study from south India. Indian J Dermatol Venereol Leprol. 2008;74:600-6.
40. Gaikwad R, Deshpande S, Raje S, Dhamdhere DV, Ghate MR. Evaluation of functional impairment in psoriasis. Indian J Dermatol Venereol Leprol. 2006;72:37-40.
41. Matto SK, Handa S, Kaur I, Gupta N, Malhotra R. Psychiatric morbidity in vitiligo and psoriasis: A comparative study from India. J Dermatol. 2001;28:424-32.
42. Assouly P and Reygagne P. Lichen planopilaris: update on diagnosis and treatment. Semin Cutan Med Surg. 2009;28:3-10.
43. Walsh SRA, Graham-Little-Piccardi-Lasseur syndrome. Medscape Reference. [Internet] [updated 2012, January 17, cited 2012, June 7] Available from: http://emedicine.medscape.com/article/1073743-overview.
44. Misery L, Touboul S, Vincot C, Dutray S, Rolland-Jacob G, Consoli SG, et al. [Stress and seborrheic dermatitis] Ann Dermatol Venereol. 2007;134:833-7. [article in French].
45. Oztas P, Cahkoglu E, Cetin I. Psychiatric tests in seborrheic dermatitis. [internet] [accessed on September 7, 2012] Available from: www.medicaljournals.se/acta/content/download.php?doi=10.1080.
46. Bleehen, S.S. and Anstey, A.V. (2004) Disorders of skin colour. In: Burns T, Breathnach S, Cox N, Griffiths C (eds.) Rook's Textbook of Dermatology. volume 2, 7th edn. Oxford: Blackwell Publishing. Chapter 39.
47. Pichaimuthu R, Ramaswamy P, Bikash K, Joseph R. A measurement of the stigma among vitiligo and psoriasis patients in India. Ind J Dermatol Venereol Leprol. 2011;77:300-6.
48. Parsad D, Dogra S, Kanwar AJ. Quality of life in patients with vitiligo. Health Qual Life Outcomes. 2003;1:58. Published online 2003 October 23. doi: 10.1186/1477-7525-1-58.

22

Shampoos and Conditioners

Anil Abraham

"Take care of your body; it's the only place where you live."
—*Emmanuel James "Jim rohn"*

Introduction

"Which shampoo should I use?" This seems to be an often repeated question by patients to their dermatologists and with the average female having 4-8 m^2 surface area to apply the shampoo on; it seems a rather apt question. Gone are the days where just a couple of shampoos and conditioners ruled the market. This makes the choice of product tough for both the consumer and the prescribing doctor! Hence a good knowledge of shampoo ingredients and their function is vital for accurate prescribing.

'Genealogy' of the Current Day Shampoo (Figure 22.1)

Shampoos (derived from the Hindustani word 'champo') date back to the 18th century where it was initially used in the Mughal Empire and by the Nawabs of Bengal as products for head massage. It was commercially popularized by Shaykh Din Muhammad, an Indian immigrant to the United Kingdom, a surgeon and entrepreneur, who was subsequently appointed as the 'Shampooing Surgeon' to Kings George IV and William IV. A century later, the concept of using a shampoo changed from that of a massage to one that was used primarily for its role as a detergent for cleansing the hair and scalp. Since ancient times, extracts from boiled soapnut and gooseberry have been used as an efficient hair cleanser in India. Similarly shikakai, mustard cakes and hibiscus flowers have also been used. Native American tribes used extracts from coastal woodfern and in Indonesia, ashes of husk and straw of rice were mixed with water and used as equivalents of shampoo with coconut oil used thereafter as a conditioner. The current day shampoo was a creation of a British stylist Kasey Hebert. It began to be commercially marketed at the turn of the 20th century in Britain and the US. Initially these shampoos contained soaps admixed with fragrant flowers, herbs and water. The first shampoo which contained synthetic surfactants 'Drene' was introduced in the 1930's.

Definition (Box 22.1)

Shampoos are hair care products aimed at clearing off sebum, sweat, desquamated stratum corneum, environmental pollutants, contaminants and styling products that gradually build up on the hair and scalp. They are thus liquid cleansing agents for washing hair and scalp and consist of a cocktail of various ingredients.

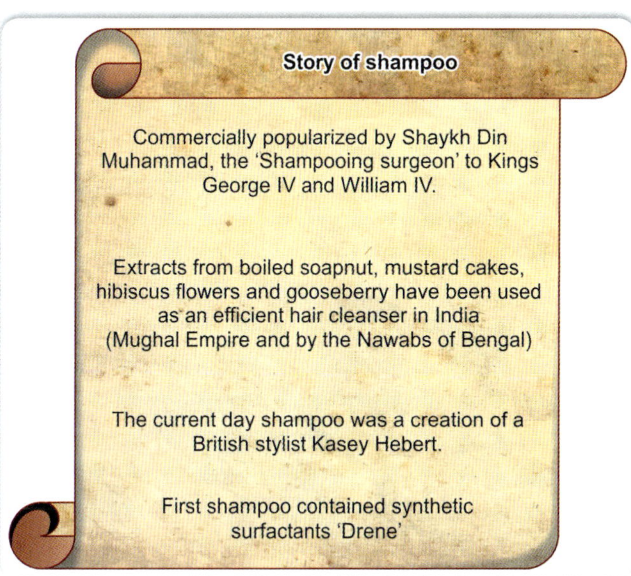

Fig. 22.1: Genealogy of shampoo

Box 22.1: Definition of a shampoo

Hair care products aimed at clearing off sebum, sweat, desquamated stratum corneum, environmental pollutants, contaminants and styling products that gradually build up on the hair and scalp

Ingredients of a basic shampoo include:
1. Detergents
2. Foaming agents
3. Conditioners
4. Sequestering agents
5. Thickeners and opacifiers
6. pH adjusters
7. Fragrances and preservatives.

Detergents: These are surfactants that are amphiphilic or amphipathic. This implies that they have a lipophilic portion that binds to sebum and a hydrophilic portion that permits rinsing off with water. When a shampoo contains more than one detergent, the one listed first is the primary agent which is present in higher concentration than the ones that follow. Detergents may be classified as follows **(Figure 22.2)**:

I. *Anionic detergents:* These are derived from fatty alcohols and have a negative polar group. They function as powerful detergents. Chemically, they are classified into the following, which decide how powerful a detergent they are **(Table 22.1)**.

II. *Nonionic detergents:* They have no polar group. Known for their mild cleansing action, they generally serve as secondary detergents in shampoo formulations. Examples include polyoxyethylene fatty alcohols, polyethylene sorbitol esters and alkanolamides.

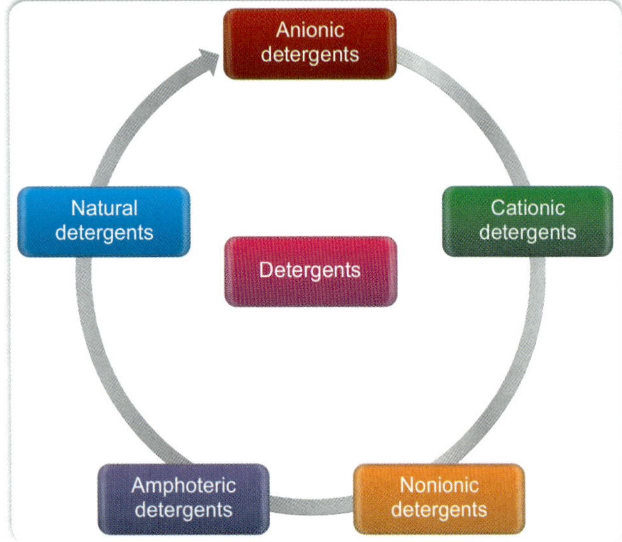

Fig. 22.2: Classification of detergents

Table 22.1: Classification of anionic detergents

Chemical Class	Feature	Examples
Lauryl sulfates	Potent detergents Harsher on hair Suitable for oily scalp/hair	Sodium lauryl sulfate Ammonium lauryl sulfate Triethanolamine lauryl sulfate
Laureth sulfates	Good detergents Less hair shaft damage Suitable for normal-dry hair	Sodium laureth sulfate Ammonium laureth sulfate Triethanolamine laureth sulfate
Sulfosuccinates	Potent detergents Used as secondary detergents Useful for oily scalp/hair	Disodium oleamine sulfosuccinate Sodium dioctyl sulfosuccinate
Sarcosines	Inefficient detergents Good conditioners Suitable for very dry hair	Lauryl sarcosine Sodium lauryl sarcosinate

III. *Cationic detergents:* These have a positive polar group. They do not produce adequate lather and are less effective cleansers. They cannot be mixed with anionic detergents. Cationic detergents are ideal for use on chemically treated hair as they are not harsh on the hair shaft and can even be used on a daily basis.

IV. *Amphoteric detergents:* These are so named because they act as anionic detergents at higher pH and cationic detergents at lower pH. They are common ingredients in baby shampoos as they do not irritate the eyes and are not harsh on hair. Examples include cocamidopropyl betaine and sodium lauraminopropionate.

V. *Natural detergents:* These include a host of botanicals. Despite having fair lathering properties, they have poor cleansing property and are used as adjuncts in shampoo formulations. Examples include soapwort, sarsaparilla, ivy, agave and soap bark.

***Foaming agents*:** These help by better spreadability of the shampoo formulation and act by introducing air bubbles into the water.

***Conditioners*:** Sebum is the perfect hair conditioner **(Box 22.2)**. While shampoos aim to cleanse hair, conditioners are meant to enhance its appearance, once cleansed. Hair lacking in sebum appears dull, harsh and is subject to static electricity. This occurs typically after the use of potent detergents in shampoos. Conditioners also decrease hair shaft combing friction by nearly 50% contributing to disentangling. This led to the emergence of conditioners to restore hair manageability and to impart softness and gloss to cleansed hair. They also decrease brittleness, increase

Box 22.2: Physiological hair conditioner

- Sebum is the perfect conditioner
- Hair lacking in sebum appears dull, harsh and is subject to static electricity

porosity and prevents degradation of hair. Examples of conditioning agents include dimethicone, simethicone, glycerin, hydrolysed animal protein, polyvinylpyrrolidone, propylene glycol and stearalkonium chloride.

There are 3 chemical categories of conditioners **(Figure 22.3)**.

1. *Cationic detergent conditioners:* These are quaternary ammonium compounds that deposit a positively charged film over the negatively charged damaged hair shaft resulting in neutralization of surface charge reducing static electricity forces. The coating of the conditioner on the shaft also restores softness and shine.
2. *Film forming conditioners:* These are positively charged polymers that fill surface cuticle defects.
3. *Protein based conditioners:* These contain amino acids and small chain polypeptide fragments of hydrolyzed proteins which get cross linked with keratin in damaged shaft. The hydrolyzed protein is more efficient in penetrating the hair shaft and approximating frayed remnants, enhancing its tensile strength by 5%. Though they claim to repair split ends and lost protein, one must be wary of the fact that these changes are temporary and will at the most last until the next shampooing. The sources of protein include animal protein, eggs, placenta, collagen, keratin and beer.

Based on their usage properties, conditioners may be 'leave in' conditioners or 'rinse' conditioners which have an added advantage of preventing hair dryer damage. Another way of categorising them is depicted in **Table 22.2**.

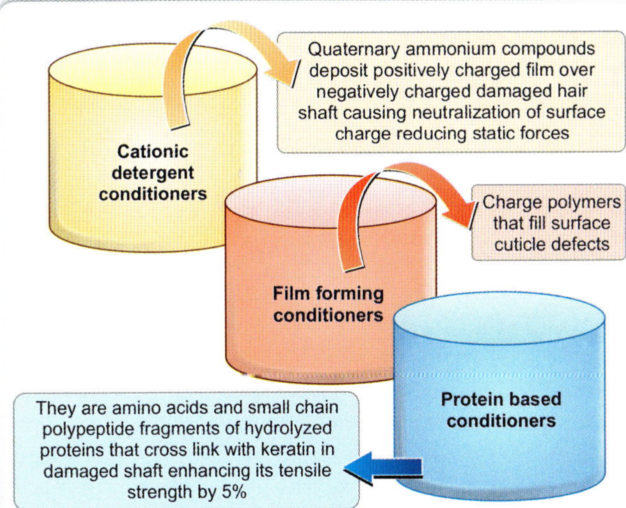

Fig. 22.3: Schematic representation of characteristics of conditioners

Sequestering agents: Insoluble soaps (scum) formation on the scalp and hair result in dull hair. Sequestering agents chelate calcium and magnesium ions, thus preventing the formation of 'scum'. The addition of sequestering agents is what distinguishes a shampoo from soap.

Thickeners and opacifiers: They alter the physical and optical properties of the shampoo.

pH adjusters: Detergents are essentially alkaline in nature. This can predispose the hair shaft to forces of weathering. Hence agents such as glycolic acid are added as pH adjusters and the resultant product is labelled as being 'pH balanced'.

Speciality additives: To improve its market value, a shampoo may contain certain add-ons such as vitamins and a host of botanicals notably tea tree oil, jojoba oil, chamomile, rosemary and lavender. This is particularly relevant in today's market where consumers are always on the lookout for products that are 'organic' and 'all-natural'. **Table 22.3** highlights the features of an ideal shampoo.

Shampoos that Address Specific Needs (Figure 22.4)

1. *Dry and damaged hair shampoo:* Also called '2-in-1 shampoos', these contain a shampoo and a conditioner

Table 22.2: Classification of conditioners

Instant conditioners	Most popular; useful for minimally damaged hair and aids wet combing Applied after shampooing, left for 5 minutes and rinsed off
Blow drying lotions/ hair thickeners/ hair glazes	To be applied after towel drying hair
Deep conditioners	Used every week to fortnight; applied on cleansed hair and left on for 20–30 minutes with or without application of heat and then removed
Fillers	Used prior to chemical hair treatment

Table 22.3: Features of an ideal shampoo

Features of an ideal shampoo
❑ Pleasant fragrance
❑ Suitable color and formulation
❑ Adequate lather formation
❑ Easily rinsable
❑ Minimal weathering to hair, slightly acidic in pH
❑ Minimal to absent ocular and cutaneous irritation
❑ Low toxicity
❑ Added conditioning property
❑ Economical

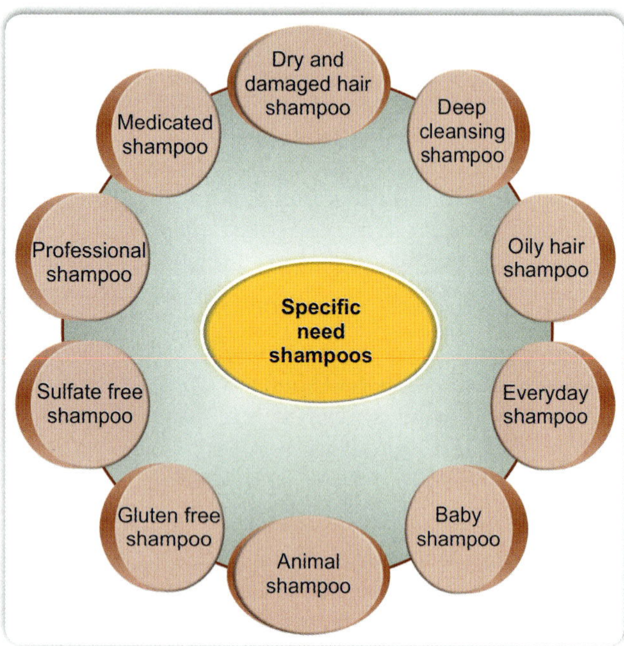

Fig. 22.4: Schematic representation of specific need shampoos

Box 22.3: 2 in 1 shampoos

These contain a detergent that degreases and a conditioner like silicone – dimethicone that coats hair shaft, wrapped in a single product used for dry and damaged hair

wrapped in a single product. The mild detergent in them degreses the scalp and rids it of dirt while the silicone (dimethicone) forms a thin coat over the hair shaft imparting a conditioned look **(Box 22.3)**.

2. *Oily hair shampoo:* These contain potent surfactants such as lauryl sulfates with minimal conditioning property as oily hair rarely requires additional conditioners.
3. *Everyday shampoos:* Though experts do not recommend daily shampooing due to increased weathering, there are people who still prefer it, especially in a country like India due to personal, cultural, religious and social reasons. Everyday shampoos contain mild detergents and an instant conditioner may be combined with it use.
4. *Deep cleansing shampoos (clarifying shampoos):* These contain strong detergents and are recommended for use in individuals who use hair styling products such as gels or mousse **(Box 22.4)**.
5. *Baby shampoo:* Mild detergents from the amphoteric group are used while formulating baby shampoos since their skin has limited sebum. These have an added advantage of having a mild anesthetic property which makes them non-irritant to the ocular mucosa.
6. *Medicated shampoo:* These aim at delivering topical medications to the scalp in addition to cleansing. They

Box 22.4: Clarifying shampoos

Contain strong detergents and are recommended for use in individuals who use hair styling product

Box 22.5: Pharmaceuticals in medicated shampoos used in scalp dermatoses

- Salicylic acid, tar derivatives, selenium sulfide, ketoconazole
- Ciclopirox olamine, zinc pyrithione, flucinolone
- Polyvinylpyrrolidone: Iodine complex, menthol and chlorinated phenols

are used in conditions such as seborrheic dermatitis, tinea capitis, scalp psoriasis and scalp pruritus. Medications such as salicylic acid, tar derivatives, selenium sulfide, ketoconazole, ciclopirox olamine, zinc pyrithione, flucinolone, polyvinylpyrrolidone-iodine complex, menthol and chlorinated phenols have been incorporated into shampoo formulations **(Box 22.5)**.

7. *Professional shampoos:* These are meant for use in salons and are generally sold at beauty stores. The two types of professional shampoos are those meant for cleansing prior to cutting or styling hair and those meant for use after chemically treating hair. These are more concentrated than commonly available shampoos and need to be diluted eight to ten times before use.
8. *Sulfate free shampoos:* These lack sulfates hence making them gentle on hair especially that which has been previously chemically treated.
9. *Gluten free shampoos:* Gluten containing grains such as wheat, barley, rye and oats are used in shampoo formulations as binding agents and also as emollients. These may require to be avoided in individuals who are gluten sensitive.
10. *Animal shampoos:* Designed for use in pets, these shampoos contain ingredients such as insecticides (pyrethrin and pyrethroids), antibacterials, antifungals, anti-seborrheic agents, anti-pruritic agents, emulsifiers, emollients and humectants.

Adverse Reactions to Shampoos

These have rarely been reported with shampoo use as the contact period is very short. The most common adverse effect is irritation to mucosa—ocular, nasal and oral. Sudden irreversible matting of hair has been reported which clinically resembles a 'bird's nest' **(Box 22.6)**. Electron microscopy revealed 'welding of hair'. Ingredients such as formalin, fragrances, triclosan, parabens, hexachlorophene and miranols have been incriminated in causing allergic contact dermatitis. If patch testing is desired, either the ingredients are tested individually or a 1-2% aqueous solution is used as a closed patch test.

Box 22.6: Bird's nest

- Sudden irreversible matting of hair as a consequence of adverse effect of use of shampoo and conditioners
- Electron microscopy reveals 'welding of hair'

Alternatively, a 5% solution of the shampoo may be used in an open patch test.

Though methylisothiazolinone, one of the shampoo ingredients is known to be neurotoxic, cytotoxic and allergenic, its use in shampoos is considered safe as its concentration is very low.

Common shampoo myths busted:

1. Shampoos that foam better are superior
2. Shampoos cause hair loss from the root
3. Salon brand shampoos are superior to common brands
4. Shampoos can nourish and repair damaged hair
5. You need to keep changing your brand of shampoo regularly
6. Baby shampoo being mild, can be used on adult hair as a daily shampoo

23

Follicular Unit Transplantation

Manoj Khanna, Dolly Gupta

"Success is not final, failure is not fatal; it is the courage to continue that counts."

—*Winston Churchill*

Introduction

It is found that over 50% of men and 25% of women suffer from some degree of hair loss.[1-3] With hair loss being a multibillion dollar industry, there is a plethora of products available in market claiming to restore hair loss. However, hair transplantation is the only definite method to correct male pattern baldness (MPB) permanently. It is one of the most rapidly evolving procedures in aesthetic surgery. There has been considerable improvement in its techniques at regular intervals. The recent advances in technology and the concept of using "follicular unit grafts" have made this procedure to reach a new height. The ability to provide very natural appearing-results has encouraged larger number of balding men and women to opt for this surgical solution, which leaves a marked impact not only in their appearance but also in their psychosocial aspect.

History and Evolution of Hair Transplantation

As early as 1804, Baromio had demonstrated the possibility of successful hair-bearing transplants in animals.[4] Hair-bearing autografts for the correction of traumatic alopecia have been carried out with varying success since 1893. Flaps and relatively larger free grafts were the methods used.[5] In 1939, Okuda, a Japanese dermatologist actually gave the first description of hair transplantation. He used small full-thickness autografts of hair-bearing skin for the correction of alopecia of the scalp, eyebrow and moustache area in burn victims during World War II. Unfortunately, records of Okuda's work were lost due to the war and this original procedure was not acknowledged until recently.[6,7] In 1943, Tamura, who was very advanced for his time, described the use of single-hair grafts (which would later become known as micrografts) to transplant pubic hair using a technique very similar to that used today. However, none of the Japanese authors mentioned the usefulness of these techniques in the treatment of androgenic alopecia.[8] In 1950, Norman Orentreich, a dermatologist from New York rediscovered the technique and performed the first hair transplant successfully in the United States for patients with male pattern baldness (MPB) **(Box 23.1)**.[9]

Theory of Donor Dominance: Basis of Hair Transplantation

Autosomal dominant genetic linkage is believed to be responsible in androgenetic alopecia or MPB, which is the commonest cause of baldness in men. It is known that the male hormone, testosterone, gets converted to 5 dihydroxy testosterone (5-DHT). In genetically susceptible men under the influence of 5-DHT, the hair follicles on the front and top of the scalp bearing the receptor for 5-DHT, become finer gradually over the years. The hair growth also gets restricted and eventually the hair disappears completely.

Box 23.1: History of hair transplantation

- 1804—Baromio demonstrated successful hair-bearing transplants in animals
- 1893—Autografts for the correction of traumatic alopecia
- 1939—Okuda gave the first description of hair transplantation in burn victims
- 1943—Tamura described the use of single-hair grafts
- 1950—Norman Orentreich performed the first hair transplant for MPB
- 1994—Bobby Limmer described follicular unit transplantation (FUT)

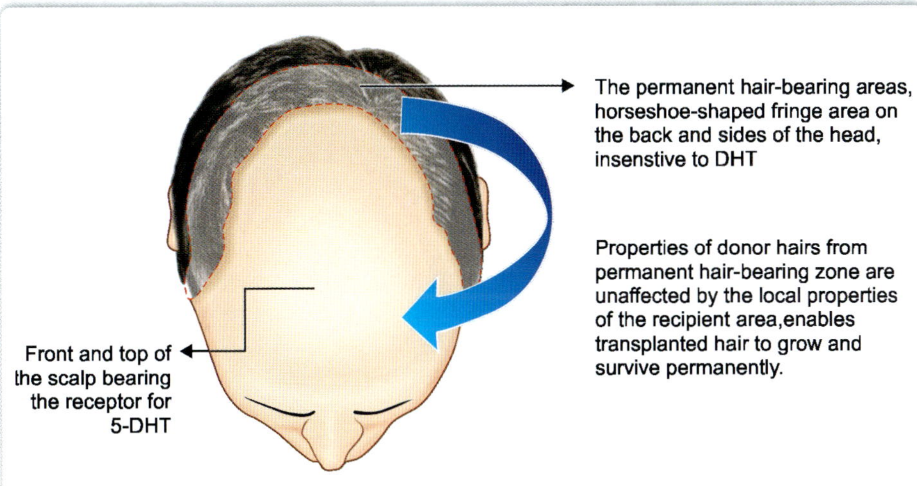

Fig. 23.1: Theory of donor dominance

Box 23.2: Disadvantages of using large circular grafts

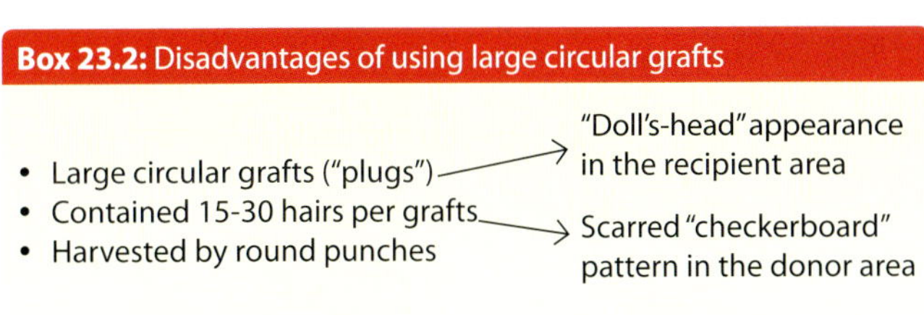

Table 23.1: Types of grafts used in hair transplantation

Hair plugs	15–30 hair per graft
Single hair graft	One hair
Minigraft	3–8 hair per graft
Micrograft	1–2 hair per graft
Follicular unit	1, 2, 3, or 4 hair surrounded by single arrector pili

In 1959, Orentreich suggested the term "donor dominance" in androgenetic alopecia, which formed the scientific basis of hair transplantation. If hairs taken from the permanent hair-bearing areas, which is a horseshoe-shaped fringe area on the back and sides of the head, are transplanted to the area of alopecia (the recipient area), they would continue to grow for as long as it would have survived in its original site. Donor hairs from this permanent hair-bearing zone are insensitive to DHT. This property of donor hair, unaffected by the local properties of the recipient area, enables transplanted hair to grow and survive permanently. These hairs maintain the same texture and color and apparently grow at the same rate with the same period of anagen that governed them in the donor site **(Figure 23.1)**.[9,10]

Although Orentreich's discovery gave a new way to the possibility of hair transplantation but the results were unnatural and disappointing due to the use of large circular grafts (called "plugs") containing 15–30 hairs per grafts, harvested by round punches. This used to give the "doll's-head" appearance in the recipient area and often left a scarred "checkerboard" pattern in the donor area **(Box 23.2)**.

Mini-micro Grafting

The above-mentioned method continued until early 1980s, when the concept of relatively smaller grafts, called "minigrafts" and "micrografts" came into being to disguise the unesthetic frontal hairline. The grafts to be transplanted were separated as three to eight hair units from the original punch grafts and called "minigrafts". They were called 'micrografts" when they were trimmed to one or two hair units. Gradually the concept of combination of mini-micro grafting was adopted. Instead of small round punches, small slit incisions were used for the recipient area, which increased the yield of grafts per session. Use of round punches for the donor tissue harvesting was switched to strip harvesting technique. A single strip of donor tissue was extracted, which were subsequently trimmed into individual grafts. Although, this mini-micro grafting significantly reduced the drawbacks associated with Orentreich's original method, the results were still not completely natural.

Bobby Limmer's publication in 1994 brought a major positive change in the hair transplantation technique. It described the use of the stereomicroscope in the dissection of the donor strip. Limmer did not dissect the grafts based on size, but rather on the basis of follicle groupings that usually contained 1, 2, 3 or 4 hairs. While he did not use the term follicular unit, it is he who in fact described the concept of follicular unit hair transplantation.[11] Finally in the 1990s, Bernstein and Rassmann defined the concept and surgical techniques further and popularized this method **(Table 23.1)**.[12,13]

Follicular Units and Follicular Unit Transplantation

Scalp hair tends to grow in tiny bundles, called "follicular units," rather than individually.[14] The *follicular units* as described by Headington includes one to four terminal hairs, one to two vellus hairs, their associated sebaceous glands, neurovascular plexus, an arrector pilorum muscle, and a circumferential band of adventitial collagen, the perifolliculum **(Box 23.3)**.[15]

This definition suggests that the unit is a physiological entity rather than an anatomical one. The density of follicular units varies significantly in different races. The relative constancy of the follicular unit density at 1/mm^2 has been observed after performing densitometry measurements on thousands of patients and also observed histologically by Headington as early as 1982.[12,15] It is significantly less in the dark skinned races and decreases in everyone's scalp as one moves laterally from the densest part over the occiput, towards the temples. It is best to describe a *follicular unit* for all practical purposes as an aggregation of hair shafts emerging from the scalp in which the distance between the hairs is less than the distance to the nearest aggregation of hairs. This pattern has to be kept in mind while harvesting, dissecting and transplanting hair to achieve maximal efficiency and to give a natural appearance to the patient.

In *follicular unit transplantation (FUT),* these naturally occurring units are used exclusively. Here once a strip of donor tissue has been removed, follicular units are separated out intact through careful stereomicroscopic dissection, avoiding injury to the follicles.[16-18] The recipient site in FUT always consist of small incisional slits.

Advantages of Follicular Unit Transplantation (FUT)

The FUT procedure has the following advantages over the traditional micrografting technique due to anatomic proximity of the hairs within each unit:[13,14,19,20]

1. Keeps the recipient site wound size to a minimum.
2. Virtually eliminates any skin surface change in the recipient area.
3. Enables grafts to be placed very close together to achieve better density.
4. Permits large numbers of grafts to be safely transplanted in a single session (because of the small recipient wound size).
5. The ability to insert upto four hairs in a tiny recipient site is especially valuable cosmetically and has been instrumental in eliminating the see-through quality of micrografting.

Box 23.3: Follicular unit

- The *follicular unit* includes:
  - One to four terminal hairs
  - One to two vellus hairs
  - Associated sebaceous glands
  - Neurovascular plexus
  - An arrector pilorum muscles
- Circumferential band of adventitial collagen—the perifolliculum

Thus, the transplanted hair will look natural, as long as the transplant surgeon makes the right esthetic decisions about graft placement, angling and distribution.

Follicular unit extraction (FUE): It is a technique that involves the removal of the intact follicular unit directly from the donor area using a 0.8–1 mm punch. The yield by this technique of harvesting can diminish due to transection and avulsion injury to the follicular unit. Also, although marketed as a technique that leaves no scar in the donor area, it leaves multiple 'dot-scars' in the donor area, which in its entirety is larger than in the strip method (Refer to Chapter 24).[21]

Indications of FUT or Candidates for Hair Transplantation

- Realistic expectations
- Patient aged more than 25 years with androgenic alopecia. There is no upper age limit, so long the patient is in good health
- Adequate density and thickness of donor hairs
- Stable condition or unresponsive to initial medical treatment (Finasteride and minoxidil)
- MPB with clinically visible bald patches in the recipient area (Norwood II–VI). The author prefers patients beyond Grade III unless there is professional or psychosocial urgency on the part of the patient
- It is important to distinguish between diffuse-patterned alopecia (DPA)—which has a stable donor area and the less common diffuse unpatterned alopecia (DUPA)—where the donor fringe continues to thin significantly over time. DUPA advance faster to Norwood VII, however unlike the Norwood VII, the DUPA horseshoe can look almost transparent because of the low density of the back and sides. DUPA are not the candidates for hair transplantation. The chance of missing the diagnosis of diffuse-patterned alopecia argues strongly against performing hair transplantation at an early age **(Table 23.2)**[22]
- Female pattern androgenic alopecia in Grade II or III on the Ludwig scale, provided the patient has good donor density
- Other common indications of hair transplantation in females are the lowering of extremely high hairlines due to heredity or following brow lift

- Reconstruction of eyebrows, eyelashes, beard, moustache, pubic hair or correction of scars due to trauma or surgery are other possible indications of hair transplantation.

Surgical Planning and Organization

- ***Proper counseling and patient education***: Patient should have a realistic expectation, which is probably the most important pre-requisite. They should have a thorough understanding of the procedure, its benefits and associated risks. The physician must emphasize that the goal of transplantation is to cover the bald areas and that the procedure will not prevent existing nontransplanted hair from continuing to miniaturize and suffer the consequences of androgenic alopecia and further hair loss.
- ***Selection of candidates:*** Although, there is no specific age bar for hair transplantation, the pros and cons of a transplant need to be carefully evaluated in the younger age group. Patients between 20 to 30 years of age should have a stabilized rate of hair loss before they are considered for hair transplantation. A detailed family history is useful in assessing hair loss and planning a new hairline. Non-compliant patients or those with evidence of body dysmorphic disorder, any psychiatric or obsessive concerns should be avoided.
- ***Hair and scalp characteristics:*** The color, quality and density of the donor hair and the contrast between the hair color and skin color are important factors that affect the result. The lesser the contrast between the donor hair and the skin, the better is the result.[23]

  Hairs with higher caliber, frizzy, curly or wavy are advantageous characteristics, adding not only increased naturalness but also giving more fullness, density and allowing less scalp visibility between them **(Box 23.4)**.
- ***Future hair styling preference:*** Surgeon should give preference to the preferred styling pattern of the patient and create greater density in the frontal forelock, first followed by portion of the recipient area from which the hair would be combed to give an illusion of denser coverage.
- ***Evaluating patient's donor supply:*** Donor density, scalp laxity and physical size of the donor area are the three main determining factors for the total donor reserves. The number of follicular units in the mid-portion of the donor area of a normal Caucasian man, who has not had surgery, is approximately one unit per mm^2 of scalp.[20] The average yield declines when longer strips are taken because density decreases towards the sides. Follicular unit density also varies according to race, therefore the number of grafts obtained per unit area of donor tissue will exhibit racial variability and must be accounted for in the surgical planning.[13] Final yield would also depend on degree of presence of one, two or three follicles in the individual unit, any scarring from previous surgeries, stretching of scalp from previous transplants, scalp reductions, or scalp lifts which would space the follicular units further apart, making it necessary to actually measure the density of follicular units to accurately estimate the number of grafts obtainable from the strip.

  Patients with very loose and very tight scalp often make poor candidates for strip method FUT as they tend to heal with widened scar where FUE is considered to be a better option.[21]

  Donor dimensions horizontally measures approximately 32-34 cms and extends from the mid-portion of the harvestable donor zone, which generally lies over the occipital protuberance and extends laterally to within 3 cm of the temple hairline on either side. The height of permanent zone varies in different individuals and hair should be harvested from only where it is stable and lacks significant miniaturization. An often overlooked condition is the ascending hairline, where miniaturization occurs in the lower margin of the permanent zone. Both receding temples and an ascending posterior hairline are

Table 23.2: Differences between DPA and DUPA

DPA	*DUPA*
Diffuse-patterned alopecia	Diffuse un-patterned alopecia
Common	Rare
Stable donor area	Unstable donor area
Slow progress	Advances faster to type VII
Grade VII—donor area is dense	Grade VII—transparent donor area

Box 23.4: Hair characteristics favorable for transplantation

- Less contrast between hair and scalp color
- Higher caliber
- Frizzy
- Curly
- Wavy

Box 23.5: Evaluation of donor area

Check for:
- Donor density—density per cm^2, hair in each unit
- Scalp laxity—avoid very loose or very tight scalp
- Physical size of the donor area
- Miniaturization of hair in donor area
- Ascending hairline, receding temples

alarming sign of shrinking donor zone and necessitate conservative surgical planning **(Box 23.5)**.

- ***Area of transplantation:*** This can be divided into two parts:
  a. Establishing the hairline zone with designing an effective frame of the face.
  b. Coverage of areas of baldness, which in order of priority includes frontal area, vertex and lastly the crown.

  Crown coverage should not be the primary goal because it is the least visible of the balding regions, occupying a very large surface area and thus consumes inexhaustible demand of donor supply **(Box 23.6)**. A useful alternative to covering the crown with transplanted hair is to end the transplant at the vertex transition point.[24,25] The patient can then groom the hair back to conceal the remaining bald area. Final aim should be to create sufficient density so that the results will look natural after one session, though additional sessions may be desired.[13]
- ***Hairline and its importance:*** Designing hairline is the most important step in hair restoration and thus must be accurately planned to give a natural look. It is the most highly visible feature and the quality of work of a surgeon is often judged by the quality of the hairline. It is probably best to follow the rule proposed by Leonardo Da Vinci dividing the face into three equal thirds from the trichion to the glabella, from the glabella to the subnasale, and from the subnasale to menton.[26] The superior border of the upper third is not actually the hairline but is the point to which the hair falls when it is styled. The height is adjusted based on age, gender, hair loss progression and availability of donor grafts, etc. In the midline the hairline starts from at least 8 cm or more from the glabella. A curve sweeps around to the lateral side of the forehead from the center. At this point, the sides of the hairline should be oriented parallel to the curve when the subject is looking straight ahead. The lateral hairlines are usually 9.5 to 11.5 cm above the lateral canthii of the eyes. The temporal angles should form relatively sharp right angles or acute angles in most men but in women these angles should be more rounded. The hairline shape also varies according to the variation of the shape of the face—round, oval or triangular. The patient's desires and constraints are also other factors that can affect the shape of the hairline.

Many patients prefer a "widow peak" in the center, which fits better in men with somewhat more elongated, more vertical facial structures. This conserves a lot of grafts as it allows to slightly raise the height of the hairline.

Box 23.6: Crown area transplantation

- Should not be the primary goal
- Least visible area
- Occupying a very large surface area
- Consumes inexhaustible demand of donor supply

Box 23.7: Hairline creation

- In the midline, the hairline starts from at least 8 cm or more from the glabella
- The lateral hairlines are usually 9.5 to 11.5 cm above the lateral canthii of the eyes
- The temporal angles form relatively sharp right angles or acute angles in men, but rounded in women
- Single hair grafts, 250-300 micrografts are used to create hairline
- Behind the hairline, two hairs FUGs are used to provide new hair
- Three or four hairs FUGs are used just further behind

Single hair grafts are used to create a natural hairline. Usually 250 to 300 micrografts will be necessary to create a new hairline in any individual. The micrografts in the hairline should be placed in an irregular saw-toothed pattern of macro- and micro-irregularity to give a natural appearance.[27] Behind the hairline, two hairs FUGs are used to provide new hair. Three or four hairs FUGs are used just further behind **(Box 23.7)**.

Preoperative Preparation

- Patients using topical minoxidil are advised to discontinue its use at least two days before surgery (because of its vasodilator properties) and wait a couple of days after the procedure before resuming (to avoid the irritating effects of the alcohol or the propylene glycol in the solution)
- Use of finasteride unless contraindicated is encouraged from at least one month prior to surgery as it is believed to minimize post-surgical effluvium as well as retard progression of baldness of non-transplanted areas
- If the patient has dandruff, it must be controlled with ketoconazole shampoo
- Patient is advised not to shave the hairs of donor area and allow them to grow at least 2 cms (to cover suture)
- Stop smoking and alcohol intake preferably one week before the surgery as they cause intraoperative bleeding, interfere with healing and heighten the chances of wound infection and scarring
- Do not take anticoagulant medication such as aspirin, plavix or their derivatives, vitamin B or E from 7 days before the procedure
- Wear clothes that do not need to be pulled on over the head as this will help avoiding any damage to the grafts after the surgery

- Ask the patients with gray hairs to dye them one or two days before the procedure as it helps in easy visualization of follicles avoiding their transection
- Allow light meal before the surgery
- Inform the patient, that as they would be receiving medications during the procedure that would make them drowsy, they cannot drive home following the surgery
- The day before and the morning of the procedure wash hair with an antiseptic shampoo, such as Povidone iodine
- Like any other surgery, all patients of hair transplantation must be treated with universal precautions
- The preoperative workup includes: Complete blood count, blood sugar (random), coagulation profile, serology for human immunodeficiency virus, hepatitis B and C viruses
- Consent form must be read thoroughly and signed by the patient prior to surgery.

Steps of Follicular Hair Transplantation (Box 23.8)

Step 1: Anesthesia of Donor Area

Local anesthesia is used for the entire procedure. A solution is made of 2% xylocaine- 30 cc in 100 cc normal saline, and 1 ampoule of adrenaline 1:1000 is added. The hair in the donor area is trimmed to about 2 mm in length and the unbuffered local anesthetic solution is injected just below the donor area using 26 size needles. The donor area is then tumesced by injecting normal saline, about 50 mL into the entire zone and one should wait for at least 10 minutes to minimize bleeding. The donor area should be turgid at the completion of infiltration, as tumescence provides excellent anesthesia and results in minimum bleeding.

Step 2: Donor Strip Dissection

Donor site hairs are trimmed to 2 to 4 mm. Strip of about 1 to 1.5 cm width is taken from just above the occipital protuberance extending from one ear to the other avoiding temporal hairs to prevent visibility of the scar. Total length of the strip depends on the area of baldness and the number of grafts required, which can vary from 500 to 4,000 **(Figure 23.2)**. The donor strip can be harvested using a single bladed knife or a multiple bladed knife containing 3 to 7 blades. The multibladed knife harvests numerous (2 to 6) parallel strips of thickness varying according to the spacer used which may be 1.5, 2 or 2.5 mm but this blind incision increases the chance of follicular damage, and it is better to use a single or double-bladed knife. It is very important that while harvesting the donor area the blades remain parallel to the direction of the hair so that the hair roots are not damaged. The hair in the lower part of the occipital area and the temporal area are finer and these should be used to create a new hairline. Dissecting donor hair which is white or light coloured is more difficult. Thus instructing the patient to dye his hair a few days before the procedure may be helpful. In addition, patients undergoing a second procedure need extra caution. The scar distorts the direction of the hair in the donor area and the surgeon must be cautious while harvesting the strip.

After the strip has been harvested, the gap can be closed either by using sutures or staples. The authors prefer giving interrupted deep sutures in the galea or subcutaneous tissue with 2-0 nylon to reduce the tension and width of the scar while many other surgeons prefer continuous or interrupted sutures using 3-0 vicryl or silk. The skin can be opposed by a running suture with 4-0 nylon or prolene. Care is taken to take the bites not too far away from the margin lest you damage more tissue. Also it is important to take a bite only up to the dermis so that the roots which are deeper below are not damaged, and can be utilised in subsequent surgery. The sutured donor area is then covered with padded dressing and fixed with a head band. Suture removal is done on the 10th postoperative day.

Trichophytic donor closure: The trichophytic closure of donor area is a way of improving the appearance of the linear donor scar from strip harvesting. A trichophytic closure involves trimming the lower edge of the incision and then closing the wound in such a way that the hair near the edge can grow towards or through the scar. Removal of the inferior skin edge is preferred over the superior as the beveled cut of the donor wound favors a natural overhang of the superior flap over the cut skin edge and thereby allows hair follicles to grow through the scar **(Figure 23.3)**.

Box 23.8: Steps of follicular unit transplantation

1. Anesthesia of donor area
2. Donor strip dissection
3. Preparing grafts
4. Anesthesia of recipient area
5. Creation of recipient sites or punching
6. Graft insertion

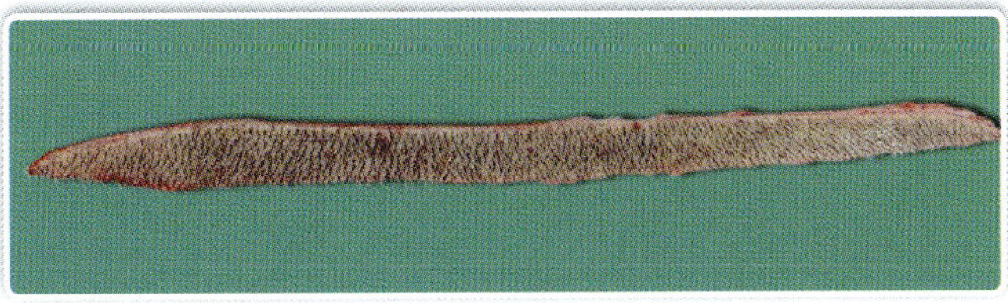

Fig. 23.2: Harvested strip from donor area (*Courtesy:* Department of Dermatology, STD and Leprosy, BMCRI, Bengaluru)

This has the potential to produce a donor scar that is virtually undetectable and thus proving to be a boon in FUT technique.[28]

Step 3: Preparing Grafts

The harvested donor strips are immediately immersed in chilled normal saline. Proper hydration of the donor grafts along with maintenance of a cold temperature of saline is very important throughout the surgery as it influences the survival rate of the grafts. In case, a single large strip has been harvested, it can be divided into thin slices or "slivers" each about the width of one FU which are further dissected into individual 1 to 4 hairs FU grafts **(Figures 23.4A and B)**.[29] The subcutaneous fatty tissue below the hair roots or bulbs is stripped leaving up to 2 mm of fat below the hair bulb. FUGs are made having 1 to 4 hairs.

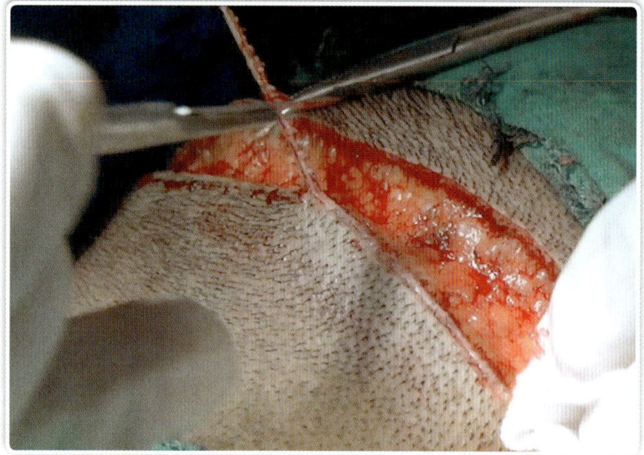

Fig. 23.3: Trichophytic trimming of the lower edge (*Courtesy:* Department of Dermatology, STD and Leprosy, BMCRI, Bengaluru)

Grafts are immersed in chilled saline in a Petri dish or kept on moist stockinet in kidney trays in bunches of fixed numbers **(Figure 23.5)**.

Grafts are very susceptible for drying and hence desiccation of the grafts must be avoided under all cost by proper immersion of the the grafts in cold saline throughout the procedure. Limmer has shown a high survival rate for grafts kept in chilled saline for up to 8 hours.[30] More exotic solutions with potential graft-sustaining properties, such as platelet rich plasma, have been developed, but they are not widely used.[31-33] Good illumination is essential during the cutting of the grafts. The grafts may be cut on wooden tongue depressors or on a clear vinyl dissecting surface with a backlighting system. It is important that no pieces of wood stick to the grafts when they have been cut, for these foreign bodies can later cause epidermal cysts which may be troublesome. Loupe magnifications of 2X or 3X is useful but most of the hair restoration surgeons these days prefer using dissecting stereomicroscope, which has become the standard practice in most centers. This makes the dissection a little slower, but is much more accurate and minimizes transection of hairs significantly.

Step 4: Anesthesia of Recipient Area

A supratrochlear block and a supraorbital block along with a ring shaped infiltration along the margin of the hairline beyond the zone of hair transplantation is given with the prepared local anesthetic mixture. The entire recipient area is then tumesced with saline solution. The authors avoid use of adrenaline in the recipient area for this has shown to diminish the uptake of the grafts and also increase telogen effluvium in the immediate post-operative period. Adrenaline must definitely be avoided in the recipient area in women where severe effluvium may be seen after its use.[34]

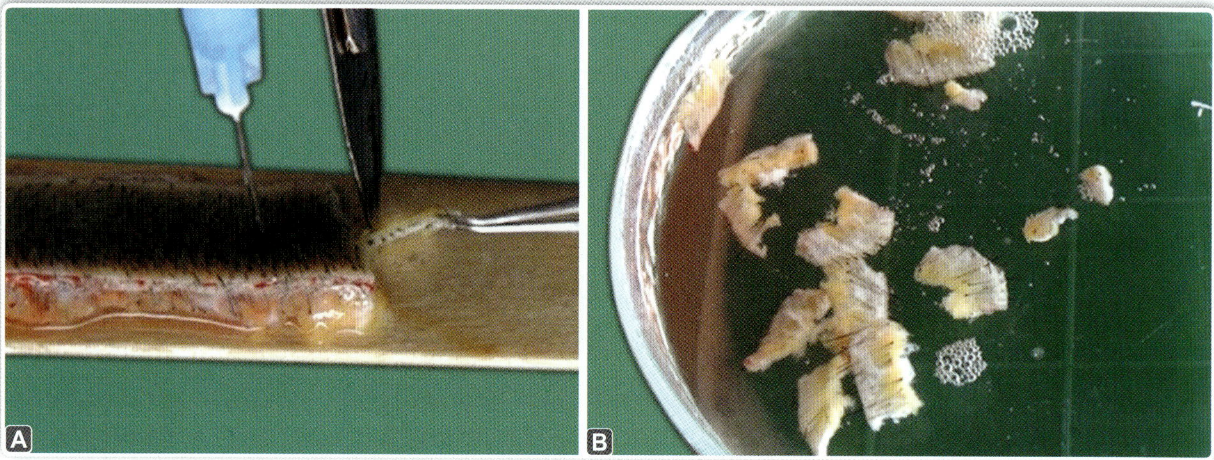

Figs 23.4A and B: (A) Slivering, (B) Slivered grafts
(*Courtesy:* Department of Dermatology, STD and Leprosy, BMCRI, Bengaluru)

Step 5: Creation of Recipient Sites or Punching

The recipient sites should provide a snug fit for the graft: Just large enough to accommodate a follicular unit, but not so small that insertion is difficult or traumatic.[14] Numerous instruments have been developed to create recipient sites. The main aspect to consider in choosing one is its diameter.[35] While making gaps, it is very important to follow the direction of the existing hair. The hairline should have a ragged saw-toothed natural look. Holes are made in a pattern of organized disorganization. About 250 to 300 micrografts are necessary to create a normal hairline and the authors use 19 or 20 gauze needle. Behind the hairline, slits can be made by using Nokor needles or 18 gauze needle. Depth of the punching should be 4 to 5 mm, to avoid damage to deeper vessels, slits can have coronal (horizontal) or sagittal (vertical) orientation but because coronal incisions provide better coverage and a slightly more natural look, they are currently preferred by the majority of hair transplant surgeons. An instrument is devised by the author, which is being patented as "Kolkata slit" **(Figure 23.6)**. It can be re-used in a number of cases, has different sizes and creates a gap just about the size of the graft to be inserted, also taking care of the direction of orientation of the graft. The slit can be used in bald areas as well as in areas where there are existing hairs in an attempt to increase density. The direction and angle of punching should follow the existing hairs and is generally made at 45 degree to the scalp with gradual downward direction towards the temporal sides.

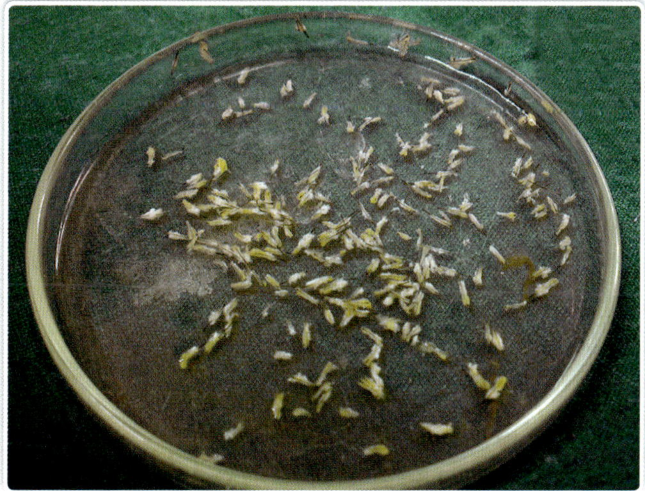

Fig. 23.5: Separated follicular units placed in a Petri dish

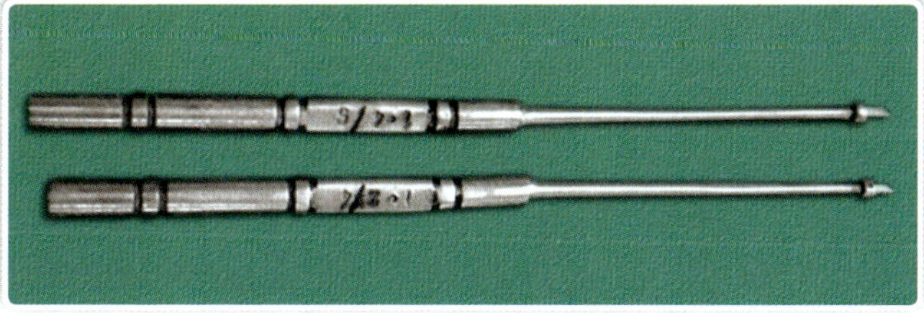

Fig. 23.6: Kolkata Slits

It has been noted that there is increased bleeding in the recipient area in patient undergoing secondary or tertiary procedures. Some amount of fibrosis is expected from the earlier procedures and this also makes the tissue tougher while making recipient gaps. Increased bleeding is also seen in patients who have been using minoxidil in the pre-operative period. Good tumescence, and waiting for 10 to 15 minutes before making gaps can reduce this disturbing ooze.

Step 6: Graft Insertion

The grafts may be inserted using either the simultaneous "Stick and Place method", or the separated "Stick and then Place technique". The grafts are placed into the recipient sites using fine forceps that are usually angled. It is important to be extremely atraumatic while placing the grafts. Preferably the 2 mm of subcutaneous tissue left below the hair bulbs is used in grasping these grafts and placing them into the recipient sites. The grafts should not be grasped by the follicle end to avoid damaging the hair bulbs. Steady pressure is applied to control any bleeding in the area and ensure that the grafts are flushed with the surrounding skin. Burying the grafts beneath the level of the skin must be avoided. It is probably better to leave a graft protruding slightly above the level of the skin than below it for epidermal cysts may result from the latter. Maintaining the grafts as close to the level of the surface of the skin is important for if they are sunk too deep, they get a pitted appearance which is very difficult to correct while being too elevated from the surface creates cobble stone appearance. Two or even three persons can insert grafts at the same time, which make the procedure faster and more efficient. It is again emphasized to keep the graft moist at all times during the procedure. Mega sessions can last upto 5 or 6 hours and upto 2,000 to 4,000 FU's grafts may be transplanted in one such session.

Postoperative Instruction (Box 23.9)

- At the end of the procedure, the patient is discharged usually without any bandage. The autors prefer use of a bandana or a loose cap from next day. Bandaging is still preferred by some surgeons but must be done very carefully to avoid any shearing, which can dislodge the grafts. The bandage must be removed very meticulously

Box 23.9: Postoperative instructions

- Post operative medications like antibiotics and analgesics
- A headband worn immediately postoperatively is useful to prevent the swelling
- Sleep with head end slightly elevated
- Moisten the recipient area with saline drops every 6 hourly for next 24 hours
- Mild shampoo from the 2nd or 3rd day after the surgery
- Avoid wearing clothes like T-shirts or pullovers
- Avoid hair oils, stronger shampoos, heavy exercises, smoking, alcohol intake and use of helmets for 3 weeks
- Use of minoxidil 5% in the areas of hair transplant 7 days after surgery

for grafts may stick under the surface of the bandage and may be inadvertently removed

- Postoperative medications like antibiotics (levofloxacin 500 mg once daily for 5 days), analgesics for pain and other supportive therapy are given
- Some swelling is obvious after a hair transplantation surgery and the patient should be informed of this prior to the procedure. A head-band worn immediately post-operatively is useful to prevent the swelling from coming down on to the face and creating puffy eyelids which may be unsightly although temporary. Patient must sleep with head end slightly raised using one or preferably two pillows for a period of three weeks
- Patients are instructed to moisten the recipient area with saline drops every 6 hours for next 24 hours to prevent desiccation of grafts
- The patient may be allowed to shampoo his hair using a mild shampoo from the 2nd or 3rd day after the surgery
- While combing his hair in the transplanted area, the tooth of the comb should not strike against the transplanted plugs for three weeks
- Wearing clothes like T-shirts or pullovers which have to be taken off over the head should also be avoided for 3 weeks
- Hair oils or other stronger shampoos, heavy exercises, smoking, alcohol intake and use of helmets are also avoided for the same period
- Use of minoxidil 5% in the areas of hair transplant 7 days after surgery for a period of 6 months is advised as this promotes earlier growth of the transplanted hair. In women, minoxidil 2% is used.

Sequelae Following Hair Transplantation

The epidermis and dermis along with the shaft of the transplanted hair outside the skin fall-off as scabs in the next 2 to 3 weeks after the surgery but, the follicles remain and go into the resting phase. New hairs start growing about 3 months after the procedure. Use of minoxidil 5% (2% in females) accelerates this process. It usually takes 6 to 9 months to appreciate the result of a hair transplant **(Figure 23.7)**.

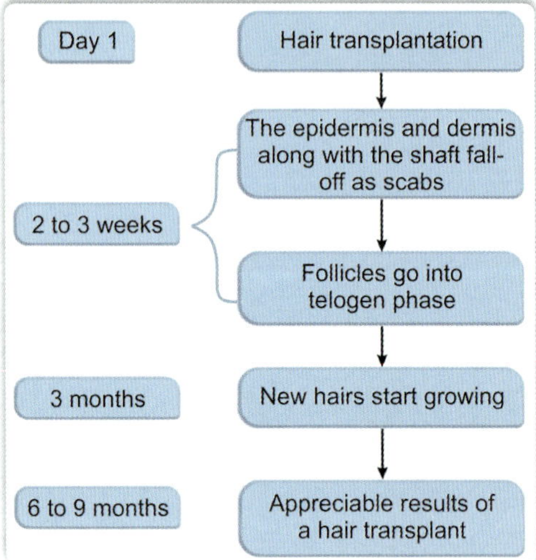

Fig. 23.7: Post-transplantation sequence

If a second procedure has been planned, it must be at least 6 months after the first sitting. Some patients may complain of hypoesthesia of the scalp in the donor area. It is usually temporary but may persist for as long as 18 months in some cases. The density of transplanted hair is usually thinner, especially in areas that are totally bald. The patient should be informed of this preoperatively, and a second sitting can be undertaken to increase this density **(Figures 23.8 and 23.9)**.

Postoperative Complications (Box 23.10)[36-38]

- Complications are few and rarely encountered. Most common complication is postoperative pain which is well managed with analgesics
- Sweling over forehead due to injection of large amount of saline during anesthesia occasionally occurs which can be controlled with use of ice compresses and short course of oral steroids. This begins usually 1–3 days after surgery typically lasting for 7–10 days
- In 10–20% of patients, more common in females a complication called as shock loss or telogen effluvium occurs where a percentage of existing hairs in the donor or recipient area gets traumatized during the procedure and goes into telogen effluvium. Usually, these are temporary and grow back
- True infections in the recipient areas occur infrequently. In the donor areas, infection around sutures may be seen but usually resolves upon their removal

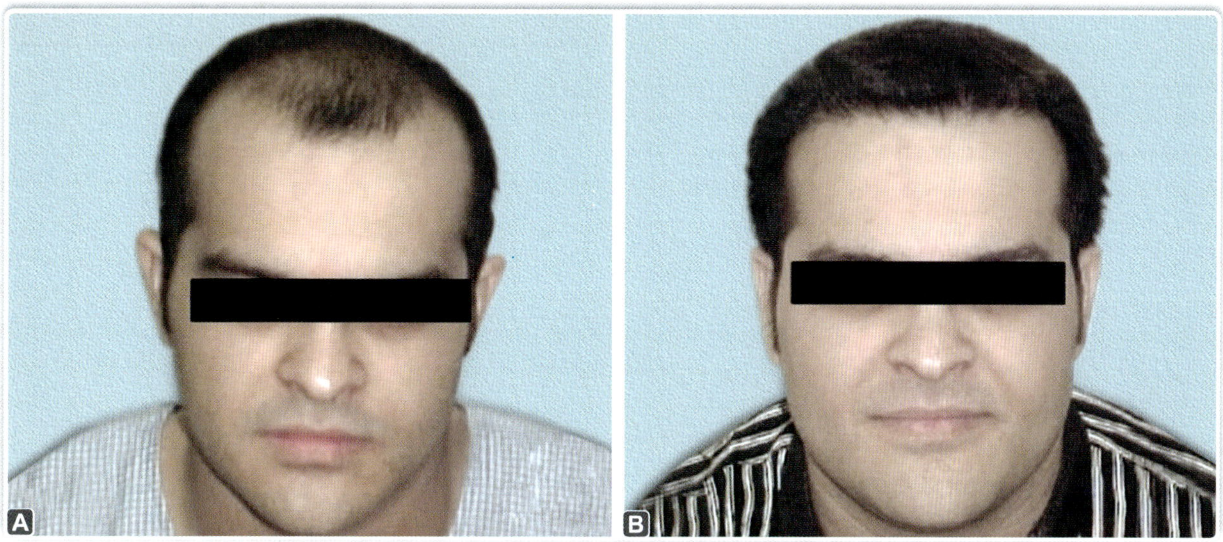

Figs 23.8A and B: (A) Pretransplantation; (B) Post-transplantation

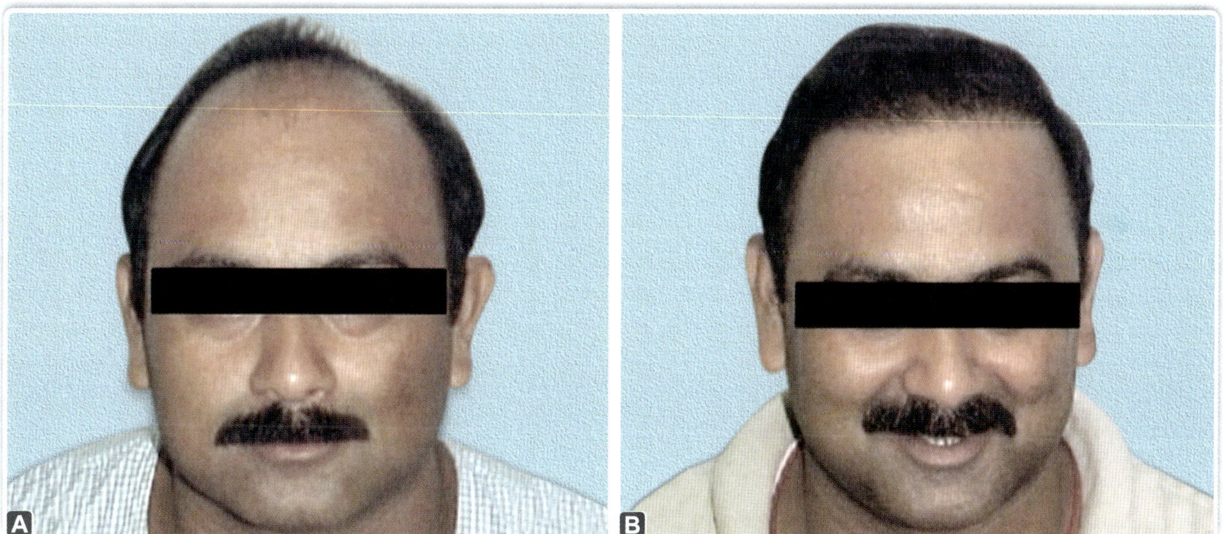

Figs 23.9A and B: (A) Pretransplantation; (B) Post-transplantation

Box 23.10: Complications of hair transplantation

- Postoperative pain
- Swelling over forehead
- Shock loss or telogen effluvlum
- True infections in the recipient areas and donor area
- Epidermal cysts
- Sterile pustules
- Hypo- or hyperesthesia
- Donor area—wound dehiscence, necrosis, wide scar, keloid formation
- Less growth than expected

- Epidermal cysts may be seen where small pieces of skin of the minigraft recipient holes have been left behind, or "piggy backing" one graft on top of another has occurred, or grafts have slipped beneath the skin surface
- Sterile pustules caused by irritant reaction of hair growth sometimes occur during the second month
- Hypo- or hyperesthesia resulting from injury to nerves in the donor and/or recipient area. It usually lasts for 3–6 months but rarely persists as long as 18 months

- A permanent small area of hypoesthesia occurs in approximately 1% of patients
- It is important that not to harvest too wide donor strip for tension on the suture line. At times it lead to dehiscence and even necrosis leaving a wide scar. Keloid formation and central frontal necrosis are rare occurrences
- Less growth than expected from the grafts. This is mostly attributed to improper handling of grafts and injury due to desiccation and hypoxia.

Hair Transplantation in Females[34,39]

Hair loss is not as socially acceptable in females as in males, which make them feel really uncomfortable. Hair transplantation can be done successfully in females too and the number is on the rise. Fortunately in female pattern alopecia in contrast to male pattern alopecia, the hair line is usually not affected. Instead there occurs a diffuse thinning in the central scalp behind the hairline. Following issues are to be known by a surgeon before planning for hair transplantation in a female:

- Before deciding if they are good candidates for surgery, all possible causes of hair loss in females must be ruled out after detailed history, examination and proper investigation. Only those females who have had little success or failed to respond despite adequate treatment should be considered for hair transplantation
- Many females often have unrealistic and high expectations desiring full head of thick hairs. They are not good candidates and hair transplantation surgery in them must be avoided
- They need to be well counseled that the surgeons are not changing the number of hairs on the head, but only redistributing them giving fullness in the area of cosmetic importance for proper styling
- Females, who are Ludwig type 3 having severe hair loss, are not good candidates as their thinning extends to the entire scalp including the parietal and occipital donor areas and thus have insufficient donor hairs to perform the surgery
- Postoperative complication of shock loss or telogen effluvium of existing hairs is much more common in females (30-50%) compared to males (10-20%). Usually they are temporary starting about 2-3 months after surgery and resolves in about 4-6 months. Rarely hair may not grow back completely. So females undergoing surgery needs to be warned about this rarest possibility.
- Hair transplantation is found to be an excellent tool and gaining popularity in females for lowering of abnormally high hairlines which gives the appearance of a large forehead **(Box 23.11)**.

Box 23.11: Issues for transplantation in females

- Muliple etiologies for hair loss other than patterned hair loss
- Many females have unrealistic and high expectations
- Females who are Ludwig type 3 are not suitable as thinning extends to the entire scalp including donor areas
- Postoperative complication of shock loss or telogen effluvium more common in females (30–50%) compared to males (10–20%)
- Hair has to grow a considerable length to appreciate results which might take up to 2 years

Hair Transplantation under Special Situation

- ***Eyebrow transplantation:*** This is done to improve or recreate eyebrows. It is an esthetic essentiality to follow the direction of the eyebrow hairs while creating one. Around 150-200 single hair micrografts are usually required for an eyebrow of one side. The donor site for eyebrow transplantation should be of finer hair preferably taken from the nape of the neck or the temporal region.[40] A 20 or 21-gauge needle is used to make the recipient incisions. Cynoacrylate glue may be placed over the grafted areas to keep the grafts in place during the immediate postoperative period.
- ***Grafting eyelashes:*** Placing grafts in the recipient wounds just above the tarsus in the skin is a more challenging procedure. Fortunately few lashes are necessary to produce a good result. Six to twelve one-hair micrografts per lid may satisfy most patients. The cyanoacrylate glue is also very useful here. The rate of hair growth of the scalp hair is much faster than those of the eyebrows and elsewhere. Patients must be informed preoperatively that this transplanted hair will need trimming from time to time.
- ***Moustache and beard transplanting:*** This is especially useful in patients who have had a cleft lip or a scar following trauma. The hair in the moustache and beard areas are single hair units and much more wiry and coarser than hair in the scalp. Therefore, two hair grafts are usually used to match its quality. Harvesting hair from the beard area just inferior to the jaw line also provides better donor hair, which can be transplanted as micrografts.[41]
- ***Corrective surgery for old technique:*** Patients who have undergone hair transplantation using older techniques have larger plugs. This gives the hairline a pluggy cornrow appearance, which needs correction. The current approach is by plug reduction and recycling

(PR and R), and is applied aggressively at least to the front two rows.[42]

- ***Transplantation into cicatricial or scarring areas:*** Hair transplantation can be successfully used to treat areas of scarring on the scalp, eyebrow, moustache or beard area caused by various reasons such as trauma, burns, radiation therapy, inflammatory skin conditions etc. Special considerations are needed when transplanting into areas of scarring. Scar tissues have inadequate blood supply and thus in addition to poor graft survival; there are increased possibility of infection, ischaemia and necrosis. If feasible, scar tissues are always serially excised into smaller area where hairs are transplanted without dense packing.[43]
- ***Long hair transplantation:*** Instead of the traditional 1 to 2 mm clipped hairs, long hairs are transplanted which allows patients to temporarily see the actual results immediately following the surgery. In this technique, the donor hair is left long (upto 25 cm) throughout the harvesting, dissecting, and plantation. As with traditional hair transplants, the hair is shed about 4 weeks after surgery. Although the procedure gives the patient an early view of the results and eliminates the problems of piggy-backing and buried grafts, it is technically more laborious and requires more meticulous post-operative care.[44,45]

Limitations of Follicular Unit Transplantation

Although blessed with several advantages, FUT has certain limitations:[46]

- It needs adequate special surgical skill
- Follicular units are delicate and needs special handling
- Needs microscopic dissection of hairs and thus needs precision
- It needs more assistants and thus more expensive
- Body hair transplantation cannot be done with FUT
- FUT is labor intensive causing muscle fatigue and eye strain for the operative team.

Conclusion

Recent advances in technology have made hair replacement surgery a viable option for many people but we must utilize this technique prudently. It is very important to form an efficient well-trained team because one individual cannot perform the entire procedure single-handedly.

Fine tuning and accuracy in all steps of the surgery beginning from harvesting of the donor area, cutting of plugs, making recipient sites, inserting the grafts and postoperative care all are essential in getting satisfactory results. No compromize should be made with proper lighting in the operating room and instruments. A comfortable ambience in the operating room, and use of audio-visual means break the monotony, both for the patient and the surgical team. Poor hair replacement surgery is much worse than being bald and brings disrepute to the surgeon as well as the technique. There is no single best approach in hair restoration surgery. Various surgeons employ their skill and experience gained over time and follow different routes to achieve very similar results. If done judiciously, hair transplantation can be a very rewarding procedure, both for the surgeons and the patients.

References

1. Norwood OT. Male pattern baldness: Classification and incidence. South Med J. 1975;68:1359-65.
2. Hamilton JB. Patterned loss of hair in man: Types and incidence. Ann NY Acad Sci. 1951;53:708-28.
3. Venning VA, Dawber, RPR. Patterned androgenetic alopecia in women. J Am Acad Dermatol. 18:173-7,1988.
4. Dieffenbach JF. Nonnulla de Regeneratione et transplantatione. Dissertation inauguralis. 1822.
5. Lamont ES. A plastic surgery transformation. West J Surg Obstet Gynecol. 1957;65:164.
6. Okuda S. Klinische und experimentelle Untersuchungenuber die Transplantation von lebenden Haaren, Jpn J Dermatol [Japanese]. 1939;40:537.
7. Okuda S. Clinical and experimental studies of transplantation of living hairs, Jpn J Dermatol [Japanese]. 1939;46:135-8.
8. Tamura H. Pubic hair transplantation. Jpn J Dermatol. 1943;53:76.
9. Orientreich N. Autografts in alopecias and other selected dermatological conditions. Ann NY Acad Sci. 1959;83:463-79.
10. Orentreich N. Pathogenesis of alopecia. J Soc Cosmet Chem. 1960;11:479-99.
11. Limmer BL. Ellipitical donor stereoscopically assisted micrografting as an approach to further refinement in hair transplantation. Dermatol Surg. 1994;20:789-93.
12. Bernstein RM, Rassman WR, Szaniawski W, Halperin A. Follicular transplantation. Int J Aest Rest Surg. 1995;3:119-32.
13. Bernstein RM, Rassman WR. Follicular transplantation: patient evaluation and surgical planning. Dermatol Surg. 1997;23:771-84.
14. Bernstein RM, Rassman WR, Szaniawski W, Halperin A. Follicular transplantation. Intl J Aesthetic Rest Surg. 1995; 3:119-32.

15. Headington JT. Transverse microscopic anatomy of the human scalp. Arch Dermatol. 1984;120:449-56.
16. Limmer BL. Elliptical donor stereoscopically assisted micrografting as an approach to further refinement in hair transplantation. Dermatol Surg. 1994;20:789-93.
17. Bernstein RM, Rassman WR, Seager D, Shapiro R, et al. Standardizing the classification and description of follicular unit transplantation and mini-micrografting techniques. Dermatol Surg. 1998; 24:957-63.
18. Seager D. Binocular stereoscopic dissecting microscopes: should we use them? Hair Transplant Forum Intl 1996;6(4): 2-5.
19. Bernstein RM, Rassman WR: The logic of follicular unit transplantation. Dermatologic Clinics. 1999;17(2):277-95.
20. Bernstein RM, Rassman WR: The esthetics of follicular transplantation. Dermatol Surg. 1997;23:785-99.
21. Rassman WR, Bernstein RM, McClellan R, et al. Follicular unit extraction: minimally invasive surgery for hair transplantation. Dermatol Surg. 2002;28:720-8.
22. Bernstein RM. Follicular unit hair transplantation. In: Robinson JK, Hanke CW, Siegel DM, et al (Eds). Surgery of the skin. London7 Mosby; 2005.
23. Haber RS, Stough DB. In: Stough DB, Haber RS (Eds): Hair Replacement, Surgical and Medical. St Louis, Mosby. 1997. pp. 390-2.
24. Beehner M. Nomenclature proposal for the zones and landmarks of the balding scalp. Dermatol Surg. 2001;27:375-80.
25. Beehner M. Where is thy crown, your majesty? Hair Transplant Forum Int. 1998;8:18-9.
26. Khan S, Stough DB. In: Stough DB, Haber RS (Eds). Hair Replacement, Surgical and Medical. St Louis, Mosby, 1997. pp. 425
27. Martinick JH. Hairline placement: getting it right the first time. Hair Transplant Forum International. 1999;9(3):65-71.
28. Marzola M. Trichophytic closure of the donor area. Hair Transplant Forum Int. 2005;15(4):113,116-7.
29. Harris JH. Follicular Unit Transplantation; dissecting and planting techniques. Facial Plastic Surgery clinics of North America. 2004;12(4):225-32.
30. Limmer BL. Micrograft survival. In: Stough DB, Haber, RS (Eds). Hair replacement: surgical and medical. St Louis: Mosby; 1996:147-9.
31. Raposio E, Cella A, Panarese P, et al. Power boosting the grafts in hair transplantation surgery. Evaluation of a new storage medium. Dermatol Surg. 1998;24:1342-6.
32. Krugluger W, Moser K, Hugeneck J, Laciak K, Moser C. New storage buffers for micrografts enhance graft survival and clinical outcome in hair restoration surgery. Hair Transplant Forum Int. 2003;13:325;333-4;343.
33. Greco J, Brandt RJ. Preliminary experience and extended applications for the use of autologous platelet-rich plasma in hair transplantation surgery. Hair Transplant Forum Int. 2007;17(4):131-2.
34. Epstein JS. Surgical Hair Restoration in Women. Hair Transplant Forum International. 1999;25-6.
35. Arnold J. Mini-blades and a mini-blade handle for hair transplantation. Am J Cosm Surg. 1997;14:195-200.
36. Unger WP. Complication of hair transplantation. In: Unger WP (Ed). Hair transplantation, 3rd edn. Marcel Dekker, New York. 1995;pp. 363-374.
37. Gandelman M, Mota AL, Abrahamsohn PA, et al. Light and electron microscopic analysis of controlled injury to follicular unit grafts. Dermatol Surg. 2000;26:25-30 [discussion 31].
38. Greco J. The H-factor in micrografting procedures. Hair Transplant Forum International. 1996;6:8-9.
39. Unger R. Transplanting in women. Unger W, Shapiro R(eds) Hair Transplantation. 4th Edition. Marcel Decker, New York 2004:516-24.
40. Gandelman M. Eyebrow and eyelash transplantation. In: Unger WP (Ed). Hair Transplantation. New York: Marcel Deker. 1995;p. 294.
41. Unger WP. Moustache transplants. In: Unger WP (Ed). Hair Transplantation. New York: Marcel Deker. 1995;p. 311.
42. Vogel JE. Correction of the cornrow hair transplant and other common problems in surgical hair restoration. Plast Reconstr Surg. 2000;105:4.
43. Shapiro R, Rose P. Transplanting into scar tissue and other areas of cicatricial alopecia. Unger W, Shapiro R (Ed). Hair Transplantation 4th edn. Mercel Decker, New York. 2004:606-9.
44. Bouhanna P. Long hair grafts: 20 years of experience. Hair Transplant Forum Int. 2007;17(4):127-8.
45. Pitchon M. Preview Long-hair follicular unit transplantation: An immediate temporary vision of the best possible final result. Hair Transplant Forum Int. 2006;16(4):114,118-9.
46. Stough D, Whitworth JM. Methodology of follicular unit hair transplantation. Dermatol Clin. 1999;17:297-306.

24

Recent Advances in Hair Transplantation

Venkataram Mysore, Raghini Ghiya

"The seeker embarks on a journey to find what he wants and discovers along the way, what he needs."

—*Wally Lamb*

Introduction

There have been several efforts in the last decade to improve the outcome of hair transplantation.[1] These include:

- Efforts to minimize donor scarring, by methods such as trichophytic closure and follicular unit extraction[2]
- Efforts to increase the number of grafts transplanted in one session- Giga sessions
- Efforts to preserve grafts better, by using holding solutions
- Efforts to find alternate source of donor hairs—body hair transplantation
- Efforts at automation, use of robotics.

Improving Donor Scar

With increasing tendency for keeping hairs shorter, visibility of donor scar is a major cosmetic problem and patients have demanded better scars. This demand for pencil line scar, coupled with the demand for larger mega and giga sessions, has proven challenging for surgeons. This is particularly so in patients who have lesser quality donor such as Asian populations, who have less follicular unit density, less elasticity and smaller head width. The efforts to produce a less visible scar have concentrated on three areas as given in **Box 24.1**.

Box 24.1: Donor scar reduction methods in hair transplantation

- Trichophytic closure
- Better suturing techniques of donor strip
- Follicular unit extraction (FUE)

Trichophytic Closure

When hair transplant surgeons meticulously close the edges of a donor wound, they generally end up with a fine, linear scar that is approximately 1-2 mm in width. Sometimes, the scar can be a bit wider and every once in a while, when the person's connective tissue is weak, or the edges of the scar are closed too roughly or have too much tension, the scar can be a cosmetic problem. The educated patient, who has expectations of a thin scar, or the patient who is likely to wear his hair very short, hopes that their hair transplant doctor can produce scars that are practically invisible.

A trichophytic closure[2] is a way of improving the linear donor scars of hair transplant patients. A trichophytic incision in hair transplantation involves trimming off the upper or lower edge of the incision by cutting 0.5 mm deep, 1-2 mm wide strip, and then closing the wound in such a way the hairs near the edge can grow through the scar. This has the potential to produce a scar that is virtually undetectable **(Figures 24.1A and B)**.

However, it needs to be understood that attending to basic principles of suturing, avoiding tension, avoiding postoperative edema are vital and trichophytic closure can not compensate for poor closure techniques.

Follicular Unit Extraction (FUE)

FUE was first described by Bernstein and Rassman,[3] who referred to it as the FOX procedure. However, it has been described by other workers under different names such as Wood's technique,[4] FU Isolation method.[5] It has been also referred to as sutureless method of transplantation **(Box 24.2)**.

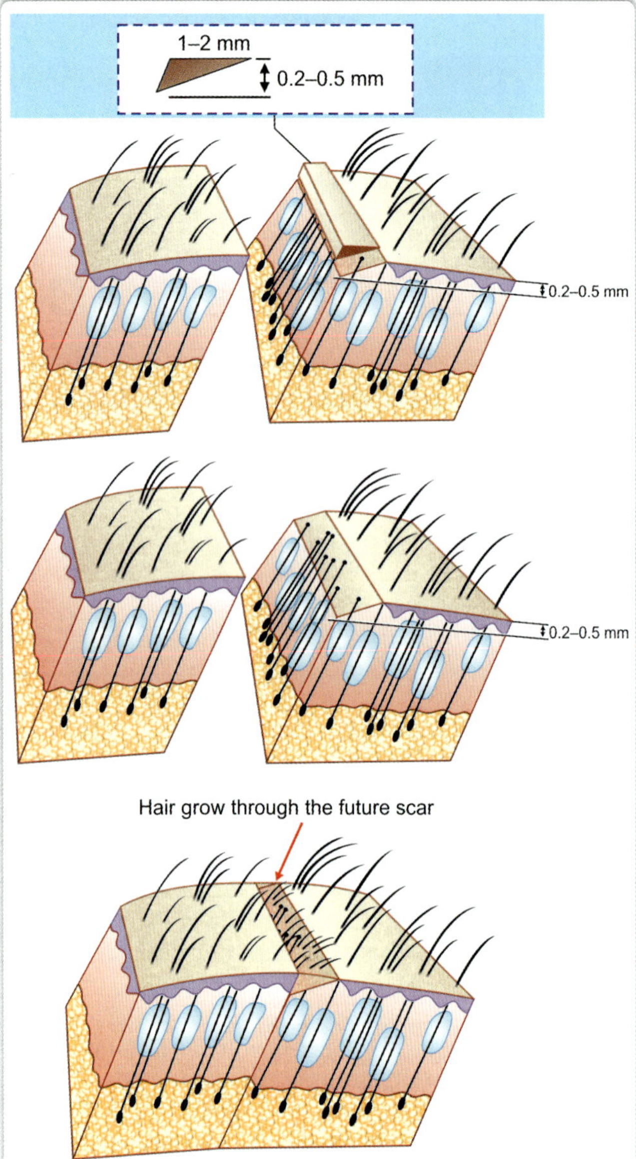

Fig. 24.1A: Trichophytic closure

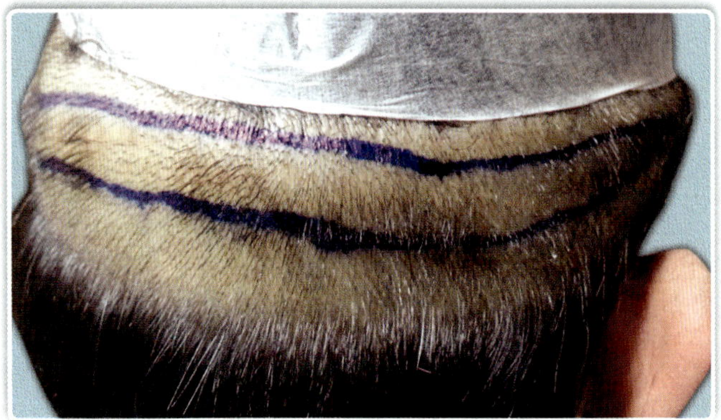

Fig. 24.1B: A very fine scar after trichophytic closure

Principle

In a follicular unit, it is the arrectores pilorum which holds the hairs together in a bunch. The bulge area, is the narrowest part of the unit, with the hairs splaying below, resulting in a pyramid shaped unit **(Figure 24.2)**.

The site of attachment of arrector muscle to the follicular unit is the zone where the hairs are held at their tightest. Below this site is the inferior segment, which is temporary and disappears cyclically, in the telogen phase of the hair cycle. The inferior segment is therefore held loosely and once the hold of the arrectores in the unit is weakened, the inferior segment can be extracted easily. Because the follicular unit is narrow at the surface, one needs to make a small opening, of size 0.8–1.0 mm, to reach the bulge area, through which the unit can be extracted.[3,6] This small opening heals easily and quickly with a very inconspicuous scar. Thus, the basic principle of the FUE is to extract an intact unit through a hole, which is as small as possible, which would then heal with minimal and inconspicuous scarring **(Figures 24.3A to C)**.[6]

However, there have been many limitations and difficulties in implementing the above principle:[1,3,6]

a. The main anatomical limitation is that it is a blind technique, as it is not possible to identify the level of the bulge from outside.
b. Also, the inferior segments of the hairs splay at the lower end in different directions **(Figure 24.2)**, making the follicular unit pyramid shaped-wider at bottom and narrower at the top, rendering the process of extraction difficult.
c. Further, the tightness with which the unit is held together by arrectores and the perifollicular collagen may vary greatly from person to person, from area to area.

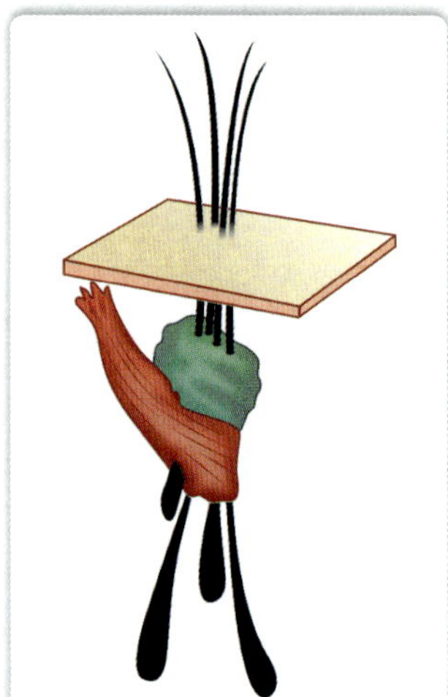

Fig. 24.2: Pyramid shaped follicular unit

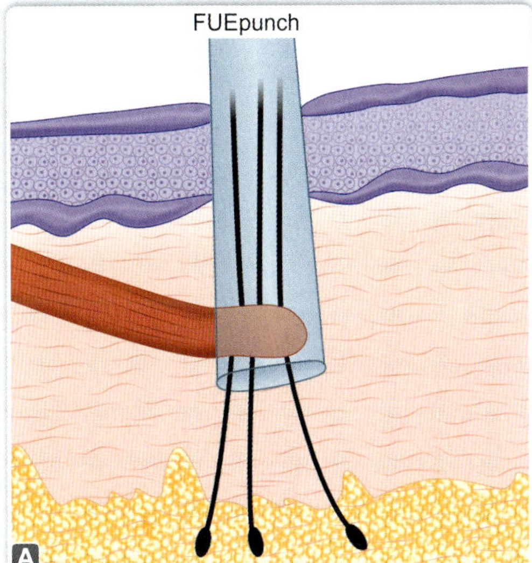

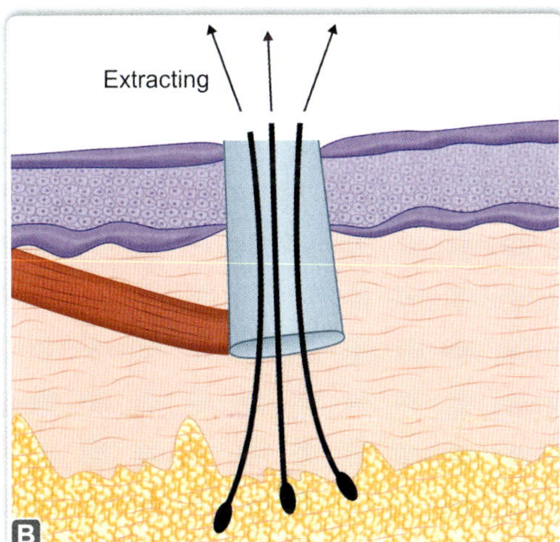

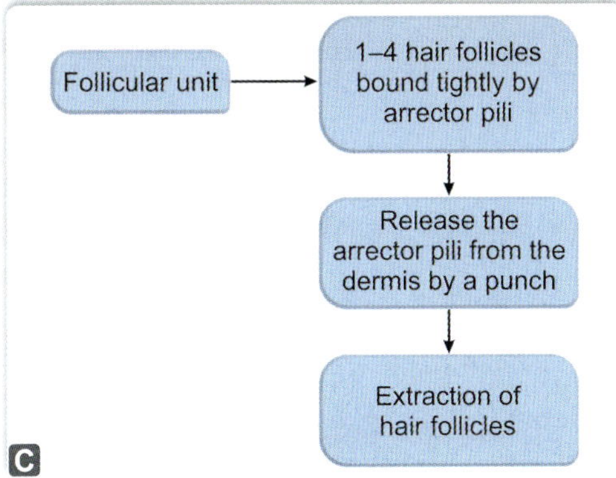

Figs 24.3A to C: Principle of FUE

d. The direction of emergence of hairs varies from area to area. Particularly in lower occipital scalp, the hairs emerge and run parallel to the surface, making extraction difficult.

All these factors have made the technique of extraction slow, difficult and associated with a higher level of transection.[7] Because of the slow process, the procedure is also more expensive. Another criticism of the technique has been that this is a throwback to the olden days of punch grafting. However, the results of the past few years have shown that the scar in FUE is indeed very small and the cosmetic result of the donor area after FUE is excellent.

Over the last few years, surgeons have developed increasing experience and techniques to perform the procedure rapidly and with lesser transection rates to overcome the above criticisms to some extent. The procedure now accounts for about 25% of all transplants and is likely to become more popular in future. It is now possible to perform FUE mega sessions, with about 1500–2000 grafts in a day and hence cover larger areas.[8] Surgeons have developed ingenious methods of harvesting from new areas, which were previously never considered, such as temporal area, beard area etc and larger areas are being covered by this technique. The method is also very suitable for automation and robotic machines have been developed for extraction.[8]

Table 24.1 gives the relative advantages and disadvantages of FUE technique and **Table 24.2** gives the comparison of the two techniques follicular unit transplantation (FUT) and follicular unit extraction (FUE).

Indications for FUE include[3]

- Patients who want to cut their hair very short (and hence even a very thin linear donor scar is unacceptable) and therefore specifically request for FUE
- In patients with limited hair loss or those who require relatively small sessions. However, this indication is changing as mentioned above and large areas are being covered by FUE mega sessions
- For second/third session, in patients with widened scars resulting from traditional strip excision
- FUE technique is the only technique useful in body hair transplantation[9]
- Of late, FUE (on day 1) has been used along with FUT (day 2) to perform larger sessions (Giga sessions).[9] A 1200–1500 graft FUE can be combined with a 3000 graft FUT to cover a large area.

Contraindications for FUE include[3]

- Patients with tightly held units (FOX grade 4 and 5-see below)
- Unrealistic patient expectations: It must be mentioned here that this technique has received somewhat exaggerated publicity over internet sites as a scarless hair transplantation. Patients have to be properly

Table 24.1: Advantages and disadvantages of follicular unit extraction (FUE)

Advantage of FUE	*Disadvantage of FUE*
1. Needs less manpower than FUT; one doctor with one or two assistants can run a centre 2. The procedure is less aggressive and advanced surgical experience is not essential 3. Graft dissection and preparation is minimal 4. Less space and equipment are needed 5. Patient can cut hairs short 6. Minimal postoperative pain and recovery time 7. Small scars in donor area are almost invisible 8. The technique can be used for extracting body hair, as additional source of donor hair 9. Can be used for grey/white hair where accurate dissection with strip surgery is difficult 10. Can be combined with strip surgery to achieve maximum yield of grafts (e.g. Giga sessions)	1. Slow and tedious 2. There is a long learning curve in FUE 3. Higher transection rate 4. The procedure is long and hence tiring for the patient 5. Number of grafts extracted per day is limited 6. Very fine trimming of donor hair which may be unacceptable to many people 7. Because of the time consumed, the procedure is more costly, almost two times that of FUT 8. The total number of grafts that can be harvested without having noticeable thinning of donor area is limited (2500 to 3000 grafts) so not suitable for large cases in need of more grafts

Table 24.2: Comparison of strip harvesting and follicular unit extraction (FUE)

Strip harvesting	*FUE*
❑ Strip excision of donor skin with suturing	❑ Extraction of individual units one by one through small punch holes; each alternate hair unit is removed. No suturing
❑ Heals with a single linear scar which is 1–3 mms wide, hidden under hairs	❑ Heals with multiple tiny scars in between hairs
❑ Healing over 1 week	❑ Healing over 2–3 days
❑ Donor hairs not trimmed; suture completely hidden	❑ Donor hairs trimmed
❑ Quicker; 4–5 hours for 2000 grafts	❑ Slower, 6–7 hours for 2000 grafts
❑ More precise because of microscopic dissection	❑ Less precise as units are pulled blindly
❑ Transection rate 1–2%	❑ Transection rate 2–5%
❑ More comfortable as patient is mostly sleeping face up watching TV	❑ Patient in head down position for several hours—more uncomfortable
❑ Operation site over donor hidden completely hidden on the day of surgery	❑ Operation site shaven and hence visible
❑ Large sessions, up to 3000 grafts possible	❑ Large sessions difficult—so suitable for smaller areas
❑ Less expensive	❑ More expensive because of the prolonged procedure
❑ 90% of world's transplants are done by this method	❑ 25% of transplants by this method- suitable for small areas, people who are afraid of suture and people who want to keep short hair
❑ Grafts separated are relatively thicker with more adventitial tissue surrounding and easier to handle	❑ Grafts are very thin and delicate with very little adventitial tissue. So more chances of injury while handling. Needs to be handled with care
❑ 2nd hair transplant session can be carried out with minimum difficulty as it doesn't disturb the remaining donor area	❑ 2nd hair transplant session becomes difficult due to scarring from previous session all over the donor area

counseled that the method is a sutureless method, not really a scarless method

- Patient who is not willing to cut his hair short and for this reason women are not good candidates for FUE
- Large bald areas needing more than 2500 grafts.

Procedure of FUE

Preparation

The entire donor area from the occipital scalp is trimmed to 1-2 mm length. It is not possible to perform FUE on long hairs. However, total shaving is not preferred as a small length of hair is needed to mark the direction of emergence of the hair. In patients who want to hide the trimmed operated area, horizontal strips of long hairs are left alternating with extracted areas, so that the long hairs (at least one inch long) hide the operated area (also known as Microstrip shave). The patient lies in the prone or lateral position on the operating table. Local anesthesia with Xylocaine 1% diluted with saline is administered slowly over the entire donor area. The use of tumescence has been controversial .While deep tumescence helps by decreasing bleeding during extraction, it may also distort the directing of emergence of hairs.

The grafts are then extracted from the donor area with the help of 0.8, 0.9 and 1 mm micropunches.

The extraction of follicles is done under 2.5-5X magnification. Extraction process starts from distal to proximal and is done row by row. This helps in an assistant extracting the hairs as the holes are being made. Punches of different types have been introduced. While some surgeons prefer sharp punches, others use a shaper punch to score the skin, followed by a dull punch to reach the bulge level. The size of the punch varies from 0.8-1 mm, depending on the expertise of the surgeon and the type of unit being extracted. The punch is introduced along the direction of hair, up to a depth of about 2–3 mms, until a sensation of give in is felt. While this is being done, traction is applied downwards by the assistant, to render the hair as vertical as possible to facilitate smooth entry of punch. Alternate units are extracted so that the density after extraction is not less than 50% of original density. If the level of bulge is reached properly, the unit just pops out and can be easily picked up. The extracted grafts are then preserved in saline or cool Ringer's lactate solution.[10]

This is the most time consuming and tedious part of the whole procedure and time taken depends on the skill and experience of the surgeon. After the extraction is over, the grafts are implanted in a similar way as in the rest of FUT. The extraction has been greatly facilitated by introduction of automated machines, which helps speed up the process and reduces surgeon fatigue. It is now possible to extract up to 1200 grafts in three hours **(Figures 24.4 and 24.5)**.

Techniques of extracting the grafts:

1. *One-step procedure:* In this method, a single punch is used to mark the skin and then rotated in one direction by 2–3 turns till it suddenly gives way (when the bulge level is reached). At the same time, assistant pushes the skin down in the direction opposite to that in which hair is being pulled. Single step procedure, though the quickest, is often associated with higher transection rates than two and three step procedures.[7]

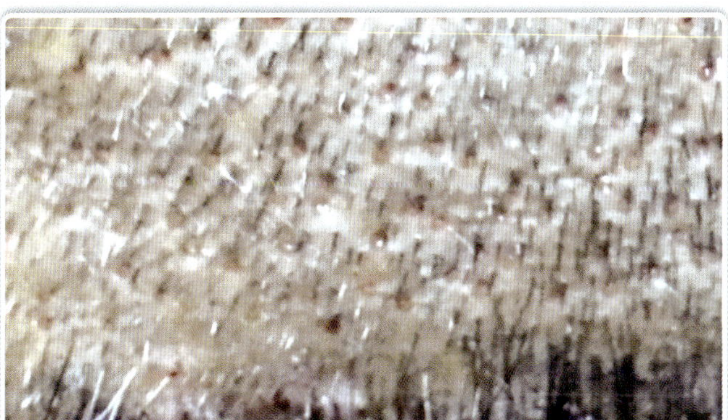

Fig. 24.4A: Donor area immediately after FUE

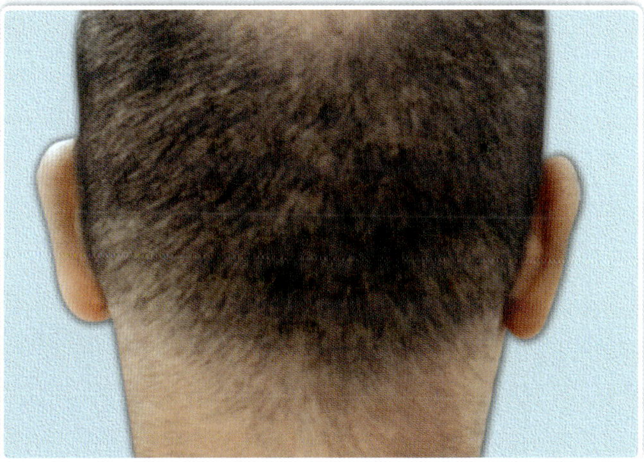

Fig. 24.4B: Donor area two months after FUE

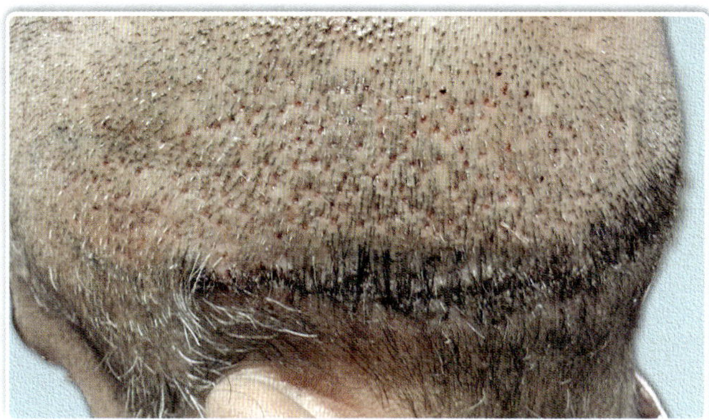

Fig. 24.5: Donor scar after giga session

2. *Two-step procedure:* If the unit does not pop out as above after introduction of the punch, a fine forceps is used to apply gentle upward traction to the top of follicular unit (FU) while another forceps is used to push it up form below the bulge level.[11] (Two forcep technique of Lorenzo). Care should be taken not to hold the unit at the bulge level, where stem cells are located.
3. *Three-step procedure:* The three-step technique for FUE is advocated by Harris who used an instrument with a sharp punch on one side and dull punch on the other side.[12] The sharp punch is used to score the epidermis, and then dull punch is used to bluntly dissect the follicular unit with twisting movement from the surrounding epidermis and dermis. Lastly, the graft is held with forceps and pulled out. This variation may be more accurate, but is considerably slower.

Tips to Avoid Transection

The main criticism against FUE has been that, being a blind process, the percentage of transection is higher than in FUT. As mentioned earlier, the transection rate can come down significantly, to less than 5%, by adopting the tips[13] given in **Box 24.2**.

FOX Test

As mentioned already, the extraction is a variable process and FOX test has been introduced to determine whether the patient is a suitable candidate for FUE or not. In FOX test, the surgeon takes out a few (about 100) grafts from the donor area and then evaluates how many complete/incomplete follicular units are extracted. According to the ease and completeness of extracted grafts, Bernstein and

Box 24.2: Tips to avoid transection

- Use of blunt punches minimizes risk of transection
- FU's are more vertical than the exit angle, so giving gentle traction to the skin while using the punch can make hair more vertical and easy to extract.
- Reduce the depth of insertion of punch for thin skin and acutely emerging hair
- Accentric placement of the follicle inside the punch, away from the follicular direction, can minimize chances of damage to the follicle.

Box 24.3: FOX grading

Grade 1-	Intact follicular units literally pop out of the scalp	Suitable for FUE
Grade 2-	Transection rate is 20%	
Grade 3-	Neutral	
Grade 4-	Most of the surrounding fat is avulsed	FUE contraindicated
Grade 5-	Damage in virtually all the grafts	

Rassman[3] classified FOX test into five grades depending the ease with which units can be extracted. Grade 1 is when intact follicular units literally pop out of the scalp or when there is only occasional transection of individual hairs in the unit. In Fox grade 4-5, when the extraction process is too slow and transection rate is too high, FUE cannot be performed **(Box 24.3)**.

Complications in FUE

It is a minor procedure, but is not without complications. Like any surgery, infection can occur and hence proper antibiotic cover is advocated. Burial of graft is another complication, which can delay the procedure. It can be avoided by avoiding the nuchal area where the angle of the hair is very acute and clipping the hair very short (less than 1 mm). The buried graft can be removed by exerting pressure on the buried graft by a comedone extractor. While the extraction site heals without any incidents usually, occasional bleeding may occur postoperatively, which may be alarming to the patient. Extraction of too many units without adequate gaps may lead to thinned out appearance or a moth eaten or Swiss cheese appearance of the donor area.[14]

Automated FUE Hair Transplantation

Several machines have been recently introduced. The FUE Matic machine is an automated hair transplant machine that seeks to assist the doctor in performing a hair transplant using the FUE technique. It is claimed to give a faster extraction rate of grafts in a limited time. Several machines have been introduced which use a motorized equipment to make punches and then use suction to suck the loosened units.[11,14-16] These have been made to make the process faster and more accurate.

Transplantation in Difficult Areas

Vertex transplantation: Vertex (back of head) is generally a difficult area-this area is large, circular in shape, and therefore hairs emerge in a radiating pattern, like spokes of a wheel. It also has whorls. Therefore, it needs a large no. of grafts and these have to be arranged in different directions. This takes more time, and more importantly, because the baldness is circular, in future, it could expand in a centrifugal pattern. Hair transplantation in the central circular area could result in a situation in future wherein, grafted hairs remain in the centre and new area of baldness is seen all around it. This is cosmetically unacceptable. For these reasons, it is always preferable not to operate vertex area early, to always try drugs first in this area, and operate in the front of the head first. Only experienced transplant surgeons should perform vertex surgeries.

Hair transplantation in other areas—eye brow, moustache, beard, eyelashes: Hair transplantation can be done, not only for baldness over scalp, but also over other areas such as eyebrows, eyelashes, moustache, beard, etc. These need special considerations as they are mobile areas. They are also more expensive.

Eyebrows: Eyebrows are transplanted with only single hair units, which are extracted either by strip of FUE technique.[17] It is important to observe the direction of the eyebrows properly. In the median part of the eyebrow, hairs emerge vertically, while in lateral part, they emerge parallel to the skin. This is an area where a properly done transplantation can yield gratifying results.

Eyelashes: Eyelash transplantation is difficult and time consuming.[18] The donor hair used in an eyelash restoration must match, as closely as possible, the original eyelash. Hair suited for this purpose includes the fine short hairs at the nape of the neck, hair from behind the ears or the eyebrows. The incision made into the lid margin should be made with a curved instrument and the hair should be rotated to follow the curvature of the original lashes.[19] Corneal protection and proper anesthesia is vital. Only single hairs are to be used. It is important to place the direction of the hairs to emerge away from the eyeball, to avoid districhiasis. This can be performed by any of the following techniques:

- Using slit and place as in scalp hair transplantation
- Using KNU implanters
- Using long hairs which are inserted into the eye of curved needles. The needles are then inserted in the conjunctival side of the eyelid and then pushed to emerge on the skin side.

Moustache area can also be transplanted. Since it is a mobile area, proper immobilization is important. Transplantation for cleft repair scar is commonly sought. Postoperative edema is common as it is a vascular area.

Transplantation in women: Hair transplantation in women, presents several challenges, which should be discussed in person with the patient.[20]

1. In women, there are multiple causes for hair loss. These should be investigated and treated before transplantation.
2. In female pattern hairloss, hair loss is more diffuse and widespread. Hence, a proper discussion about which area should be transplanted is necessary. Counseling about possible progression of baldness, need for concurrent drug therapy should be thorough.
3. Women have long hairs and do not accept trimming of hairs. Hence, transplantation should be done amidst these hairs. This is more time consuming and needs experience.
4. Since women wants hairs to be long, results take almost 1½ years, to grow to required length, in contrast to the 9 months needed in men.
5. Since grafting has to be done in between existing hairs, possibility of post transplantation telogen effluvium is high and needs to be explained during counseling.
6. Finally, women often have exaggerated expectations about their results and hence need proper counseling.

Body Hair Transplantation (BHT)

Due to the continuous need and larger amount of hair to cover the bald area, more cases with Norwood V, VI, VII are opting for hair transplant and with increase in hair density that can be provided in one session, the body hair has emerged as an important source of hair. Body hair transplantation, first reported by Woods[4] depends on the principle of recipient influence demonstrated by Tommy Hwang.[21] Tommy Hwang showed that in pattern hairloss, in addition to donor dominance, there is also the recipient influence, which determines the response in a transplant of hairs from another area. He demonstrated that body hair when transplanted to scalp would grow longer and thicker. This principle along with the introduction of the FUE technique paved the way for body hair transplantation, which has the following characteristics:

- Body hair has to be extracted by FUE technique and hence is very slow; it may take 12–14 hours for a 2000 graft session **(Figure 24.6)**
- Body hair are thin, short and acutely placed with variable directions
- For anesthesia, blocks are difficult and need to give local anesthesia to individual area necessitating large doses of anesthesia
- Body hair occurs mostly as single hair units and hence gives less density
- Body hair diameter is less and so gives less volume

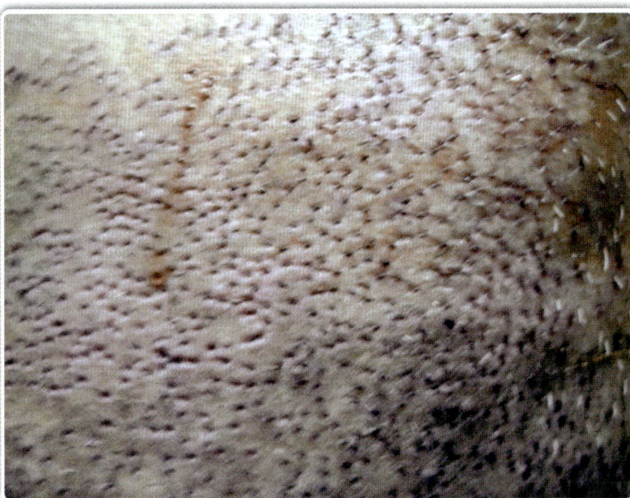

Fig. 24.6: Body hair FUE

- Long term behavior of body hair is still not known as the technique is new
- Body hair may grow long when transplanted on to scalp, but not as long and as thick as scalp hair, so it is inferior to scalp hair in quality. Body hair takes longer time to grow as compared to scalp hair
- Lastly and most importantly, body hair transplantation is possible only for patients who have good body hair on chest, shoulder and other areas
- BHT is associated with tiny scars on chest.

Hence, BHT is performed only when scalp donor is exhausted. Beard hair being 2.5 times thicker than scalp hair, can be a good option to BHT.

Long Hair Transplantation

The usual length of grafted hair is 0.5 cm. Some patients want long hairs after transplantation, to look natural and to get a preview of how they would look after transplantation. This is called long hair or preview transplantation in which hairs are left long, 4–6 cm. However, it is technically more difficult to do and therefore is more expensive. Further, it should be remembered that whether hairs are transplanted long or short, they will fall off in the second week.

Holding Solutions for Graft Storage

The optimal holding solution should reduce the trauma to tissue from reperfusion injury and free radical formation as well as from ion and osmolarity abnormalities created by the ischemic phase soon after grafting.

The storage solutions are of two kinds—intracellular and extracellular.

Intracellular storage solutions are hypertonic solutions with elevated K^+ levels and reduced Na levels more similar to the intracellular space along with a larger anion that is unable to cross the cell membrane and will therefore provide osmotic support. Examples of intracellular storage solutions include Hypothermosol, Collins, Euro Collins, Viaspan (University of Wisconsin Solution), CryoStor, Celsior, HTK-Custodial, Unisol, and KPS I.

The extracellular storage solution is an isotonic solution having a plasma-like complement of ions that mimics the normal extracellular environment of cells. Examples include normal saline, Ringer's lactate, BSS, and tissue culture media that mimic the extracellular composition of plasma and other body fluids. Despite the research to date, there is no conclusive evidence to guide which solution is best for graft survival and which can help to prevent anagen effluvium.[22]

Robotics

Since the hair transplant surgery is repetitive, it has been thought the procedure is ideally suited for a robotic application.[22] Recently, a machine called ARTAS has been introduced to perform robotic assisted follicular unit extraction. The robot has mirror-assisted calculation of hair emergence angles to enable smooth extraction and it has been claimed that it can extract up to one thousand units in an hour.[23] While the claims are to yet to be proven, robotic hair transplantation remains an exciting option.

Conclusion

The field of hair transplantation has seen several important advancements. FUE technique is an important advance, which caters to specific needs of selected patients. Body hair offers an alternative source, but should be undertaken only after proper counseling and in selected patients. In skilled hands, areas such as moustache, eyebrows can be transplanted with gratifying results.

References

1. Shiell RC. A review of modern surgical hair restoration techniques. J Cutan Aesthet Surg. 2008;1:12-6.
2. Marzola M.Trichophytic closure of the donor area. Hair Transplant Forum Int. 2005;15:113-6.
3. Rassman WR, Bernstein RM, McClellan R, Jones R, Worton E, Uyttendaele H. Follicular Unit Extraction: Minimally invasive surgery for hair transplantation. Dermatol Surg. 2002;28:720-7.
4. Woods A. Chest hair micrografts display extended growth in scalp tissue: A case report. Br J Plast Surg. 2004;57:789-91.
5. Kingsley S. Sharing experiences of follicular isolation technique? Follicular Unit Extraction. Hair Transplant Forum Int. 2004;14:15.
6. Bernstein RM. A neighbor's view of the "follicular family unit." Hair Transplant Forum Int. 1998;8:23-5.
7. Yamamoto K. Intraoperative monitoring of the follicular transection rate in follicular unit extraction. Hair Transplant Forum Int. 2008;18:175.
8. Bernstein RM, Rassman WR, Anderson KW. Follicular unit extraction mega sessions: Evolution of a technique. Hair Transplant Forum Int. 2004;14:97-9.
9. Poswal A. Body hair transplant: An additional source of donor hair in hair restoration surgery. Indian J Dermatol. 2007;52:104-5.
10. Serdar G, Nessin B, Gurcan A. Follicular Unit Extraction in hair transplantation: Personal experience. Ann Plast Surg. 2008;60:127-33.
11. Bernstein RM, Rassman WR. New instrumentation for three step Follicular Unit Extraction. Hair Transplant Forum Int. 2006;16:229-37.
12. Harris JA. The SAFE System: New instrumentation and methodology to improve follicular unit extraction (FUE). Hair Transplant Forum Int. 2004;14:163-4.
13. Bertram NG, Damkemg P. Follicular Unit Extraction; experience in Chinese population. Hair Transplant Forum Intl. 2009;19:14.
14. Unger W. Commentary follicular unit extraction. Dermatol Surg. 2002;28:727-8.
15. Ekrem C, Aksoy M, Koc E, Aksoy B. Evaluation of three instruments used in FUE. Hair Transplant Forum Intl. 2009;14-5.
16. Onda M, Igawa HH, Inoue K, Tanino R. Novel Technique of Follicular Unit Extraction Hair Transplantation with a Powered Punching Device. Dermatol Surg. 2008;34:1683-8.
17. Epstein J. Eyebrow Transplantation. Hair Transplant Forum Int. 2006;16:121.
18. Breeling JL. Eyelash Transplantation: Who Why and How. Hair Transplant Forum Int. 2007;1:17-20.
19. Rassman WR, Bernstein RM. Plastic surgery products. Jan 2006;34-8.
20. Beehner M. A Perspective on Transplanting Females. Hair Transplant Forum Int. 2005;15:113-6.
21. Sungjoo, Hwang T. Long-term Evaluation of Hair Transplantation into Various Recipient Sites. Hair Transplant Forum Int. 2006;16:37.
22. Cole John. The optimal holding solution and temperature for hair follicle.www. The optimal holding solution and temperature for hair follicle. Cole Hair Transplant.webarchive. last visited on 28-10-2012.
23. Rassman WR, Bernstein RM. Automation of hair transplantation past, present and future. In: Harahap M, editor. Innovative techniques in skin surgeon. New York: Marcel Dekker, Inc. 2002;489-502.

25

Laser Hair Removal

Sanjeev J Aurangabadkar

"I hear and I forget, I see and I remember, I do and I understand."

—*Confucius*

Introduction

The removal of unwanted hair by lasers and light devices is one of the most commonly performed cosmetic procedures in the world and the demand continues to grow. Lasers and light devices offer excellent long-term hair reduction, and along with electrolysis is the only permanent method of hair reduction.[1]

Though laser hair reduction (LHR) is an established modality for reducing unwanted hair, certain limitations exist. These include treatment of darker skin phototypes due to the risk of post inflammatory hyper and hypo pigmentation, the need for multiple sessions, long total treatment duration, variable results depending on the system used and the skill of the operator and hormonal profile of the patient. With proper patient selection and use of established standards of care, excellent outcomes can be achieved with minimal side effects. This chapter will enumerate the basics of LHR, patient selection, choice of the machines and the protocol of LHR and its associated adverse effects **(Box 25.1)**.

Patients seek hair removal for unwanted hair that may be in a normal distribution, termed hypertrichosis or in a male pattern distribution, termed hirsutism. Hypertrichosis may be constitutional or related to ethnicity of the patient. Hirsutism is often associated with endocrinopathies such as polycystic ovaries, hyperandrogenism, etc. Patients may also seek LHR for social, cultural and cosmetic reasons and it is not uncommon for male patients seeking LHR on areas, such as the body, ears, beard, nose, etc.

Definition

Temporary hair reduction: It is defined as a delay in hair regrowth, lasting 1-3 months, consistent with the induction of telogen. Temporary methods of hair reduction include plucking, shaving, waxing and chemical depilatories.[2]

Permanent hair reduction: It is significant reduction in the number of terminal hairs after a given treatment, which is stable for a period of time, longer than the complete growth cycle of the hair follicles at the given body site **(Figure 25.1)**. Laser treatment often produces complete but temporary hair loss lasting 1–3 months, followed by partial but permanent hair loss.[1]

Box 25.1: Limitations of laser hair reduction

- Risk of postinflammatory pigmentation in dark skin
- The need for multiple sessions
- Long total treatment duration
- System dependent results
- Operator dependent results

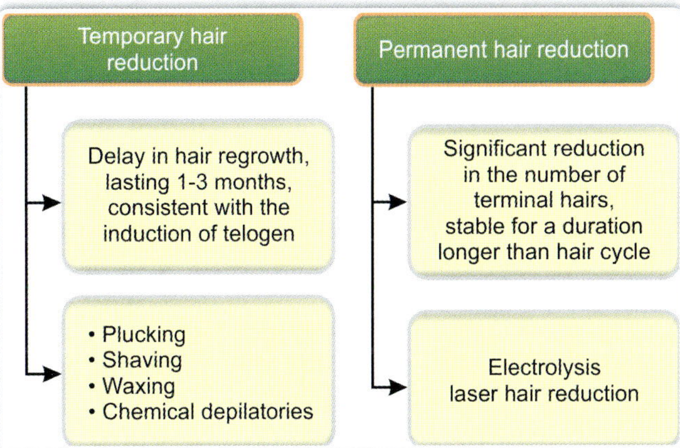

Fig. 25.1: Hair reduction methods

Histologically, laser treatment shows damage predominantly in hair follicles with large, pigmented hair shafts, where as those with small (<25 μm) hypopigmented shafts do not show any morphological changes.

Hair Growth Cycle

There are three types of hair—lanugo, vellus, and terminal hairs:

1. Lanugo hairs are fetal-type, soft fine hairs
2. Vellus hairs are non-pigmented, superficial and have a diameter of 30 μm
3. Terminal hairs are usually 40 μm and vary widely in thickness with the size of the hair bulb.

Hair growth cycle involves the following stages:

1. Anagen (period of active synthesis)
2. Catagen (regression)
3. Telogen (rest)
4. Exogen (shedding).

Hair undergoes asynchronous cycling between these stages thus controlling the growth and length of the hair shaft. The duration of anagen determines the length of the hair shaft. The catagen phase lasts about 3 weeks and is constant at different locations of the body. The anagen and telogen phases differ significantly at different body sites[3] (Refer to Chapter 2). **Table 25.1** shows the duration of anagen at various body sites.[4, 5]

Principle of Laser Kinetics and Dynamics for Hair Reduction

LHR is based on the principle of selective photothermolysis, which was introduced by Anderson and Parrish.[6] Selective destruction of the hair follicle can be achieved by choosing the correct wavelength of laser light (which is absorbed by melanin in the hair shaft) at a pulse duration that is equal to or shorter than the thermal relaxation time (TRT) of the target along with the right amount of energy delivered to the chromophore (target absorbing the laser light) **(Box 25.2)**.[7,8]

This laser-tissue interaction leads to the energy being confined to the hair follicle and its surrounding bulb and bulge region. The light energy is converted to heat thus leading to destruction of the selected target **(Figure 25.2)**. The conventional laser systems utilize high peak fluences with short pulse duration, to maximize efficacy and selectivity. Melanin absorption lies in the visible light to infrared wavelengths of the electromagnetic spectrum and any laser between the wavelengths of 600–1,000 nm may be effective for the removal of unwanted hairs. This therapeutic window forms the basis of choosing the wavelength for LHR. The competing chromophores in the skin and hair, oxyhemoglobin and water, have a decreased absorption between 690 nm and 1,000 nm, thus making this an ideal range for laser and light sources.[9,10]

Table 25.1: Hair cycle duration at various sites

Body site	*Duration of anagen (months)*	*Duration of telogen (months)*	*Percentage of hairs in telogen*
Scalp	48–72	3–4	10–15
Eyebrows	1–2	3–4	85–94
Moustache	2–5	1.5	34
Beard	12	2–3	15–20
Axillae	3–6	3–6	31–79
Arms	1–3	2–4	72–86
Pubic area	3–6	0.5	65–81
Thighs	1–2	2–3	64–83
Lower legs	4–6	3–6	62–88

Types of Lasers for Hair Removal

Hair removal lasers emit a monochromatic beam of light and are highly selective for the chromophore melanin. The lasers that are used for hair reduction include the long pulse alexandrite 755 nm, the long pulse diode 810 nm and long pulse Nd: YAG 1,064 nm **(Box 25.3)**. These lasers have proved to be safe and effective even in darker skin types and have well documented evidence base.[11]

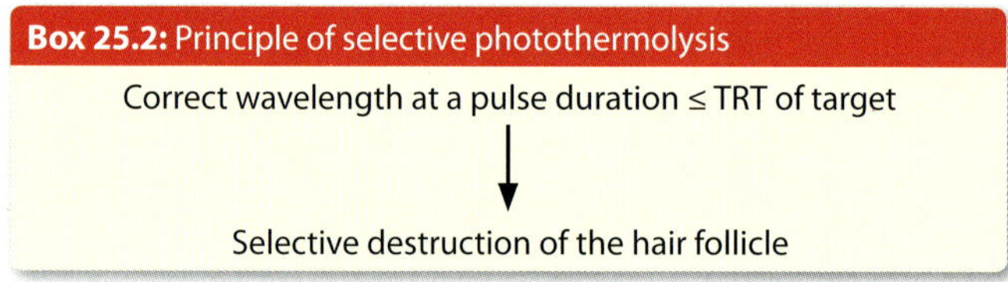
Box 25.2: Principle of selective photothermolysis

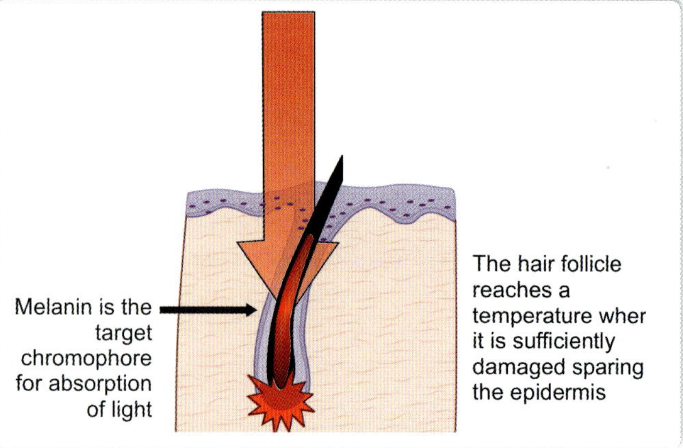

Fig. 25.2: Selective photothermolysis

Box 25.3: Types of lasers used for hair reduction

- **Lasers**
  - 694 nm Ruby Long pulsed laser
  - 755 nm Alexandrite Long pulsed laser
  - 810 nm Diode laser
  - 1,064 nm Nd: YAG laser
- **IPL Systems**
  - Intense pulse light (IPL) and Variable pulse light (VPL) 610 nm-950 nm
- **Low fluence and in-motion HR systems**
  - 810 nm Diode
  - Intense Pulse Light systems 610-950 nm
- **IPL+radiofrequency systems**
  - ELOS (electro-optical synergy) systems

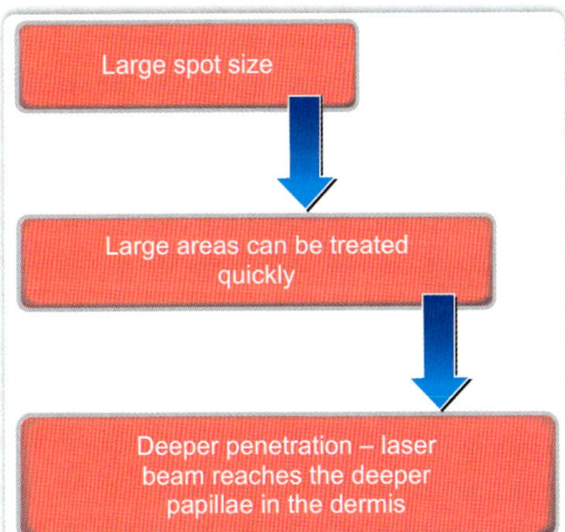

Fig. 25.3: Advantages of large spot size

Most lasers for hair removal have a large spot size (10 mm and above) so that large areas can be treated quickly. The large spot size allows deeper penetration thus allowing the laser beam to reach the deeper papillae in the dermis **(Figure 25.3)**.[12]

Most lasers have some sort of inbuilt cooling devices into the system. The cooling can be in the form of sapphire chill tips, air cooling or a dynamic cooling device that delivers a cryogen spray to the treated area. Cooling of the skin is critical while treating the darker skin types so as to prevent epidermal injury, which is a associated sequelae.[13] This is the key to successful therapy in Fitzpatrick IV, V and VI and also minimizes side effects considerably.[14,15] Ideally, the cooling should be pre-, parallel and post-laser delivery to get the best results **(Box 25.4)**.

Intense pulse light (IPL) systems deliver polychromatic light and use cut off filters to emit light in the red to infrared spectrum and have variable pulse duration with on times and off times to achieve effective and safe hair reduction. The IPLs have a large spot size and have chill tips. Large areas can be treated in relatively short duration and are generally cheaper than lasers.[16,17]

Box 25.4: Cooling system

Cooling prevents epidermal injury, which is advantageous in Fitzpatrick IV, V and VI skin type:

- Sapphire chill tips
- Air cooling
- Dynamic cooling device that delivers a cryogen spray

Newer systems utilizing low fluence and in motion technologies have been introduced with the primary objective of making the treatments more tolerable and pain-free for the patients. These systems offer the added benefit of greater safety due to the lower fluences used and the built-in cooling mechanisms. These systems also use a large spot size for faster treatment times and to cover large surface areas rapidly. The low fluence systems may be either diode or IPL based systems. Instead of delivering high energy pulses in a short time, these devices deliver power energies over a longer period of time typically in seconds to gradually heat up the hair follicle, thus delivering a cumulative dose of energy measured in kilo Joules/KJ. Since the targeted hair follicles and its immediate surroundings (including the bulb and bulge region) are uniformly heated, destruction of the hair follicle occurs with reduction of unwanted hairs. Because the TRT of the hair shafts is not so important, theoretically even fine hairs can be targeted with these systems.[18]

Recently, radiofrequency (RF) has been combined with lasers or broad band light sources theoretically offering a synergistic benefit. This combination is called electro-optical synergy or ELOS. The devices have electrodes placed on each side of a sapphire window 8 mm apart, generating heat to a depth of 4 mm thus targeting the hair follicle. The hand piece has a chilled tip allowing protection of the epidermis and the laser and RF pulse are delivered simultaneously. The laser causes selective heating of the hair follicle thus lowering the impedance of the follicle. This allows the RF current to preferentially pass though the hair follicle, causing thermal coagulation.[19] Since RF current does not require a chromophore, theoretically even blond or white hair can be treated.

Indications[15,20,21]

- Hirsutism
- Cosmetic removal of unwanted body hair
- Therapeutic hair removal to address an underlying disease, e.g. Sycosis barbae/pseudofolliculitis where hairs are removed for therapeutic reasons
- Hair removal from donor site after skin grafting

Contraindications[13,22]

Absolute

- Prepubertal patient
- Less than 15 years of age
- Uncooperative, noncompliant or unrealistic patient
- Associated photoaggravated skin diseases and medical illness, e.g. SLE
- Treatment area with active cutaneous infections, e.g. herpes labialis, staphylococci infections etc.

As recommended by taskforce on laser hair removal, no age limit is imposed for laser hair removal. One can consider LHR in younger patients for appropriate indications after adequate counseling of parents and patients.

Relative

The clinician must exert due caution and use best medical judgment before selecting following patients for hair removal.

a. Patient having keloids over area to be lased are best avoided, for those who have keloidal tendencies utmost caution has to be exercized and preferable to conduct a patch test first.
b. Patient on long-term photosensitizing drugs, e.g. doxycycline, minocyclines, isotretinoin, etc. Patients who were on above drugs in past can be taken for treatment after proper explanations to them. Sun protection is mandatory.
c. Unrealistic patients.
d. Patients with underlying chronic dermatoses like psoriasis and vitiligo should be treated cautiously as there is increased risk of koebnerization of the treated area.
e. Previous history of herpes simplex is a relative contraindication for laser hair removal because of risk of precipitation of active lesions. Laser hair removal being a cosmetic procedure, this risk should be seriously considered prior to performing the procedure. If the treating physician decides to perform the procedure, the risk and benefit should be explained to the patient, and the procedure should be performed, after proper informed consent and only after a course of oral acyclovir.

History and Examination

A detailed history to rule out any associated illnesses is essential before taking up a patient for laser hair removal **(Box 25.5)**. Female patients must be thoroughly evaluated for underlying causes of hirsutism. A gynecology and/or endocrinology opinion should be sought if deemed necessary. Specific tests that may be carried out are listed in **Table 25.2**.

Preprocedure Workup[13,22,23]

1. Patients are instructed to avoid bleaching, threading, plucking, thermolysis or electrolysis, waxing of the treatment area 2 weeks prior to starting LHR
2. Sun avoidance and sun protection to avoid tanning of the treatment area
3. It is preferable to avoid any herbal products, over the counter (OTC) products, homeopathic treatments prior to LHR procedure
4. Counseling and written informed consent
5. Pretreatment photographs
6. Use of topical skin lightening creams prior to LHR if the patient is excessively tanned.

Test Patch

Test patches may be performed to define the precise treatment parameters and to determine the pain threshold of the patient.[13,22]

Laser Hair Removal Procedure[13]

The hair is trimmed with an electric trimmer or the patient can shave the treatment area a day prior to the procedure.

Box 25.5: History taking prior to laser hair removal (LHR)

- Use of photosensitizing drugs
- Recent sun exposure and tanning
- Keloidal and hypertrophic scarring
- History of herpes simplex
- Prior hair removal methods used and their outcomes
- Menstrual history
- Thyroid disorders
- Diabetes
- Hypertension
- Obesity

Table 25.2: List of investigations in a patient for laser hair removal

Complete blood counts
Fasting blood sugars
Urine analysis
Serum LH, FSH
Serum prolactin
Serum DHEAS
Free and total testosterone
T3, T4, TSH
RBS, serum insulin
USG—abdomen and pelvis

Any make up should be removed and the area is cleaned thoroughly before the treatment is commenced. Local anesthesia is generally not required but topical EMLA (Eutectic mixture of lidocaine and prilocaine) can be used 45 minutes to 1 hour before the procedure in apprehensive patients and those with poor pain tolerance.[24-26] It is important to ensure adequate illumination of the treatment area.

Pre, parallel and post-cooling of the treated area during the laser procedure is preferable as it minimizes discomfort and protects the epidermis from thermal injury. Most lasers today have built-in cooling devices either in the form of contact cooling, air cooling or cryogen spray. Cooling is essential especially while treating darker skin types as it minimizes the chances of epidermal injury and burns. Ice packs may also be used before and after treatment.

Standard laser protocol should be followed, such as eye protection for the patient and the treating physician, such as eye shields and eye goggles provided by the manufacturer.[27] Treatment area should not have any metallic objects, such as jewelry, chains etc. Emergency hazard switch may be used in case of an emergency or sudden unauthorized entry.

Treatment parameters should be individualized and a record of each session is maintained for future references. Cooled gel is applied to the prepared area prior to LHR (except in case where a light heat energy (LHE) device is used). The hand piece is placed perpendicular to the treatment area and laser is delivered in a single pass with minimum overlap (approx 10%) to prevent any skipped areas. In the low fluence technique, laser light is delivered in motion and with repeated passes in a circular or to and fro motion until the desired cumulative energy is delivered to the specified marked out area. The end point is usually erythema and perifollicular edema.

After the completion of the treatment, the area is cleaned and ice packs is applied to cool the area. Mild topical steroid with antibiotic may be used for a short time post-procedure to minimize redness, sweling and any erosions/scabs that may arise after treatment. The patient is encouraged to use sunscreen post-procedure.

The laser treatment is repeated at 4–8 weekly intervals (depending on the site and re-growth of the hairs). Multiple sessions are generally necessary to achieve sufficient reduction of the unwanted hairs.

Written instructions on post-treatment care and follow-up is suggested. Patient is encouraged to report any adverse effects, such as blistering, crusting, scabbing, herpetic lesions on the treatment area **(Box 25.6)**.

Use of Eflornithine Cream Along with Laser

Eflornithine cream when combined with lasers has documented benefits and can be started immediately after lasers and continued in the interim phase between sittings.[28-31]

Box 25.6: Procedure of hair removal

- The hair is trimmed or shaved
- Remove makeup and cleanse the area
- Local anesthesia is optional
- Cooling of the area
- Eye protection for the patient and the operator
- The hand piece is placed perpendicular to the treatment area and laser is delivered in a single pass with minimum overlap (approx 10%). The end point is usually erythema and perifollicular edema
- After treatment, the area is cleaned and ice packs applied to cool the area
- Mild-topical steroid with antibiotic may be used for a short time post-procedure
- The patient is encouraged to use sun block post-procedure
- Written instructions on post-treatment care and follow-up is suggested

Hair Reduction Systems (Table 25.3)

The laser and light-based devices used today target the melanin in the hair follicleto produce selective destruction of the hair follicle, bulb and bulge region. These include Ruby, Alexandrite, Diode, Nd: YAG laser and intense pulse-light devices. The ruby has the shortest wavelength (WL) and the Nd: YAG, the longest. The shorter WL is better absorbed by melanin but has lesser penetration and the longer WL have deeper penetration but weaker absorption in melanin. The diode and alexandrite lie between these extremes and are more balanced with good absorption and reasonable penetration. The addition of cooling and a large spot size aid in safe and effective treatment in darker individuals **(Table 25.3)**.[32]

Table 25.3: Various types of lasers used for hair reduction

Laser	Wavelength	
Ruby laser	694 nm	High melanin absorption and lesser penetration into the dermis—increased risk of pigmentation
Long-pulsed Alexandrite laser	755 nm	Penetrates deeper in the dermis, has good absorption in melanin leading to effective targeting of the melanin in the hair shaft, while sparing the epidermis
Diode laser	800–810 nm	Sufficient penetration into the dermis, adequate absorption by melanin, minimal adverse effects even in skin of color and is considered the gold standard for laser hair reduction
Long pulse ND: YAG laser	1,064 nm	Allows deeper penetration than the diode and alexandrite, less absorbed by epidermal melanin, considered safe for treatment of darker skin photo types and tanned skin
Intense pulse light	550–1200 nm	Pulse of an IPL can be altered or split into micropulses with on-times and off-times allowing epidermal cooling thus minimizing the side effects

No recommendation can be made on the best laser device as all systems have their advantages and drawbacks. Choice should be made based on the skin type of the patient, the experience and training of the user.

Ruby Laser

The pulsed ruby laser has a WL of 694 nm and is highly absorbed by melanin. The active medium is a ruby crystal and emits light in the red portion of the visible spectrum. Due to the high melanin absorption and lesser penetration into the dermis, it is not recommended in darker skin types due to risk of post inflammatory hyper and hypo pigmentation.[15]

Long-Pulsed Alexandrite Laser

The long-pulse alexandrite laser emits a 755 nm beam in the near infrared portion of the electromagnetic spectrum. This WL penetrates deeper in the dermis compared to the ruby laser and has good absorption in melanin leading to effective targeting of the melanin in the hair shaft, while sparing the epidermis. The addition of parallel effective epidermal cooling such as cold air or cryogen spray makes these systems safer even in relatively dark skin types. In the author's experience, the use of long-pulse alexandrite is effective and safe upto Fitzpatrick skin type V. The laser has a pulse duration ranging from 5 ms to 40 ms allowing flexibility in targeting fine or thick hairs. The laser has a large spot size of up to 15 mm thereby enhancing deeper penetration and allowing rapid treatment times. Side effects include, epidermal crusting, blistering, dyspigmentation but is usually transient. Numerous studies have validated the efficacy and safety of this laser for hair reduction **(Figures 25.4 to 25.7)**.[33-36]

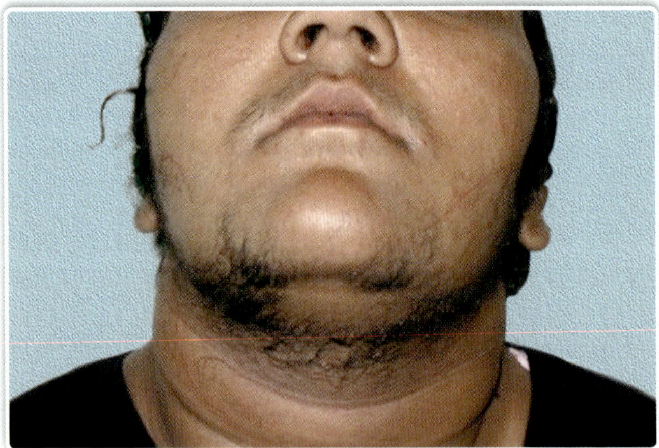

Fig. 25.4: Severe hirsutism in a young female with polycystic ovary syndrome

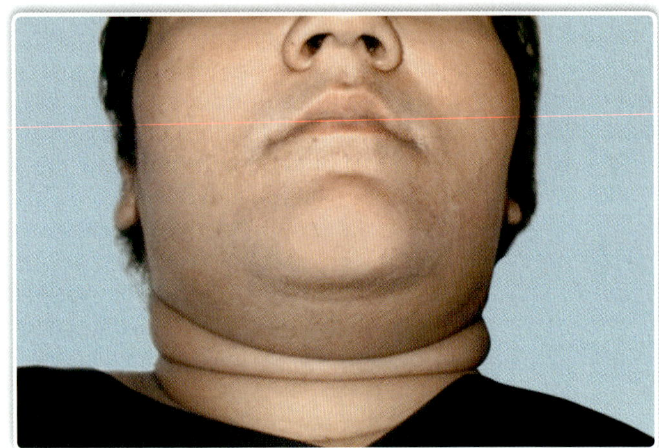

Fig. 25.5: After six long pulse alexandrite hair removal laser sessions

Diode Laser

The diode laser emits a WL of 800-810 nm in the near infrared spectrum. This WL allows sufficient penetration into the dermis and adequate absorption by melanin aiding in-effective hair removal with minimal adverse effects even in skin of color and is considered the gold standard for laser hair reduction. Many studies have documented its effectiveness and safety.[37,38]

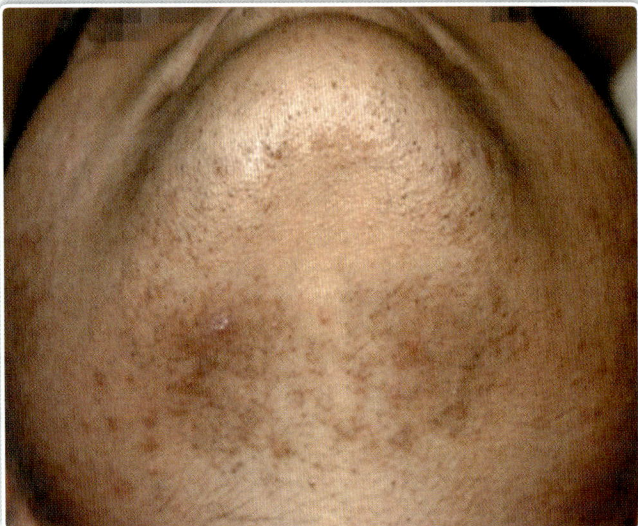

Fig. 25.6: Hirsutism with pseudofolliculitis and postinflammatory hyperpigmentation

Long-Pulse Nd: YAG Laser

The active medium in the Nd: YAG laser is the yttrium-aluminum-garnet crystal that is doped with neodymium ions. This laser produces a WL of 1,064 nm. The long-pulse Nd: YAG laser is used for laser hair removal. The longer WL allows deeper penetration than the diode and alexandrite, and the WL is less absorbed by epidermal melanin as is

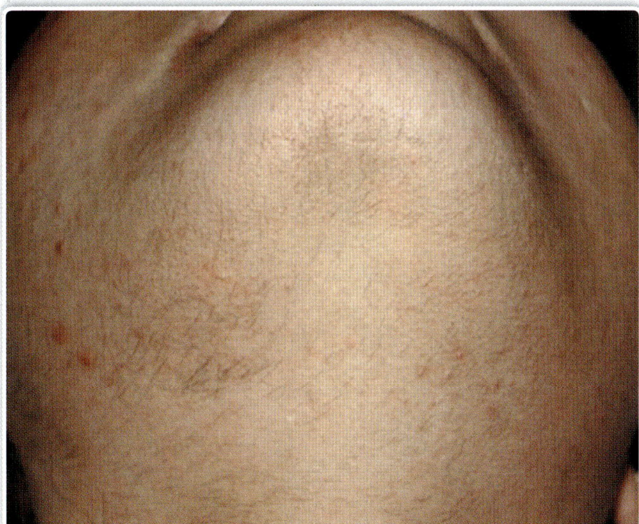

Fig. 25.7: Post four long pulse alexandrite laser sessions—at 3 months follow-up

considered safe for treatment of darker skin phototypes and tanned skin. Most Nd: YAG lasers also employ some form of epidermal cooling thereby providing added safety and comfort during the treatment. Several studies have shown the safety and long-term efficacy of the long-pulse Nd: YAG laser in skin types III, IV, V and even VI.[39-41]

Intense Pulse Light

Intense pulse light (IPL) is a poly-chromatic light source that uses cut-off filters to produce the desired WL of light. IPLs with a range of 550–1,200 nm can be used for LHR. The pulse of an IPL can be altered or split into micro-pulses with on-times and off-times allowing epidermal cooling thus minimizing the side effects. Most IPL systems have in-built cooling to provide additional safety. The IPLs generally have a large spot size allowing large areas to be covered in a short time. Multiple treatment sessions are needed to achieve sufficient hair reduction, as has been documented by various clinical studies.[42-44]

Newer Concepts in Laser Hair Removal

With evolving concepts and better understanding of the hair biology, newer low-fluence lasers and light devices are being developed that may offer better safety and tolerability of LHR along with satisfactory hair reduction. The effectiveness of LHR not only depends on the fluence and pulse duration but also on the spot size of the laser beam. Studies have shown that larger spot size is more effective for LHR. This can be explained in part by the phenomenon of dermal scattering. Thus, a larger spot size allows deeper penetration of the laser beam. A larger spot size allows more effective dermal heating, allowing the use of lower fluencies.[45, 46] This is the basis of low-fluence laser hair removal that is in vogue today.

Box 25.7: Factors governing optimum hair reduction

- Body site
- Hair color
- Hair shaft diameter
- Hormonal profile/endocrine status
- Laser system: WL, spot size, number of sessions, energy/fluence used

Low-fluence, in-motion hair removal (super hair removal) claims pain free and more efficient hair removal by employing the technique of repetitive pulses of low energy applied over a given area with high average power and multiple passes. A high cumulative energy is delivered over time there by heating the dermis and the hair follicle. The WL employed is 650–950 nm for the IPL based system and 810 nm Diode for the laser-based systems. The device also features an additional contact cooling to safeguard the epidermis. The procedure is done in-motion, in a circular or to and fro pattern (vertical or horizontal paint brush like pattern) with multiple overlap passes. These passes are delivered in grids of 10 × 10 or 10 × 15 cms on the skin after applying cooled gel on the surface. The chilled-tip handpiece is in contact with the skin during the procedure. The end point is perifollicular erythema and/or edema. Repeated sessions are performed once every 4–8 weeks to achieve sufficient hair reduction.

Factors governing optimum hair reduction are enumerated in **Box 25.7.**

Choosing Appropriate Patients[32]

Proper patient selection is of paramount importance for LHR. For optimal outcome, a light skinned patient with coarse dark hair is ideal, but many times this may not be the case. Coarse terminal hairs respond best to LHR and if possible, it is best to avoid patients with fine, vellus hairs. A patient with unrealistic expectations is also best avoided. Proper counseling of the patient is the key to patient compliance and satisfactory results. Darker patients seeking hair removal should be evaluated for excessive tanning and ideally test patch should be done to gauge the results before taking up the case for LHR. The risk of adverse effects increases with darker phototypes and adequate care should be taken for priming these individuals before LHR and also a longer wavelength laser should be chosen in such situations. Adequate cooling of the skin during laser treatment is essential to minimize epidermal damage and the risk of post inflammatory hyperpigmentation (PIH). It is best to avoid treating very young patients, though many times adolescents may seek HR for subtle hypertrichosis. Hypertrichosis may be related to ethnicity and constitution of a given patient and may not necessitate LHR.

Complications

The most common complications are pain and discomfort, usually transient and respond well to analgesics.[47] While treating darker skin types vesicles and blistering are most commonly seen with high fluence usage.[48,49] These generally resolve with steroid and antibiotic creams applied topically. Reactivation of herpes can be prevented by prophylactic acyclovir. In case reactivation of herpes occurs, oral acyclovir should be started. Secondary bacterial infections can be treated with topical therapy or oral antibiotics if severe. Post-laser hyperpigmentation is usually transient and resolves with topical lightening agents and sun protection.[50] Paradoxical hypertrichosis is associated with suboptimal laser energy and should be treated with higher fluencies **(Box 25.8)**.[51,52]

Box 25.8: Complications

- Pain and discomfort
- Vesicles and blistering
- Reactivation of herpes infections
- Secondary bacterial infections
- Post-laser hyperpigmentation
- Paradoxical hypertrichosis

Conclusion

Significant advancements have been made in laser and light-bases technologies over the past decade and LHR remains one of the most commonly performed and popular cosmetic dermatology procedures worldwide. Despite this, many limitations still exist, such as long-term hair reduction and not permanent hair loss, need for multiple sessions to achieve this, prolonged treatment times and potential risk of adverse effects if due precautions are not observed. To get the best results, the physicians have to familiarize themselves with the system, individualize the treatment parameters, observe the correct protocol for a given system and employ proper patient-selection criteria. Thorough counseling of the patient is mandatory to satisfy the individual post-laser therapy. With better understanding of the hair growth cycle and cutaneous biology, further advances in laser physics we hope to find the perfect solution to the problem of unwanted hairs.

References

1. Haedersdal M, Wulf HC. Evidence-based review of hair removal using lasers and light sources. J Eur Acad Dermatol Venereol. 2006 Jan;20(1):9-20.
2. Olsen EA. Methods of hair removal J Am Acad Dermatol. 1999;40:143-55.
3. Lin TD, Manuskiatti W, Dierickx CC, et al. Hair growth cycle affects hair follicle destruction by ruby laser pulses. J Invest Dermatol. 1998;111:107-13.
4. Dierickx C, Alora MB, Dover JS. A clinical overview of hair removal using lasers and light sources. Dermatol Clin. 1999;17:357-66.
5. Goldberg DJ. Laser Dermatology—pearls and problems. Year 2008;40. Blackwell Publishing.
6. Anderson RR, Parrish JA. Selective photothermolysis: precise microsurgery by selective absorption of pulsed radiation. Science. 1983;220:524.
7. Arndt KA, Noe JM, Northam DBC. Laser therapy: basic concepts and nomenclature. J Am Acad Dermatol. 1981;5:649-54.
8. O'Shea DC, Callen WR, Rhodes WT. Introduction to lasers and their applications. Menlo Park (CA): Addison-Wesley Publishing Co. 1978.
9. Nelson AA, Lask GP. Principles and practice of cutaneous laser and light therapy. Clin Plast Surg. 2011 Jul;38(3):427-36.
10. Choudhary S, Elsaie ML, Nouri K. Laser assisted hair-removal. G Ital Dermatol Venereol. 2009 Oct;144(5):595-602.
11. Tanzi EL, Jason R, Lupton M, Alster TS. Lasers in dermatology: Four decades of progress J Am Acad Dermatol. 2003;49:1-31.
12. Richard J. Barlow, George J. Hruza, " Lasers and Light tissue Interactions" Lasers and Light Volume-I, Year 2005,Page-1/ Saunders (Elsevier India Pvt Limited). 978-81.
13. Christine C. Dierickx and Melanie C. Grossman, Chapter 4 -Laser Hair Removal , Lasers and Lights Volume 2, Edited by David J Goldberg (ISBN 1 4160 2360 7) year 2005, Page 61-6.
14. Liew SH. Laser hair removal: guidelines for management. Am J Clin Dermatol. 2002;3:107-15.
15. Jackson BA. Lasers in ethnic skin: A review J Am Acad Dermatol. 2003;48:S134-8.
16. Weiss RA, Weiss MA, Marwaha S, Harrington AC. Hair removal with a non-coherent filtered flashlamp intense pulsed light source. Lasers Surg Med. 1999;24:128-32.
17. Gold MH, Bell MW, Foster TD, Street S. Long-term epilation using the EpiLight broad band, intense pulsed light hair removal system. Dermatol Surg. 1997;23:909-13.
18. Goldberg DJ. Laser- and light-based hair removal: an update. Expert Rev Med Devices. 2007 Mar;4(2):253-60.
19. Sadick NS. Combination radiofrequency and light energies: electro-optical technology in esthetic medicine. Dermatol Surg. 2005;31:1211-17.
20. Kelly AP. Pseudofolliculitis barbae. In: Arndt KA, LeBiot PR, Robinson JK, Wintroub BU, editors. Cutaneous medicine and surgery:an integrated program in dermatology. Philadelphia (PA):WB Saunders. 1996;p. 499-502.
21. Satish S Savant. Laser Hair Removal Chapter 55 : Text book of Dermatosurgery and Cosmetology. 2005;55:454-5.
22. Satish S Savant. Laser Hair Removal: Text book of Dermatosurgery and Cosmetology. 2005;55:457.

23. Dover JS, Arndt AK, Dinehart SM, Fitzpatrick RK, Gonzalez E. Task force: Guidelines of care for laser surgery. J Am Acad Dermatol. 1999;41:484-95.
24. Koay J, Orengo I. Application of local anesthetics in dermatologic surgery. Dermatol Surg. 2002;28:143-8.
25. Epstein RH, Halmi B, Lask GP. Anesthesia for cutaneous laser therapy. Clin Dermatol. 1995;13:21-4.
26. Drake LA, Dinehart SM, Goltz RW, et al. Guidelines of care for local and regional anesthesia in cutaneous surgery. J Am Acad Dermatol. 1995;33:504-9.
27. Russell SH, Dinehart SM, Davis I, Flock ST. Efficacy of corneal eye shields in protecting patients eyes from laser irradiation. Dermatol Surg. 1996;22:613-6.
28. Hamzavi I, Tan E, Shapiro J, Lui H. A randomized bilateral vehicle-controlled study of eflornithine cream combined with laser treatment versus laser treatment alone for facial hirsutism in women. J Am Acad Dermatol. 2007 Jul; 57(1): 54-9. Epub 2007 Jan 30.
29. Tan E, Hamzavi I, Shapiro J, Lui H. Combined treatment with laser and topical eflornithine is more effective than laser treatment alone for removing unwanted facial hair - a placebo controlled trial. Presented at: The 4th Intercontinental Meeting of Hair Research Societies; June 17-19, 2004; Berlin, Germany. Abstract #P10.144.
30. Smith SR, Piacquadio D, Beger B. A randomized, double-blind, vehicle controlled, bilateral comparison study of the efficacy and safety of eflornithine HCl 13.9% cream in combination with laser in the treatment of unwanted facial hair in women. Presented at: The 61st Annual Meeting of the American Academy of Dermatology; March 21-26, 2003; San Francisco, CA. Abstract #P649.
31. Xia Y, Cho S, Howard RS, Maggio KL. Topical eflornithine hydrochloride improves the effectiveness of standard laser hair removal for treating pseudofolliculitis barbae: A randomized, double-blinded, placebo-controlled trial. J Am Acad Dermatol. 2012 Jan 6. [Epub ahead of print].
32. Battle EF Jr. Advances in laser hair removal in skin of color. J Drugs Dermatol. 2011 Nov;10(11):1235-9.
33. Eremia S, Li CY, Umar SH, Newman N. Laser hair removal: long-term results with a 755 nm alexandrite laser. Dermatol Surg. 2001 Nov;27(11):920-4.
34. Rao J, Goldman MP. Prospective, comparative evaluation of three laser systems used individually and in combination for axillary hair removal. Dermatol Surg. 2005 Dec;31(12):1671-6; discussion 1677.
35. Davoudi SM, Behnia F, Gorouhi F, Keshavarz S, Nassiri Kashani M, Rashighi Firoozabadi M, et al. Comparison of long-pulsed alexandrite and Nd:YAG lasers, individually and in combination, for leg hair reduction: an assessor-blinded, randomized trial with 18 months of follow-up. Arch Dermatol. 2008 Oct;144(10):1323-7.
36. Uyar B, Saklamaz A. Effects of the 755-nm Alexandrite laser on fine dark facial hair: Review of 90 cases. J Dermatol. 2012 May;39(5):430-2.
37. Handrick C, Alster TS. Comparison of long-pulsed diode and long-pulsed alexandrite lasers for hair removal: a long-term clinical and histologic study. Dermatol Surg. 2001 Jul;27(7):622-6.
38. Ibrahimi OA, Kilmer SL. Long-term clinical evaluation of a 800-nm long-pulsed diode laser with a large spot size and vacuum-assisted suction for hair removal. Dermatol Surg. 2012 Jun;38(6):912-7.
39. Wanner M. Laser hair removal. Dermatol Ther. 2005 May-Jun;18(3):209-16.
40. Goh CL. Comparative study on a single treatment response to long pulse Nd:YAG lasers and intense pulse light therapy for hair removal on skin type IV to VI—is longer wavelengths lasers preferred over shorter wavelengths lights for assisted hair removal. J Dermatolog Treat. 2003 Dec;14(4): 243-7.
41. Alster TS, Bryan H, Williams CM. Long-pulsed Nd:YAG laser-assisted hair removal in pigmented skin: a clinical and histological evaluation. Arch Dermatol. 2001 Jul;137(7): 885-9.
42. Mohanan S, Basheerahmed P, Priyavathani R, Nellainayagam G. New intense pulse light device with square pulse technology for hirsutism in Indian patients: a pilot study. J Cosmet Laser Ther. 2012 Feb;14(1):14-7.
43. Ismail SA. Long-pulsed Nd:YAG laser vs. intense pulsed light for hair removal in dark skin: a randomized controlled trial. Br J Dermatol. 2012 Feb;166(2):317-21.
44. Feng YM, Zhou ZC, Gold MH. Hair removal using a new intense pulsed light source in Chinese patients. J Cosmet Laser Ther. 2009 Jun;11(2):94-7.
45. Shlomit Halachmi and Moshe Lapidoth. Low-fluence vs. standard fluence hair removal: A contralateral control non-inferiority study J Cosmet Laser Ther. 2012 February; 14(1):2-6.
46. Barolet D. Low fluence-high repetition rate diode laser hair removal 12-month evaluation: reducing pain and risks while keeping clinical efficacy. Lasers Surg Med. 2012 Apr;44(4):277-81.
47. Nanni CA, Alster TS. Laser assisted hair removal: side effects of Q-switched Nd:YAG, long-pulsed ruby, and alexandrite lasers. J Am Acad Dermatol. 1999;41:165-71.
48. Lanigan, SW. Incidence of side effects after laser hair removal. J Am Acad Dermatol. 2003;49(5):882-6.
49. Breadon JY, Barnes CA. Comparison of adverse events of laser and light-assisted hair removal systems in skin types IV-VI. J Drugs Dermatol. 2007 Jan;6(1):40-6.
50. Buddhadev RM. Standard guidelines of care: Laser and IPL hair reduction. Indian J Dermatol. Venereol Leprol. 2008;74:68-74
51. Kontoes P, Vlachos S, Konstantinos M, et al. Hair induction after laser-assisted hair removal and its treatment. J Am Acad Dermatol. 2006;54:64.
52. Lolis MS, Marmur ES. Paradoxical effects of hair removal systems: a review. J Cosmet Dermatol. 2006;5:274.

26

Mesotherapy for Hair and Scalp Disorders

Maya Vedamurthy

"No great discovery was ever made without a bold guess."
—*Isaac Newton*

Introduction

Mesotherapy also known as intradermotherapy. It is a procedure invented by Dr. Micheal Pistor in 1958 to treat a variety of medical conditions, mainly as a pain-relieving technique.[1] But now mesotherapy has undergone revolutionary changes and has found a place in a variety of aesthetic conditions including hair regrowth.

Mesotherapy is a technique which involves micro-injections of conventional homeopathic medication/allopathic medication and/or vitamins into the mesoderm or middle layer of the skin to promote healing or corrective treatment to a specific area of the body **(Box 26.1)**.[2]

Principle of Mesotherapy

The principle behind mesotherapy is application by intradermal injections of pharmacological agents in small amounts directly into the region to be treated.[3]

A study of cintilography has helped to understand the theory of practicing and standardizing mesotherapy. This explains the mechanism of the activity that occurs over short distances (by stimulating dermal receptors in situ) and the activity occurs over long distances (by reaching other organs by way of circulation).[4]

It has been postulated that by this technique the local activity of the product could last longer as there is a persistent reservoir effect with a weak local diffusion in the dermis. On the basis of this theory, a concept has been developed known as the concept of meso-interface, which is the surface of contact established between the injected products and the tissue injected **(Box 26.2)**.

The more fragmented the substance delivered, greater the meso-interface and the greater number of activated dermal receptors.

Several studies including those by Kaplan and Coutris have stressed the importance of the depth of injection in the diffusion of medications used in mesotherapy **(Box 26.3)**.

For products to remain longer at the site of injection, it has been suggested that injections involving mesotherapy be given at a depth of 4 mm or less.

For best results, the injections should be limited to the region of the superficial papillary dermis.[5]

The therapeutic end result occurs both from the effect of the chemical action of the products used and the reflex stimulation by the multiple punctures made in different sites.

Box 26.1: Principle of mesotherapy

Direct application on intradermal injections of pharmacological agents in small amounts into the region to be treated, so local activity of the product lasts longer, i.e a persistent reservoir effect with a weak local diffusion in the dermis

Box 26.2: Concept of mesointerface

- It is the surface of contact established between the injected products and the tissue injected
- The more fragmented substance delivered, greater the meso-interface and the greater number of activated dermal receptors

Box 26.3: Factors affecting efficacy of mesotherapy

- Injections to be given at a depth of 4 mm or less to allow products to remain at site
- Injections should be limited to the region of the superficial papillary dermis
- Chemical action of the products used
- Reflex stimulation by the multiple punctures made in different sites

Techniques used in Mesotherapy for Hair

- Manual
- Mesogun
- Roller
- Dermoelectroporation

Mesotherapy for hair involves intradermal injections of the pharmacological products at the level of hair follicle. Typically this would involve injecting at about a depth of 4 mm to get the desired effect.

Manual Injections

Manual injections are made using sterile syringes of 1–2 mL and mesoneedles also known as Lebel needles.

Injection Techniques (Figure 26.1)

Nappage: This technique involves holding the syringe at 30–60° angle from the skin and by applying light and constant pressure on the syringe's plunger, the physician flicks the wrist to infuse a drop of the solution.

Point by point: This technique involves an injection of 0.02–0.05 mL spaced 1 cm apart by inserting the entire length of a 4 mm needle.

Multi-injector Plates

Manual injections on the scalp can be made promptly and effectively by using multi-injector plates mounted on a Luer Lock syringe. The multi-injector plates come without needles and come in a circular configuration suitable for scalp injection. Suitable needles appropriate for the thickness of the scalp is chosen and manually mounted before the treatment by the operator as shown in **Figure 26.2**. A standard female luer connector allows an easy connection to the syringe containing the injectable drug.

Injection of 0.2 mL–0.05 mL spaced 1 cm apart by inserting the entire length of a 4 mm needle

Nappage technique

Point by point technique

Syringe held at 30°–60° angle from the skin and by light and constant pressure on the syringe's plunger the physician flicks the wrist to infuse a drop of the solution

Fig. 26.1: Injection techniques

Mesogun

Mesotherapy guns are programmed to penetrate the skin at various depths. Mesotherapy guns are useful to deliver injectables rapidly and accurately at the desired depth and help to cover large areas in a short time **(Figure 26.3)**. A syringe filled with the mesotherapy product is mounted on the mesogun and is programmed to deliver the product as required.

Mesopen

Also known as auto-micro needle therapy system involves piercing on the skin along with vibrating function, which helps to reduce pain and discomfort along with increasing the absorption of products **(Figure 26.4)**.

Procedure

The scalp is anesthetized using topical anesthetic cream. The area is disinfected thoroughly. A mesopen is used to

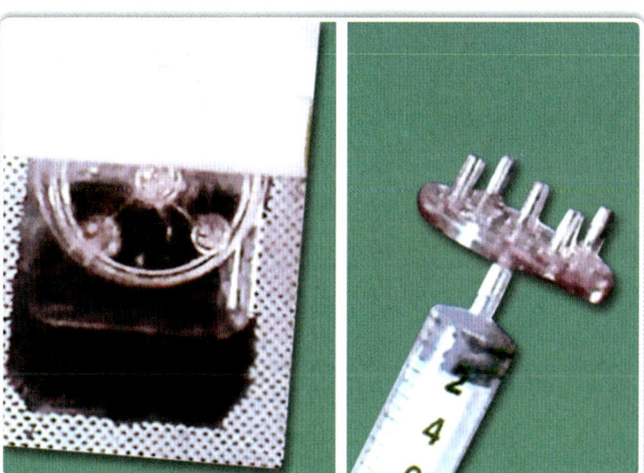

Fig. 26.2: Multi-injector plates

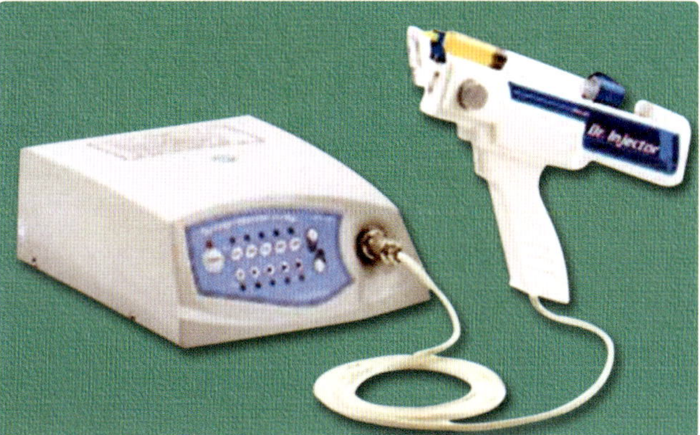

Fig. 26.3: Mesogun

deliver the products. The depth of the needle and the speed are adjusted by making the necessary changes.

Mesotherapy with Dermaroller

Dermaroller also known as microneedling, is a novel way of delivering mesoproducts at the desired sites. Dermarollers are designed to be used as rollers or as stamps for the purpose of creating microchannels **(Figure 26.5)**. This helps in better penetration of topical anti-hair loss products.

Procedure

The scalp is anesthetized using topical anesthetic cream like eutectic mixture of local anesthetics (EMLA) to decrease pain sensitivity although the procedure is usually associated with minimal or no pain. The scalp is then cleaned thoroughly with an antiseptic solution. The topical anti-hair loss solution is applied first. A dermaroller with 1.5 mm needle size is used with light-to-medium pressure. The roller is rolled only in one direction in the direction of hair growth to avoid tangling and thereby hair fall **(Figure 26.6)**. It is rolled three times in one area. This area is again covered with anti-hair loss solution, which will now enter the micro-perforation created in the upper layers of the scalp.

Dermoelectroporation

It involves needless mesotherapy technique to deliver the mesoproducts. Here an electrical wave pushes them painlessly through the skin without any harm to the cell membranes, based on a technology known as isophoresis **(Figure 26.7 and Box 26.4)**.

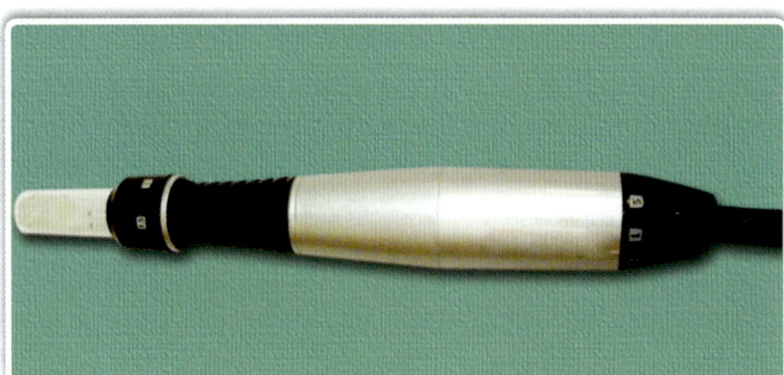

Fig. 26.4: Mesopen

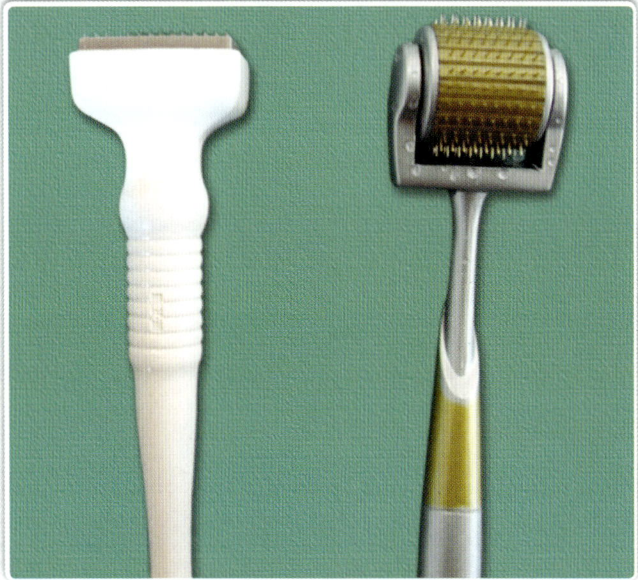

Fig. 26.5: Dermarollers

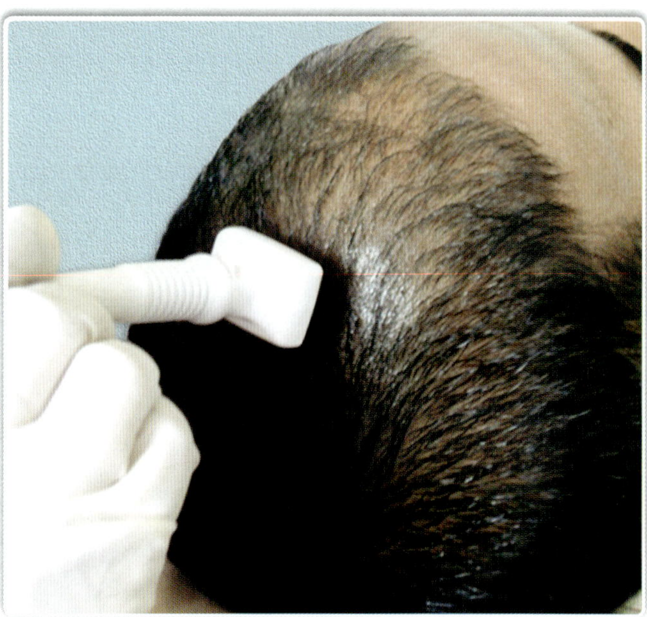

Fig. 26.6: Dermarollers in use

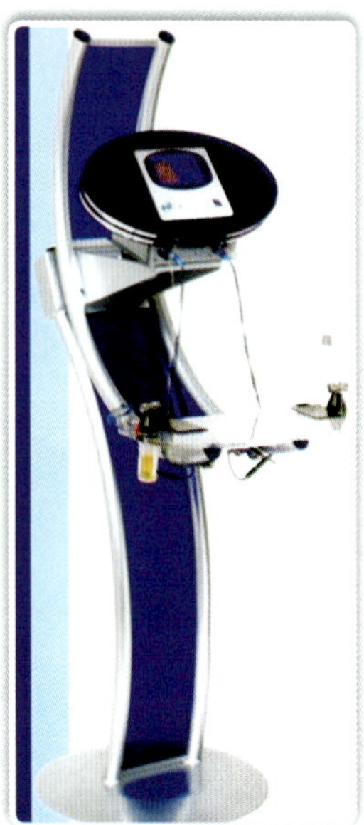

Fig. 26.7: Needleless mesotherapy

Box 26.4: Isophoresis

Refers to process by which an electrical wave pushes mesoproduct painlessly through the skin without any harm to the cell membranes

Ingredients used in Mesotherapy for Hair Loss

- *Minoxidil*: Stimulates blood flow to the hair follicle. It can be used both in men and women to stop hair loss.
- *Finasteride/Dutasteride*: It inhibits the conversion of testosterone to DHT and thereby prevents premature hair loss. Most useful in men with androgenetic alopecia.
- *Biotin*: Combined with vitamin B complex prevents hair loss and seborrhea.
- *Amino acids (L Dopa)* strengthens the hair follicles
- *Co-enzymes*: Co-enzyme A.
- *Buflomedil*: Produces vasodilation and thereby improves blood microcirculation around hair follicles.

Indications

- Androgenetic alopecia
- Telogen effluvium
- Seborrhea
- Pre- and post-hair transplantation.

Treatment Protocol and Procedure (Box 26.5)

Candidate selection is important for treatment of hairloss with mesotherapy. Careful history-taking is essential to avoid side effects. Proper documentation is necessary in view of the current position of mesotherapy. A proper counseling with regard to the current status of mesotherapy, with full information about the products, techniques, and side effects is mandatory. A well informed written consent should be obtained prior to procedure. Photographic documentation before, during and after treatment is useful. A good case sheet with details of treatment like products used, number of visits and outcome of treatment should be maintained. Side effects if any, should be attended to immediately and mesotherapy should be discontinued if warranted. The patient should be evaluated at each visit and treatment options should be discussed at regular intervals.

Box 26.5: Mesotherapy protocol

- Candidate selection
- Proper documentation of history
- Counseling of techniques, products and side effects
- Maintenance of a detailed case sheet about product used, number of treatment visits, outcome, side effects if any
- Photographic documentation

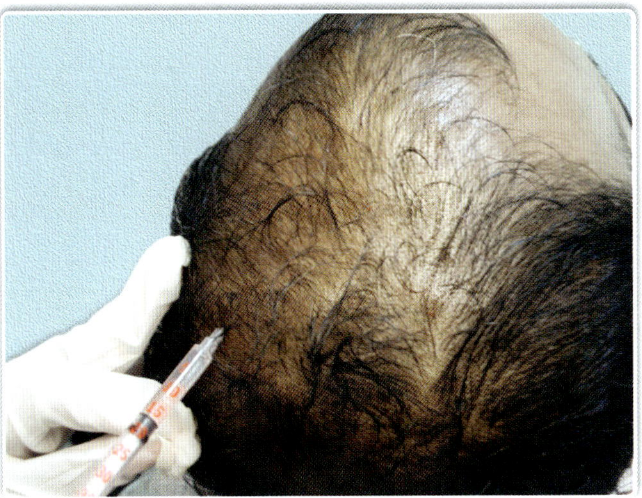

Fig. 26.8: Mesoinjection

The patient is made to lie comfortably. The scalp is cleaned thoroughly with a suitable disinfectant. Usually about 2 mL of the product selected based on the indication is drawn in a syringe. Using a 30 g needle, the product is injected in rows, 1 cm apart and at an injection depth of 1.5–2 mm **(Figure 26.8)**.

Protocol and Formulas (Table 26.1)

Protocol

Injections are usually given once every week for 8–10 treatments, followed by once every two weeks till recovery and then once a month as maintenance if needed.

Postmesotherapy Instructions/Care

1. Not to take a shower or undertake any activity that causes perspiration for atleast 8 hours postprocedure.
2. No excessive sun exposure for 2 days after the treatments.
3. Not to wash the hair for atleast 12 hours after the treatment or apply any other haircare products.

As mesotherapy procedure is noninvasive and requires little downtime, it is convenient for the physician and patient.

Contraindications

Contraindications to mesotherapy includes:

- Pregnancy
- Insulin dependent diabetes
- History of strokes
- History of recent cancer
- Thromboembolic phenomena
- History of allergies to products used in mesotherapy cocktail.

Table 26.1: Protocols and formulas

Cellular activator Vitamin C Ginkgo biloba Lidocaine	2 cc 2.5 cc 2.5 cc 2 cc	Dexapanthenol Minoxidil Procaine 2%	1 cc 1 cc 1 cc	Dexapanthenol Biotin	1 cc 1 cc 1 vial
Cellular activator Hyaluronidase Organic silicium	2 cc 2 cc 5 cc	Buflomedil Dexapanthenol Lidocaine	3 cc 1 cc 2 cc	Cytokines—growth peptides Vitamins Amino acids Minerals Co-enzymes	
Minoxidil Dutasteride					

Adverse Effects

Adverse effects are mainly based on the products used for treatment. Bruising and edema of the injected area can occur due to the inflammation response provoked by some of the chemicals used in mesotherapy. Icepacks may be used to reduce pain, bruise and swelling.

Skin necrosis can occur due to the irritant effect of the chemicals used.

There have been reports of development of alopecia following use of mesotherapy for hairloss.[6]

Atypical mycobacterial infections have been reported at sites of injections necessitating antimycobacterial therapy.[7]

Position of Mesotherapy

There has been a lot of controversy regarding the techniques and use of mesotherapy products for hair loss.[8,9]

At present there is a need for more scientific data for its effectiveness and safety.[10]

The CDC has recommended that providers should adhere to recommend standard precautions, follow safe injection practices with appropriate aseptic techniques, and inject only FDA approved products that are prepared following guidelines to ensure sterility as described in the FDA's good manufacturing practices **(Box 26.6)**.[11]

Advantages of Mesotherapy

Interlesional therapy is a well known technique in dermatology, e.g. intralesional steroids in alopecia areata. So technique of mesotherapy which is similar and easy to perform by dermatologists can be offered as a simple office procedure.

It is a noninvasive procedure with no down time and relatively painless. It does not require hospitalization or general anesthesia.

As per mesotherapy rule of "Little - Seldom - at the right place" the therapeutic product is injected in small quantities and therefore there is lack of systemic side effects. The target area is addressed directly and effectively with mesotherapy. With judicious use and proper scientific approach, mesotherapy can be a useful tool in therapeutic armamentarium **(Box 26.7)**.

Box 26.6: CDC recommendation

- Adhere to standard precautions
- Follow safe injection practices
- Aseptic techniques
- Inject FDA approved products

Box 26.7: "Little – Seldom – at the right place"

- Therapeutic product is injected in small quantities and therefore there is lack of systemic side effects
- The target area is addressed directly and effectively with mesotherapy

References

1. Brown SA. The science of mesotherapy chemical anarchy. Aesthet surg. J. 2006;26(1):95-8.
2. Vedamurthy M. Mesotherapy; Indian J Dermatol Venereol Leprol. 2007;76:60-2.
3. Pistor M. What is mesotherapy; Chir Dent Fr. 1976;46:59-60.
4. Herreros FOC, Moraes AM, Velbo PENF, Mesotherapy; a bibliographical review. An Bras Dermatol. 2011;86(1):91-101.
5. Fabbrocini G, Forgione P, Capasso C. methodologies. In Tosti A, Padova MPD (eds). Atlas of mesotherapy in skin rejuvenation. UK: Informa Healthcare. 2007;pp. 15-23.
6. Duque-Estrada B, Vincenzi C, Misciali C, Tosti A. Alopecia secondary to mesotherapy. J Am Acad Dermatol. 2009;61:707-9.
7. Nagore E, Ramos P, Botella Estrada R, Ramoz - Niguez JA, Sanmritan O, Castejon P. Cutaneous infection with Mycobacterium fortuitum after localized microinjections (Mesotherapy) treated successfully with a triple drug regimen. Acta Derm veneol. 2001;81:291-3.
8. Bryant R. controversial mesotherapy; could it be the next Botox? Derm times. 2004;125:1.
9. Mysore; Mesotherapy in alopecia. International Journal of Trichology. Jan-Jun 2010;2(1):pp. 45-46.
10. Sarkar R,Garg VK,Mysore V.Position paper on mesotherapy. Indian Dermatol, Venereol Leprol. Mar-Apr 2011;77(2):232-7.
11. Rotunda AM, Kolodney MS. Mesotherapy and phosphatidylcholine injections; Historical classification and review. Dermatol Surg. 2006;S2:456-80.

27

Hair Cosmetics

Malavika Kohli, Sheena Bansal

"Beauty is the pilot of the young soul."

—*Ralph Waldo Emerson*

Introduction

Beauty is the harmonious balance of face, hair and body. A lustrous head of hair changes and enhances overall features of an individual. Nothing makes as dramatic a statement as healthy, shiny and silky hair.

Hair plays a significant role in every individual's life. Every individual wants to know about hair care products and hair styling products suitable for their hair type and to enhance their hair health and looks. There can be different concerns for different individuals. Common concerns seen now a days are diffuse hair loss, androgenetic alopecia, dry frizzy hair, pityriasis sicca, premature graying of hair.

For any patient who comes with hair problems, one has to ask for duration of the problem, nutritional history, lifestyle, family history, hair treatments such as artificially straightened or curled hair, hair coloring and bleaching, routine hair care products and use of styling devices (**Box 27.1**).

Common sources of mechanical and thermal damage include excessive brushing, hot blow drying and hair ironing. Examine the hair for hair quality and texture, hair shaft problems, thinning, hair line and scaling of the scalp. As the hair grows away from the scalp it degenerates to some degree and this can be exaggerated by physical and chemical procedures such as overzealous brushing, bleaching, permanent waving and trichotillomania. Hair shaft damage also occurs due to environmental factors such as sunlight, air pollution, wind, seawater, and chlorinated swimming pool water. This kind of hair damage is called as 'weathering'.[1]

Box 27.1: History to be taken for any patient who comes with hair problems

- Duration of the problem—acute or chronic
- Nutritional history
- Lifestyle
- Family history
- Artificially straightened or curled hair
- Hair coloring
- Bleaching
- Routine hair care products
- Use of styling devices

Hair cosmetics are products designed for maintaining the integrity of the hair and also, to beautify the appearance. This chapter deals with hair cleansers, moisturizers, and products that chemically alter hair color and physically alter hair shape.

Throughout history, people have worn their hair in a wide variety of ways, largely determined by the fashions of the culture they live in. Hairstyles are markers and signifiers of social class, age, marital status, racial identification, political beliefs and attitudes about gender. Hairstyling in part is dictated by available technology in hair styling products.

In ancient civilizations, women's hair was often elaborately and carefully dressed in special ways. Women colored their hair, curled it, and pinned it up in a variety of ways. They set their hair in waves and curls using wet clay, which they dried in the sun and then combed out, or else by using a jelly made of quince seeds soaked in water, or curling tongs and curling irons of various kinds.[2,3]

Hair Treatments

Keratin complex is a specially formulated protein complex designed to eliminate frizz and out of control curls and leaves hair shiny, healthy and radiant. As proteins infuse into the hair, it penetrates deep into the damaged cuticle, giving the hair a naturally straight and smooth look. The products are applied onto the hair and washed out after 24–30 hours. The products mainly employ keratin, wheat germ oil, olive fruit oil, shea butter, acai berry extracts, chestnut extract, vitamin A and vitamin E for healthy nourished hair. Traditionally keratin treatments had more than 2% formaldehyde, which was damaging to the hands of the salon personnel. Newer products are designed with less than 2% formaldehyde for increased safety.

Other treatments with cysteine complex are available for softening the curls, to leave hair straighter and more manageable. Cysteine is a compound already found in the hair, and it makes up to 40% of hair's natural protein composition. Cysteine also has antioxidant properties and gives increased stability on bonding into the hair shaft. This treatment is free of formaldehyde and can be washed on the same day as compared to the keratin infusion treatment. It manages to reduce 70% curl volume on Caucasian hair and 50–60% curl volume on ethnic hair. The effect of the treatment lasts for about 3–5 months **(Box 27.2)**.

These treatments are a natural, effective way of naturally restoring and transforming chemically treated as well as virgin hair to a manageable, luxurious finish.

Styling Aids (Table 27.1)

Hair Spray

Hair spray also called as hair lacquer or spritz is an aerosolized liquid applied to the finished hair style to set it in desired position.[4,5] Hair sprays consist of copolymers such as polyvinylpyrrolidone (PVP). It is a water-soluble resin, which creates temporary bonds between the hair shafts leaving the hairstyle stiff. It gets easily washed away with shampoo. However, since the resin also absorbs water, it may become sticky due to humidity and perspiration. Vinyl acteate can be added to PVP to make it water-resistant, however, it also makes the spray harder to remove with the shampooing.[6] The newest flexible-hold hair sprays containing polyvinyl pyrrolidone dimethylaminoethyl methacrylate are available which provide high hold with reduced stiffness.[7]

Box 27.2: Products used for hair treatment

- Keratin
- Wheat germ oil
- Olive fruit oil
- Shea butter
- Acai berry extracts
- Chestnut extract
- Vitamin A
- Vitamin E
- Cysteine

Gel

Hair gels are same as hair spray as they contain same PVP-type co-polymers. It is applied to towel-dried, damp hair and hand combed to form a thin film on hair shafts. The gel gives enhanced hold to the hairstyle with increased shine. When applied in large amounts, hair will have a wet, spiky look and feel stiff. Hair gels are available in two types: styling gels and sculpturing gels. Styling gels offer moderate hold whereas sculpturing gels are ideal for gravity-defying hair styles due to their stronger hold. Hair gels can hold the hair away from the scalp, creating illusion of fullness. This is especially important in people with thinning hair.[8]

Wax

Hair waxes are again based on copolymers as hair sprays and gels, designed to give increased hold to hair. The waxes are designed to soften at body temperature and again can be re-formed, providing styling products that can be reshaped frequently yet, allow the hair to remain in the same position. Some looks that can be created are 'bed-head' look; hair standing on the end away from the scalp but has a rather greasy look. The product has to be scooped from the can and softened on the palm before application. It is massaged along the length of hair shafts to provide a thin coating.[7]

Mousse

Hair mousse comes as foam in aerosolized can and is applied on towel-dried hair. It can also be applied on dry hair to create wet spiky look. Hair mousse employs lighter co-polymers and does not provide as strong a hold as a gel. It also produces less flaking and stickiness than a gel under moist conditions. Women usually prefer mousse to other styling products.[7]

Table 27.1: Hair styling aids

1.	Hair spray	Aerosolized liquid applied to the finished hair style to set it in desired position and consist of polyvinylpyrrolidone(PVP), which is water soluble
2.	Gel	Contain PVP-type co-polymers, applied to towel-dried, damp hair and hand combed to form a thin film on hair shafts. Gels can hold the hair away from the scalp, creating illusion of fullness
3.	Wax	Contain PVP-type co-polymers, soften at body temperature and again can be reformed, providing styling products that can be reshaped frequently yet allow the hair to remain in the same position
4.	Mousse	Foam in aerosolized can and is applied on towel-dried hair, contains lighter co-polymers and does not provide as strong a hold as a gel
5.	Pomade	Are designed to straighten, moisturize, and condition kinky hair. Pomade is an anhydrous ointment containing petrolatum, waxes, lanolin, and vegetable or mineral oils which are comedogenic

Pomade (Cream Brilliantine)

Hair pomades are designed to straighten, moisturize and condition kinky hair. Pomade is an anhydrous ointment containing petrolatum, waxes, lanolin and vegetable or mineral oils.[9] They help by minimizing hair breakage due to combing friction in tightly kinked hair through lubrication. It also allows hair to remain close to the scalp with some curl reduction. It is especially useful for African-American men and women with curled, kinky hair.[7]

Brilliantine

Hair brilliantines are liquids designed to style and maintain natural kinky hairstyles without oil build up. They employ mineral and vegetable oils and are comedogenic. Newer formulations are available that contain silicone, castor oil and soluble glycoproteins for enhanced shine and lubrication.[7]

Permanent Hair Waving Agent

Permanent waving is a method of transforming straight hair to curly hair. It requires three chemical steps[10] **(Box 27.3)**:

1. Chemical softening of keratin disulfide bond (kSSk) with a thiol compound to form symmetrical disulfide of the thiol waving agent (RSSR).
   kSSk + RSH ↔ kSH + kSSR
   kSSR + RSH ↔ kSH + RSSR
2. Rearrangement of hair protein structure to relieve internal stress determined by curler size and hair wrapping tension.
3. Fixation with an oxidizing agent as a catalyst to reform the keratin disulfide bond.
   kSH + HSk ↔ kSSk + H_2O

There are different types of permanent waves depending on the waving solution used. The waving solution is a reducing agent such as thioglycolic acid, thiolactic acid, glycerol monothioglycolate, sodium sulfite in an alkaline solution of ammonium hydroxide or triethanolamine, to break the keratin disulfide cross-links. Chelating agent such as tetrasodium EDTA is added to remove trace metals. Wetting agents are added for better penetration of the reducing agent into the hair shaft. The most common wetting agents used are fatty alcohols, sodium lauryl sulfate, sodium laureth sulfate, disodium laureth sulfosuccinate, cocoamphodiacetate. Other ingredients used are antioxidants, opacifiers, conditioners and buffers **(Figure 27.1)**.[7,11]

Box 27.3: Chemical steps in hair waving

- Chemical softening of keratin disulfide bond
- Rearrangement of hair protein structure
- Fixation to reform the keratin disulfide bond

Permanent waving products can be classified as follows **(Box 27.4)**:

1. Alkaline permanent waves utilize ammonium thioglycolate or ethanolamine thioglycolate as the active reducing agent. The pH is adjusted to pH 9–10 because thioglycolates are inactive at acidic pH. They have short processing time and produce tight, long-lasting curls rapidly. However, they are not so popular since the hair is left inelastic and harsh.
2. Buffered alkaline waves use ammonium bicarbonate in addition to alkaline wave ingredients to adjust pH to 7–8.5. They are preferred over alkaline waves because they produce tight curls like alkaline waves but are less harsh on the hair.
3. Exothermic permanent waves are so called because the chemical reaction between thioglycolate and peroxide to produce dithiodiglycolate releases heat. Heat released is comforting to the patient; however, the ingredients should be properly mixed to avoid hair damage due to excessive heat.
4. Self-regulated solutions, which utilize dithioglycolic acid and thioglycolate at pH of 6.5-7, stop processing

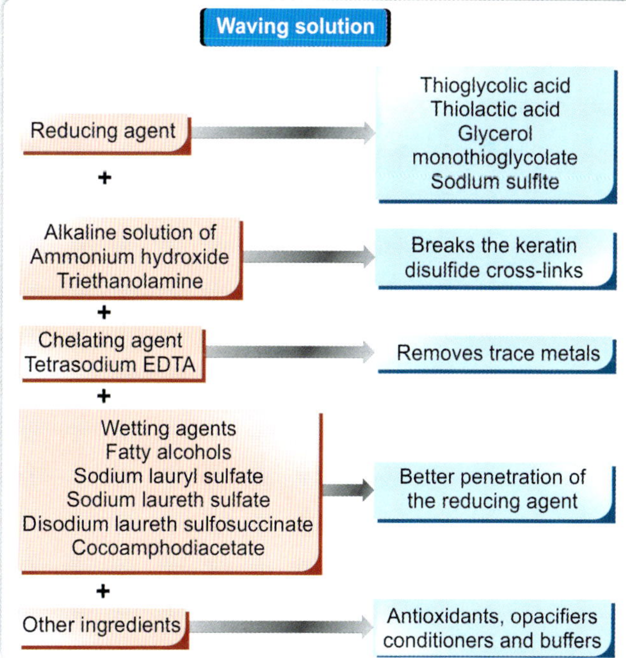

Fig. 27.1: Waving solution

Box 27.4: Classification of permanent waving products

- Alkaline
- Buffered alkaline
- Exothermic
- Self-regulated acid
- Acid
- Sulfite

automatically once equilibrium is achieved. They produce loose curls but cannot be used for hard to perm hair.

5. Acid waves are the most common waves used in the salon. The active ingredients used are thioglycolate esters, such as glycerol monothioglycolate at pH of 6.5–7 to produce loose, shorter lasting curls. The lower pH leaves the hair soft with minimal damage because less hair shaft swelling occurs at acidic pH.[7,10] However, glycerol monothioglycolate may cause allergic contact dermatitis, and surprisingly, hair may continue to be allergenic even after all products have been rinsed off from the hair.[12]
6. Sulfite waves are not preferred since they produce loose curls but with harsh and inelastic hair and have a long processing time.[13]

Hair Straightening Agent

Chemical hair straightening is similar to permanent hair waving, except that keratin disulfide cross-links are reformed with the hair straight rather than curved around the curler. Hair straightening agents are as follows **(Box 27.5)**:

1. Lye-based, or sodium hydroxide straighteners are generally restricted to salon use. The straightening occurs as one-third of the hair cystine content is changed to lanthionine along with minor hydrolysis of the peptide bonds.[15] Sodium hydroxide is a caustic substance that can damage hair, produce scalp burns, and cause blindness if exposed to eye.
2. Lye-free chemical straightening uses other strong alkalis such as guanidine hydroxide or lithium hydroxide as the active agent. The kit contains 4% to 7% calcium hydroxide and liquid guanidine carbonate, which are mixed to produce calcium carbonate and guanidine hydroxide, the active agent.
3. Thioglycolate straighteners are same as permanent wave solutions except that they are formulated as thick creams, rather than lotions, to add weight to the hair and hold them straight. However, they are extremely harsh on the hair due to the high pH of 9–9.5 that removes the protective sebum.
4. Bisulfite straighteners are least damaging to the hair. They contain a mixture of bisulfite and sulfite in different ratios, depending on pH of the lotion. They are usually used for at-home chemical straightening but they produce least permanent straightening.[10]

Box 27.5: Hair straightening agents[14]

- Lye-based
- Lye-free
- Ammonium thioglycolate
- Bisulfite creams

Hair Coloring Agents

Hair color is the most important cosmetic aspect of the hair, although pigment comprises only 3% of the fiber mass of hair. Hair coloring is a technique used to alter the natural color of hair or to camouflage gray hair. The tradition of dyeing hair with Henna, dates to third dynasty of Egypt 4000 years ago.[10] Modern hair coloring began in 1863 when Hoffman discovered that p-phenylenediamine on oxidation produces brown-black discoloration of hair. Eugene Schuller, the founder of L'Oréal, marketed the first commercial brand of hair color in 1907.[7] Since that day, the hair coloring industry has grown bigger and bigger, adding a new dimension to hair cosmetics.

Three pigments namely eumelanin, pheomelanin and oxymelanin produce the extensive variety of color seen in human hair. Based on their formulation and the longevity, hair dyes are usually divided into four types—gradual, temporary, semipermanent, and permanent **(Table 27.2)**.[10]

1. Gradual or progressive hair dyes change the color of hair shaft gradually from gray to yellow-brown to black after repeated applications. The principle is the deposition of oxides, suboxides, and sulfides of water-soluble metal salts on the hair shaft. The most common metal used is lead, rarely iron, copper, silver, bismuth, manganese and

Table 27.2: Hair coloring agents

	Type of dye	*Constituent dye*	
1.	Gradual or progressive hair dyes	Lead, iron, copper, silver, bismuth, manganese and nickel	Changes the color of hair shaft gradually from gray to yellow-brown to black after repeated applications
2.	Temporary hair dyes	Azo, anthraquinone, triphenylmethane, phenazinic, xanthene, or benzoquinone classes	Based on textile dyes, the particles are used to coat the hair shaft, removed after a single wash
3.	Semi-permanent hair dyes	Nitroanilines, nitrophenylenediamines, nitroaminophenols, azos, anthraquinones	Used for natural, unbleached hair to cover gray hair and add highlights. Dyes are retained in the hair shaft by weak polar and van der Waals forces. Dyes are removed in four to six shampooings
4.	Permanent hair dyes	P-phenylenediamine, p-toluenediamine, p-aminophenol with hydrogen peroxide	Cover gray hair and to change the existing hair color for 4 to 6 weeks

nickel have been used. However, hair color lightening is not possible with these kind of metallic dyes.[16]

2. Temporary hair dyes are based on textile dyes belonging to azo, anthraquinone, triphenylmethane, phenazinic, xanthene, or benzoquinone classes. The particles are used to coat the hair shaft, so as to add a slight tint to natural color or improve an existing dye shade. The particle size is too large to penetrate through the cuticle of the hair shaft and gets removed in one shampooing.[17]
3. Semi-permanent hair dyes are used for natural, unbleached hair to cover gray hair and add highlights. The formulation consists of dyes (nitroanilines, nitrophenylenediamines, nitroaminophenols, azos, anthraquinones), alkalinizing agent, solvent, surfactant, thickener, fragrance, and water. The dyes are retained in the hair shaft by weak polar and van der Waals forces. Due to their intermediate sized particles that can both enter and exit hair shaft, the dyes are removed in four to six shampooings. Recently, the longer lasting products containing hydrogen peroxide have become available.[18] They are available as lotions, shampoos, and mousses. The shampoo-in process dyes combine colored molecules with alkaline detergent shampoo to promote the hair shaft swelling so that the dye penetrates the hair and a foam stabilizer so that product does not stain the facial skin. The mousse dyes contain the colored molecules in aerosolized foam; which is applied to wet, freshly shampooed hair and are rinsed in 20 to 40 minutes.[19]
4. Permanent hair dyes are designed to cover gray hair and to change the existing hair color for 4 to 6 weeks, where after redyeing is necessary because on new hair growth at the scalp. Permanent dyes incorporate colorless dye precursors; such as p-phenylenediamine, p-toluenediamine, p-aminophenol that undergo oxidation with hydrogen peroxide inside the hair shaft. These intermediates are then exposed to couplers (resorcinol, 1-naphthol, m-aminophenol, and so on) to result in a wide variety of dyes.[20] Different colors can be produced by variations in the concentration of hydrogen peroxide, chemicals selected for primary intermediates and the couplers. Red is produced by using nitroparaphenylenediamine alone or in combination with mixtures of paraaminophenol with metaphenylenediamine, alphanaphthol, or 1,5-dihydroxynaphthalene. Yellow is produced by mixtures of orthoaminophenol, orthophenylenediamine, and nitro-orthophenylenediamine. Combinations of p-phenylenediamine, phenylenediamine, methyltoluenediamine, or 2,4-diaminoanisol without any oxidation dye intermediate produce blue.[21] Permanent hair dyes can be designed to produce both lighter and darker shades than one's original hair color. Boosters such as ammonium persulfate or potassium sulfate, can be added to color lightening. However, individuals with dark hair who choose to dye their hair a light blonde color can notice the appearance of reddish hues with time.[10]

Hair Bleaching Agents

Hair bleaching involves lightening of natural hair color through use of oxidizing agents at an alkaline pH. The most common oxidizer used is hydrogen peroxide, which releases oxygen from hair keratin in proportion to hair color lightening achieved. The hydrogen peroxide solution is alkalinized to a pH between 9 and 11 by mixing with ammonia just before application. The chemical reaction occurs more rapidly in presence of body heat, thus hair near the scalp lightens with greater speed than the hair shaft. The amount of hair lightening achieved is in direct proportion to the volume of peroxide used.[22]

About 15 to 25% of hair disulfide bonds are degraded during moderate bleaching, resulting in 2 to 3% weight loss of hair shaft.[23] The weakening of hair shaft with the bleaching agent is more when the hair is wet, thus hair must be dried before grooming to prevent the damage. Bleached hair is also more porous, absorbs water readily, requires longer time to dry, difficult to detangle, and is more susceptible to further chemical damage **(Box 27.6)**.[10]

Hair Shampoos

Shampoos are designed to remove sebum,dirt, dandruff, environmental pollutants and other contaminant particles that gradually build up in hair, so as to leave the hair manageable with volume and luster.[24] Detergents or surfactants most often sodium lauryl sulfate and/or sodium laureth sulfate are the primary ingredients in the shampoo to remove dirt and sebum. However, excessive removal of sebum leaves the hair dull, susceptible to static electricity, and difficult to comb.[10]

The detergents have to be properly chosen keeping both the cleansing and cosmetic properties of a shampoo. The foaming agent is added to provide lather, which consumers equate with cleansing; however, the two are unrelated. Conditioners leave the hair manageable after shampooing. Thickeners, opacifiers, softeners, and fragrance are added for the look, feel and smell of the product. Sequestering

Box 27.6: Disadvantages of bleaching

- Loss of hair shaft
- Longer time to dry
- Difficult to detangle
- More susceptible to damage

agents prevent scum formation on the hair in presence of hard water, which can lead to scalp pruritus and leave hair dull. This is why shampoos and not the bar soaps should be used to cleanse the hair. Lastly, preservative like DMDM hydantoin and imidazolidinyl urea are necessary to prevent fungal and bacterial spoilage **(Figure 27.2)**.[7,25]

Shampoo detergents can be chemically classified as anionics, cationics, amphoterics, and nonionics **(Table 27.3)**. The anionics are excellent cleansers but harsh on hair, whereas nonionics and cationics are mild cleansers and leave the hair more manageable.[10] Cationic detergents are primarily used in daily wash shampoos, designed to restructure and protect colored and chemically treated, porous hair. They are popular as detergent less shampoos as they don't contain strong detergents such as laurel or laureth sulfates. Amphoteric detergents produce mild cleansing and are nonirritating to the eye since they anesthetize the conjunctiva. Amphoteric detergents such as cocamidopropylbetaine and sodium lauraminopropionate, are found in baby shampoos. They are also used in shampoos for fine and chemically treated hair. The detergents from different groups can be combined to meet consumer needs.[7,10] Natural surfactants such as sarsaparilla, soapwort, soap bark, ivy, agave can also be combined with synthetic detergents. However, they are poor cleansers but produce excellent lather.

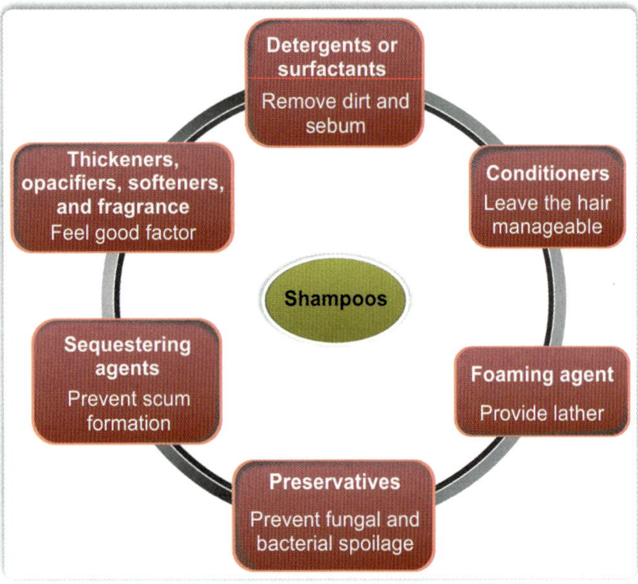

Fig. 27.2: Shampoo constituents

Table 27.3: Shampoo detergents[10]

Surfactant type	*Chemical class*	*Properties*
Anionics	Lauryl sulfates Laureth sulfates Sarcosines Sulfosuccinates	Deep cleansers Leave hair harsh
Cationics	Long chain aminoesters Ammonioesters	Poor cleansing Poor lather
Nonionics	Polysorbate Nonoxynols Poloxamers Alkanolamides	Mild cleanser Leave hair manageable
Amphoterics	Glucinates Propionates Betaines	Mild cleansing Non-irritating to the eyes

Different shampoos are available in market for oily hair, dry hair, dandruff, colored hair, etc. They differ from each other by their specific ingredients and formulations, e.g. creamy moisturizing shampoos with ingredients like nut oils, shea butter, and wheat germ oil are especially good at bonding to parched strands of dry hair and clear gel based shampoos with tea tree oil, citrus oil, rosemary, sage, stinging nettle, and chamomile help degreasing the fatty scalp in oily hair. Dry hair shampoos containing milder surfactants such as sodium laureth sulfate provide mild cleansing and excellent conditioning. Shampoos for oily hair have strong surfactants such as sodium lauryl sulfate and sulfosuccinates, which provide excellent cleansing but minimal conditioning. Conditioning shampoos contain added hydrolyzed proteins, to minimize static electricity, taking away the need for extra conditioners. Muru Muru butter is a natural conditioner in newer shampoos for frizzy hair. Oleic and linoleic acids in Muru Muru plant allow for a richer lather, while emollients deliver a natural vibrant glossiness that quickly eliminates frizz and repairs split ends. Panthenol is the best volumizing ingredient for the fine hair; it swells the hair shaft and adheres to individual strands to make them thicker. For people with fatty scalp who cannot wash hair daily, dry shampoos can be a solution. The new formulas with oatmeal, semolina flour, talcum powder, cornstarch, cottonseed oil and aloe vera extracts very gently degrease hair, however, they cannot replace wet shampooing. Professional shampoos are available which are cationic acidic shampoos designed for use in salon following hair dyeing to reduce hair shaft swelling in response to residual hair shaft alkalinity. Specialized products for colored hair are available in the market, which incorporates color enhancing emollient beads, silk proteins and amino acids to lock in the color and UV protectants to prevent color fading. Newer formulations with peppermint, sunflower seed extract and ginger extracts are available which claim to stimulate and dilate blood vessels creating an increased blood flow to the scalp for faster healthier hair growth.

Hair Conditioners (Box 27.7)

Current practice of shampooing daily or every other day removes the natural conditioner; sebum of the hair.

Box 27.7: Functions of a conditioner

- Maintain static electricity by neutralizing negative change on a sebum washed off hair shaft
- Improve manageability by reducing friction by 50%
- Increases shine
- Helps in maintaining the hairstyle
- Temporarily revitalizes damaged hair

Excessive removal of sebum leaves hair dull, dry and unmanageable; which created the need for synthetic sebum-like substance to maintain static electricity, improve manageability, increase shine and helps in maintaining the hairstyle. Following brushing or combing, hair shafts become negatively charged, causing hair to repel each other. Conditioners deposit positively charged ions on the hair shaft, neutralizing the charge. They also reduce combing friction by about 50%. They also attempt to rescue and revitalize the hair damaged due to chemical and mechanical trauma and bring them back to life. Any conditioner is minimal and temporary until the next wash.

Most common ingredient used in hair conditioner is silicone. Silicone is lightweight oil used to form a thin film on the hair shaft. The amount of silicone left behind on the hair determines whether the product is designed to add volume to fine hair which requires minimal conditioning or straighten the curly hair which needs maximal conditioning.

Moisturizers and lubricants are required to hold moisture in the hair. Reconstructors containing hydrolyzed protein are added to strengthen hair structure through polymer crosslinking. Thermal protectors, usually heat-absorbing polymers, shield the hair against excessive heat caused by, e.g. blow-drying, curling irons or hot rollers. Glossers like dimethicone or cyclomethicone are the light-reflecting chemicals added for esthetic value **(Table 27.4)**.

There are various types of conditioners available in the market to meet consumer demands. Instant conditioners are left in contact with hair for brief time immediately after hair wash. They are most suitable for minimally damaged hair and aids wet combing. Deep conditioners have same ingredients but are more concentrated. They are left on hair after a wash for 20–30 minutes and then rinsed off. The extended application helps more coating and they are specially meant for dry and chemically damaged hair. Leave-in conditioners are applied to towel dried hair and not rinsed off. They remain on till next shampooing, prevent damage due to blow-drying and aid styling. Rinse conditioners are applied after shampooing and removed prior to drying the hair. Clear rinse is used to remove the soap residue and cream rinse aids in disentangling dry hair.[7] Newer formulations containing plant-derived products such as Argon oil, Moroccan oil and avocado oil, Acai oil are available which when applied to damp hair before blow-drying, prevent thermal damage to the hair shaft and can also be applied to dry hair as and when needed to improve manageability and reduce the frizz.These plant extracts act as strong antioxidants to renew and restore even the most porous hair, giving damaged hair a healthy, elegant texture. Special conditioners for colored hair are available with vitamin E, amino acids, silk proteins and UV protecting agents to lock in the hair color and the shine.

Hair Prosthesis

Hair prosthesis are commonly used now-a days to camouflage the scalp defects. These include hair pieces, and hair forms. A dermatologist should be aware of the hair prosthesis available in the market.

Hair Pieces

Wig is the traditional hair piece that covers the entire scalp.

Wiglets are the pieces made to cover only the defect or the involved area of the scalp.

Hair weaving involves the procedure of attaching the wiglet to the scalp by sewing it to the braided hair on the scalp margin.

When a wiglet is attached to the scalp by adhesive paste in the front and by clips on the sides, it is called as hair bonding **(Box 27.8)**.

For women with long tresses, falls and cascades can be attached to the vertex and occipital area of the scalp , these are known as hair extensions.

Switch is a plait or ponytail tied to the scalp margin.

Table 27.4: Hair conditioners[7]

Category	*Primary ingredients*	*Advantage*	*Grooming benefits*
Cationic detergent	Quarternary ammonium compound	Smoothen cuticle, decrease static electricity	For damaged and chemically processed hair
Film formers	Polymers	Fill hair shaft defects	Improve the appearance of dry, kinky hair
Protein containing	Hydrolyzed proteins	Penetrate hair shaft to increase strength	Mend split ends temporarily
Silicones	Dimethicone, cyclomethicone, amodimethicone	Thin coating on hair shafts	Add shine, decrease combing friction

Box 27.8: Hair bonding vs hair weaving

- Hair weaving involves the procedure of attaching wiglet to the scalp by sewing it to the braided hair on the scalp margin
- When a wiglet is attached to the scalp by adhesive paste in the front and by clips on the sides, it is called as hair bonding

Silicon system is a hair integration system, which employs a loose elastic mesh of hair over the scalp through the wide gaps of which existing hair is pulled, so as to create an appearance of dense hair.

Hair Forms

Hair forms are vacuum attached hair pieces most ideal for alopecia universalis. The thin synthetic form is sized appropriately using a plaster mold.

References

1. Dawber R. Cosmetic and medical causes of hair weathering. J Cosmet Dermatol. 2002;1(4):196-201.
2. Yarwood, Doreen. The Encyclopedia of World Costume. Scribner. New York. 1978;216-20.
3. Sherrow, Victoria. For Appearance' Sake: The Historical Encyclopedia of Good Looks, Beauty, and Grooming. Greenwood. 2001:142.
4. Guth J, Russo J, Kay T, et al. Addressing the low VOC hair spray issue. Cosmet Toilet. 1993;108:97-103.
5. Jachowicz J, Yao K. Dynamic hair spray analysis. I. Instrumentation and preliminary results. J Soc Cosmet Chem. 1996;47:73-84.
6. Pavlichko J. Aqueous dispersion hair-spray resin. Cosmet Toilet. 1995;110:63-7.
7. Zoe Diana Draelos. Hair Cosmetics. In: Ulrike Blume-Peytav (ed). Hair Growth and Disorders. Springer. 2008:498-513.
8. Wood C, Nguyen-Kim S, Hoessel P. A dimension in hair styling- VP/methacrylamide/Vinyl imidazole copolymer. Cosmet Toilet. 2004;119:59-66.
9. Goode ST. Hair pomades. Cosmet Toilet. 1979;94:71-4.
10. Zoe Diana Draelos. Cosmetic therapy. In: Stephen E Wolverton (ed). Comprehensive Dermatologic Drug Therapy. Saunders. Elsevier Science. 2002:695-709.
11. Lee AE, Bozza JB, Huff S, et al. Permanent waves: an overview. Cosmet Toilet. 1988;103:37-56.
12. Wickett RR. Disulfide bond reduction in permanent waving. Cosmet Toilet. 1991;106:37-47.
13. Draelos ZK. Hair cosmetics. Dermatol Clin. 1991;9:19-27.
14. Cannell DW. Permanent waving and hair straightening. Clin Dermatol. 1988;6:71-82.
15. Hsuing DY. Hair straightening. In: deNavarre M (ed). The chemistry and manufacture of cosmetics. Wheaton IL, Allured publishing. 1975;2:1155.
16. Spoor HJ. Part II: metals. Cutis. 1977;19:37-40.
17. Spoor HJ. Hair dyes: temporary colorings. Cutis. 1976;18:341-4.
18. Spoor HJ. Semi-permanent hair color. Cutis. 1976;18:506-8.
19. Zviak C. Hair coloring, non oxidation coloring. In: Zviak C, editor. The science of hair care. New York. Marcel Dekker. 1986;235-61.
20. Ticker HH. Formulation of oxidation hair dyes. Am J Perfum Cosmet. 1968;83:69.
21. Zviak C. Oxidation coloring. In: Zviak C (ed). The science of hair care. New York. Marcel Dekker. 1986;263-86.
22. Zviak C. Hair bleaching. In: Zviak C (ed). The science of hair care. New York. Marcel Dekker. 1986;213-33.
23. Corbett JF. Hair coloring processes. Cosmet Toilet. 1991;106:53-7.
24. Bouillon C. Shampoos and hair conditioners. Clin dermatol. 1998;6:83-92.
25. Markland WR. Shampoos. In: deNavarre M (ed). The chemistry and manufacture of cosmetics. Wheaton IL, Allured publishing. 1988;2:1283-312.
26. Corbett JF. The chemistry of hair care products. J Soc Dyers Colour. 1976;98:285-303.

28

Platelet Rich Plasma in Trichology

S Sacchidanand, Lakshmi DV

"We have to continually be jumping off cliffs and developing our wings on the way down."

—*Kurt Vonnegut*

Introduction

There has been continuous and accelerating progress in the basic understanding of platelet functions and its utilization in various bleeding disorders, since platelets were first identified in 1881.[1] Platelet rich plasma (PRP) is being widely used in a number of medical and surgical specialties to enhance tissue repair and healing. It was first promoted by M Ferrari in 1987 as an autologous transfusion component after an open heart operation to avoid homologous blood product transfusion.[2] PRP has emerged as a new treatment modality in dermatology. Its potentiality to promote hair growth in areas containing hair follicles is known since 1900.[3]

Definition

Platelet rich plasma (PRP) is an autologous concentration of human platelets in a small volume of plasma that has a higher platelet concentration (4–7-times) above baseline.[4] It contains growth factors (GFs) derived of platelets alone (stored as α-granules in platelets) and/or plasma proteins, namely fibrin, fibronectin and vitronectin.[5]

Working Definition of Platelet Rich Plasma (PRP)

Normal platelet counts in blood range between 150,000/μL to 350,000/μL and average about 200,000/μL. Because the scientific proof of bone and soft tissue healing enhancement has been shown using PRP with 1,000,000 platelets/μL, it is this concentration of platelets in a 5-mL volume of plasma which is the working definition of PRP, a therapeutically effective concentration.[6]

Mechanism of Action[5]

PRP is an organically based therapy that enables healing through the use of one's own natural growth factors. Plasma proteins act as a scaffold for epithelial migration and connective tissue regeneration. There is degranulation of GFs when platelets come in contact with coagulation factors. Later GFs bind to transmembrane receptors expressed over adult mesenchymal stem cells, osteoblasts, fibroblasts, endothelial cells, and epidermal cells. A cascade of intracellular signaling pathways are activated that leads to cellular proliferation, matrix formation, osteoid production, collagen synthesis, etc. thereby augmenting the natural wound-healing process **(Figure 28.1)**.

Growth Factors of Platelet Rich Plasma

The various growth factors present in PRP is illustrated in **Table 28.1** with their respective mechanism of actions.

Classification of Platelet Concentrates

Ehrenfest, et al. have proposed a classification of platelet concentrates into four categories depending upon their leukocyte and fibrin content.[8] It consists of:

- P-PRP (Pure platelet rich plasma)
- L-PRP (Leukocyte and platelet rich plasma)
- P-PRF (Pure platelet rich fibrin)
- L-PRF (Leukocyte and platelet rich fibrin)

The various mechanisms involved in obtaining these different types of platelet concentrates are tabulated in **Table 28.2**.

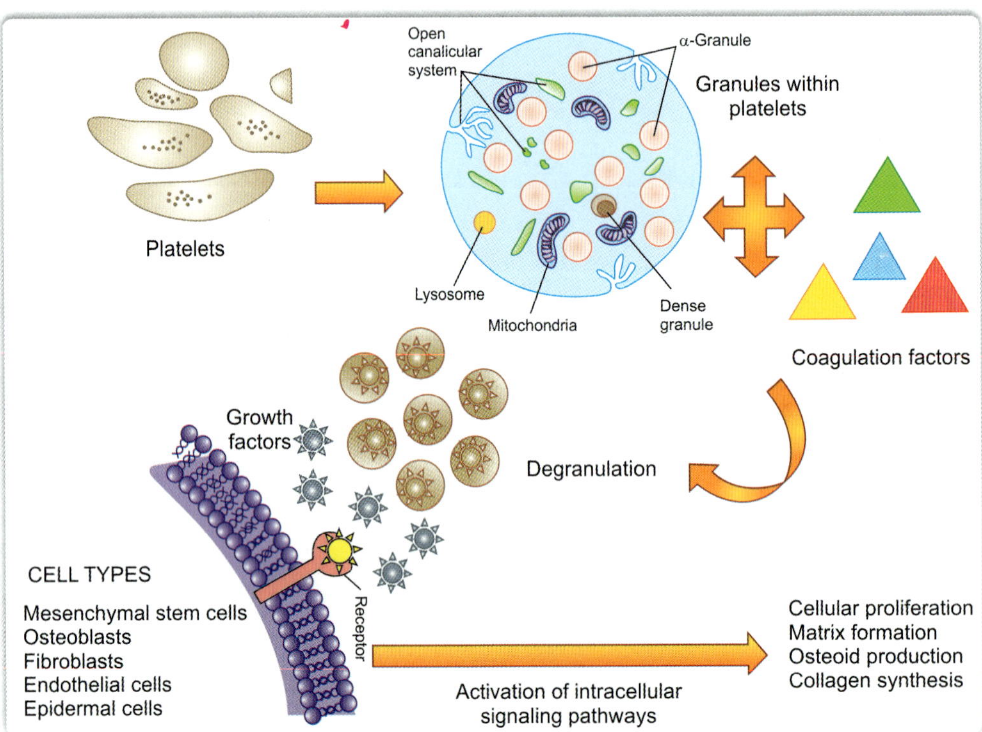

Fig. 28.1: Schematic representation of mechanism of action of platelet rich plasma

Table 28.1: Growth factors present in platelet rich plasma with their mechanism of action[5,7]

Growth factors	Mechanism of action
PDGF	❑ Chemotactic for fibroblasts and macrophages ❑ Mitogenic for fibroblasts, smooth muscle cells and endothelial cells
TGF	❑ Mediates angiogenesis ❑ Chemotactic for fibroblasts, keratinocytes and macrophages ❑ Mitogenic for fibroblasts and smooth muscle cells ❑ Inhibits endothelial cells, keratinocytes and lymphocytes ❑ Regulates matrix proteins, including collagen, proteoglycans, fibronectin and matrix-degrading proteins
VEGF	❑ Chemotactic and mitogenic for endothelial cells ❑ Mediates angiogenesis
EGF	❑ Mediates angiogenesis ❑ Mitogenic for fibroblasts, endothelial cells and keratinocytes
HGF	❑ Mediates regeneration
FGF	❑ Mediates tissue organization and regeneration
FGF-9	❑ Aids generation of new follicles

Abbreviation: PDGF: Platelet derived growth factor, TGF: Transforming growth factor, EGF: Epidermal growth factor, FGF: Fibroblast growth factor, VEGF: Vascular endothelial growth factor, HGF: Hepatocyte growth factor

Table 28.2: Types of platelet concentrates and their composition

Types	Composition	Examples
P-PRP	Consists of an undetermined fraction of buffy coat and platelets obtained when superficial buffy coat layer is pipetted out and prepared for next centrifugation	Anitua's plasma rich in growth factors (PRGF)
L-PRP	Consists of platelets, along with leukocytes and some residual RBCs, suspended in fibrin-rich plasma obtained when, platelet poor plasma (PPP) along with the entire buffy coat layer and superficial 1–2 mm layer of RBCs are pipetted out and centrifuged	Plateltex and Regen ACR kit Automated systems for L-PRP are PCCS and Smart PReP
P-PRF	P-PRP is mixed with activator and allowed to incubate, a stable PRFM clot is obtained	Fibrinet PRFM kit
PRF	Blood is collected without any anticoagulant and immediately centrifuged to obtain RBC base layer, acellular plasma top layer and L-PRF clot in the middle	Choukroun's PRF

Method of Preparation of Platelet Rich Plasma (PRP)

PRP can be prepared by two techniques:
- Manual double spin method
- Automated devices.

Manual Double Spin Method

The American Association of Blood Banks technical manual states that "platelet-rich plasma is separated from whole blood by 'light-spin' centrifugation and subsequently the platelets are concentrated by 'heavy-spin' centrifugation with removal of the supernatant plasma."[9]

The basic principle behind the PRP separation procedure is shown in **Box 28.1**.

Technique

Under aseptic precautions, 40–75 mL venous blood is drawn and is added to a test tube containing acid citrate dextrose in a ratio of 9:1 (blood: acid citrate dextrose- ACDA). The first spin called the hard spin (5000 rotation per minute for 15 minutes/160 g for 10 minutes at 20°C[10]) will separate the red blood cells from the plasma, which contains the platelets, the white blood cells, and the clotting factors. The plasma is then aspirated with a micropipette and transferred to a sterile test tube without an anticoagulant which is subjected to a second centrifugation (soft spin) at 2000 rotation per minute for 10 minutes/400 g for 10 minutes at 20°C[10], which allows the precipitation of the platelets (0.8 to 1.2 mL) to fall onto the bottom, while the surface platelet poor plasma is discarded using a micropipette.[11,12]

The PRP is then transferred to a sterile dish and stored at room temperature until further use. Just before placing the PRP in the dish, a few drops of 10% calcium chloride (obtained by mixing 1 g of calcium chloride in 10 mL of distilled water) is added to the PRP. Within 10 minutes they secrete 70% of their stored growth factors and close to 100% within the first hour.[13] Later additional amounts of growth factors are synthesized for about 8 days until they are depleted and die.[13] Hence, PRP should be activated just prior to the procedure, not in advance.

The procedure is illustrated in a simplified flowchart in **Figure 28.2**.

Box 28.1: The basic principle behind the PRP[5]

- Depending on the different specific gravities, components of whole blood gets separated
- RBCs being the heaviest settles down first, followed by WBCs, whereas platelets are the lightest
- First centrifugation is slow to avoid spinning down platelets and to isolate plasma, which concentrates on the top of the buffy coat layer
- Second centrifugation is faster, so that platelets are spundown and separate as a pellet at the bottom of the tube from platelet-poor plasma (PPP) above
- The final platelet concentration depends on the volume reduction of PPP
- Approximately 3/4 of the supernatant is discarded and the platelet-rich pellet is resuspended in remaining amount of plasma. The resulting suspension is used as PRP
- Calcium chloride or thrombin can be used as an "activator" to trigger coagulation and hence degranulation of GFs to yield "activated PRP"

Automated Devices

Numerous automated devices are available which are advantageous in being less time consuming, but viability, concentration and activation of platelets are of unknown relative efficacy, also being expensive with inconsistent reproducibility. Various FDA approved automated devices include Smart PReP, PCCS and BioMet GPSII.

Factors Affecting Platelet Yield and Viability

The platelet yield depends mainly on conditional parameters like size and shape of the container used, rate and time of spin and anticoagulant used. The viability of the platelets is assured by carrying out the process in a refrigerated centrifuge at 20°C. Trypan blue staining can confirm the viable state of the platelet concentrate. PRP must be used on the treated site within 10 minutes of activation.[13] The concentrated platelets remain viable for up to 8 hours.[14]

Double Spin Method vs Single Spin Method

Double spin is preferred over single spin method as therapeutic concentration is not obtained in the single spin method.[15] To attempt PRP with a single spin would not produce a true PRP. Instead, it would produce a mixture of PRP and platelet poor plasma and have disappointingly low platelet counts. Regardless of the rate of centrifugation or the time of centrifugation, a single spin cannot adequately concentrate platelets, because the red blood cells will interfere with the fine separation of the platelets.[13]

Indications for Platelet Rich Plasma

Dermatological indications are enumerated in **Box 28.2**.

Androgenetic Alopecia (AGA)

The angiogenic role of PRP has pointed towards its usefulness as a hair growth modality.

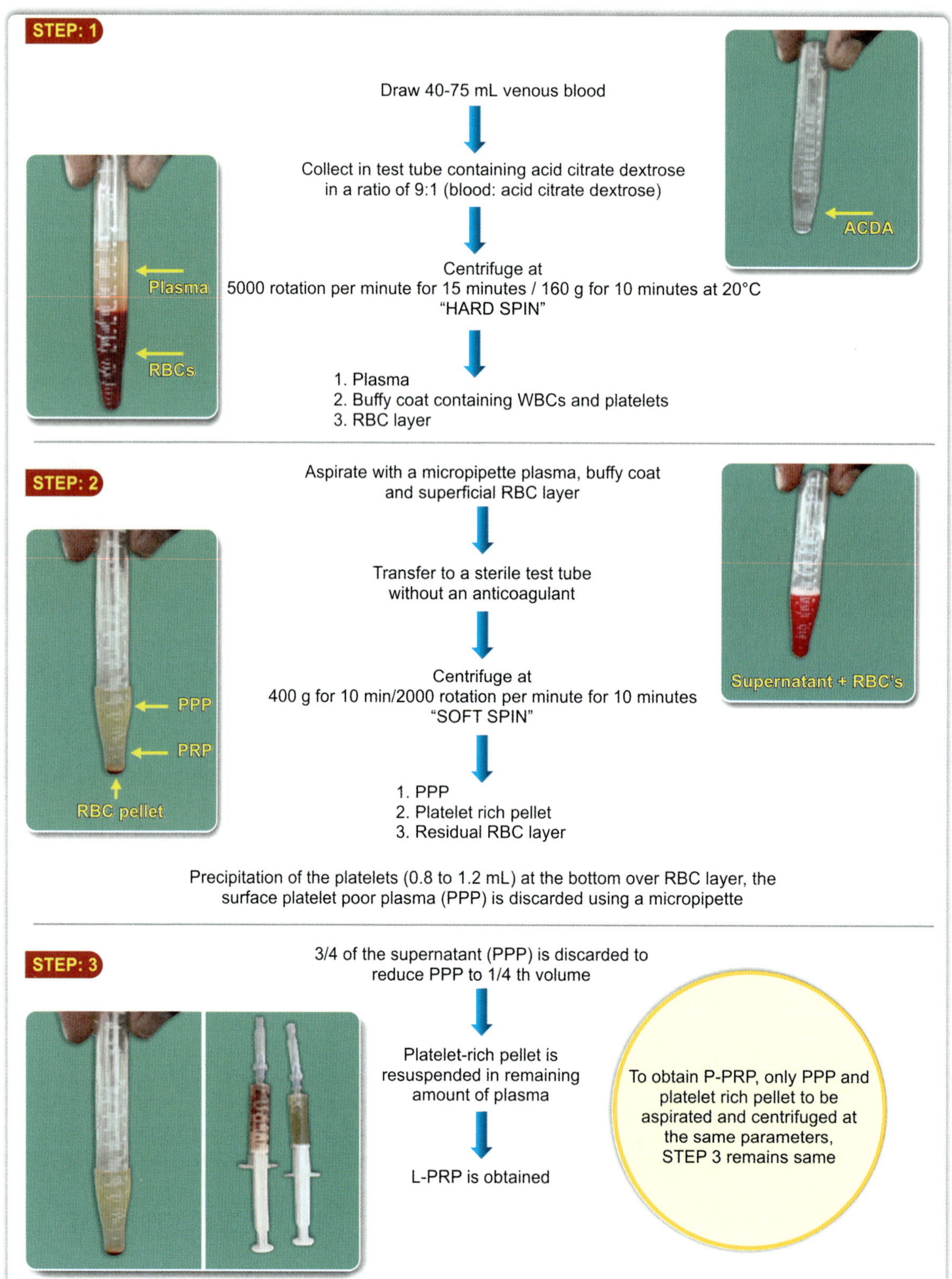

Fig. 28.2: Schematic representation of steps involved in preparation of platelet rich plasma

Box 28.2: Indications of PRP[5]

Indications

- Androgenetic alopecia
- Alopecia areata
- Skin rejuvenation
- Acne scars and contour defects
- Wound ulcers
- Striae distensae
- Lichen sclerosus
- Lipodermatosclerosis

Rinaldi et al, found that growth factors from PRP could prevent dermal papilla apoptosis, prolong anagen phase, delay catagen and telogen, eventually reducing diffuse hair loss and stimulating hair regrowth in androgenetic alopecia, without side effects during the treatment period and after 12 months from the end of treatment.[16] Uebel et al, in 2005, showed that area treated with PRP demonstrated a yield of 18.7 FU/cm^2 v/s 16.4 FU/cm^2 of the placebo group, an increase in follicular density of 15.1%.[17] Greco et al. and Lopez et al. observed a significant increase in hair diameter and hair density respectively, with PRP.[18,19]

Mechanism of Action of PRP in AGA

Multiple molecular mechanisms are proposed to be responsible for hair growth. VEGF8 and PDGF4 found in PRP are known to facilitate angiogenesis around the hair follicle, and this may be one mechanism underlying observations that PRP can foster robust hair growth.[20]

Figure 28.3 shows the various mechanisms by which PRP induces hair growth in AGA.

Box 28.3: Modes of PRP in AGA

- Inter-follicular injection
- PRP mesotherapy
- PRP as an adjunct to hair transplantation

Various Modes of PRP therapy for AGA[5] (Box 28.3):

They are as follows:

1. Inter-follicular injection of PRP at a concentration of 0.05–0.1 mL/cm, at every centimeter, throughout the treated site.
2. PRP mesotherapy: Microneedle roller of 1 mm fine needles are used initially, followed by interfollicular injections of PRP over the treated area. It is usually done in 3 monthly sessions **(Figure 28.4)**.
3. PRP as an adjunct to hair transplantation:
   a. The follicular grafts are dipped into PRP for about 15 minutes, before implantation so as to increase their survival rate after implantation.
   b. PRP is injected into the recipient area of scalp prior to or just after implantation of grafts.
   c. PRP is injected at and around the donor strip excision line, in follicular unit transplantation (FUT), to minimize bleeding, stimulate wound healing and reduce scarring.

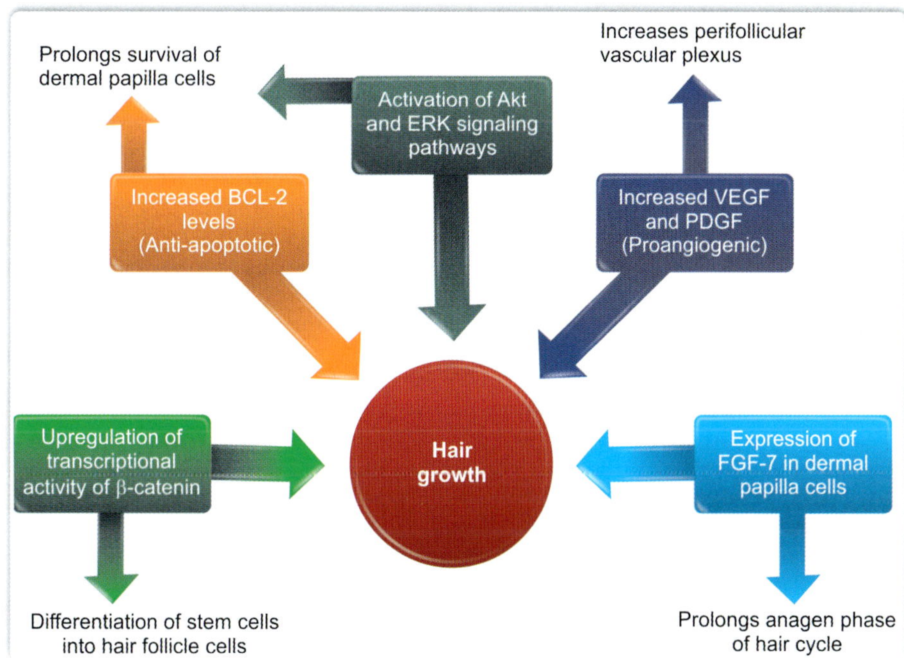

Fig. 28.3: Schematic representation of mechanism of action of platelet rich plasma in androgenetic alopecia

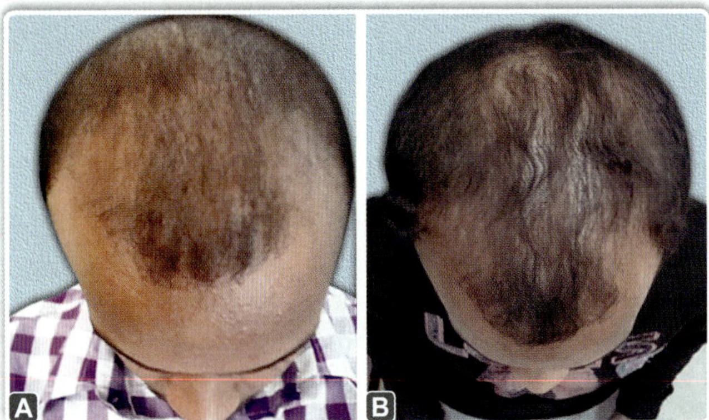

Fig. 28.4: PRP showing good response after 6 months of therapy by microneedle roller technique

Modification of PRP

A study conducted by Takikawa et al. showed that dalteparin in PRP could further improve the hair thickness as compared to PRP alone without any side effects.[21] A low-molecular weight heparin, dalteparin can act as a carrier for PRP, helps to adsorb, stabilize and gradually release the GFs in PRP.

Alopecia Areata

Greco et al, tried it in a single patient of alopecia areata as mesotherapy, with good subjective results at 10-months follow-up.[18] A randomized double bind, placebo and active controlled, half-head study evaluated PRP in 45 patients of alopecia areata. Ki-67 analysis revealed that PRP administration led to a significant increase in Ki-67 levels in AA patches. Levels of Ki-67, a marker for cell proliferation was considered in the study. Both Ki-67 and SALT score parameters were significantly better than with triamcinolone administration. It was a monthly regimen for three sessions that showed significant increase in hair regrowth and decrease in hair dystrophy and burning/itching sensation at 1-year follow-up.[22]

Telogen Effluvium

There is a clear paucity of published data in support of PRP in telogen effluvium. Patients may have spontaneous remissions and respond well to commonly used medications, so it is difficult to attribute the regrowth of hair to PRP.

Advantages of Platelet Rich Plasma

1. PRP is autologous preparation, hence its non-antigenic.
2. Devoid of any serious adverse effects, apart from local injection site reactions like pain or secondary infection.
3. The mitogenic effects of PRP are only limited to augmentation of the normal healing process and is theoretically not mutagenic, as the GFs released do not enter the cell or its nucleus, but only bind to the membrane receptors and induce signal transduction mechanisms.[23]
4. The inclusion of leukocytes in PRP as in L-PRP with a potential benefit to combat infection and regulate immune function, they also produce additional angiogenic factors.[24]
5. Economical preparation.

Conclusion

PRP represents a relatively new biotechnology that is part of the growing interest in tissue engineering and cellular therapy today. Method of promoting hair growth by application of a blood extract is an interesting and upcoming safe, easy and inexpensive modality to treat hair loss, with no danger of allergic reactions. But, there is lack of double blind, randomized, placebo controlled trials. Further research is awaited to unfold its long term efficacy and safety.

Acknowledgment

We would like to thank Dr Shruthi Gupta, Resident, Department of Dermatology, BMCRI, Bengaluru for her contribution in this chapter.

References

1. Michelsen AD. Flow cytometry: A clinical test of platelet function. Blood. 1996;87:4925-36.
2. Ferrari M, et al. A new technique for hemodilution, preparation of autologous platelet-rich plasma and intraoperative blood salvage in cardiac surgery. Int J Artif Organs. 1987;10(1):47-50.
3. Knighton DR, Hudson, Wis, inventors. Regents of the University of Minnesota, Minneapolis, Minn, Curative Technologies. Method For Promoting Hair Growth. 1990 (September 18). US Patent 4957742.
4. Marx RE, Garg AK. Dental and Craniofacial Applications of Platelet-Rich Plasma. Chicago: Quintessence Publishing; 2005.
5. Arshdeep M, Sendhil K. Platelet - rich plasma in dermatology: Boon or bane? Indian J Dermatol Venereol. 2014;80(1):5-14.
6. Mc Aleer JP, Kaolan E, Persich G. Efficacy of concentrated autologous platelet derived growth factor in chronic lower extremity wounds. J Am Podiatar Med Assoc. 2006;96(6):482-8.
7. Steed DL. The role of growth factors in wound healing. Surg Clin North Am. 1997;77:575-86.
8. Dohan Ehrenfest DM, Rasmusson L, Albrektsson T. Classification of platelet concentrates: from pure platelet-

rich plasma (P-PRP) to leukocyte- and platelet-rich fibrin (L-PRF). Trends Biotechnol. 2009;27:158-67.
9. American Association of Blood Banks technical manual committee. Method 6.11: Preparation of platelets from whole blood. In: Vengelen-Tyler V, editor. AABB Technical Manual, 13th ed. Bethesda (MD): American Association of Blood Banks. 1999;p. 725.
10. Gonshor A. Technique for producing platelet-rich plasma and platelet concentrate: Background and process. Int J Periodontics Restorative Dent. 2002;22:547-57.
11. Marx RE. Platelet-rich plasma (PRP): What is PRP and what is not PRP. Implant Dent. 2001;10(4):225-8.
12. Sanchez AR, Sheridan PJ, Kupp LI. Is platelet-rich plasma the perfect enhancement factor? A current review. Int J Oral Maxillofac Implants. 2003;18:93-103.
13. Bhanot S, Alex JC. Current applications of platelet gels in facial plastic surgery. Facial Plast Surg. 2002;18(1):27-33.
14. Marx RE. Platelet-rich plasma: Evidence to support its use J Oral Maxillofac Surg. 2004;62:489-96.
15. Kurita M, Aiba-Kojima E, Shigeura T, Matsumoto D, Suga H, Inoue K, et al. Differential effects of three preparations of human serum on expansion of various types of human cells. Plast Reconstr Surg. 2008;122:438-48.
16. Rinaldi F, Sorbellini E, Coscera T. The role of platelet rich plasma to control anagen phase: Evaluation in vitro and in vivo in hair transplant and hair treatment. Int J Trichol. 2011;3:S14-5.
17. Uebel CO, da Silva JB, Cantarelli D, Martins P. The role of platelet plasma growth factors in male pattern baldness surgery. Plast Reconstr Surg. 2006;118:1458-66.
18. Greco J, Brandt R. The effects of autologous platelet rich plasma and various growth factors on non-transplanted miniaturized hair. Hair Transplant Forum Int. 2009;19: 49-50.
19. Lopez V, Vaya A, Bautista D, Ricart JM. Autologous platelet-rich plasma as a potential therapeutic tool in androgenetic alopecia. J Am Acad Dermatol. 2013;68:103.
20. Reese RJ. Autologous Platelet Rich Plasma: What do we know? Important concepts relevant to Hair Restoration Surgery. Hair Transplant Forum Intl. 2010 (Jan-Feb);20(1):14-7.
21. Takikawa M, Nakamura S, Nakamura S, Ishirara M, Kishimoto S, Sasaki K, et al. Enhanced effect of platelet-rich plasma containing a new carrier on hair growth. Dermatol Surg. 2011;37:1721-9.
22. Trink A, Sorbellini E, Bezzola P, Rodella L, Rezzani R, Ramot Y, et al. A randomized, double-blind, placebo and active-controlled, half-head study to evaluate the effects of platelet rich plasma on alopecia areata. Br J Dermatol. 2013.
23. Schmitz JP, Hollinger JO. The biology of platelet-rich plasma. J Oral Maxillofac Surg. 2001;59:1119-21.
24. Anitua E, Alonso R, Girbau C, Aguirre JJ, Muruzabal F, Orive G. Antibacterial effect of plasma rich in growth factors (PRGF ®-Endoret) against *Staphylococcus aureus* and *Staphylococcus epidermidis* strains. Clin Exp Dermatol. 2012;37:652-7.

29

Stem Cell Therapy in Hair Restoration

Eswari L, S Sacchidanand

"Man's mind stretched to a new idea never goes back to its original dimensions."

—*Oliver Wendell Holmes Jr*

Introduction

Androgenetic alopecia (AGA) has become a plaguing condition giving an impetus to constant research with respect to its cause and management. Drugs and hair transplantations are the widely known treatment options for AGA. Drugs are not permanent solution in AGA because discontinuing medications may progress the hair loss. Hair transplantation gives limited results because it depends on the transplanted hair. To overcome these problems, introducing external source of stem cells to regenerate hair can prove to be a much solicited therapeutic boon.

Stem cells

Stem cells have the capacity to self-renew and to give rise to cells of various lineages. Broadly speaking, there are two main types of stem cells, embryonic and non-embryonic **(Box 29.1)**. Embryonic stem cells (ESCs) are derived from the inner cell mass of the blastocyst and can differentiate into cells of all three germ layers.[1] However, teratoma formation and ethical controversy hamper their research and clinical application.[1] On the other hand, non-embryonic stem cells also known as mesenchymal stem cells or adult stem cells, are already somewhat specialized and have limited differentiation potential.[1] They may be derived from adult tissues like bone marrow, adipose tissue, or derived from neonatal tissues like umbilical cord, cord blood, amnion or placenta. They are potential candidates in regenerative medicine.

Box 29.1: Types of stem cells

- Embryonic stem cells (ESCs) are derived from the inner cell mass of the blastocyst and can differentiate into cells of all three germ layers
- Non-embryonic stem cells (mesenchymal stem cells or adult stem cells) are derived from adult tissue like bone marrow, adipose tissue, or derived from neonatal tissues like umbilical cord, cord blood, amnion or placenta

Hair and Stem Cells

The hair follicle is a mini-organ that is totally distinct from other tissues in the human body, as it is characterized by cycles, in which all of the hair growth machinery is lost, then fully reconstituted from its pool of intrinsic stem cells.[2] Embryogenesis of hair is an excellent example of epithelio-mesenchymal interaction. The salient events of hair follicle morphogenesis can be summarized as follows:[3]

1. Formation of dermal condensations
2. Epithelial invagination to form the follicular wall
3. Formation of dermal papilla (DP) at the base of the follicle
4. Topologic arrangement of localized stem cells, transient amplifying (TA)/proliferating cells, and differentiated cell clusters
5. Morphogenesis to build the architecture of different hair types in the differentiating zone
6. Molecular differentiation of hair-shaft components
7. Ability to shed hairs while preserving stem cells and DP for the next cycle
8. Ability to regenerate.

Failure of any of these events will lead to disrupted hair-follicle structures, resulting in various degrees of incomplete hair-follicle formation. Hair follicles are also believed to be involved in regeneration of the epidermis and play a crucial role in wound healing. Despite this regenerative capacity, often the degree of degeneration is so severe that the permanent portion of the follicle is lost, the adult human body being unable to regenerate the hair follicle and restore homeostasis. In these cases, hair transplantation may no longer be a viable option for treatment, as there might not be sufficient donor hair follicles (available from the scalp or other areas) that can be transplanted without causing collateral damage elsewhere. Moreover, type and quality of follicle from other body parts than the scalp do not give rise to the same type of hair, with long shafts that usually grow on the scalp. Thus, stem-cell therapy to restore bald scalp areas has become an emerging focus in addressing this medical condition.[4]

Stem-cell therapy provides a powerful concept for regenerative medicine. However, in reality, it is often limited by (lack of) availability of multipotential stem cells that could be introduced, either systemically or directly to a site of injury. Stem cell therapy for hair restoration is still in its infant stage of research and based on the available limited literature stem cell therapy for hair loss can be classified as two types **(Figure 29.1)**:

1. **Autologous mesenchymal stem cell therapy:**
   - Human induced pluripotent stem cells (hiPSCs)
   - Human hair follicle stem cells (HFSCs)
   - Stem cells derived from adipose tissue, bone marrow, etc.
2. **Heterologous mesenchymal stem cell therapy:** Derived from neonatal tissues like umbilical cord, cord blood, amnion or placenta.

Human Induced Pluripotent Stem Cells

Induced pluripotent stem cells (iPSCs) cells, which are created through genetic modification of adult cells by viral transfection, or as recently reported, by direct delivery of reprogramming proteins, circumvent ethical issues surrounding embryonic ES cells. Yang et al[5] developed a strategy to differentiate human iPSCs into $CD200^+/ITGA6^+$ epithelial stem cells (EpSCs) that can reconstitute the epithelial components of the hair follicle and interfollicular epidermis. The human iPSC-derived $CD200^+/ITGA6^+$ cells show a similar gene expression signature as EpSCs directly isolated from human hair follicles. Human iPSC-derived $CD200^+/ITGA6^+$ cells are capable of generating all hair follicle lineages including the hair shaft, and the inner and outer root sheaths in skin reconstitution assays. The regenerated hair follicles possess a $KRT15^+$ stem cell population and produce hair shafts expressing hair-specific keratins **(Box 29.2)**. These results suggest an approach for generating large numbers of human EpSCs for tissue engineering and new treatments for hair loss, wound healing and other degenerative skin disorders. However, iPS cells currently face their own challenges concerning

Box 29.2: Human iPSC-derived CD200+/ITGA6+ epithelial stem cells (EpSCs)

- Can reconstitute the epithelial components of the hair follicle and interfollicular epidermis
- Cells are capable of generating all hair follicle lineages including the hair shaft, and the inner and outer root sheaths in skin reconstitution assays
- The regenerated hair follicles possess a KRT15+ stem cell population and produce hair shafts expressing hair-specific keratins

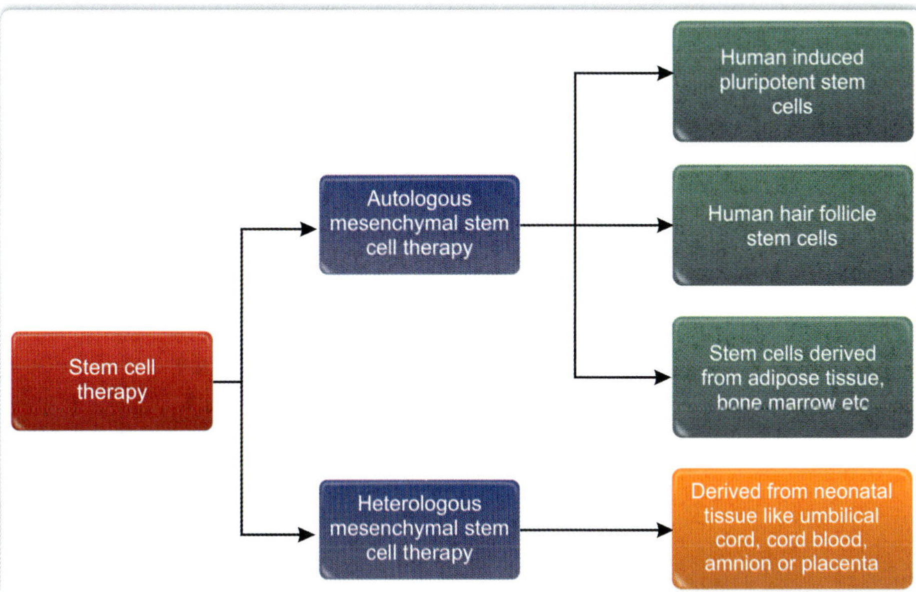

Fig. 29.1: Schematic representation of types of stem cell therapy

therapeutic application and may not be available for clinical use in the near future.

Human Hair Follicle Stem cells (HFSCs)

HFSCs[4]

- Do not bear any known risk of oncogenesis
- Are immune-privileged as autologous cells
- Are located in well-known and easily accessible locations of the human body.

Furthermore, beyond their innate capabilities for complete self-renewal, these cells have been characterized by their multipotency to differentiate into various lineages.[6] This important attribute makes HFSCs valuable candidates for regenerative medicine beyond hair and skin regeneration, and topical wound healing.[4]

Localization of the bulge area of human hair follicles has proved to be challenging, due to lack of obvious anatomical features that can be visualized using light microscopy.[7] For this reason, along with relatively small size of the hair follicle, manual dissection of HFSCs from hair follicles has been difficult, and research into human HFSCs has been limited.[4] As a solution, Ohyama et al,[8] suggested utilizing flow cytometry for sorting of cells from the bulge area, and isolating human HFSCs using CD200, mostly known for its role in autoimmunity as the putative cell surface marker.

Oh JH et al, have made efforts to expand human hair follicle stem cells in vitro to become numbers suitable for purposes of stem-cell therapy, usually introduced through direct injection into the site of application. Number of cells injected, as reported for such treatment have been in the magnitude of millions of cells.[9,10] As an individual intact hair follicle contains putative stem cells in the order of hundreds of cells, an important consideration was to obtain numbers of multipotential cells needed for regenerative medicine, while causing the least amount of collateral damage; in other words, while it would also be possible to extract cells from eventually several thousands of intact hair follicles, an attractive therapy should not lead to significantly more follicle-depleted areas on the scalp beyond the occipital region. For this reason, they focused only on a limited quantity of starting material, to stay within the scope of medical demand. Hair follicle stem cells, were isolated from intact human hair follicles obtained from superfluous material after hair transplant surgery, and as such, amounts of starting material were limited (60–100 hair follicles per session). HFSCs are well-known to be highly concentrated in the bulge region of the hair follicle, and therefore, this area was targeted by manual dissection, followed by cell extraction and enrichment for CD200+ cells.

Another important factor in attempts to expand numbers of hair follicle stem cells was to prevent differentiation. Hair follicle stem cells have previously been differentiated into various lineages other than cells involved in the hair growth mechanism. These include neuronal, glial and smooth muscle cells, as well as keratinocytes and melanocytes.[11,12,13] As many reports indicate, this multipotency may become significantly reduced, if cells begin to differentiate into precursor cells of a particular lineage. Thus, in the search for an appropriate medium for non-differentiating propagation of hair follicle-derived stem cells, a culture medium closely related to maintenance media for human embryonic stem cells was developed.[4]

Heterologous Mesenchymal Stem Cells

Researchers have used, culture-expanded mesenchymal stem cells (MSCs) to produce self-aggregated spheroidal dermal papilla like tissues (DPLTs) with the aid of a special culture condition in vitro.[14] Hair inducing activity of self-aggregated DPLTs employing MSCs was tested in athymic mice and was found to have the same hair bulb structure inductive ability as natural DPLTs in vitro.[14] As a result, umbilical cord derived (UC-MSCs) and bone marrow derived (BM-MSCs) may be an applicable and novel cell source for the generation of human hair **(Box 29.3)**.[14]

The MSCs can be isolated from various tissues such as adipose tissue, peripheral blood, umbilical cord, amnion and placenta and there by classified into adult derived and neonatal derived mesenchymal stem cells.

Criteria to Define Mesenchymal Stem Cells

In 2006, the International Society of Cellular Therapy defined MSCs by the following three criteria:[15]

- MSCs must be adherent to plastic under standard tissue culture conditions
- MSCs must express certain cell surface markers such as CD73, CD90, and CD105, and lack expression of other markers including CD45, CD34, CD14, or CD11b, CD79 alpha or CD19 and HLA-DR surface molecules
- MSCs must have the capacity to differentiate into osteoblasts, adipocytes, and chondroblasts under in vitro conditions.

Box 29.3: Types of mesenchymal stem cells

- Culture-expanded mesenchymal stem cells (MSCs)
- Umbilical cord derived (UC-MSCs)
- Bone marrow derived (BM-MSCs)

Therapeutic Effects of Mesenchymal Stem Cells

The therapeutic effects of MSCs are mainly attributed to their four important biological properties **(Figure 29.2)**:[16]

- Ability to home to sites of inflammation following tissue injury when injected intravenously
- Ability to differentiate into various cell types
- Ability to secrete multiple bioactive molecules capable of stimulating recovery of injured cells and inhibiting inflammation
- Lack of immunogenicity and the ability to perform immunomodulatory functions

Based on these properties we can speculate how injecting neonatal derived mesenchymal stem cells can stimulate hair growth in androgenetic alopecia.

- They home to the hair follicle bulge or the dermal papilla where the pathogenesis of AGA is centered.
- Hair follicle development being an excellent example of epitheliomesenchymal development, they are capable of differentiating into all components of hair follicle.
- By secreting multiple bioactive molecules like growth factors, cytokines, chemokines which may help in sending signals for hair growth, there by stimulating the existing stem cells in the bulge.
- There are no adverse reactions like immune rejection seen after mesotherapy with stem cells.
- They have known anti-apoptotic and regeneration-stimulating effects.[17]

These effects can be either direct or indirect or both: direct by causing intracellular signaling or indirect by causing another cell in the microenvironment to secrete functionally active agent.[16] In mesotherapy repeated multiple injections there by stimulating the dermal papilla cells is given. The dermal papilla (DP), a cluster of specialized fibroblasts, regulates the growth and activity of the various cells in the follicle, thereby, plays a key role in the regulation of hair cycle and growth.[18] Hair follicle regeneration begins when signals from the mesenchyme derived DP cells reach multipotent epidermal stem cells in the bulge region.[19]

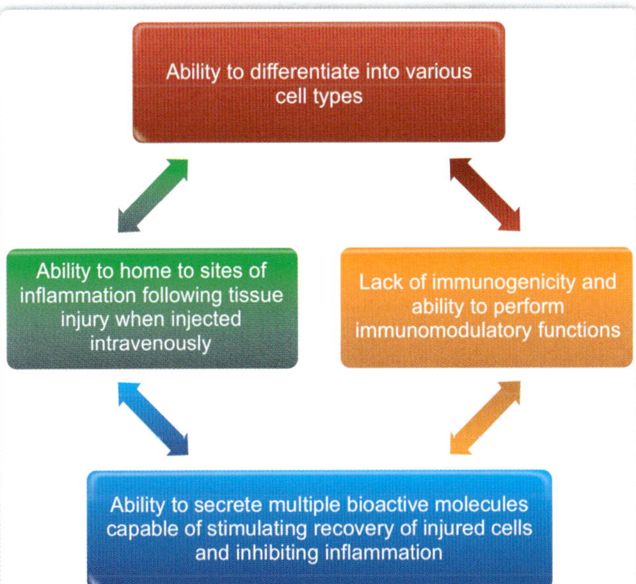

Fig. 29.2: Schematic representation of biological properties of mesenchymal stem cells

A significant advantage of these neonatal tissues is their ready availability, thus avoiding invasive procedures and ethical problems. Moreover, birth-associated tissues harbor a variety of embryonic or premature cell populations including MSC, endothelial stem/progenitor cells and hematopoietic stem cells (CD34+, CD133+).[20] It is also suggested that MSC from these neonatal tissues may have additional capacities in comparison to MSC derived from adult sources with respect to improved proliferative capacity, life span and differentiation potential.[20]

Limits of Mesenchymal Stem Cells

At the same time there are many challenges posed by the MSCs:[16]

- They have been reported to promote tumor growth and metastasis.
- There may be risk of microbial contamination during the various phases of harvesting the stem cells.
- During in vitro expansion of MSC, continuous passaging of MSCs could lead to cell transformation. To reduce malignant transformation of human MSCs, meticulous attention must be taken to prevent cell senescence and limit the number of passaging.
- They are immune privileged cells because of low expression of MHC-I molecules. Thus both autologous and allogeneic MSCs can be used in the clinical setting. However, which one to prefer needs further investigation.
- Methods and criteria for the culture, storage, shipping, and administration of MSCs must be standardized and regularized.

Conclusion

Research related to the role of stem cells in AGA is likely to open up newer therapeutic options. While stem cell therapy is already being used in many centers, there is no significant data in support of clinical use at present. The use of bio-engineered hair follicles derived from stem cells has found to be effective in animal studies and in future this could be a definite option for AGA.

References

1. Wang S, Qu X, Zhao RC. Clinical applications of mesenchymal stem cells. J Hematol Oncol. 2012;5:19.
2. Paus R, Cotsarelis G. The biology of hair follicle. N. Engl. J. Med.1999;341:491-7.
3. Chuong CM, Cotsarelis G, Stenn K. Defining Hair Follicles in the Age of Stem Cell Bioengineering. Journal of Investigative Dermatology. 2007;127:2098-100.
4. Oh JH, Mohebi P, Farkas DL,Tajbakhsh K. Towards expansion of human hair follicle stem cells in vitro. Cell Prolif. 2011;44:244-53.
5. Yang R, Zheng Y, Burrows M, et al. Generation of folliculogenic human epithelial stem cells from induced pluripotent stem cells. Nature Communications. Published online January 28, 2014.
6. Blanpain C, Lowry W, Geoghegan A, Polak L, Fuchs E. Self renewal, multipotency, and the existence of two cell populations within an epithelial stem cell niche. Cell. 2004;118:635-48.
7. Tiede S, Kloepper J, Whiting D, Paus R. The 'follicular trochanter': an epithelial compartment of the human hair follicle bulge region in need of further characterization. Br. J. Dermatol. 2007;157:1013-6.
8. Ohyama M, Terunuma A, Tock C, Radonovich M, Pise-Masison C, Hopping S, et al. Characterization and isolation of stem cell enriched human hair follicle bulge cells. J. Clin. Invest. 2006;116:249-60.
9. Hui J, Aiyer A, Su J, Borgstrom P, Stupack D, Friedlander M, et al. A homing mechanism for bone marrow-derived progenitor cell recruitment to the neovasculature. J. Clin. Invest. 2006;116:652-62.
10. Hare J. Translational development of mesenchymal stem cell therapy for cardiovascular diseases. Tex. Heart Inst. J. 2009;36:145-7.
11. Oshima H, Rochat A, Kedzia C, Kobayashi K, Barrandon Y. Morphogenesis and renewal of hair follicles from adult multipotent stem cells. Cell. 2001;104:233-45.
12. Amoh Y, Li L, Katsuoka K, Hoffman R. Multipotent nestinexpressing hair follicle stem cells. J. Dermatol. 2008;36:1-9.
13. Yu H, Fang D, Kumar S, Ling L, Ngueyn T, Acs G, et al. Isolation of a novel population of multipotent adult stem cells from human hair follicles. Am. J. Pathol. 2006;168:1879-88.
14. Yoo BY, Shin YH, Yoon HH, Seo YK, Song KY, Park JK. Application of mesenchymal stem cells derived from bone marrow and umbilical cord in human hair multiplication. J Dermatol Sci. 2010;60(2):74-83.
15. Dominici M, Le Blanc K, Mueller I, Slaper-Cortenbach I, Marini F, Krause D, et al. Minimal criteria for defining multipotent mesenchymal stromal cells. The International Society for Cellular Therapy position statement. Cytotherapy. 2006;8:315-7.
16. Wang S, Qu X, Zhao RC. Clinical applications of mesenchymal stem cells. J Hematol Oncol. 2012;5:19.
17. Parekkadan B, van Poll D, Suganuma K, Carter EA, Berthiaume F, Tilles AW, et al. Mesenchymal stem cell-derived molecules reverse fulminant hepatic failure. PLoS One 2007, 2:e941.
18. Kwack MH, Sung YK, Chung EJ, Im SU, Ahn JS, Kim MK, et al. Dihydrotestosterone-inducible dickkopf 1 from balding dermal papilla cells causes apoptosis in follicular keratinocytes. J Invest Dermatol. 2008;128:262-9.
19. Dhurat R, Sukesh MS, Avhad G, Dandale A, Pal A, Pund P. A randomized evaluator blinded study of effect of microneedling in androgenetic alopecia: A pilot study. Int J Trichol. 2013;5:6-11.
20. Hass R, Kasper C, Böhm S, Jacobs R. Different populations and sources of human mesenchymal stem cells (MSC): A comparison of adult and neonatal tissue-derived MSC. Cell Commun Signal. 2011;9:12.

30

Overview of Management of Disorders of Hair and Scalp

Prabhakar M Sangolli

"Medicine rests upon four pillars—Philosophy, Astronomy, Alchemy and Ethics."

—*Phillipus Von Hohenheim*

Disorders of hair and scalp can be broadly classified as:

I. Alopecia which include androgenetic alopecia, telogen effluvium, alopecia areata, cicatricial alopecia, artefactual alopecia

II. Scaling disorders of scalp

III. Inflammatory diseases of scalp

IV. Disorders of hair pigmentation

V. Abnormalities of hair shaft.

Alopecia

Alopecia Areata

- Single or few lesions (AA simplex/multiplex) spontaneously recover in nearly 80 % cases
- Detailed history, physical examination and few appropriate investigations are necessary before starting the treatment
- Investigations are carried out to rule out.
  - Syphilis
  - Auto immune thyroid disorder
  - Other infections (HepB)
  - Iron and zinc deficiency.
- Dermatoscopic evaluation includes demonstration of yellow dots, black dots, exclamation hair, hair diameter. Volume estimation is a very important diagnostic and prognostic tool.
- Biopsy with transverse section may be needed to rule out telogen effluvium, acute diffuse type alopecia of female scalp (ADTAFS).

Treatment

a. ***Contact immunotherapy*** - 1 to 2 % diphencyprone (DPC) is applied over scalp lesion. 3 weeks later 10^{-4} dilution is reapplied just to induce mild inflammation. Treatment is continued at 2 weekly intervals till acceptable hair growth is seen.[1] Adverse effects include irritant dermatitis, contact sensitization, lymphadenopathy and vitiligo.

b. ***Intralesional steroids*** are useful in acute phase. 4 to 5 mg/mL of triamcinolone acetonide is employed at 3 weekly interval. Some patients exhibit steroid resistance due to deficiency of thioredoxin reductase enzyme.[2]

c. ***Turban PUVA***: Dose of 6-12 J/cm^2/week till satisfactory hair growth is effective in few cases.[3]

d. ***Topical minoxidil (5%)*** is a very effective topical agent to induce hair growth. However, the disease relapses on discontinuation as it does not reduce peribulbar infiltration.[4]

e. ***Oral dexamethasone mini pulse (OMP)*** is a commonly employed successful treatment modality in acute phase of diffuse hair loss.[5]

f. ***PUVA therapy with OMP*** has been used as a combination therapy with good remission rate.

g. ***Oral anti histamine ebastine*** (10 mg/d) is effective in few cases as it decreases perifollicular infiltration of CD3 cells.[6]

f. ***Miscellaneous*** treatment modalities[7]

- Topical cryotherapy with liquid nitrogen
- Topical carpunomium cream, a parasympathomimetic agent.

Telogen Effluvium

In telogen effluvium (TE) more than 7 % anagen hairs shift into telogen phase.[8] Management entails detailed history taking
- Duration of hair loss
- Stress
- Recent surgery
- Blood loss
- Drugs
- Systemic illness
- Crash dieting.

Detailed examination of scalp is the next step to look for:
- Scaling
- Perifollicular scaling
- Pustules.

Diagnostic tests include:
- Hair pull test
- Hair pluck test
- Wood's light
- Dermatoscopy
- Scalp biopsy.

Nail involvement will give clue to period of onset of hair damage.[9]

The following investigations may be necessary to assess the probable cause of TE.
- Complete blood count
- Metabolic and thyroid profile
- Serum ferritin- Baseline, 6 week and 6 month serum ferritin estimation is carried out to assess iron storage[10]
- Zinc estimation
- Total testosterone.

Treatment

a. ***Balanced diet*** with adequate calories, proteins, vitamins and minerals is advised. Lactating women should take multivitamin and iron supplements on regular basis.

b. ***OCP:*** If patients need OCP, combination of ethinyl estradiol with progesterone with least androgenic activity like desogestrel is prescribed.

c. ***Thyroid replacement*** therapy will help.

d. ***Zinc:*** Since zinc helps in iron absorption and has anti androgen property, recommended daily allowance (RDA) of 15 mg/d is adequate.[11]

e. ***Vitamin A:*** It assists in cell maturation, cell differentiation and has immune stimulating property. The RDA of vitamin A is about 4000 units/d.

f. ***Biotin:*** It is an essential vitamin which plays an important role in normal growth of hairs and nails. About 0.3 mg/d is RDA and therapeutic dose is 3–5 mg/d.

g. ***Vitamin D*** helps to maintain cell cycle. The RDA of vitamin D is 400 U/d which is prescribed with one gram/d of calcium supplements.[12]

h. ***Essential amino acid supplements*** definitely boost hair growth. Deficiency of essential fatty acids (EFA) can induce TE which can be reversed by EFA supplementation.[13]

i. ***Treatment of systemic illnesses*** can slow down TE.

j. ***Avoidance of drugs*** like coumarin, carbamazepine, fluoxetine, NSAIDs, enalapril, metoprolol can reverse drug induced hair loss.[14]

k. ***Adequate management of underlying inflammatory dermatoses*** like psoriasis, seborrheic dermatitis will be helpful in restoring normal hair cycle.

l. ***Minoxidil:*** Concomitant treatment with minoxidil (5 % in males and 2% in females) will enhance hair growth by above mentioned treatment.[15]

m. ***Co-cyprindiol or spironolactone:*** In patients suffering from SAHA, co-cyprindiol or spironolactone administration helps.

n. ***Finasteride*** (1 mg/d) is an approved drug in male patients.[16]

o. ***Miscellaneous:*** Other agents which have been tried are botanicals which inhibit DHT activities. Examples include saw palmetto, azelaic acid, etc.

Androgenetic Alopecia

Treatment of AGA in Men

a. ***Counseling*** is necessary for assessment of patient's perception of his condition and his knowledge of various treatment options available as of today.

b. ***Minoxidil (5%)*** has a preventive role in slowing down the progression of hair loss and to some extent restores lost hair.[17] Twice daily application of 1 mL for 2 years can give satisfactory results. Side effects include scalp irritation, allergic contact dermatitis to minoxidil or propylene glycol.

c. ***Finasteride***: Type II alpha reductase inhibitor is administered in the dose of 1 mg/d for 1 year. It reduces serum and scalp levels of DHT by 70%.[18] It can cause sexual dysfunction, gynecomastia and carcinoma of breast in minority of patients.
   Combination of minoxidil and finasteride may not offer added advantage even though both have different modes of action.

d. ***Dutasteride:*** Higher doses of dutasteride (2.5 mg/d) may have a role in the future.[19]

e. ***Surgery:*** Surgical outcome depends on the age of the patient (25 years), sufficient hairs in the donor area, graft in frontal area, thick hairs. Follicular unit transplantation (FUT) is a popular procedure.

f. ***Hair replacements:*** Weaving, bonding, wig and toupee are the non-surgical options in the management of AGA.

Treatment of AGA in Women

Investigations
- Complete blood count
- Serum ferritin
- Total iron
- Total testosterone
- DHEAS
- TSH.

Dermatoscopy reveals peripilar casts and miniaturized hairs.

a. ***Minoxidil*** (2 %) is prescribed. Hair count and hair weight show definite increase in nearly 40 % of women treated with minoxidil. Even though 5 % minoxidil gives better results, frontotemporal and side burns hypertrichosis is seen which can be minimized by once daily application.[20]

b. ***Antiandrogens*** may have role in FAGA if patient has signs of hyperandrogenism. Co-cyprindiol, spironolactone, flutamide are useful in patients having androgenetic alopecia with hirsutism.[21] Finasteride (2.5 mg/d) has given conflicting results in post-menopausal and infertile women. Loss of libido, weight gain, mastodynia and depression are reported with cyproterone. Hepatotoxicity is seen in patients on flutamide and cyproterone. Spironolactone can cause hyperkalemia, mastalgia and break through bleeding.

c. ***Iron supplements*** definitely help women who have serum ferritin level less than 40 mcg/L.[22]

d. ***Surgery*** may be necessary in women who have major hair loss in limited area.[23]

e. ***Future:*** Hair follicular culture methods may hold promise.[24]

Cicatricial Alopecia

In cicatricial alopecia (CAs) hair follicles are destroyed and are replaced by scar tissue.

Treatments aim at alleviating symptoms and arrest the progression of the disease.

Lymphocytic CAs

a. ***Topical steroid:*** Topical therapy consists of long-term use, followed by application of calcineurin inhibitors like tacrolimus (0.1 %).

b. ***Intralesional steroids*** (10 mg/mL triamcinolone acetonide) is effective as bridge therapy till main treatment demonstrates its efficacy.

c. ***Hydroxychloroquine*** is effective in the treatment of LE, LPP in the dosage of 200 mg twice a day for 6–12 months with close monitoring of ophthalmic and hematological parameters.[25]

d. ***Antibiotics*** like doxycycline or minocycline are used in antimalarial non-responsive patients.

c. ***Acitretin*** is the first line drug in the management of LE and can be tried in LPP also.[26]

d. ***Mycophenolate mofetil*** in the dosage of 1 to 2 g/d in 2 divided doses can be prescribed in antimalarial unresponsive patients.

e. ***Cyclosporin A*** (3–5 mg/kg/d) is an useful drug in the initial inflammatory phase.[27]

f. ***Prednisolone*** is employed during early phase till other immunosuppressive drugs start showing results.

Neutrophilic CAs

a. ***Oral clindamycin*** (300 mg bid) in combination with Rifampicin (300 mg bid) for 10 weeks is the treatment of choice.[28]

b. ***Nasal topical mupirocin*** is employed to prevent recurrence.

c. ***Isotretinoin:*** Isotretinoin (1 mg/kg/d) gives excellent results in resistant cases.[25]

Mixed CAs

a. ***Oral quinolones*** are combined with topical clindamycin.

b. ***Intralesional steroids*** are utilized to treat inflammatory papules and hypertrophic scars.

Surgical Management

Surgical modalitics include incision and drainage for boggy swellings, scalp reduction with or without tissue expanders, flap and hair transplant which though widely used can be limited by donor reservoir and atrophic recipient site. In treated or burnt out cases , a waiting period of 6–9 months is employed before performing surgical modalities.[29] Various techniques like test grafts, larger plugs and using Er:YAG laser[30] to create holes in donor site are adopted to enhance success rate of autologous transplants.

Factitial Hairloss

Trichotillomania is an impulse control disorder characterized by hair pulling. It has a genetic basis with mutations in SLITRK1 gene.[31]

Treatment includes pharmacotherapy and non-pharmacological intervention:

- Drugs used are
  - Fluoxetine
  - Sertraline
  - Paroxetine
  - Escitalopram (SSRIs)[32]

Combination with atypical antipsychotics like olanzapine and risperidone is rewarding.[33] At least 4 week therapy is necessary to obtain visual improvement.

Gastrointestinal (nausea, vomiting, diarrhea), CNS (tremors, restlessness) are the commonly observed adverse effects of SSRI and typical antipsychotics cause extrapyramidal symptoms and prolongation of QT interval.[34]

Non-pharmacological therapy involves habit reversal therapy[35] which is combined with pharmacotherapy to augment treatment efficacy.

Scaling disorders

Dandruff and Seborrheic Dermatitis

Dandruff is a visible flaking of scalp. In seborrheic dermatitis scaling is more pronounced with signs of inflammation such as erythema and itching. Management should address inflammation, scaling, Malassezia overgrowth and bacterial infection.

a. ***General measures*** include
   - Regular shampooing
   - Avoidance of oil based hair products
   - Nutritious food
   - Stress avoidance
   - Proper use of topical treatment

b. ***Antifungal shampoos:*** Regular use of antifungal shampoos containing 2 % ketoconazole,/1% ciclopirox olamine/climbazole is sufficient.[36]

c. ***Thick scales:*** In the presence of thick scales, salicylic acid, coal tar shampoos are advocated.[37]

d. ***In more severe cases*** topical antifungal/anti-bacterial creams are prescribed.[38]

e. ***Topical steroids:*** If inflammatory component is prominent, night application of topical steroid ointments is advised with daily shampooing in the morning.[39]

f. ***Combination of 2% ketoconazole with 2% pyrithione zinc*** (ZPT) is a popular measure.[40]

g. ***Calcineurin inhibitors*** like tacrolimus and pimecrolimus can be used on face.

Scalp Psoriasis

Nearly 50% of patients with psoriasis have scalp involvement. Severity varies with mild to severe degree with lesions extending beyond scalp margins.

Medications for scalp psoriasis include those to be left on the scalp and the wash off products. Left on products are:

- Gels
- Lotions
- Ointments containing steroids, coal tar, and salicylic acid or vitamin D_3 analogs.

Wash off products are shampoos containing:

- Coal tar
- Salicylic acid
- Sulfur
- Selenium
- Ketoconazole
- Zinc pyrithione.

Treatment needs to be individualized and period of 8 to 10 weeks may be necessary.

a. ***Coal tar and salicylic acid*** lotions and shampoos are popularly used. Coal tar preparations can be left overnight and washed in the morning.[41]

b. ***Dithranol:*** Short contact therapy (SCAT) with dithranol (0.5 %) is effective. It is an irritant and can stain skin.[42]

c. ***Topical antibiotic*** may be necessary to treat secondary infection.

d. ***Topical calcipotriol*** is left overnight and is quite effective. It causes facial dermatitis. Short course of therapy with calcipotriol and betamethasone dipropionate is a useful modality. Calcitriol and clobetasol combination is another alternative.[43]

d. ***Topical tazarotene*** can be prescribed for overnight application with due precautions to prevent facial irritation.[44]

e. ***Potent topical steroids*** (Gels, foam, lotions, shampoo) are popularly employed for 2 weeks, to obtain quicker relief. To prevent adverse effects, rotational therapy with coal tar, dithranol and tazarotene is practiced.[45]

f. ***UVA:*** To deliver UVA, hand held UVA combs are prescribed.

g. ***Targeted phototherapy*** with Excimer laser with high local dose of NBUVB is gaining popularity.[46]

h. ***Systemic therapy*** with methotrexate, acitretin and cyclosporine is necessary when scalp is involved in patients with moderate to severe psoriasis.[47]

i. ***Pityriasis amiantacea:*** Nearly 15 % patients with psoriasis can develop pityriasis amiantacea. Oil based products containing coal tar and salicylic acid loosen up the scales. Later coal tar based shampoos are used to prevent recurrence.[48]

Tinea Capitis

Even though tinea capitis is seen in children aged between 4–7 years, it is common in younger age because of prevailing practice of tonsuring. Trichophyton and Microsporum genera are the causative organisms.

Diagnosis

- Detailed clinical examination with examination of occipital and posterior cervical lymphadenopathy
- Wood's lamp examination
- Potassium hydroxide mount (KOH 10 to 30 %)
- 40 percent DMSO can be added to penetrate keratin
- Staining of hyphae can be done with chlorazol black or calcofluor white (0.1 %)

- Fungal culture remains the gold standard. Water moistened cotton tipped bud is effective in collecting samples which can be inoculated into bacterial culture media for transportation or can be directly inoculated into Sabouraud's dextrose agar (SDA) or dermatophyte test medium (DTM)[49]
- PCR is a new diagnostic tool which helps in identification of species.

Treatment

a. ***Topical therapy*** has no role as active drugs do not penetrate hair shaft.
b. ***Ultra micronized griseofulvin*** (10 to 15 mg/kg/d) for 8 weeks gives satisfactory clinicomycological cure. It is advisable to take with fatty meal. Head ache, gastrointestinal discomfort are the commonly reported side effects.
c. ***Terbinafine:*** It is administered in the dose of 5 mg/kg/d for 4 weeks. 3-4 pulses of weekly therapy also has been practiced with good results.[50] Gastrointestinal disturbances, transient elevation of serum liver enzymes and rashes are the reported side effects.
d. ***Itraconazole:*** Usual dosage is 5 mg/kg/d for 4 weeks. It should be taken with food. After the medication is discontinued, therapeutic drug levels persist up to 9 months in the hairs.[51] Pulse therapy similar to terbinafine has also been advocated. It inhibits cyt P 450 enzymes. Caution is exercised when co-prescribed with anticonvulsants, anticoagulants and antidepressants. Adverse effects reported are headache, rash, dysgeusia and transiently elevated liver enzymes. Dose adjustment is not necessary in patients with renal failure.
e. ***Fluconazole:*** It is a hydrophilic triazole which is prescribed in the dosage of 5–8 mg/kg/d for 3–4 weeks.[52] It also inhibits cyt P 450 enzymes. Dose adjustment is necessary in patients with renal failure. Elevated liver enzymes, rashes, hypoglycemia, headache are reported adverse events.
f. ***Voriconazole:*** It works well against *T.tonsurans* and *M.canis*. Dosage is 6 mg/kg/d twice a day on day 1, followed by 4 mg/kg twice a day subsequently.[53] It should be taken 1 hour before or 2 hours after food. It is an expensive drug. It should be reserved for serious infections. Visual disturbance, rash and liver toxicity are the reported side effects.

   For systemic antifungals, drugs need to be continued for 2 weeks after clinical cure. Culture may be necessary in relapsing cases.
g. ***For kerion***, systemic antifungal therapy suffices. Steroids offer little advantage.
h. ***Adjunctive therapy***

   Frequent shampooing with ketoconazole 2% and zinc pyrithione 1% may prevent transmission among contacts.[54] Fomites like comb, brush should be disinfected. In zoophilc infection, pets need veterinary referral.

Piedra

It is an asymptomatic hair shaft infection. Black piedra is caused by *Piedraia hortai* and white piedra is due to *Trichosporon biegelii*. Black piedra involves scalp and white piedra can involve pubic area, nails.

- KOH mount aids in diagnosis.
- Black piedra is treated with shaving and oral griseofulvin.
- White piedra is managed with oral itraconazole.
- Systemic therapy is combined topical imidazoles and ciclopiroxolamine in both conditions.

Pediculosis capitis

CDC says that many nits seen 6.5 mm from scalp is diagnostic of head lice infestation.

Diagnostic methods include:

- Detailed examination with magnifying lens
- Use of transparent adhesive tape.

Management

Drug resistance is increasing with 2 possible mechanisms

A. Increased glutathione-s -tranferase activity (malathion resistance) and enhanced MAO activity
B. Nerve insensitivity (pyrethroid resistance)

a. ***Topical 1% permethrin:*** Permethrin should be repeated after one week. 5% permethrin may be tried to counteract pyrethroid resistance.[55]
b. ***Topical 0.5% malathion***, kills adults and is ovicidal also. Malathion works well within 2 hours of application when 5 % permethrin fails.[56] It causes conjunctival and scalp erythema and dandruff.
c. ***Topical 1% lindane***, which is neurotoxic.
d. ***Topical 10% crotamiton*** lotion.[57]
e. ***Topical 0.9% spinosad***
f. ***Topical 0.5% ivermectin***
g. ***Topical 5% benzyl alcohol (under occlusion)***
h. ***Oral ivermectin***
i. ***Albendazole*** 400 mg single dose, repeated after one week.
j. ***Thiabendazole***
k. ***Levamisole***
l. ***Co-trimoxazole***
m. ***Soaking nit comb:*** Various methods are used to remove nits. Soaking nit comb in equal mixture of water and

white vinegar and removing nits every other day for 10 days is very effective.

g. ***Formic acid 8%:*** Though 8% formic acid dissolves nit, it may damage the hairs also.

h. ***Fomites*** need to be disinfected with water at 55 degrees for 30 minutes, or hot air for 30 minutes. Fomites which cannot be exposed to hot water or hot air can be kept sealed in a plastic bag for 10 days.

Hair Dyes

Hair coloring is commonly used to change color or disguise gray hair.

Permanent hair dyes containing para phenylene diamine (PPD), para toluidine diamine (PTD) are formed within hair cortex and can withstand 10 washings. They contain color intermediates with hydrogen peroxide. Nearly 10% of hair dye users develop allergic contact dermatitis (ACD) involving scalp, hairline face, eye lids, ears and shoulders.[58] Even contact urticaria and anaphylaxis are reported. Extensive and irreversible hair loss is another rare complication.[59] Semi-permanent and temporary dyes contain derivatives of nitro anilines, nitrophenylendiamines and nitroaminophenols. They can withstand 4-5 hair washes. Very rarely ACD is reported.[60]

Temporary hair dyes contain mild organic acids and dyes and dyes that coat hair shaft like Basic Red 22 and HC Yellow are incorporated. They last till one wash only.[61]

Hair restorers (Metallic dyes) are used to conceal graying. They contain lead acetate with colloidal sulfur or sodium thiosulfate. Other chemicals used are basic dye, bismuth citrate, indolamine and indophenols.[62]

Vegetable hair dyes include henna, indigo leaves, chamomile flowers and powdered walnuts. Basic ingredient of henna is lawsonia. Henna is applied alone (application time- 5-6 hours) or can be mixed with PPD and used (application time—30 minutes).[6] Eventhough ACD to henna is rare, incidence increases when combined with PPD.[63]

References

1. Hoffman R, Happle R. Topical immunotherapy in alopecia areata. what: how and why? Dermatol Clinic. 1996;14:739-44.
2. Kubeyinje EP. Intralesional triamcinolone acetonide in alopecia areata among 62 Saudi Arabs. East Afr Med J. 1994;71:675.
3. Taylor CR, Hawk JL. PUVA treatment of alopecia areata partialis, totalis and universalis: audit of 10 years experience at St.John's Institute of Dermatology. Br J Dermatol. 1995;133:9118.
4. Fiedler Weiss. Topical minoxidil (1% and 5 %) in the treatment of alopecia areata. J Am Acad Dermatol. 1987;16:745-8.
5. SieterS, Ugurel S, Tilgen W, Reinhold U. High dose pulse steroid therapy in the treatment of severe alopecia areata. Dermatology. 2001;202:230-4.
6. Yoshizawa Y, Kawana S. Efficacy of ebastine in the treatment of alopecia areata. Jap J Dermatol. 2005;115:1473-80.
7. Taisuke Ito. Advances in the treatment of alopecia areata. J of Dermatol. 2012;39:11-7.
8. Fiedler VC, Gray VC. Diffuse alopecia: teolgen hair loss. In: Olsen EA (ed). Disorders of Hair Growth: Diagnosis and Treatment. McGraw Hill. 2003;303-20.
9. Trueb RM. Idiopathic chronic telogen effluvium in the women. Hautarzt. 2001;51:899-906.
10. Trost LB, Bergfield WB, Calogeras E. The diagnosis and treatment of iron deficiency and its potential relationship to hair loss. J Am Acad Dermatol. 2006;54:824-34.
11. Arnaud J, Beani FC, Favier A, Embliard R. Zinc status in patients with telogen effluvium. Acta Derm Venereol. 1995;75:248-9.
12. Sutton AL, McDonald PN. Vitamin D, more than a bone -a-fide hormone (A review) Molecular Endocrinol. 2003;17:777-91.
13. Riella MC, Broviac J, Wells M, Scribbner BH. Essential fatty acid deficiency in human adults during total parenteral nutrition. Ann Intern Med. 1975;83:786-9.
14. Tosti A, Misciali C, Piracinni BM, Peluso AM, Bardazzi F. Drug induced hair loss and hair growth: Incidence, management and avoidance. Drug Saf. 1994;10;310-17.
15. Arck PC, Hanjiski Peter EM et al. Topical minoxidil counteracts stress induced hair growth inhibition in mice. Exp Dermatol. 2003;12:580-90.
16. Ross E, Shapiro J. Management of hair loss. Dermatol Clin. 2005;23:222-43.
17. Olsen EA, Weiner MS, Amara IA, Delong ER. Five year follow-up of men with androgenic alopecia treated with topical minoxidil. J Am Acad Dermatol. 1990;22:643-6.
18. Drake L, Hordinski M, Fiedler V, et al. The effect of finasteride on scalp and serum androgen levels in men with androgenetic alopecia. J Am Acad Dermatol. 1999;41:550-54.
19. Olsen EA, Hordinski M, Whiting D. The importance of duel 5 alpha reductase inhibition in the male pattern hair loss: results of randomized placebo controlled study of dutasteride. J Am Acad Dermatol. 2006;55:1014-23.
20. Ulrike BP, Kathrin H, Ekhart D, Douglas C, Natalie GB.A randomized single blind trial of 5% minoxidil foam in the treatment of androgenetic treatment of women. J Am Acad Dermatol. 2011;65:1126-34.
21. Sinclair R, Wewerinke M, Jolley D. Treatment of female pattern hair loss with oral anti androgens.Br J Dermatol. 2005;152:466-73.
22. Rushton DH, Ramsay ID. The importance of adequate serum ferritin levels during oral cyproterone acetate and ethinyl estradiol treatment of diffuse androgen dependent alopecia in women. Clin Endocrinol. 1992;36:421-7.
23. Olsen A, Messenger AG, Shapiro J. Evaluation and treatment of male and female pattern hair loss. J Am Acad Dermatol. 2005;52:301-11.
24. Cooley J. Follicular cell implantation: an update on hair follicle cloning. Facial Plast Surg Clin North Am. 2004;12:219-34.

25. Price VH. The medical treatment of CA. Semin Cut Med Surg. 2006;25(1):56-9.
26. Laurbeg G, Geiger JM, Hjorth N, et al. Treatment of lichen planus with acitretin. A double blind placebo controlled study in 65 patients. J Am Acad Dermatol. 1991;24:434-7.
27. Mirmirani P, Willey A, Pricey VH. Short course of cyclosporine in lichen plano pilaris. J Am Acad Dermatol. 2003;49:667-71.
28. Powell J, Dawber RP. Successful treatment regime for folliculitis decalvans despite uncertainty of all aetiological factors. Br J Dermatol. 2001;144:428-9.
29. Callender VD, McMichael AJ, Cohen GF. Medical and surgical therapies for alopecias in black women. Dermatol Ther. 2004;17:164-76.
30. Podda M, Spieth K, Kauffman R. Er:YAG laser assisted hair transplantation in CA. Dermatol Surg. 2000;26:1010-4.
31. Zuchner S., et al. SLITRK1 mutations in trichotillomania. Mol Psychiatry. 2006;11:887-9.
32. Waksh KH, McDougle CJ. Pharmacological strategies for trichotillomania. Expert Opin Pharmacother. 2005;6:975-8.
33. Potenza MN, et al. Olanzapine augmentation of fluoxetine in the treatment of trichotillomania. Am J Psychiatry. 1998;155:1192-6.
34. Physician Desk Reference, 61st edn. Montvale NJ. Medical Economics Data 2007.
35. Woods DW, et al. Understanding and treating trichotillomania: what we know and what we don't know. Psychiatr Clin North Am. 2006;29:487-501.
36. Arresse JE, Pierard -Frenchimont C, De Donekar P, et al. Effect of ketoconazole-medicated shampoo on squamometry and Malssezia ovalis load in Pityriasis capitis. Cutis. 1996;58:235-7.
37. Lowe NJ, Breding JH, Wortzman MS. New coal tar extract and coal tar shampoos: evaluation by epidermal cell DNA synthesis suppression assay. Arch Dermatol. 1982;118:487-9.
38. Dandruff, seborrheic dermatitis and psoriasis drug products for over counter human use; Amendment to monograph. Federal Registry. 1994;59:4000-1.
39. Milani M, MolfettaADS, Gramazio R, et al. Efficacy of betamethasone valerate 0.1% thermophobic foam in seborrheic dermatitis of scalp: an open label multi centre prospective trial on 180 patients. Curr Med Opin. 2003;19: 342-5.
40. Pierard-Franchmont C, Goffin V, Decroix j, et al. A muticentre randomized trial of ketoconazole and 2 % ketoconazole shampoos in severe dandruff and seborrheic dermatitis. Skin Pharmacol Appl Skin Physiol. 2002;15:434-41.
41. Paghdal KV, Schwartz RA. Topical tar: Back to the future. J Am Acad Dermatol. 2009;61:294-302.
42. Chan CS, Van Voorhees AS, Lebwohl MG, Korman NJ, Young M, Bebo Jr BF, et al. Treatment of severe scalp psoriasis: From the Medical Board of the National Psoriasis Foundation. J Am Acad Dermatol. 2009;60:962-71.
43. Thaci D, Daiber W, Boehncke WH, Kaufmann R. Calcipotriol solution for the treatment of scalp psoriasis: Evaluation of efficacy, safety and acceptance in 3,396 patients. Dermatology. 2001;203:153-6.
44. Lebwohl MG, Breneman DL, Goffe BS, Grossman JR, Ling MR, Milbauer J, et al. Tazarotene 0.1% gel plus corticosteroid cream in the treatment of plaque psoriasis. J Am Acad Dermatol. 1998;39:590-6.
45. Mazzotta A, Esposito M, Carboni I, Schipani C, Climenti S. Clobetasol propionate foam 0.05% as a novel topical formulation for plaque-type and scalp psoriasis. J Derm Treat. 2007;18:84-7.
46. Morison WL, Atkinson DF, Werthman L. Effective treatment of scalp psoriasis using the excimer (308 nm) laser. Photodermatol Photoimmunol Photomed. 2006;22:181-3.
47. Sanjeev Handa. Newer trends in the management of psoriasis at difficult to treat locations. Scalp,palmoplantar disease and nails. Ind J Dermatol Venereol Leprol. 2010;76:633-4.
48. HanstedK, Lindskow R. Pityriasis amiantacea and psoriasis. A follow up study. Dermatologica. 1983;166:314-5.
49. Friedlander SF, Pickering B, Cunningham BB, et al. The use cotton swab method in diagnosing tinea capitis. Paediatrics. 1999;104:276-9.
50. Gupta AK, Adam P. Terbinafine pulse therapy is effective in tinea capitis. Pediatric Dermatol. 1998;15:66-8.
51. Lleyden J. Pharmacokinetics and pharmacology of terbinafine and itraconazole . J Am Acad Dermatol. 1998;38 (5 pt 3)S42-47.Review.
52. Solomon BA, Collins R, Sharma R. Fluconazole for the treatment of tinea capitis in children. J Am Acad Dermatol. 1997;37(2 pt 1):274-5.
53. Leveque D, Niviox Y, Jehl F. Clinical pharmacokinetics of Voriconazole. Int J Antimicrob Agents. 2006;27(4):474-84.
54. McGinley KJ, Leyden JJ. Antifungal activity of dermatological shampoos. Arch Dermatol. 1982; 272(3-4):339-42.
55. Jones KN, English KC. Review of common therapeutic options in the United States for the treatment of pediculosis capitis. Clin Infect Dis. 2003;36:1355-61.
56. Abramowitz M. Malthion in the treatment of head lice. Med Let Drugs Ther. 1999;41:73-4.
57. Karacic I, Yawalkar SJ. A single application of crotamiton lotion in the treatment of patients with pediculosis capitis. Int J Dermatol. 1982;21:611-3.
58. Oritz KJ, Yiannias JA. Cotact Dermatitis to cosmetics, fragrances and botanicals. Dermatol Therap. 2004;17:264-71.
59. Brown AC, Crounse RC. In: Hair, Trace Elements and Human illness. New York:Praegar. 1980.
60. PernoP, Lisi P. Psoriasis like contact dermatitis from a hair nitro dye. Contact Dermatitis. 1990;23:123-4.
61. Groot ACD, WeylandJW, Nater JP. In: Unwanted effects of Cosmetics and Drugs used in Dermatology, 3rd edn. Amsterdam, New York: Elsevier,1994.
62. Fitzpatric TB, Freedberg IM. In: Fitzpatrick's Dermatology in General Medicine, 6th edn. NewYork McGraw-ill Medical Pub. Division, 2003.
63. Oztas MO, Onder M, Oztas P, Atahan C. Contact allergy to henna. J Eur Acad Dermatol Venereol. 2001;40:577-9.

Index

Note: Page numbers followed by *f*, *b* and *t* indicate figures, boxes and tables respectively.

T

U

V

W

Z